INTERNATIONAL ENCYCLOPEDIA OF PHARMACOLOGY AND THERAPEUTICS

Sponsored by the International Union of Pharmacology (IUPHAR)
(Chairman: B. Uvnäs, Stockholm)

Executive Editor: G. Peters, *Lausanne*

Section 39B

PHARMACOLOGY OF INTESTINAL ABSORPTION: GASTROINTESTINAL ABSORPTION OF DRUGS

Section Editors

W. FORTH
Bochum
and
W. RUMMEL
Homburg/Saar

Volume II

INTERNATIONAL ENCYCLOPEDIA OF
PHARMACOLOGY AND THERAPEUTICS

PHARMACOLOGY OF INTESTINAL ABSORPTION: GASTROINTESTINAL ABSORPTION OF DRUGS

VOLUME II

CONTRIBUTORS

T. W. CLARKSON
A. G. F. DAVIDSON
A. DAWSON
A. FANCONI
W. FORTH
A. D. KENNY
K. R. KERRY
D. S. LAYNE
K. PFLEGER
G. SLADEN
W. RUMMEL

PERGAMON PRESS

OXFORD · NEW YORK · TORONTO
SYDNEY · BRAUNSCHWEIG

Pergamon Press Offices:

U.K.	Pergamon Press Ltd., Headington Hill Hall, Oxford, England
U.S.A.	Pergamon Press Inc., Maxwell House, Fairview Park, Elmsford, New York 10523, U.S.A.
CANADA	Pergamon of Canada Ltd., 207 Queen's Quay West, Toronto 1, Canada
AUSTRALIA	Pergamon Press (Aust.) Pty. Ltd., 19a Boundary Street, Rushcutters Bay, N.S.W. 2011, Australia
FRANCE	Pergamon Press SARL, 24 rue des Ecoles, 75240 Paris, Cedex 05, France
WEST GERMANY	Pergamon Press GmbH, 3300 Braunschweig, Postfach 2923, Burgplatz 1, West Germany

---

First edition 1975

Library of Congress Cataloging in Publication Data

Main entry under title:

Pharmacology of intestinal absorption.

(International encyclopedia of pharmacology and therapeutics, Section 39B)

1. Drug metabolism. 2. Intestinal absorption.
I. Aguiar, A. J. II. Forth, W., ed. III. Rummel, Walter, 1921– ed. IV. Series. [DNLM: 1. Drugs-Metabolism. 2. Intestinal absorption. QV4 I58 section 39B]
RM301.P46 615'.7 74–8652

ISBN 0-08-016210-X

Printed in Great Britain by A. Wheaton & Co. Exeter

CONTENTS

CONTENTS OF VOLUME I

LIST OF CONTRIBUTORS

CLARKSON, T. W., Departments of Radiation Biology and Biophysics and Pharmacology and Toxicology, University of Rochester, Rochester, N.Y., U.S.A.

DAVIDSON, A. G. F., Department of Paediatrics, University of British Columbia, Vancouver, Canada.

DAWSON, A., St. Bartholomew's Hospital and Medical College, London EC1A 7BE, U.K.

FANCONI, A., Kinderklinik, Kantonsspital, S–8400 Winterthur, Switzerland.

FORTH, W., Institut für Pharmakologie und Toxikologie der Ruhr-Universität, D–463 Bochum, F.R.G.

KENNY, A. D. Department of Pharmacology and Space Sciences Research Center, University of Missouri, Columbia, Missouri, 65201, U.S.A.

KERRY, K. R., Antarctic Division, Department of Science, Commonwealth of Australia, 568 St. Kilda Rd., Melbourne, Victoria, Australia.

LAYNE, D. S., Department of Biochemistry, Faculty of Medicine, University of Ottawa, Ottawa, Ontario, Canada.

PFLEGER, K., Institut für Pharmakologie und Toxikologie der Universität des Saarlandes, D–665 Homburg/Saar, F.R.G.

RUMMEL, W., Institut für Pharmakologie und Toxikologie der Universität des Saarlandes, D–665 Homburg/Saar, F.R.G.

SLADEN, G., St. Bartholomew's Hospital and Medical College, London, EC1A 7BE, U.K.

PREFACE

SECTION 39B of IEPT covers that part of gastrointestinal pharmacology which deals with (a) absorption processes in the gastrointestinal tract and (b) the influence of drugs on these processes. The details can be taken from the list of contents. It must be emphasized that each chapter may be read as a review *per se*.

First of all, the editors wish to thank the authors for dedication and cooperation during the preparation of Section 39B, the concept of which was born in early 1967. Only a few chapters can be read now as submitted in 1969–70; most of the chapters cover literature at least up to 1972. Not all authors were able to revise their manuscripts and enrich them by references of recent literature. The editors, therefore, added short footnotes where it appeared to be necessary.

The editors also hope that most of the information delivered in these two volumes of Section 39B of IEPT is derived from compartments of science where the half-life of knowledge is not too short.

W. FORTH
Bochum

W. RUMMEL
Homburg/Saar

CHAPTER 8

ABSORPTION OF FAT-SOLUBLE VITAMINS

W. Forth, *Bochum*, and W. Rummel, *Homburg/Saar*

Federal Republic of Germany

INTRODUCTION

Since in the preceding chapter only the principles of absorption of water-soluble vitamins have been dealt with the absorption of fat-soluble vitamins has to be discussed briefly. The evaluation of published data may not be sufficiently critical, because the editors have no personal experience in this field.

The *daily requirements* for man of the fat-soluble vitamins A, D, E and K can be taken from Table 1. As far as the wide range of requirements of different species is concerned the readers are referred to Doisy and Matschiner (1970), Draper (1970), Hartles (1970), Moore (1970) and Selby and Green (1970). The fat-soluble vitamin content of food can be taken from the authors cited above, also from Selby and Green (1970) and from "Geigy-Tables" (*Wissenschaftliche Tabellen-Geigy*, 1968).

The absorption of the fat-soluble vitamins A, D, E and K have at least two common features:

(1) The amount absorbed depends on the presence of bile: references for vitamin A: cf. Olson (1964); Wiseman (1964); vitamin D: Wiseman (1964); vitamin E: Akerib and Sterner (1971); Gallo-Torres (1970a); Harris and Muller (1971); Pearson and Legge (1972); Wiseman (1964); vitamin K: Quick *et al.* (1954); Wiseman (1964).

Bile is important for the formation of micelles in which fat-soluble vitamins can most easily be taken up into the mucosal cells. Consequently, trapping of bile acids by cholestyramin impairs the absorption as was shown for vitamins A and K in chicks (Whiteside *et al.*, 1965). The lack of bile in pathological conditions has deleterious consequences for the absorption of fat-soluble vitamins as was shown by Kasper (1967) for

TABLE 1. DAILY REQUIREMENTS OF VITAMINS IN FOOD OF MAN (daily doses in mg)

Vitamin	Daily dose		1 iu =	Chemical name
	adults	babies		
Vitamin A_1	1.5–2[a][b]	0.5–1.0[a]	0.000344 mg	Retinol-acetate
Vitamin D_3	0.04[a][c]	0.04[a]	0.000025 mg	Cholecalciferol
Vitamin E_1	10–30[a]	0.5/kg[a]	1.0 mg	DL-α-Tocopherol-acetate
Vitamin K_1	0.002[d]	0.3/kg[d]	1.0 mg	Phylloquinone

[a]Taken from *Geigy-Wissenschaftliche Tabellen* (1968) and Wiseman (1964).
[b]Requirement in pregnancy and during lactation 1.5–2 times higher.
[c]In pregnancy and lactation only; for adults 0.025 mg are recommended but not necessary provided biosynthesis in the organisms is sufficient.
[d]Doisy and Matschiner (1970); according to these authors the requirement for mothers amounts to 7 mg/day.

vitamin A, by Thompson *et al.* (1966) for vitamin D and by Kelleher and Losowsky (1968) for vitamin E. For the role of bile in malabsorption of vitamin K see also Deutsch (1966) and Vest (1966).

(2) Fat-soluble vitamins enter the organism primarily via the lymph. This was proven experimentally in many species, e.g. in man, rat, sheep, bullock and guinea pig; older references may be taken from Wiseman (1964). The lymphatic route for absorption of fat-soluble vitamins was confirmed recently by the group of Blomstrand (for references see Blomstrand, 1972).

Fat-soluble vitamins are released into lymph mainly within chylomicrons. Since the formation of chylomicrons, which depends on intact cellular metabolism, requires time, the absorption of a single dose of fat-soluble vitamins takes in general several hours (Wiseman, 1964). In rats the uptake of vitamin D into the mucosal cells is a rapid process; it takes place within 30–60 min. The release of vitamin D into the lymph, however, is not completed for 12–18 hr (Schachter *et al.*, 1964).

The properties which determine whether a substance enters the organism via the portal blood or via lymph are far from being completely understood. The substances recovered in lymph are not exclusively in the chylomicron fraction; at present, however, there appears to be no exception to the rule that a compound found in lymph after oral administration is taken up by the chylomicrons formed in the cells of the mucosal epithelium (Blomstrand, 1972).

8.1. VITAMIN A

The chemical structure of retinol and its provitamin, β-carotene, can be taken from Fig. 1. For further details of the chemistry as well as biochemistry of vitamin A and β-carotene see Moore (1970).

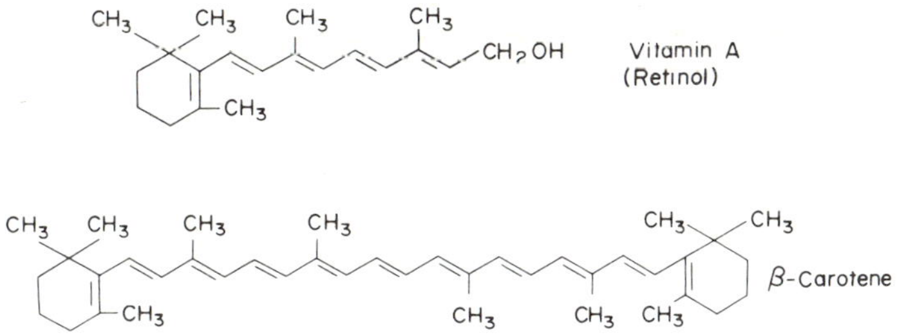

FIG. 1. Vitamin A and β-carotene.

8.1.1. SITE OF ABSORPTION

The site of absorption of vitamin A in man is still unknown. In the rat the highest activity for absorption of vitamin A is recorded for the proximal half of the small intestine (Booth, 1968). This also holds true for sheep, bullocks, guinea pigs (Wiseman, 1964) and chicks (Shellenberger *et al.*, 1964). However, one has to bear in mind that due to the different residence time in the different sections of the intestinal tract the part with highest absorptive rate is not necessarily the part in which the greatest fraction of the total amount absorbed is taken up (cf. p. 275, Chapter 4).

Vitamin A can be absorbed from the stomach (Kasper and Richter, 1971) as well as from the colon (Kasper, 1970). The proximal small intestine also appears to be the site of maximum absorptive activity for β-carotene (cf. Wiseman, 1964).

8.1.2. MODE OF TRANSFER; FATE OF VITAMIN A DURING ABSORPTION

Loran and Althausen (1959) suggested an active transfer mechanism of vitamin A across the mucosal epithelium. In rat jejunal segments *in vitro* transfer of vitamin A is inhibited by the withdrawal of oxygen and by the addition of 2,4-dinitrophenol whereas iodoacetate and sodium fluoride were ineffective. Skala and Hruba (1964) showed Michaelis–Menten-type kinetics for the uptake of vitamin A into the tissues of rat small intestine. The uptake of vitamin A is inhibited by potassium cyanide and sodium fluoride.

In vitamin A-deficient rats the amount of the vitamin absorbed is smaller than in normal animals (Baumann *et al.*, 1934). The decrease may be due to a defect of the absorbing epithelium caused by the vitamin deficiency. In rats vitamin A administered either as alcohol or aldehyde (retinal) is taken up unchanged into the mucosal cells of the intestine (Deshmukh *et al.*, 1965; Mahadevan *et al.*, 1963a); retinal is then reduced in the mucosal cells (Fidge and Goodman, 1968). Before the uptake into the mucosal cells vitamin A esters are split intraluminally (Lawrence *et al.*, 1966) and within the mucosal cells vitamin A is mostly re-esterified prior to its release into the lymph vessels (Mahadevan *et al.*, 1963b). In the lymph more than 90% of the total vitamin A present is in the form of retinyl-esters (Huang and Goodman, 1965). This also holds true for man (Goodman *et al.*, 1966). The composition of retinyl-esters in the lymph of man and rat is nearly the same (Table 2). In both species the palmitate predominates. In rats 3-dehydro-vitamin A is absorbed in the same way as vitamin A (John *et al.*, 1966).

In man and rat β-carotene is absorbed to a smaller extent than vitamin A (cf. Blomstrand, 1972; Goodman *et al.*, 1966; Huang and Goodman, 1965) and is split in the mucosal tissue into vitamin A (for references see Moore, 1970). In the lymph of rats only small amounts of unchanged β-carotene were found (Huang and Goodman, 1965). In man the intestine exhibits only a limited capacity to absorb unchanged dietary β-carotene (Goodman *et al.*, 1966). The difference in absorption of vitamin A and β-carotene is probably due to differences in their availability for absorption; the solubility of carotene in fat is limited whereas vitamin A is highly miscible with fat (cf. Moore, 1970).

TABLE 2. RETINYL-ESTER COMPOSITION IN LYMPH OF RAT AND MAN AFTER TEST MEALS CONTAINING LABELED β-CAROTENE OR RETINOL
(Taken from Huang and Goodman, 1965 and from Goodman *et al.*, 1966)
Mean values; for details see original references

Labeled-compound fed	Species	Percentage distribution of labeled retinyl-esters			
		Palmitate	Stearate	Oleate	Linoleate
β-Carotene (^{14}C)	rat	45	24	21	10
Retinol (^{14}C)	rat	48	23	14	16
β-Carotene (^{3}H)	man	56	25	13	6
Retinol (^{3}H)	man	56	19	16	9

8.1.3. FACTORS INFLUENCING THE AVAILABILITY OF VITAMIN A FOR ABSORPTION

In man the absorption of β-carotene is increased with increasing fat content of food (cf. Cornwell *et al.*, 1962; Gershoff, 1964; Kasper and Ernst, 1969). This also holds true for cats (Gershoff, 1964). There are differences of absorption between carotenes from different sources. β–Carotene from carrots is absorbed to a greater extent than α–carotene (Rao and Rao, 1970). Fat content of food has little effect on the absorption of vitamin A in man, hens and rats (cf. Gershoff, 1964).

Protein content of food influences the absorption of vitamin A (Gershoff, 1964; Ascarelli, 1969). This may be due to the activity of enzymes (esterases) of either pancreas or mucosal epithelium which are involved in the metabolic conversion of vitamin A derivatives. Splitting of vitamin A-palmitate is reduced in protein-deficient rats (Adhikari *et al.*, 1972). The activity of the ester splitting enzymes decreases with low protein intake (Deshmukh *et al.*, 1964). Also the reduction of retinal to retinol in the mucosal tissue is decreased in protein-deficient rats (Deshmukh *et al.*, 1965). High protein intake unspecifically raises the vitamin A requirements (Gershoff, 1964).

There is an increased absorption of vitamin A in the presence of vitamin E (cf. Moore, 1970); this may be due to an unspecific effect rather than the stabilizing effect of vitamin E for vitamin A (Mitchell *et al.*, 1968b).

The addition of vanadium (15–20 ppm), molybdenum (200 ppm), selenium (10 ppm), copper (600 ppm), DDT (10 and 100 ppm) to the diet of rats for a 2-week period was without an effect on the disappearance of β–carotene from ligated intestinal segments (Mitchell *et al.*, 1968a).

8.2. D-VITAMINS*

Very little is known about the absorption mechanism of D-vitamins (cf. Avioli, 1969; Blomstrand, 1972). The chemical structure of the commonly used D-vitamins can be taken from Fig. 2. Biochemical details are to be found in Hartles' review (1970).

*Here, the conventional nomenclature is used (cf. Chapter 11, pp. 545–547). At present, 25-hydroxycholecalciferol and 1,25-dihydroxycholecalciferol (25-(OH)-D_3; 1,25-$(OH)_2$-D_3) are considered to be the active forms of Vitamin D. 1,25-$(OH)_2$-D_3 is well absorbed from the GI-tract; its efficiency, however, decreases when having been administered repeatedly in oil solutions (Tanaka and DeLuca (1972) *J. Nutr.* **102:** 1569) (Eds.).

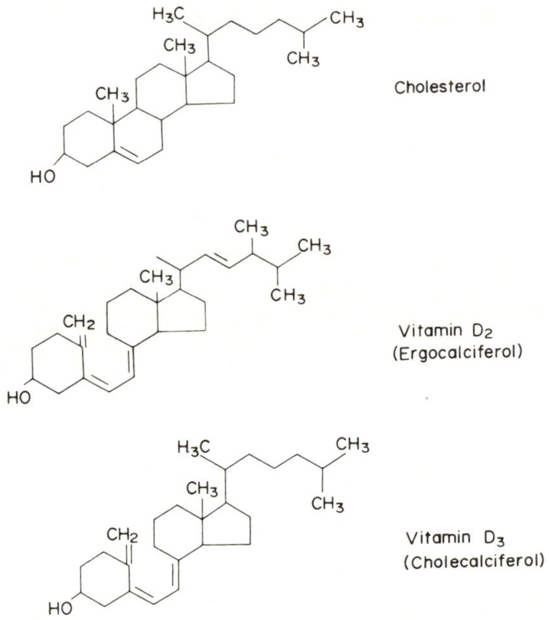

FIG. 2. Vitamins D_2, D_3 and cholesterol.

8.2.1. SITE OF ABSORPTION

In rats maximum absorption activity was demonstrated in the mid jejunum (Schachter *et al.*, 1964). In man the amount of vitamin D_3 absorbed in the duodenum was slightly greater than that in the jejunum (Hollander *et al.*, 1971). The proximal part of the small intestine is most important for the absorption of vitamin D_3 in man. This may be derived from investigations on patients subjected to resections of the distal part of the small intestine (Thompson *et al.*, 1966).

8.2.2. MODE OF TRANSFER; FATE OF D-VITAMINS DURING THE TRANSFER

The transfer of vitamins D_2 and D_3 was investigated in rat intestine by Schachter *et al.* (1964) *in vitro* and *in vivo*. The bulk of vitamin D_3 appears in the lymph as the free vitamin; only a small fraction is esterified in the mucosal epithelium with oleic acid. This is true for man (cf. Blomstrand,

1972) as well as for rats (Bell and Bryan, 1969). In contrast to vitamin D_3, most of cholesterol in lymph is in the form of the oleic acid ester (cf. Blomstrand, 1972).

Vitamin D_3 administered orally as the oleic acid ester is split intraluminally. In rats the oleic acid ester of vitamin D_3 is absorbed to a smaller extent than is the free vitamin (Bell and Bryan, 1969).

Intraluminal administration of "mixed micellar solutions" of either linoleic or palmitic acid increases the appearance of both free cholesterol and vitamin D_3 in lymph, whereas the fractions of esterified cholesterol remain the same as in control experiments with taurocholate solutions (Thompson *et al.*, 1969). In these experiments the uptake of cholesterol

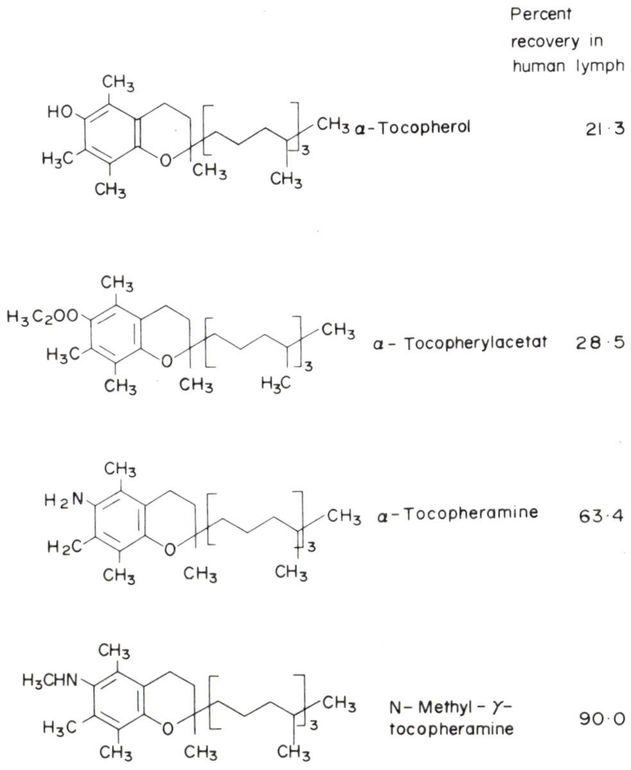

FIG. 3. Tocopherols (taken from Blomstrand, 1972). The compounds which were labeled either with ^{14}C or ^{3}H were administered in a formula diet. Radioactivity was determined in lymph collected during 24 hr.

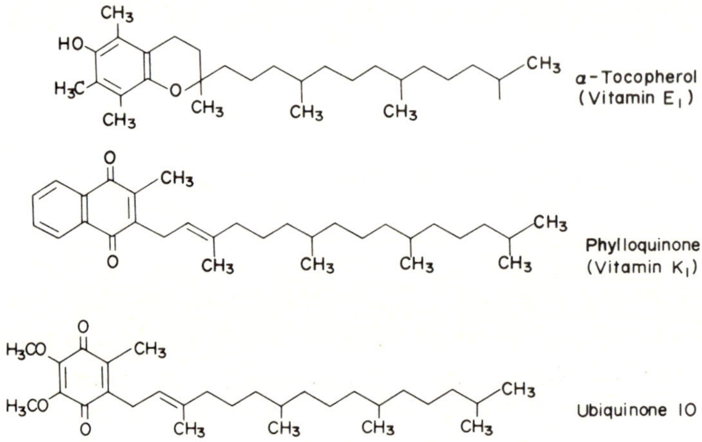

FIG. 4. Structural similarities between vitamins E, K and ubiquinone 10.

and vitamin D_3 into the mucosal cells was the same regardless of whether mixed micellar lipid or taurocholate solutions were administered intraluminally. These findings suggest that mixed micellar lipids increase the release of free cholesterol and vitamin D_3 from the mucosal cells into the lymph.

8.2.3. EXCRETION INTO THE INTESTINAL TRACT

Vitamin D_3 administered parenterally appears in the feces. Besides excretion via the bile an excretion across the gut wall is discussed. The proximal third of the small intestine is considered to be most active in this respect (cf. Wiseman, 1964).

8.3. E-VITAMINS (TOCOPHEROLS)

Some tocopherols commonly used in therapeutics are listed in Fig. 3. There are structural similarities between tocopherols, K-vitamins and ubiquinones (Fig. 4).

8.3.1. SITE OF ABSORPTION

No systematic investigations are available (Booth, 1968). When comparing the amount of α-tocopherol absorbed after feeding by stomach tube and after intracecal injections Schmandke (1964) found that the proximal sections of the intestinal tract are nearly 6 times as active as the distal ones. Since an enterohepatic circulation of vitamin E occurs (cf. Wiseman, 1964) the distal sections of the intestinal tract are not unimportant for absorption. Phytylubiquinone is excreted into bile as a conjugate hydrolyzable by glucuronidase (Blomstrand and Gürtler, 1971).

8.3.2. MODE OF TRANSFER; FATE OF E-VITAMINS DURING THE TRANSFER

A linear relationship between concentration of α–tocopherol administered in the incubation medium and the uptake by rat jejunal slices *in vitro* was obtained from 6.25–200 mcg/ml (Pearson and Legge, 1972). In man Schmandke *et al.* (1969) reported a decrease of the amount absorbed by about 40% between doses of 10 mcg and 2 mg of α–tocopherol. No systematic investigations of the transfer process of α–tocopherol across the mucosal epithelium were published.

In the lymph of man tocopheramine and tocopherol appear unchanged. Tocopheryl-acetate (Blomstrand, 1972; Blomstrand and Forsgren, 1968b) and -nicotinate (Gallo-Torres, 1970b) are split on the way from the intestinal lumen into lymph.

Tocopheramine and *N*-methyl-tocopheramine are absorbed to a greater extent than α–tocopherol and its acetic acid ester (Fig. 4); the authors (Blomstrand, 1972; Blomstrand and Forsgren, 1968b) interpret this observation by the different availability of tocopherols for absorption due to the composition of food. The difference of absorption between α–tocopherol and its acetic acid ester has also been found in rats (Underwood *et al.*, 1968).

The absorption of 8 different naturally occurring tocochromanols was investigated in rats after feeding by stomach tube by Pearson and Barnes (1970a). The same authors (1970b) found the following absorption quotas in tied-off jejunal segments of rats for α–, β–, γ– and δ–tocopherol: 32%, 18%, 30% and 1.8%.

8.3.3. FACTORS INFLUENCING THE AVAILABILITY FOR ABSORPTION

Absorption of α–tocopherol can be impaired after gastric surgery followed by steatorrhea (Kelleher and Losowsky, 1970), biliary obstruction (Macmahon and Neale, 1970; Harris and Muller, 1971) and exocrine pancreatic insufficiency (Macmahon and Neale, 1970).

Polyunsaturated fatty acids in food decrease the amount of vitamin E_1 absorbed (Akerib and Sterner, 1971; Gallo-Torres *et al.*, 1971). These fatty acids cause an oxidative destruction of vitamin E_1. Due to nutritive habits the fraction of polyunsaturated fatty acids in food of man is increasing; an increased requirement of E-vitamins of man can therefore be predicted (cf. Gershoff, 1964).

Selenium increases the absorption of vitamin E_1 in chicks by restitution of the defect exocrine pancreas function subsequent to selenium-deficiency (Thompson and Scott, 1969, 1970). For further information about the relationship between selenium and vitamin E_1 in metabolism see Draper (1970) and Underwood (1971).

8.4. K-VITAMINS

The chemical structure of K-vitamins is shown in Fig. 5. Very few systematic investigations on the absorption of K-vitamins have been

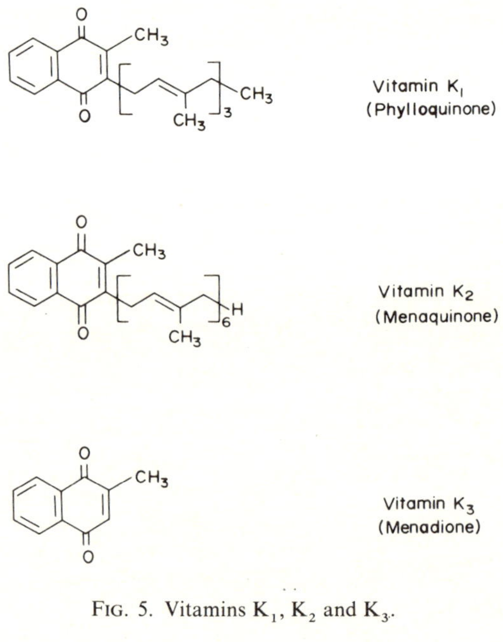

FIG. 5. Vitamins K_1, K_2 and K_3.

carried out; nothing is known about the site of absorption (Booth, 1968). In chicks vitamin K_1 and vitamin K_2 are absorbed from the rectum (Berdanier and Griminger, 1968). The colon, the site of production of K-vitamins by the microbial flora, is not necessarily also the main site of absorption (Udall, 1963). Barnes and Fiala (1959) produced prothrombin deficiency in rats by feeding a diet free of vitamins and preventing coprophagy. It is therefore doubtful whether the K-vitamins produced by the microbial flora of the gut can be absorbed directly (Doisy and Matschiner, 1965) but they may be an important nutritional source in ruminants. The list of K-vitamin analogues synthesized by bacteria can be taken from Pennock (1966).

The absorption of vitamins K_1, K_2 and K_3 was investigated in the chick *in vitro* and *in vivo*. Vitamins K_1 and K_2 are absorbed against a concentration gradient. Therefore, an active, i.e. energy dependent, process is assumed to be involved (Berdanier and Griminger, 1968). Vitamin K_3 is absorbed completely after oral administration whereas vitamin K_1 is absorbed only to 50% of the dose (Jaques *et al.*, 1954). Alkylated K-vitamins are split to menadione which is either absorbed or converted to an active form of vitamin K (menaquinone-4) prior to absorption by bacteria (Billeter *et al.*, 1964; for further ref. see Doisy and Matschiner, 1970).

Bile is prerequisite only for the absorption of vitamin K_1 and not for that of vitamin K_3 (Berdanier and Griminger, 1968; Jaques *et al.*, 1954). Vitamin K_3 enters the organism mainly by the portal route (Jaques *et al.*, 1954; Mezick *et al.*, 1968) whereas vitamin K_1 is taken up mainly by the lymph (Blomstrand, 1972; Blomstrand and Forsgren, 1968a). In the lymph the greatest part of vitamin K_1 is unchanged; only traces of unidentified metabolites were found (Blomstrand, 1972; Blomstrand and Forsgren, 1968a).

The absorption of K-vitamins is impaired by mineral oil, squalene, other oils (for references see Doisy and Matschiner, 1970) and several other lipids including vitamin A (Doisy and Matschiner, 1966; Griminger, 1965; for further ref. see Doisy and Matschiner, 1970). The hypoprothrombinemia-producing effect of vitamin A hypervitaminosis is well known (for ref. see Doisy and Matschiner, 1970). This effect is probably due to an interference of vitamin A with K-vitamins during the absorption process. In adult male rats the daily ingestion of 30 mcg of retinoic acid reduces the absorptive utilization of K-vitamins to about the same extent as does 100 mg dietary squalene; possibly, an unabsorbable complex between retinoic acid and K-vitamins is formed (Doisy and Matschiner, 1970).

Quick and Stefanini (1948) assumed an inhibition of the microbial synthesis of K-vitamins by vitamin A. However, the vitamin K content of the feces of chicks fed a low vitamin K diet revealed no differences whether retinoic acid was added to the food or not (Matschiner *et al.*, 1967). Vitamin K and vitamin A are antagonists even in germ-free rats (Wostmann and Knight, 1965).

8.5. SUMMARY

In general, the principles governing the absorption of fat-soluble vitamins are similar to those of fat absorption. The availability depends on the function of bile and the presence of pancreatic lipases. During the transfer across the mucosal cells the bulk of the fat-soluble vitamins is taken up into protein-coated chylomicrons. Prerequisite for the formation of chylomicrons is an intact cellular metabolism. The chylomicrons are released into the lymph. The portal blood plays only a minor role as route entry for fat-soluble vitamins.

The transfer mechanisms across the mucosal epithelium for fat-soluble vitamins are far from being understood well. For most of the fat-soluble vitamins even the absorption rates in the different sections of the gastro-intestinal tract are still unknown in either man and animal. Thus in man the nutritive significance of the microbial production of K-vitamins is still subject to controversy. With regard to the significance of fat-soluble vitamins in human nutrition as well as for animal production in husbandry systematic investigations are needed.

REFERENCES

Adhikari, M. R., Vakil, U. K. and Streenivasan, A. (1972) Relative rates of retinyl-palmitate and (^{3}H)-retinol absorption in protein-deficient rat. *Ind. J. Biochem. Biophys.* **9:** 89–93.

Akerib, M. and Sterner, M. (1971) Inhibition of vitamin E absorption by a lipid fraction. *Int. J. Nutr. Res.* **41:** 42–43.

Ascarelli, I. (1969) Absorption and transport of vitamin A in chicks. *Am. J. Clin. Nutr.* **22:** 913–922.

Avioli, L. V. (1969) Absorption and metabolism of vitamin D_3 in man. *Am. J. Clin. Nutr.* **22:** 437–446.

Barnes, R. H. and Fiala, J. (1959) Effects of the prevention of coprophagy in the rat. *J. Nutr.* **68:** 602–614.

Baumann, C. A., Riising, B. M. and Steenbock, H. (1934) Fat-soluble vitamins. 42. The absorption and storage of vitamin A in the rat. *J. Biol. Chem.* **107:** 705–715.

Bell, N. H. and Bryan, P. (1969) Absorption of vitamin D_3 oleate in the rat. *Am. J. Clin. Nutr.* **22:** 425–430.

BERDANIER, C. D. and GRIMINGER, P. (1968) *In vitro* and *in vivo* absorption of three vitamin K analogues by chick intestine. *Int. Z. Vit. Forschung* **38:** 376–382.

BILLETER, M., BOLLIGER, W. and MARTIUS, C. (1964) Untersuchungen über die Umwandlung von verfütterten K-Vitaminen durch Austausch der Seitenkette und die Rolle der Darmbakterien hierbei. *Biochem. Z.* **340:** 290–303.

BLOMSTRAND, R. (1972) Influence of molecular structure on the intestinal absorption of fat-soluble vitamins, pp. 231–244. In: *Transport Across the Intestine*, BURLUND, W. L. and SAMUEL, P. D. (Eds.). Churchill & Livingstone; Edinburgh and London.

BLOMSTRAND, R. and FORSGREN, L. (1968a) Vitamin K_1–^3H in man. Its intestinal absorption and transport in the thoracic duct lymph. *Int. Z. Vit. Forschung* **38:** 45–64.

BLOMSTRAND, R. and FORSGREN, L. (1968b) Labelled tocopherols in man. *Int. Z. Vit. Forschung* **38:** 328–344.

BLOMSTRAND, R. and GÜRTLER, J. (1971) Studies on the intestinal absorption and metabolism of phytylubiquinone-(1, 2, -3H) (Hexahydroubiquinone-4) in man. *Int. J. Vit. Res.* **41:** 189–203.

BOOTH, C. C. (1968) Effect of location along the small intestine on absorption of nutrients, pp. 1513–1528. In: *Handbook of Physiology*, sect. 6: *Alimentary Canal*, vol. III, *Intestinal Absorption*, CODE, C. F. and HEIDEL, W. (Eds.). Am. Phys. Soc., Washington D.C.

CORNWELL, D. G., KRUGER, F. A. and ROBINSON, H. B. (1962) Studies on the absorption of β-carotene and the distribution of total carotenoid in human serum lipoproteins after oral administration. *J. Lipid Res.* **3:** 65–70.

DESHMUKH, D. S., MALATHI, P. and GANGULY, J. (1964) Studies on metabolism of vitamin A. Dietary protein content and metabolism of vitamin A. *Biochem. J.* **90:** 98–104.

DESHMUKH, D. S., MURTHY, S. K., MAHADEVAN, S. and GANGULY, J. (1965) Studies on metabolism of vitamin A. Absorption of retinal in rats. *Biochem. J.* **96:** 377–382.

DEUTSCH, E. (1966) Vitamin K in medical practice: adults. *Vitamins and Hormones* **24:** 665–680.

DOISY, E. A. and MATSCHINER, J. T. (1966) In: *Biochemistry of Quinones*, pp. 317–353, MORTON, R. A. (Ed.). Academic Press, New York and London.

DOISY, E. A. and MATSCHINER, J. T. (1970) Biochemistry of vitamin K, pp. 293–332. In: *Fat-soluble Vitamins*, MORTON, R. A. (Ed.). Pergamon Press; Oxford.

DRAPER, H. H. (1970) The tocopherols, pp. 333–394. In: *Fat-soluble Vitamins*, MORTON, R. A. (Ed.). Pergamon Press; Oxford.

FIDGE, N. H. and GOODMAN, D. S. (1968) The enzymatic reduction of retinal to retinol in rat intestine. *J. Biol. Chem.* **243:** 4372–4379.

GALLO-TORRES, H. E. (1970a) Obligatory role of bile for the intestinal absorption of vitamin E. *Lipids* **5:** 379–384.

GALLO-TORRES, H. E. (1970b) Intestinal absorption and lymphatic transport of D,l-3-4-$^3H_2$-α-tocopheryl-acetate in the rat. *Int. J. Vit. Res.* **40:** 505–514.

GALLO-TORRES, H. E., WEBER, F. and WISS, O. (1971) The effect of different dietary lipids on the lymphatic appearance of vitamin E. *Int. J. Vit. Res.* **41:** 504–515.

GERSHOFF, ST. N. (1964) Effects of dietary levels of macronutrients on vitamin requirements. *Fed. Proc.* **23:** 1077–1082.

GOODMAN, D. S., BLOMSTRAND, R., WERNER, B., HUANG, H. S. and SHIRATORI, T. (1966) The intestinal absorption and metabolism of vitamin A and β-carotene in man. *J. Clin. Invest.* **45:** 1616–1623.

GRIMINGER, P. (1965) Vitamin K activity in chickens: phylloquinone and menadione in the presence of stress agents. *J. Nutr.* **87:** 337–343.

HARRIS, J. T. and MULLER, D. P. R. (1971) Absorption of vitamin E in children with biliary obstruction. *Gut* **12:** 579–584.

HARTLES, R. L. (1970) Biochemistry of vitamin D, pp. 279–292. In: *Fat-soluble Vitamins*, MORTON, R. A. (Ed.). Pergamon Press; Oxford.

HOLLANDER, D., ROSTENSTREICH, S. J. and VOLWIFER, W. (1971) Role of duodenum in vitamin D_3 absorption in man. *Am. J. Dig. Dis.* **16:** 145–149.

HUANG, H. S. and GOODMAN, D. S. (1965) Vitamin A and carotenoids. I. Intestinal absorption and metabolism of ^{14}C-labeled vitamin A, alcohol and β-carotene in the rat. *J. Biol. Chem.* **240:** 2839–2844.

JAQUES, L. B., MILLAR, G. J. and SPINKS, J. W. T. (1954) The metabolism of the K-vitamins. *Schweiz. Med. Wschr.* **84:** 792–796.

JOHN, K. V., LAKSHMANAN, M. R. and CAMA, H. R. (1966) Absorption, storage and distribution of 3-dehydrovitamin A in the rat. *Biochem. J.* **99:** 312–316.

KASPER, H. (1967) Vitaminresorption nach Pankreatektomie. *Gastroenterologia* **107:** 305–316.

KASPER, H. (1970) Vitamin absorption in the colon. *Am. J. Proctol.* **21:** 341–345.

KASPER, H. and ERNST, S. (1969) Effect of food fat and vitamin A on carotene resorption. *Int. Z. Vit. Forschung* **39:** 23–29.

KASPER, H. and RICHTER, E. (1971) Vitamin A absorption in the stomach. *Int. J. Vit. Res.* **41:** 472–474.

KELLEHER, J. and LOSOWSKY, M. S. (1968) The absorption of vitamin E in man. *Biochem. J.* **110:** 20P–21P.

KELLEHER, J. and LOSOWSKY, M. S. (1970) The absorption of α-tocopherol in man. *Brit. J. Nutr.* **24:** 1033–1047.

LAWRENCE, C. W., CRAIN, F. D., LOTSPEICH, F. J. and KRAUSE, R. F. (1966) Absorption, transport and storage of retinyl-15-^{14}C-palmitate-9,10-^{3}H in the rat. *J. Lipid. Res.* **7:** 226–229.

LORAN, M. R. and ALTHAUSEN, T. L. (1959) Transport of vitamin A *in vitro* across normal isolated rat intestine and intestine subjected to partial resection. *Am. J. Physiol.* **197:** 1333–1336.

MACMAHON, M. T. and NEALE, G. (1970) The absorption of α-tocopherol in control subjects and in patients with intestinal malabsorption. *Clin. Sci.* **39:** 197–210.

MAHADEVAN, S., SASTRY, P. S. and GANGULY, J. (1963a) Studies on metabolism of vitamin A. The mode of absorption of vitamin A esters in the living rat. *Biochem. J.* **88:** 531–534.

MAHADEVAN, S., SASTRY, P. S. and GANGULY, J. (1963b) Studies on metabolism of vitamin A. Studies on the mode of absorption of vitamin A by rat intestine *in vitro*. *J. Biochem.* **88:** 534–539.

MATSCHINER, J. T., AMELOTTI, J. M. and DOISY, E. A. (1967) Mechanism of the effect of ketinoic acid and squalene on vitamin K deficiency in the rat. *J. Nutr.* **91:** 303–306.

MEZICK, J. A., TOMKINS, R. K. and CORNWELL, D. G. (1968) Absorption and intestinal lymphatic transport of ^{14}C-menadione. *Life Sci.* **7:** 153–158.

MITCHELL, G. E., LITTLE, C. O. and SKERSKI, G. (1968a) Influence of subacute levels of dietary toxins on carotene disappearance from the rat intestine: *Int. Z. Vit. Forschung* **38:** 308–311.

MITCHELL, G. E., LITTLE, C. O., WARNER, R. L., KLATTE, F. J. and ALDERSON, N. E. (1968b) Influence on vitamin E on pre-intestinal disappearance of vitamin A in steers. *Int. Z. Vit. Forschung* **38:** 304–307.

MOORE, T. (1970) The biochemistry of vitamin A in the general system, pp. 223–266. In: *Fat-soluble Vitamins*, MORTON, R. A. (Ed.). Pergamon Press: Oxford.

OLSON, J. A. (1964) The effect of bile and bile salts on the uptake and cleavage of β-carotene into retinol ester by intestinal slices. *L. Lipid Res.* **5:** 402–408.

PEARSON, C. K. and BARNES, M. MCC. (1970a) Absorption of tocopherols by small intestinal loops of the rat *in vitro*. *Int. J. Vit. Res.* **40:** 19–22.

PEARSON, C. K. and BARNES, M. MCC. (1970b) The absorption and distribution of the natural occurring tocochromanols in the rat. *Brit. J. Nutr.* **24:** 581–587.

PEARSON, C. K. and LEGGE, A. M. (1972) Uptake of vitamin E by rat small intestinal slices. *Biochim. Biophys. Acta* **288:** 404–412.

PENNOCK, J. F. (1966) Occurrence of vitamins K and related quinones. *Vitamins and Hormones* **24:** 307–329.

QUICK, A. J., HUSSEY, C. V. and COLLENTINE, G. E. (1954) Vitamin K requirements of adult dogs and the influence of bile on its absorption from the intestine. *Am. J. Physiol.* **176:** 239–242.

QUICK, A. J. and STEFANINI, M. (1948) Experimentally induced changes in prothrombin level of blood; relation of vitamin K deficiency to intensity of dicumarol action and to effect of excess vitamin A intake with simplified method for vitamin K assay. *J. Biol. Chem.* **175:** 945–952.

RAO, C. M. and RAO, B. S. (1970) Absorption of dietary carotene in human subjects. *Am. J. Clin. Nutr.* **23:** 105–109.

SCHACHTER, D., FINKELSTEIN, J. D. and KOWARSKI, S. (1964) Metabolism of vitamin D. I. Preparation of radioactive vitamin D and its intestinal absorption in the rat. *J. Clin. Invest.* **43:** 787–796.

SCHMANDKE, H. (1964) Die Resorption des α-Tocopherols in den distalen Darmabschnitten der Ratte. *Int. Z. Vit. Forschung* **34:** 186–189.

SCHMANDKE, H., SIMA, C. and MAUNE, R. (1969) Absorption of α-tocopherol in man. *Int. Z. Vit. Forschung* **39:** 296–298.

SELBY, M. A. and GREEN, J. (1970) The fortification of human and animal foods with fat-soluble vitamins, pp. 485–492. In: *Fat-soluble Vitamins,* MORTON, R. A. (Ed.). Pergamon Press; Oxford.

SHELLENBERGER, T. E., PARRISH, D. B. and SANFORD, P. E. (1964) Absorption of preformed vitamin A from ligated poultry intestinal sections. *J. Nutr.* **82:** 99–105.

SKALA, I. and HRUBA, F. (1964) Accumulation of vitamin A by small intestine of the rat *in vitro. Am. J. Physiol.* **206:** 458–460.

THOMPSON, G. R., LEWIS, B. and BOOTH, C. C. (1966) Absorption of vitamin$_3$-^{3}H in control subjects and patients with intestinal malabsorption. *J. Clin. Invest.* **45:** 94–102.

THOMPSON, G. R., OCKNER, R. K. and ISSELBACHER, K. J. (1969) Effect of mixed micellar lipid on the absorption of cholesterol and vitamin D_3 into lymph. *J. Clin. Invest.* **48:** 87–95.

THOMPSON, J. N. and SCOTT, M. L. (1969) Role of selenium in the nutrition of the chick. *J. Nutr.* **97:** 335–342.

THOMPSON, J. N. and SCOTT, M. L. (1970) Impaired lipid and vitamin E absorption related to atrophy of the pancreas in selenium-deficient chicks. *J. Nutr.* **100:** 797–809.

UDALL, J. A. (1963) (letter to the editor) *New Engl. J. Med.* **268:** 274.

UNDERWOOD, B. A., ITO, Y. and DENNING, C. (1968) Effect of medium-chain triglycerides on tocopherol absorption. *Am. J. Clin. Nutr.* **21:** 538.

UNDERWOOD, E. J. (1971) Trace elements in human and animal nutrition, pp. 323–368. Academic Press; New York and London.

VEST, M. (1966) Vitamin K in medical practice: pediatrics. *Vitamins and Hormones* **24:** 649–663.

WHITESIDE, C. H., HARKINS, R. W., FLUCKIGER, H. B. and SARETT, H. P. (1965) Utilization of fat-soluble vitamins by rats and chicks fed cholestyramine, a bile acid sequestrant. *Am. J. Clin. Nutr.* **16:** 309–314.

WISEMAN, G. (1964) *Absorption from the Intestine,* pp. 329–357. Academic Press; New York, London.

Wissenschaftliche Tabellen (1968) Documenta Geigy, DIEM, K. and LENTNER, C. (Eds.). J. R. Geigy AG; Basel.

WOSTMANN, B. S. and KNIGHT, P. L. (1965) Antagonism between vitamins A and K in the germ-free rat. *J. Nutr.* **87:** 155–160.

CHAPTER 9

THE GASTROINTESTINAL ABSORPTION OF HORMONES AND RELATED COMPOUNDS

Donald S. Layne

Ottawa, Ontario, Canada

9.1. INTRODUCTION

The absorption of hormones from the intestine has little known physiological relevance, with the exception of problems related to the enterohepatic circulation of some endogenously produced compounds. However, from the therapeutic standpoint, gastrointestinal absorption of hormones and related products is of great importance. In this chapter, primary concern will be directed to the gastrointestinal absorption of the hormones of man, but, since much of the recorded information on this subject has been obtained in studies on animals, the limitations imposed by species differences on the extrapolation of this information to therapeutic uses must be borne in mind.

There are very early historical records (Paschkis *et al.*, 1958) of the use of the products of the endocrine glands of animals as therapeutic agents for clinically observed conditions, in particular to correct the effects of castration or hypogonadism in the male and to produce aphrodisia or fertility in either sex. The administration of extracts of animal glands, or of the urinary products derived from their secretions, was found to be effective. However, very few of the natural animal hormones are useful for oral therapy in the treatment of human endocrine malfunctions, since, with a few exceptions, they are either poorly absorbed from the gut or appear to be inactivated before reaching target tissues.* Accordingly, there is continuous research activity in the development of drugs which have effects similar to those of the hormones. These drugs are often, but not always, chemically related to the natural hormones,

*For a review dealing with the capacity of the gut to metabolize hormones see *Physiol Rev.* **53:** 496 (1973; K. Hartiala) (Eds.).

and a primary concern in much of this development work is that the compounds synthesized should be effective when administered by mouth.

The hormones of animals may be classified physiologically by their site of origin. However, for the purposes of the present discussion a more convenient classification is afforded by their chemical nature, since it is possible to include the synthetic compounds under the same broad categories. The hormones and their synthetic analogs will therefore be considered under the following chemical groupings.

9.1.1. PROTEINS OR PEPTIDES

These include the hormones of the pituitary and the placenta, insulin, parathyroid hormone, some of the products of the thyroid gland, thyrocalcitonin, and probably also the as yet uncharacterized entities renin, angiotensin and bradykinin. Without exception, the protein hormones are destroyed by proteolytic enzymes in the intestinal tract. If insulin is administered directly into the jejunum of rats together with inhibitors of proteolytic enzymes, some passage of the hormone through the intestinal wall can be demonstrated (Danforth and Moore, 1959). Some absorption of orally administered insulin has also been shown in newly born animals (see Pierce *et al.*, 1964), while Crane and Luntz (1968) have shown that direct administration of insulin into the small intestine of a diabetic human resulted in a lowering of blood and urinary glucose levels. However, in all these studies only a very small amount of a large dose of insulin was absorbed, and the oral route of administration has no general therapeutic importance with insulin or any of the other protein hormones.

9.1.2. STEROIDS

The hormonal products of the adrenal cortex and of the sex organs are derivatives of cyclopentanoperhydrophenanthrene, which is the parent nucleus of the steroids. The placenta also produces steroid hormones in some but not all species.

9.1.3. SMALL NON-STEROIDAL MOLECULES

The catecholamines and other non-protein neurohormones, as well as thyroxine, will be considered under this heading.

9.2. FACTORS AFFECTING GASTROINTESTINAL ABSORPTION OF HORMONES

9.2.1. DEPENDENCE OF ABSORPTION OF STEROIDS ON CHEMICAL AND PHYSICAL PROPERTIES

The biochemical class of compounds known as the steroids includes a large number of products of both animal and plant origin, notably the sterols, bile acids and cardiac glycosides, in addition to the steroid hormones. The ring structure of these compounds is shown in Fig. 1, with the conventional numbering assigned to the individual carbon atoms. This ring structure is also the basic unit of many synthetic hormone-like drugs.

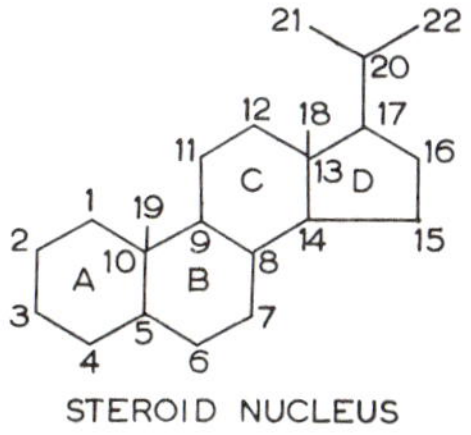

FIG. 1. Ring structure of the steroids.

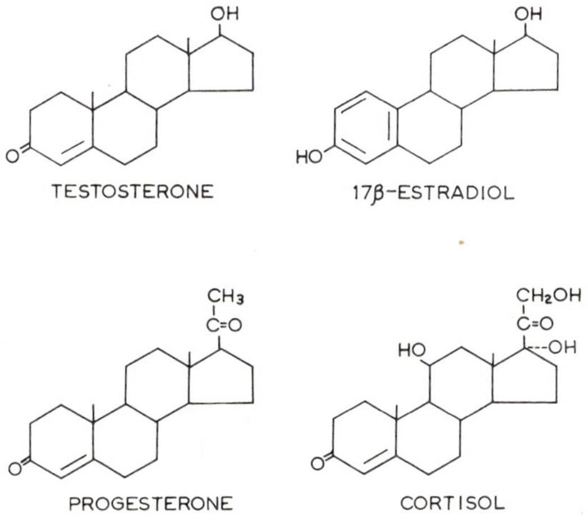

FIG. 2. Some steroid hormones secreted in humans.

TABLE 1. SYSTEMATIC NAMES OF COMPOUNDS IN THE ORDER OF THEIR OCCURRENCE IN THE TEXT

Trivial name	Systematic name
Testosterone	17β-hydroxy-4-androsten-3-one
17β-Estradiol	estra-1,3,5(10)-triene-3,17β-diol
Progesterone	pregn-4-ene-3,20-dione
Cortisol	11β,17α,21-trihydroxy-4-pregnene-3,20-dione
Prednisone	17α,21-dihydroxypregna-1,4-diene-3,11,20-trione
Triamcinolone	9-fluoro-11β,16α,17,21-tetrahydroxypregna-1,4-diene-3,20-dione
Norethynodrel	17α-ethynyl-17β-hydroxyestr-5(10)-en-3-one
Norethindrone	17α-ethinyl-17β-hydroxyestr-4-en-3-one
Mestranol	3-methoxy-17α-ethinyl-17β-hydroxyestra-1,3,5(10)-triene
Medroxyprogesterone acetate	6α-methyl-17α-acetoxy-4-pregnen-3,20-dione
17α-Hydroxyprogesterone caproate	17-caproxy-4-pregnen-3,20-dione
Diethylstilbestrol	3,4-*bis*-(*p*-hydroxyphenyl)-3-hexene
Epinephrine	3,4-dihydroxy-α[(methylamino) methyl] benzyl alcohol
Norepinephrine	3,4-dihydroxy-α(aminomethyl) benzyl alcohol
Isoproterenol	3,4-dihydroxy-α[(isopropylamino) methyl] benzyl alcohol
Amphetamine	dl-α-methylphenethylamine
Ephedrine	α [1-(methylamino) ethyl] benzyl alcohol
Thyroxine	3 [4-(4-hydroxy-3,5-diiodophenoxy)-3,5-diiodophenyl] alanine
Triiodothyronine	β[-4-(hydroxy-3-iodophenoxy)-3,5-diiodophenyl] alanine

The steroids are small molecules of a molecular weight in the region of 250 to 400. They are essentially lipophilic, or fat-soluble, in character but their hydrophilic properties may be increased by the substitution of hydroxyl groups for hydrogen atoms at various positions on the molecule. Fat solubility usually, though not always, varies with the number of double bonds between carbon atoms in the steroid.

Some steroid hormones secreted by the human are shown in Fig. 2. The systematic chemical names of all the compounds are given in Table 1. An arbitrary classification commonly used in the steroid series is based on the number of carbon atoms in the molecule. Thus, both progesterone and cortisol are C–21 steroids, and testosterone, in which the 2-carbon side chain at C–17 is absent, is a C–19 steroid. Estradiol, by virtue of the aromatic nature of ring A of the molecule, has lost the angular methyl group which is present at position 19 in the other steroids, and thus has only 18 carbon atoms.

In synthetic steroids used therapeutically the structural modifications are dictated by the desirability of increased oral potency, although they are also conditioned by the need to improve a particular therapeutic action, while simultaneously reducing one or a number of other physiological or pharmacological activities of the steroid. There has been considerable work on the development and testing of orally active testosterone derivatives, the most successful of which has been 17α-methyltestosterone. Much research has also centered on attempts to obtain steroid derivatives which are anabolic, but which do not produce marked androgenic stimulation; however, no clear pattern has emerged to indicate specific structural requirements which might be altered to dissociate these two effects.

Various alterations on the molecule can change the ratio of carbohydrate-regulating to sodium-retaining activity among the adrenal cortico-steroids. A comprehensive review of structure–activity relationships in this series of steroids is provided by Travis and Sayers (1965). A large number of orally active synthetic compounds are available which possess corticoid activity. Of the two of these depicted in Fig. 3, prednisone has predominantly carbohydrate-regulating potency, while triamcinolone is used as an anti-inflammatory drug. It is important to note that, while triamcinolone is active when given by mouth, it is not as well absorbed from the gut as some orally less potent steroids, as discussed later. Its oral potency must therefore be due to slow inactivation by the body.

An "estrogen" may be defined as any compound which, on administration to castrated rats or mice, causes cornification of the vaginal epithelium (Burrows, 1949). The naturally occurring steroid estrogens of the animal kingdom are typified by 17β-estradiol (Fig. 2). They all have a benzenoid ring A, which renders the hydroxyl group on carbon 3 phenolic. This confers weak acidic properties on the molecule, in that the phenolic hydroxyl group is ionizable and can form salts. The pK_a values of some of the phenolic steroids have been determined, and range from 10.914 for estrone to 9.079 for 6-ketoestradiol (Kirdani and Burgett,

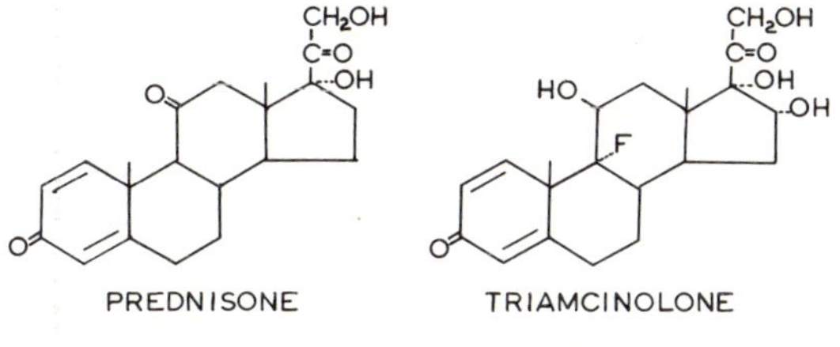

FIG. 3. Synthetic steroids with predominantly carbohydrate regulating activity (prednisone) and anti-inflammatory activity (triamcinolone).

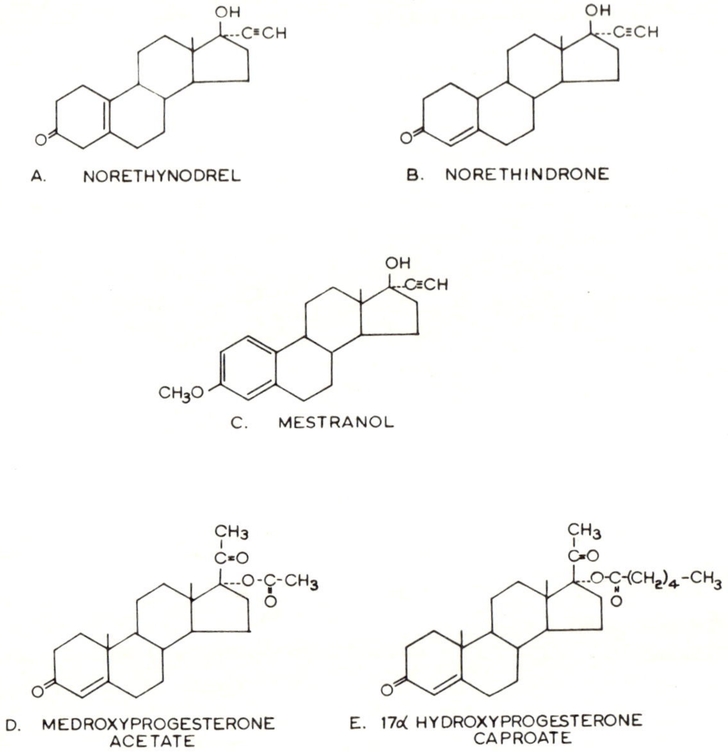

FIG. 4. Some synthetic steroids used as a contraceptive.

1967). There is, however, no evidence that the presence of the ionizable phenoxy group on these steroids confers any special properties on them, distinct from those of other steroids, with regard to absorption from the stomach or intestine.

Figure 4 shows some further representatives of the large number of synthetic steroids now available for therapeutic use. Compounds A, B and C are used for contraceptive purposes, and also for therapy in gynecologic conditions in which either progestational effect (compounds A and B), or estrogenic effect (compound C) is required. Compounds D and E (Fig. 4) are derivatives of the natural hormone progesterone (Fig. 2). They are used as oral progestational agents, both for contraception and in clinical practice. In contrast to the parent compound, progesterone, they are effective when administered orally.

It is likely that compounds A, B and C (Fig. 4) owe part of their oral efficacy to their very efficient absorption from the small intestine, a property which is conferred by the ethinyl group attached to carbon 17 of the steroid ring. However, there is evidence that the presence of the ethinyl group inhibits the metabolism of the steroids by the liver (Langecker, 1961) and this could have the effect of enhancing and prolonging their biological effect. Similarly, the chemical modifications and esterifications effected on the progesterone molecule to form compounds D and E (Fig. 4) may also have the effect of reducing hepatic inactivation of the molecule. Progesterone itself is well absorbed from the small intestine (Schedl, 1965) so that its lack of oral effectiveness appears to be due to inactivation prior to reaching its target tissues.

9.2.2. MECHANISM OF ABSORPTION OF ORALLY ADMINISTERED STEROIDS

By the incubation of steroids with everted sacs of rat intestine, evidence has been obtained (Stahl and Tapley, 1963; Smith *et al.*, 1963) that while corticosteroids appear to be absorbed by diffusion, estradiol, testosterone and androstenedione undergo metabolic transformation prior to being transferred by an active mechanism from the mucosal to the serosal side. These workers suggest that this active transfer is dependent on conjugation with glucuronic acid. In an investigation of the *in vivo* transport by rat intestine of estradiol, 17α-ethinylestradiol, and 17α-ethinylestradiol-3-cyclopentyl ether, Meli *et al.* (1968) confirmed the findings of Smith *et al.* (1963) that estradiol is converted to estrone before absorption from the intestine. 17α-ethinylestradiol was absorbed at a rapid rate equivalent to that of estradiol, but was not metabolized. Very little formation of the glucuronides of either estrone or 17α-ethinylestradiol was found, and Meli *et al.* incline to the opinion that these two compounds are absorbed *in vivo* by simple diffusion. However, in the case of 17α-ethinylestradiol-3-cyclopentyl ether, they found the absorption through the intestinal wall to be relatively slow, and suggest that this compound may be bound to material in the wall.

During the use of hydrocortisone *enemata* for the treatment of ulcerative colitis, Sampson and Brooke (1963) found that the material, administered in the form of the sodium hemisuccinate, caused elevated systemic plasma levels of cortisol, while similar enemas of saline did not cause this effect. These results indicate that the hydrocortisone was absorbed from the large bowel to some extent. Nothing is known of the mechanism of this absorption.

The work of Schedl and Clifton (1963) and Schedl (1965) has shown that absorption of steroids from the normal human small intestine is rapid, when the steroids are administered, in solution, by transintestinal intubation and steady state perfusion. The following points have been indicated by Schedl's studies:

1. The percentage absorption of one steroid tested, namely cortisol, was constant over a 2000-fold range. This suggests that the absorption of the steroid takes place by simple diffusion, rather than by means of an active transport mechanism. This result provides evidence for the absorption of this steroid by passive diffusion through the lipid phase of the mucosal membrane.

2. The oral potency of steroids bears no direct relationship to their rate of absorption by the intestine from solution. Thus progesterone, which is well absorbed, is almost inactive orally, while triamcinolone, which is much more slowly absorbed, has adequate oral potency. It seems probable that progesterone, and other compounds which are active parentally, but not orally, must undergo rapid inactivation either in the intestinal lumen, the mucosa or the liver. Whether this involves metabolism of the steroid molecule, conjugation with acids, or binding to protein, is unknown.

3. The efficiency with which a steroid is absorbed from the gut is inversely related to the number of hydroxyl groups on the steroid. Addition of hydroxyl groups renders steroids less lipophilic, indicating that the absorption of steroids is directly related to their fat solubility. Thus, the very fat-soluble steroid progesterone is well absorbed, while the tetrahydroxy compound triamcinolone is poorly absorbed throughout the small intestine. The rate of absorption of triamcinolone can be markedly increased by the formation of the acetonide, which increases the fat solubility of the molecule and masks two of its hydroxyl groups.

4. The perfusion experiments of Schedl (1965) provide no evidence that conjugation of steroids with molecules such as glucuronic acid, or any other form of metabolism in the intestinal mucosa, plays a part in the disappearance of steroids from the intestinal lumen. There is, however, ample evidence that the intestine has the ability to form steroid glucuronides (Dutton, 1966), and, indeed, the intestinal glucuronyl transferases may show a marked specificity, not only for a given steroid, but for a particular hydroxyl group on this steroid (Dahm and Breuer, 1966). It is therefore possible that, as indicated by the results of Smith *et al.* (1963), conjugation plays a role in active absorption of some steroids.

9.2.3. ENTEROHEPATIC CIRCULATION OF STEROIDS

It is well established by studies with radioactive compounds that when steroids, such as estradiol (Sandberg and Slaunwhite, 1957), progesterone (Sandberg and Slaunwhite, 1958) and norethynodrel (Layne *et al.*, 1963), are administered to humans the compounds and their oxidative metabolites undergo an extensive enterohepatic circulation. In such studies, the amounts of particular metabolites, and the types of their conjugation products, are not the same in the bile as they are in urine. Further, there is ample evidence that endogenously secreted steroids undergo enterohepatic circulation, and that conjugation in the intestinal wall, as referred to above, may play a part in facilitating this circulation. Of particular interest are recent observations of Knapstein *et al.* (1967a, b) which indicate that the sulfates of C_{19} steroids can be absorbed through the intestinal wall without hydrolysis. It is not yet possible, however, to estimate the extent to which reabsorption of an administered compound, or its metabolites after biliary excretion, may contribute to its physiological effects; while from the therapeutic viewpoint, the oral potency of the sulfates and glucuronides of steroids has not been systematically investigated.

9.2.4. NON-STEROIDAL ESTROGENS

A large number of non-steroidal compounds of animal, plant, or synthetic origin are estrogens by virtue of their physiological effects (see Emmens, 1950). The most important are diethylstilbestrol and related derivatives of stilbene. The high oral efficacy of these compounds in humans and other animals was established at an early date (see Huf, 1941; Solmmsen, 1945). After the oral administration of diethylstilbestrol to cattle, estrogenic residues are found in the tissues (Stob *et al.*, 1956; Wiberg and Stephenson, 1957). It has not, however, been shown whether these residues consist of diethylstilbestrol itself, or of a metabolite of the administered compound. Recent evidence (Fischer *et al.*, 1966) indicates that when diethylstilbestrol is administered to rats by intraduodenal infusion, it is first absorbed and converted, presumably in the liver, to the monoglucuronide, which is then excreted in the bile and hydrolyzed to free diethylstilbestrol in the gut. This free compound is then reabsorbed, so that an extensive enterohepatic circulation is maintained. The polyphosphate of diethylstilbestrol is, however, orally inactive in rodents, and appears to pass through the human intestinal tract without significant absorption (Perklev *et al.*, 1965). In general, the absorption and biliary excretion of diethylstilbestrol and related stilbenes follows the pattern expected for molecules of this size and relative polarity (Millburn *et al.*, 1967).

9.2.5. CATECHOLAMINES AND THYROXINE

No pharmacologically significant intestinal absorption of the non-protein neurohormones has been reported. Epinephrine and norepinephrine, as well as their substituted analogs, such as isoproterenol (isopropylnorepinephrine), are destroyed in the gastrointestinal tract and are also rapidly metabolized by the liver. Following oral administration, the absorption of the catecholamines is, at best, unreliable, and they do not reach pharmacologically active concentrations in the body. A large number of drugs, which possess sympathomimetic properties while lacking the catechol structure, have been studied. Some of these, for example, amphetamine and ephedrine, are active when given by mouth. Oral preparations of these drugs are usually in the form of salts, such as the sulfate or phosphate, and, as far as is known, their absorption from the gut follows the pattern usually encountered with small organic molecules.

The hormones of the thyroid gland are small molecules containing two benzenoid rings, each substituted with one or more molecules of iodine. Thyroxine was the first hormone to be isolated, but the biologically more potent compound triiodothyronine is also present in thyroid tissue. In addition, thyroid tissue contains the mono- and diiodo-derivatives of the amino acid tyrosine, which are precursors of the thyroid hormones. The hormones are normally found incorporated into a protein called thyroglobulin, from which they can be obtained by hydrolysis. A concise treatment of the steric features required for thyromimetic activity in the derivatives of 3,5-diiodo-tyrosine is presented by Astwood (1965).

It has been shown (Wiberg *et al.*, 1963) that, while at least three-quarters of an oral dose of triiodothyronine becomes available to the animal in active form, only one-sixth to one-quarter of a similar dose of thyroxine is physiologically active. There is good evidence for extensive entero-hepatic circulation of the thyroid hormones (see Jayle and Pasqualini, 1966). Following excretion in the bile as glucuronides and ester sulfates, the hormones are reabsorbed by the intestine, probably after hydrolysis of the conjugates. Several studies have been carried out on the absorption of thyroxine from the intestinal tract of the laboratory rat, making use of thyroxine labeled with ^{132}I. There is no evidence for active absorption of the molecule, which does not move across the intestinal wall against a concentration gradient (Herz *et al.*, 1961). Further, the fact that the label of D-thyroxine was as well absorbed as that of the L-isomer suggests that the mechanism of absorption does not distinguish between the optical isomers of the hormone (Cottle and Veress, 1965). Herz *et al.* (1961) showed that everted sacs of rat small intestine and colon transported the acetic, propionic and formic acid analogs of thyroxine, and the acetic and propionic acid analogs of triiodothyronine, and that these compounds accumulated in the serosal fluid in concentrations up to 14 times as great as those of the original medium. These workers found that the accumulated material was in the form of glucuronides, which were not themselves transported by the everted gut sacs. They suggested that the formation of these conjugates may explain the accumulation of the radioactivity in the serosal fluid.

Chung and Van Middlesworth (1964) obtained evidence that protein in the intestinal lumen reduced the absorption of thyroxine from washed loops of rat intestine. In a further study (1967) these workers showed that thyroxine was better absorbed from loops of large than those of small intestine. Absorption was greatest from the intestinal loops of fasting rats, being greatly inhibited by the normal contents of both the large and small intestine. When thyroxine was injected in propylene glycol into the unwashed lumen of the ileum of anesthetized rats, about 10–20% of the dose was absorbed over a 1-hr period, as compared to 40% in cases where the lumen contents had been previously removed by washing. Chung and Van Middlesworth (1967) point out that one would expect a reduced thyroxine synthesis during fasting, in order to compensate for the increased absorption and conservation of the enterohepatically circulated hormone. In both the washed and unwashed ileum, absorption over a further 3 hr was slow and, in both cases, the degree of absorption did not vary greatly over a dose range of 0.3 mcg to 30 mcg. Loops from different areas of the rat colon were shown to absorb thyroxine at a rate somewhat greater than that of the ileum.

Hays (1968) administered thyroxine labeled with ^{125}I to humans and confirmed the finding that maximal levels of absorption of orally administered thyroxine occur soon after ingestion, and that the unabsorbed fraction appears to become firmly bound by luminal contents so that no further absorption can occur. She found that the form of oral administration of thyroxine was of great importance to its absorption. When given with 0.1 g of human serum albumin about 70% of the label was absorbed, as compared to about 40% when administered in capsules with lactose. The absorption of the oral dose was not profoundly altered by diseases other than general malabsorption syndromes.

9.3. SUMMARY

The only hormones which are absorbed from the gastrointestinal tract in physiologically significant form are some of the steroids and the thyroid hormones.

The available evidence on steroid absorption by the gastrointestinal tract in the human indicates that most steroids are passively absorbed by simple diffusion, at a rate which varies directly with the lipophilic properties of the steroid. There is, however, evidence that some steroids, such as 17 β-estradiol and testosterone, are metabolized in the intestine and undergo active transfer from the mucosal to the serosal side of the wall. It is suggested that conjugation with glucuronic acid may play a role in this active transfer. In general, the rate of absorption of a steroid from the intestine is not a good index of its physiological potency after oral administration.

The thyroid hormones are conjugated as glucuronides in the intestine as well as other tissues, but there is no evidence for an active absorption mechanism for these compounds. A greater proportion of an oral dose of triiodothyronine is available to the animal in active form than is the case with thyroxine. Results obtained on rats and man strongly suggest that diet may affect the absorption of thyroxine from the intestinal tract by altering the nature and mass of the intestinal residues. This could affect the potency of oral doses of this hormone and its analogs.

Both steroids and thyroid hormones undergo enterohepatic circulation in the body. Little is known about the pharmacological relevance of this circulation.

REFERENCES

Astwood, E. B. (1965) Thyroid and antihyroid drugs, pp. 1468–1469. In *The Pharmacological Basis of Therapeutics*, Goodman, L. S. and Gilman A. (Eds.). Macmillan, New York.

Burrows, H. (1949) *The Biological Actions of Sex Hormones*, 2nd ed., p. 294. Cambridge University Press, Cambridge.

Chung, S. J. and Van Middlesworth, L. (1964) Absorption of thyroxine from the small intestine of rats. *Endocrinology* **74:** 694–700.

CHUNG, S. J. and VAN MIDDLESWORTH, L. (1967) Absorption of thyroxine from the intestine of rats. *Am. J. Physiol.* **212:** 97–105.

COTTLE, W. H. and VERESS, A. T. (1965) *Can. J. Physiol. Pharmac.* **43:** 801–807.

CRANE, C. W. and LUNTZ, G. R. W. N. (1968) Absorption of insulin from the human small intestine. *Diabetes* **17:** 625–627.

DAHM, K. and BREUER, H. (1966) Enzymatische Untersuchungen über die Glucuronidierung von Östriol beim Menschen. *Z. klin. Chem.* **4:** 153–157.

DANFORTH, E. and MOORE, R. O. (1959) Intestinal absorption of insulin in the rat. *Endocrinology* **65:** 118–123.

DUTTON, G. J. (1966) The biosynthesis of glucuronides, p. 220. In: *Glucuronic Acid, Free and Combined,* DUTTON, G. J. (Ed.). Academic Press, New York.

EMMENS, C. W. (1950) *Hormone Assay.* Academic Press, New York, pp. 392–396.

FISCHER, L. J., MILLBURN, P., SMITH, R. L. and WILLIAMS, R. T. (1966) *Biochem. J.* **100:** 69.

HAYS, M. T. (1968) Absorption of oral thyroxine in man. *J. Clin. Endocr.* **28:** 749–756.

HERZ, R. JR., TAPLEY, D. F. and ROSS, J. E. (1961) Glucuronide formation in the transport of thyroxine analogues by rat intestine. *Biochim. Biophys. Acta* **53:** 273–284.

HUF, E. (1941) Experimentelle Pharmakologie der Follikelhormon und der östrogenen Stilbene. *Klin. Wochenschr.* **20:** 755–762.

JAYLE, M. F. and PASQUALINI, J. R. (1966) Implication of conjugation of endogenous compounds. Steroids and thyroxine, p. 530. In: *Glucuronic Acid, Free and Combined,* DUTTON, G. J. (Ed.). Academic Press, New York.

KIRDANI, R. Y. and BURGETT, M. J. (1967) The pK of five estrogens in aqueous solutions. *Arch. Biochem. Biophys.* **118:** 33–36.

KNAPSTEIN, P., TREIBER, L., WENDLBERGER, F. and OERTEL, G. W. (1967a) Metabolismus und Rekonjugation von [7α-^{3}H] Androstendion, [7α-^{3}H] Androstenolon und [7α-^{3}H] Androstenolon-sulfat in der menschlichen Darmwand *in vivo. Hoppe-Seyler's Z. Physiol. Chem.* **348:** 401–404.

KNAPSTEIN, P., WENDLBERGER, F. and OERTEL, G. W. (1967b) Enterohepatic circulation of 7α-^{3}H-DHEA-^{35}S-sulfate, 7α-^{3}H-DHEA-^{14}C-glucuronoside and free 7α-^{3}H-DHEA in the human. *Experientia* **23:** 480–481.

LANGECKER, H. (1961) Die Metabolite im menschlicher Harn nach Verabreichung von 17α-aethinyl-19-nortestosteron (Noraethisteron). *Acta Endoc.* **37:** 14–18.

LAYNE, D. S., GOLAB, T., ARAI, K. and PINCUS, G. (1963). The metabolic fate of orally administered ^{3}H-norethynodrel and ^{3}H-norethindrone in humans. *Biochem. Pharmac.* **12:** 905–911.

MELI, A., CARGILL, D. I., GIANNINA, T. and STEINETZ, B. G. (1968) Studies on the transport of estrogens by the rat small intestine *in vivo. Proc. Soc. Exp. Biol. Med.* **129:** 937–939.

MILLBURN, P., SMITH, R. L. and WILLIAMS, R. T. (1967) Biliary excretion of foreign compounds. *Biochem. J.* **105:** 1275–1281.

PASCHKIS, K. E., RAKOFF, A. E. and CANTAROW, A. (1958) *Clinical Endocrinology,* 2nd ed., pp. 3–10. Paul B. Hoeber Inc., New York.

PERKLEV, T., GASSNER, F. X., MARTIN, R. P., HUSEBY, R. A. and SHIMODA, W. (1965) Excretion of radioactivity by human subjects after ingestion of liver from cattle treated with labeled polydiethylstilbestrol phosphate. *Proc. Soc. Exp. Biol. Med.* **119:** 996–998.

PIERCE, A. E., RISDALL, P. C. and SHAW, B. (1964) Absorption of orally administered insulin by the newly born calf. *J. Physiol.* **171:** 203–215.

SAMPSON, P. A. and BROOKE, B. N. (1963) Absorption of hydrocortisone from the large bowel. *Lancet* **284:** 701–702.

SANDBERG, A. A. and SLAUNWHITE, W. R. JR. (1957) Studies on phenolic steroids in human subjects. II. The metabolic fate and hepato-biliary-enteric circulation of ^{14}C-estrone and ^{14}C-estradiol in women. *J. Clin. Invest.* **37:** 1266–1273.

SANDBERG, A. A. and SLAUNWHITE, W. R. JR. (1958) The metabolic fate of ^{14}C-progesterone in human subjects. *J. Clin. Endocr. Metab.* **18:** 253–265.

SCHEDL, H. P. (1965) Absorption of steroid hormones from the human small intestine. *J. Clin. Endocr. Metab.* **25:** 1309–1316.

SCHEDL, H. P. and CLIFTON, J. A. (1963) Cortisol absorption in man. *Gastroenterology* **44:** 134–145.

SMITH, F. R., TAPLEY, D. F. and ROSS, J. E. (1963) Glucuronide formation in the transport of estradiol by rat intestine *in vitro*. *Biochim. Biophys. Acta* **69:** 68–73.

SOLMMSEN, U. V. (1945) Synthetic estrogens and the relation between their structure and their activity. *Chem. Rev.* **37:** 481–598.

STAHL, T. J. and TAPLEY, D. F. (1963) Transport of adrenal cortical steroids by rat intestine *in vitro*. *Endocrinology* **73:** 271–272.

STOB, M., PERRY, T. W., ANDREWS, F. N. and BEESON, W. M. (1956) Residual estrogen in the tissues of cattle treated with diethylstilbestrol, dienestrol, hexestrol and chlortetracycline. *J. Animal Sci.* **15:** 997–1002.

TRAVIS, R. H. and SAYERS, G. (1965) Adrenocorticotropic hormone: adrenal steroids and their synthetic analogs, pp. 1608–1648. In: *The Pharmacological Basis of Therapeutics*, GOODMAN, L. S. and GILMAN, A. (Eds.). Macmillan, New York.

WIBERG, G. S., DEVLIN, W. F., STEPHENSON, N. R. and CARTER, J. R. (1963) The relative potencies of thyroxine and liothyronine by oral and subcutaneous administration in the rat. *J. Pharm. Pharmac.* **15:** 644–651.

WIBERG, G. S. and STEPHENSON, N. R. (1957) The detection of estrogenic activity in tissues of steers which have been fed diethylstilbestrol. *Can. J. Biochem. Physiol.* **35:** 1107–1112.

CHAPTER 10

GASTROINTESTINAL ABSORPTION OF ALKALI IONS

Thomas W. Clarkson

Rochester, N.Y., U.S.A.

10.1. INTRODUCTION

This chapter reviews the published work (up to 1969) on the gastrointestinal absorption of the alkali metal cations: lithium, sodium, potassium, rubidium and cesium. Other monovalent cations, e.g. triethylammonium, will be briefly discussed. As might be expected, a great deal more attention has been directed to the physiologically important cations—sodium and potassium. In fact, information on the other monovalent cations is usually found in studies directed toward sodium and potassium. The other cations are included for comparative purposes, to help elucidate mechanisms of absorption of the physiologically important cations. This review necessarily reflects this imbalance in the literature.

10.2. SITES OF ALKALI METAL TRANSPORT

The normal dietary intake of sodium ranges from 70 to 350 mEq per day (Davidson and Passmore, 1966). Fecal excretion averages 5 mEq per day. The potassium intake varies from 50 to 150 mEq per day. Fecal excretion of this cation is slightly higher than that of sodium (7 to 15 mEq per day). Certain disease states may greatly change the fecal excretion; for example, diarrhea may increase excretion of sodium and potassium to over 90 mEq per day.

Most of the excretion of sodium and potassium occurs via the urine. Normal sweat accounts for a negligible amount. However, during profuse perspiration, people may excrete up to 8 liters per day, containing from 20 to 80 mM sodium.

The difference between oral intake and fecal excretion indicates a net sodium absorption of approximately 65 to 345 mEq per day. However, the turnover of this alkali metal in the gastrointestinal tract is much greater than these figures would suggest. Large volumes of salt solution are secreted into the upper tract. In addition to the 1.5 liters of water ingested orally, the gastrointestinal tract must absorb another 7 liters of digestive fluid (Fordtran, 1968). These secreted fluids contain substantial amounts of sodium and potassium. Salivary and stomach fluids are hypotonic, containing approximately 50 mM sodium and 6 mM potassium. Pancreatic juice and bile contain 150 mM sodium and less than 6 mM potassium.

Fordtran (1968) has reviewed radioisotope studies of sodium movement across the gastric wall and concludes that it is negligible compared to transport rates in the lower gastrointestinal tract. The sites of absorption in the small intestine have been described by Fordtran and Locklear (1966). To a limited extent, the pattern is influenced by diet. For example, following a steak meal, 120 mEq of sodium passed along the proximal duodenum, 105 arrived at the proximal jejunum and only 23 mEq actually reached the terminal ileum. Thus, a net absorption was observed in all regions. However, after a "milk and doughnut" meal, the following pattern emerged: 80 mEq of sodium at the mid-duodenum, 130 mEq at the proximal jejunum, and 32 mEq at the lower ileum. In both cases the amount of sodium arriving at the terminal ileum was about the same, but in the case of the "milk and doughnut" meal, a net entry of sodium into the lumen was observed in the duodenum–jejunum area. Fordtran explained the effect as due to the high osmolarity of the milk and doughnut meal. Thus water flowed from the plasma to the concentrated digesta in the duodenum, thereby inducing a net transport of sodium by solvent drag.

The pattern of potassium absorption is not influenced by the diet. Approximately 20 mEq of potassium passed in mid-jejunum and only 2 mEq arrived at the terminal ileum.

Absorption and secretion in the colon have been estimated by comparing the volume and composition of the fluid delivered to the colon from the small intestine with that excreted in stool water (Dempsey *et al.*, 1958; Welch *et al.*, 1936). The colon normally absorbs about 400 ml water, 55 mEq of sodium, and secretes 4 to 9 mEq of potassium per day.

In summary, most of the sodium and potassium ingested orally, plus the much larger quantities secreted into the upper gastrointestinal tract, is absorbed in the jejunal–ileal regions of the small intestine. Most of the remaining sodium is absorbed in the colon and potassium is secreted. The intestinal segments exhibit a pattern of absorption and secretion somewhat reminiscent of the renal tubule.

10.3. FACTORS INFLUENCING TRANSPORT

Studies in humans and in experimental animals have demonstrated that the rate of absorption of sodium in the small intestine is influenced by its luminal concentration. Sumers and Schedl (1968) reported that, as the luminal sodium concentration was reduced below plasma level in rats, the rate of absorption was reduced. The effect is most obvious in the jejunum where, according to observations on humans, net sodium absorption ceased when the luminal concentration was reduced to 13 mM below that of plasma (Fordtran *et al.*, 1968). Lower luminal concentrations cause net secretion of sodium across the human jejunum. Sodium transport across human ileum and colon may take place against much higher concentration gradients (Fordtran *et al.*, 1968).

Phillips and Code (1966) reported that the absorption of potassium was dependent on the concentration in the luminal fluid of the small intestine of dogs. Their findings confirm *in vitro* studies, to be discussed later, that, in the jejunum and ileum, net transport of potassium will closely follow the electrochemical potential gradient across the intestine. Potassium is usually secreted by the colon (Fordtran, 1968). *In vivo* studies on the rat indicate that the rate of secretion decreases with increasing luminal concentrations of potassium and changes to net absorption at luminal concentration above 4 mM (Edmonds, 1967a, b).

In vitro studies on jejunal and ileal segments from various experimental animals indicate that actively transported sugars and amino acids, when present in the solution bathing the luminal surface, stimulate net sodium transport (reviewed by Crane, 1968). In humans, glucose and galactose stimulate sodium absorption in the jejunum (Schedl and Clifton, 1963; Holdsworth and Dawson, 1964; Malawer *et al.*, 1965). For example, Sladen and Dawson (1968) reported that sodium absorption by human jejunum increased from 8.7 mEq per hour per 30 cm length when the intestine was infused with isotonic saline to 30 mEq per hour per 30 cm length when 56 mM glucose was present in the saline.

The presence of bicarbonate in the lumen of the jejunum has been reported to stimulate sodium absorption in man (Fordtran *et al.*, 1968;

Sladen and Dawson, 1968) and in the rat jejunum (McHardy and Parsons, 1957). The increase in sodium transport produced by bicarbonate is about the same as that observed with glucose. The bicarbonate effect is observed only in the jejunum and is not related to the influence of this anion on pH. An anion exchange process between chloride and bicarbonate cannot be involved, since this process would not lead to net anion transport, and therefore could not account for increased net sodium transport. Studies by McHardy and Parsons (1957) on the rat small intestine indicate that sodium transport is affected by the pH of the bathing solutions. To what extent pH specifically affects sodium transport, as compared to other transport and metabolic processes in the cell, has not yet been elucidated.

The role of osmotic activity gradient and net water flow (i.e., solvent drag) has been the subject of considerable discussion (for a review, see Schultz and Curran, 1968). Studies in humans indicate that sodium transport across the jejunum is closely affected by the direction and rate of water transport (Fordtran *et al.*, 1968). For example, net water secretion from plasma to lumen, induced by infusion into the lumen of solutions of high osmolarity, also causes net secretion of sodium. It has also been shown *in vivo* in rats that, when water absorption is enhanced by infusion of hypotonic solution, net sodium absorption is increased (Sumers and Schedl, 1968).

The adrenal hormones influence sodium absorption in the colon, but the effect of the hormones in the small intestine is equivocal (Fordtran, 1968). Aldosterone and 9α-fluorohydrocortisone stimulate sodium absorption and potassium secretion in the human colon (Levitan and Ingelfinger, 1965; Wrong and Metcalfe-Gibson, 1965).

Studies on the upper small intestine in humans and in experimental animals (rabbit, rats and dogs) indicate that vasopressin* increases the intestinal absorption of sodium and water (Soergel *et al.*, 1968; Blickenstaff, 1954; Dombradi *et al.*, 1960). Findings on the effects of vasopressin on colon are variable; the absorption of water, sodium and chloride by human colon is inhibited according to Levitan and Mauer (1968). Aulsebrook (1961) reported an enhancement of sodium absorption from the rat colon, while Green and Matty (1966) were unable to detect any effect on ion transport in ileum or colon of the rat, mouse and toad.

The effects of insulin have been studied on the absorptive function of the small intestine in experimental animals. *In vitro* observations on the rat and rabbit small intestine indicate that insulin stimulates the

*See also Chapter 3, p. 212.

absorption of glucose and sodium (Aulsebrook, 1965; Canavan and Love, 1969). Experimental observations on *in situ* perfused segments of rat intestine also indicate that insulin stimulates glucose absorption (Sols *et al.,* 1948).

Diarrhea is known to occur in states of bile salt malabsorption. Dawson and Isselbacher (1960) reported that free bile acids inhibited the uphill transport of glucose by the small intestine *in vitro* and subsequently Rummel and Stupp (1962) observed that water and electrolyte absorption can be inhibited by bile acids. Mekhjian *et al.* (1968) have claimed that glycine and taurine conjugates of the three major bile salts, in concentrations similar to those found in the small intestine, block net electrolyte and water transport in the human colon. However, the observed inhibition of transport was probably due to the presence of bile acid impurities since Forth, Rummel and Glasner (1964, 1966) have demonstrated that only free bile acids are able to inhibit absorption. For further details, see Chapter 3.

Certain disease states greatly affect sodium and potassium absorption by the gastrointestinal tract. All diarrhea states lead to losses of potassium in the feces and may lead to potassium deficiency. An interesting genetic abnormality has been described by Evanson and Stanbury. Congenital chloridorrhea is characterized by watery feces and metabolic alkalosis and the presence of high concentrations of chloride in fecal water. Evanson and Stanbury indicate that the primary lesion is the inability of the intestinal cells to absorb chloride ions. Consequently these ions now have the typical osmotic effect of any impermeant anion, and so cause diarrhea and a loss of potassium in the feces. The symptoms of metabolic alkalosis are probably due to the hypochloremic state but potassium deficiency may contribute.

Diarrhea produced by cholera infection is apparently not due to a specific inhibition of sodium reabsorption. Grady *et al.* (1967) could not detect any effect of cholera enterotoxin on sodium transport across isolated human ileum. This finding is consistent with previous studies, indicating that the villus capillary is the primary reactant to cholera toxin. The enhanced capillary permeability leads to leakage of water and electrolytes into the bowel lumen (Finkelstein *et al.,* 1966).

Loss of water and electrolytes from the intestinal tract may be caused by radiation doses to the whole animal of 1000 rd or more. This loss of fluid and salts has been implicated as the cause of "intestinal death" following irradiation injury (Quastler, 1956). Such effects on intestinal function, usually observed from 3 to 5 days after large X-ray doses, have usually been attributed to gross damage to the intestinal epithelium. However, Curran *et al.* (1960) observed a decrease in sodium transport in intestinal segments removed from rats only 6 hr after a radiation dose of 2500–3000 rd. Recently McKenney (1968) and Sullivan (1968) have reported effects on electrolyte transport at doses of from 1000 to 1500 rd, and Sullivan (1968) noted the protective effect of bile salts.

A wide variety of drugs and selective inhibitors have been used in *in vitro* studies of sodium transport. The effects of these compounds will be discussed later in relationship to the mechanisms of alkali metal transport.

10.4. MECHANISMS OF TRANSPORT

The small intestine is capable of absorbing a wide variety of substances. The early experiments revealed that the intestine *in vivo* and *in vitro* always transported a combination of solutes and water, amounting, in effect, to a transport of a "solution" (Ingraham *et al.,* 1938; Wilson and Wiseman, 1954; Wilson, 1954, 1956; Fisher, 1955; Parsons, 1956; Clarkson and Rothstein, 1960). The history of experimental work on this tissue indicates that, no matter how the investigator adjusts the experimental conditions, he is unable to study the transport of any single species in the absence of transport of anything else. Thus, right from the outset, the research on intestinal transport has always been concerned with the possible influence of the flow of one species on that of another. From the point of view of this article, this means that the transport of alkali metal cations cannot be considered in isolation from other processes.

The problem of interdependent flows is well illustrated by considering what happens when an isolated jejunal segment of rat small intestine is incubated in Ringer's bicarbonate-buffer containing glucose (Table 1). The tissue develops a spontaneous electrical potential difference of about 8 mV. All the principal components of the buffer are transported from mucosal to serosal sides, i.e. water, sodium, chloride, bicarbonate, and glucose. The composition of the "transported solution" (Table 1) differs slightly from that of the bathing solution. Glucose and bicarbonate are present at a higher concentration than in the solutions bathing the tissues. The composition of this solution varies for different segments of the small intestine (Clarkson and Rothstein, 1960). However, the main features remain, viz. that an approximately isotonic solution is transported—containing most, if not all, of the constituents of the bathing solution.

TABLE 1. INTESTINAL TRANSPORT[a] IN KREBS-RINGER BICARBONATE SOLUTIONS

Species transported	Transport rate micromol/hr	Composition of transported "solution" millimol/l.	Composition of bathing solutions[c] millimol/l.
Sodium	193	139	143
Potassium	4	3	4
Chloride	74	53	123
Bicarbonate	45	32	25
Lactate	83	60	—
Glucose	37	28	
Total solutes[b]	436	312	
Total solutes[b] (F.P.)	431	310	310
Water (ml/hr)	1.39		

[a]The intestinal segment, dry weight 406 mg, was removed from the upper jejunum of the rat.

[b]Total solutes are reported as the sum of the determinations of the individual solutes and also as determined from freezing point (F.P.) depression measurements. The data are taken from table 2 of the publication by Clarkson and Rothstein (1960).

[c]Ca^{++}, Mg^{++} and $H_2PO_4^-$ were also added to concentrations not exceeding 1 mM.

Similar observations were published in the 1930s and early 1940s by Visscher and coworkers from *in vivo* studies on the dog (Ingraham and Visscher, 1936; Visscher and Roepke, 1945; Visscher *et al.*, 1945). These authors proposed that the tissue possesses a fluid pump capable of transferring fluid from mucosal to serosal sides of the intestine, bringing about the absorption of solutes by entrainment in the fluid stream.

This hypothesis prevailed until the 1950s when studies on intestinal mucosa (for references see Wilson, 1962) and on other epithelia indicated that specific solutes were actively transported. Specific experimental criteria for active transport were proposed and tested (Ussing, 1963; Rosenberg, 1954). For example, studies by Ussing and Zerahn (1951) on frog skin, by Leaf *et al.* (1958) on isolated toad bladder, indicated that sodium ions were actively transported. These criteria were applied to studies of intestinal absorption (Curran and Solomon, 1957). Thus the view developed that the transport of solution by the intestine was a consequence of active solute transport (viz. sodium, glucose and possibly chloride) and that water flow was determined by the solute transport (Curran and Solomon, 1957; Smyth and Taylor, 1957; Clarkson and Rothstein, 1960; Parsons and Wingate, 1961; Parsons and Paterson, 1966).

However, it soon became clear that a simple categorization of active and passive transport processes was inadequate to fully explain transport across epithelia. Andersen and Ussing (1957) demonstrated, in toad skin, that water flow could induce net transport of solute—the "solvent drag" concept implicit in Visscher's original hypothesis. Subsequently, Kedem and Katchalsky (1961) gave a formal theoretical basis to coupling phenomena in their analysis of transport processes in terms of irreversible thermodynamics. Some attempts have been made to apply this approach to the study of intestinal transport (Ogilvie *et al.*, 1963; Clarkson, 1967). Consideration of the mechanisms of coupling between flows of different species leads to questions on the pathways of transport across the intestine (Kedem and Essig, 1965; Clarkson, 1967).

In reviewing the research studies related to the mechanism of alkali metal ion transport, it will be necessary to consider experimental evidence relating the nature of the driving forces, the question of active and passive transport, the coupling between flows of different species and the nature of the different pathways across the intestine.

10.5. ACTIVE AND PASSIVE TRANSPORT OF ALKALI METAL CATIONS

According to Rosenberg's (1954) definition, an ion is actively transported if it passes across a membrane against the prevailing electrochemical potential difference (ECPD). This, of course, assumes the absence of other potential energy differences between the two solutions. The ECPD ($\Delta\mu_i$) for any ionic species may be calculated from the relationship:

$$\Delta\mu_i = 2.303\,(RT/F)\log_{10}(C_i)_m/(C_i)_s + z_i\,(\Psi_m - \Psi_s) \tag{1}$$

where R is the gas constant and z_i is the charge on the ion, T the absolute temperature and F is Faraday's number. The value $2.303(RT/F)$ is approximately 60 mV at 38°. (C_i) and Ψ refer to the concentration of the ion, i, and the electrical potential, respectively, in the bathing solutions. The subscripts m and s refer to the solutions bathing the mucosal and serosal surfaces of the epithelial tissue. In this formulation, $\Delta\mu_i$ and $(\Psi_m - \Psi_s)$ have the units of millivolts.

Applying Rosenberg's definition to the data in Table 1, it is evident that sodium is actively transported across the isolated jejunal segment of the rat. Each surface of the tissue was bathed by solutions of identical composition such that $(C_{Na})_m = (C_{Na})_s$. The value of $(\Psi_m - \Psi_s)$ was approximately 8 mV. Thus, according to eqn. (1), sodium transport in the mucosal to serosal direction is opposed by an ECPD of 8 mV. Potassium transport was too small to be of significance. This picture is the same for other segments of the rat small intestine – the electrical potential difference is always positive on the serosal side, having the lowest value in ileal segments (4.4 mV) and the highest value in the mid-jejunal areas (9 mV) (Clarkson *et al.*, 1961).

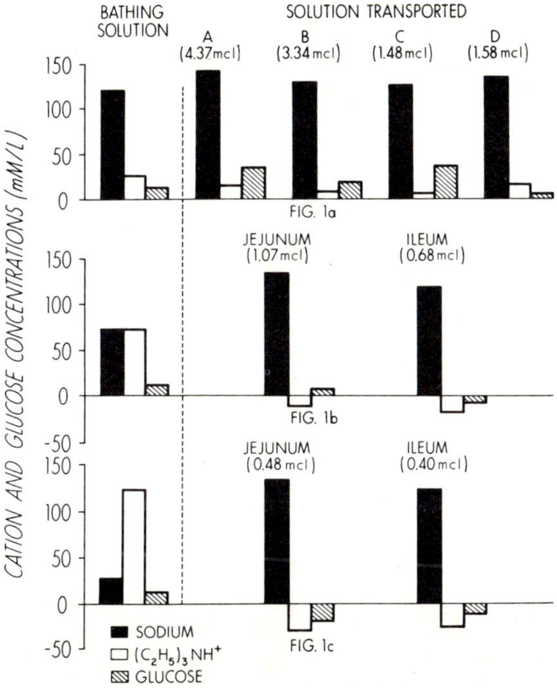

FIG. 1. Comparison of the ion composition of the moving solution and bathing solution with partial substitution of $(C_2H_5)_3NH^+$ for Na^+. The values for concentrations in the moving solution were obtained by dividing the net glucose and cation transport by the water transfer during 60 min incubation at 37°C. A positive value indicates net entry into, and a negative value a net loss from, the serosal solution. The net water transport in mcl/mg dry wt and hr is given in parentheses for each segment of intestine so that absolute values may be calculated. The letters A, B, C and D denote intestinal segments of approximately equal length consecutively removed from upper jejunum to the ileocecal valve.

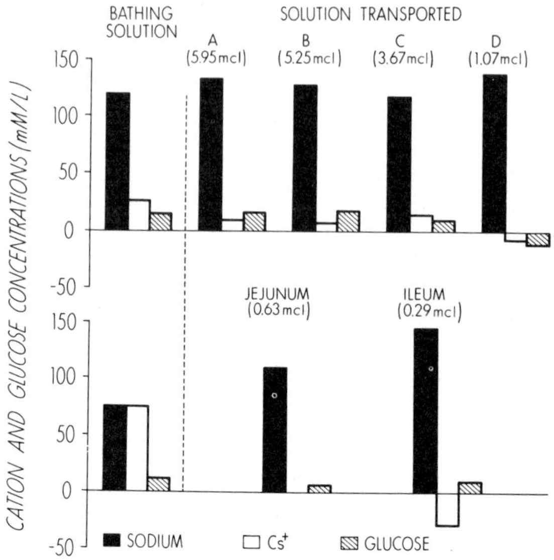

FIG. 2. Comparison of the ion composition of the moving solution and bathing solution with partial substitution of Cs^+ for Na^+. The values for concentrations in the moving solution were obtained as described in Fig. 1, with the letters A, B, C and D having their usual significance.

The question arises as to whether other alkali metal cations may be actively transported by the small intestine. To answer this question, isolated segments were exposed to Ringer's solution in which sodium was partially replaced by another monovalent cation. The results demonstrated that the active transport system is completely specific to sodium (Figs. 1, 2, 3 and 4). This point is best illustrated by comparing the concentrations of the cations in the "transported solution" to the corresponding concentrations in the bathing solution. The concentrations of sodium in the transported solution always remained high—120–140 mM—despite the fact that the concentration in the bathing solution was reduced to 72 mM by substitution of Cs^+, K^+ and Li^+. In one set of experiments (Fig. 1), the external sodium was reduced to 30 mM. Nevertheless, the concentration in the transported solution reached levels greater than 100 mM.

In contrast to the behavior of sodium, the concentration of the other monovalent cations in the transported solution was always less than the

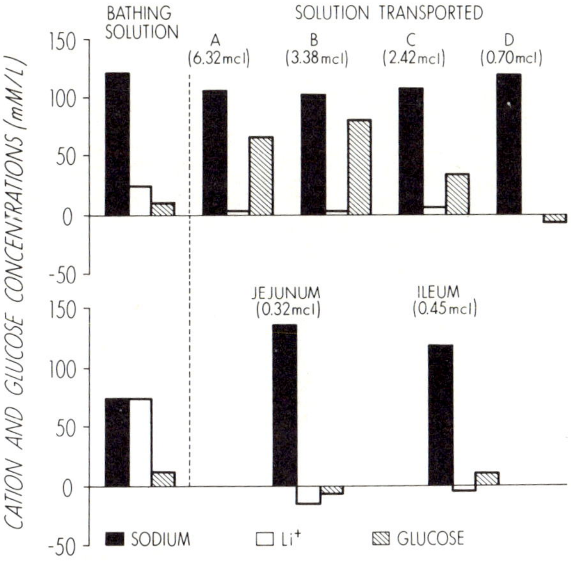

FIG. 3. Comparison of the ion composition of the moving solution and bathing solution with partial substitution of Li^+ for Na^+. The values for concentrations in the moving solutions were obtained as described in Fig. 1, with the letters A, B, C and D having their usual significance.

external concentration. When the concentration of the substituent cation was raised to 73 or to 120 mM, frequently the concentration in the moving solution was negative; that is to say, the substituent cation was transported in the serosal to mucosal direction.

In these experiments, sodium was always transported against the prevailing electrochemical potential gradient. The other cations either moved down the gradient, or exhibited no significant transport. These observations are in agreement with other reports indicating that sodium is transported against the ECPD across rat jejunum *in vitro* (Barry *et al.*, 1965) and the rat ileum *in vivo* (Curran and Solomon, 1957) and *in vitro* (Curran, 1960).

Studies by Gilman *et al.* (1962) on isolated rat jejunum and ileum indicate that potassium is transported down the electrochemical potential gradient. In these experiments the mucosal surface of the intestine was exposed to solutions containing different concentrations of potassium. Solution transported to the serosal side appeared as droplets on the

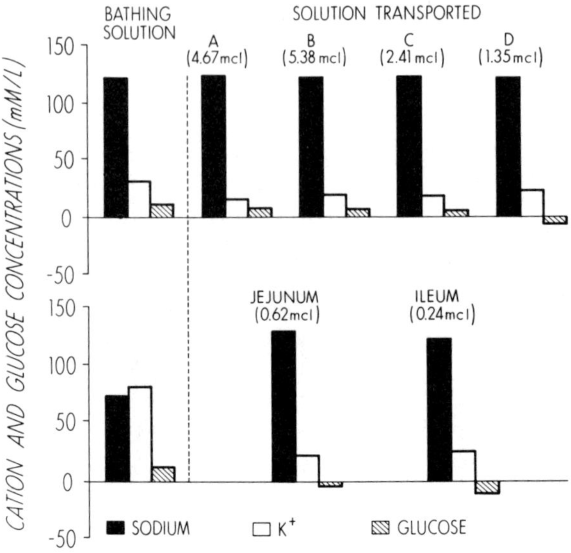

FIG. 4. Comparison of the ion composition of the moving solution and bathing solution with partial substitution of K^+ for Na^+. The values for concentrations in the moving solution were obtained as described in Fig. 1, with the letters A, B, C and D having their usual significance.

serosal surface. Measurement of potassium concentration in the serosal fluid and of the transmucosal electric potential difference indicated that potassium always moved "down hill".

There are few observations on the electrical potential difference across human intestine. The voltage across isolated human ileal mucosa has been reported as 4 mV (Grady *et al.*, 1967).

In vivo measurements have been reported by Sacher *et al.* (1969). One conducting bridge was placed in the lumen and the other bridge brought into contact with abraded skin. Voltages across the ileum ranged from 6 to 13 mV, the high values being recorded when glucose was present in the lumen. Since net absorption of sodium takes place in the ileal segment (see p. 478) and the concentration in the lumen is close to plasma level, it is clear that sodium is absorbed against the electrochemical potential gradient.

Potassium is also absorbed across human ileum (p. 478). The concentration of potassium in the luminal contents is consistently higher by about 2 mM than the concentration in plasma (Fordtran, 1968). This potassium transport would be in the direction of the electrochemical potential gradient, provided the electrical potential across human ileum does not exceed 11 mV. Thus, the ileal potential differences reported by Sacher *et al.* (1969) are consistent with a downhill movement of potassium.

Net sodium absorption across rat colon, *in vivo,* takes place against thc prevailing electrochemical potential gradient (Curran and Schwartz, 1960; Edmonds, 1967a, b). The concentration of potassium in the lumen of the colon is higher than in plasma and increases in value from cecum to anus (Edmonds, 1967a, b). The transmural potential difference is not sufficiently great to account for the concentration gradient. However, as Edmonds points out, one cannot infer an active transport process since the increase in luminal potassium concentration is mainly due to absorption of water. Potassium is not necessarily being transported against the gradient.

10.6. APPLICATIONS OF USSING'S FLUX RATIO EQUATION

The flux ratio equation first proposed by Ussing (1949) has found extensive application in studies of the mechanism of membrane transport. In its simplest form, the equation may be stated as

$$J_i^{ms}/J_i^{sm} = \alpha_i^m/\alpha_i^s\,[Z_iF\,(\Psi^m - \Psi^s)/RT] \qquad (2)$$

where J_i^{ms} and J_i^{sm} are, respectively, unidirectional fluxes of species i from mucosal to serosal solutions, and in the opposite direction, α_i^m and α_i^s the activities of species in the mucosal and serosal solutions respectively. All the other symbols are as defined for eqn. (1). Assuming that the activity coefficients for species in the mucosal and serosal solutions are the same, eqn. (2) may be written:

$$J_i^{ms}/J_i^{sm} = (C_i^m/C_i^s)\exp\,[Z_iF\,(\Psi^m - \Psi^s)/RT]. \qquad (3)$$

This equation possesses the advantage that all the measurements can be made on the bulk solutions. The restricting assumptions underlying the equation have been stated and discussed by Ussing (1949), Meares and Ussing (1959), Hoshiko and Lindley (1964) and Kedem and Essig

(1965). In brief, eqn. (3) will correctly predict the flux ratio if the ionic species crosses the membrane by simple diffusion under the influence of an electrochemical potential gradient only. Other transport mechanisms, e.g. exchange diffusion and other forces acting on the ionic species such as those related to active transport and to solvent drag, will cause deviations from the equation. Ussing and Zerahn (1951) demonstrated that eqn. (3) correctly predicted the flux ratio of chloride ions across isolated frog skin. The flux ratios of sodium ions were consistently greater from those calculated for eqn. (3). This discrepancy was interpreted as evidence for active sodium transport. Certainly, according to the assumptions implicit in the equation, an observed flux ratio greater than that calculated for the electrochemical potential gradient is consistent with an additional force causing transport of sodium.

Studies on the application of eqn. (3) to tracer fluxes of sodium across the intestinal tract have been reviewed by Schultz and Curran (1968). The observed flux ratio was always greater than the calculated ratio in rat ileum, *in vivo* and *in vitro*; rabbit ileum, *in vitro*; guinea-pig cecum, *in vitro*; and rat colon, *in vivo* and *in vitro*. Curran (1960) observed that, with glucose present in the bathing solution, the flux ratio of sodium across isolated rat ileum was always greater than predicted. However, in the absence of glucose, the flux ratio became close to that calculated from the electrochemical potential gradient.

It would be very interesting to measure the flux ratio of other alkali metal cations, especially those which may be transported by passive processes. A study of the fluxes of cesium, for example, might reveal if passive transport of alkali metal cations involved only passive diffusion, or if other mechanisms are involved, such as coupling with water flow.

The ratio of the transmural fluxes of potassium across the rat colon are greater than the value predicted from the Ussing equation, indicating an active secretion of this cation (Edmonds, 1967a, b).

10.7. APPLICATION OF USSING'S "SHORT-CIRCUIT" PRINCIPLE

The short-circuit principle is a special case of the application of Rosenberg's (1954) definition of active transport. If each surface of the biological membrane is bathed by solutions of identical composition and if an external current (called the "short-circuit current") is applied, so that the electrical potential difference across the membrane becomes zero, it follows that the electrochemical potential gradient is zero. Under these circumstances, "passively" transported ions will not exhibit any net flow across the membrane. Consequently, the short-circuit current must be carried across the membrane by all those ions undergoing "active" transport. In practice, the investigator has to identify all the ionic species transported by using isotopic tracers or by chemical analysis. The algebraic sum of the ion flows should then equal the short-circuit current.

Ussing and Zerahn (1951) were the first to make measurements of ion transport across short-circuited epithelium. Applications of this technique to the small and large intestines of a variety of experimental animals (for review, see Schultz and Curran, 1968) have revealed that sodium transport quantitatively accounts for the short-circuit current when the tissue is bathed in Ringer's glucose solution. In the study reported by Clarkson and Toole (1964), the transport of all the ions present in the bathing solution was measured, and it was found that the transport of all the ionic species was negligible compared to that of sodium. However, a significant movement of water took place. In fact, the ratio of solute to water transport was close to that observed in the normal open-circuited tissue. Thus, short-circuiting the intestine cannot exclude the possibility of solvent drag—for example, the possible entrainment of sodium ion in a stream of water as suggested by Visscher.

10.8. PATHWAYS ACROSS THE INTESTINE

The coupling of the flow of one species with that of another implies that the two species share a common pathway across the intestine or, at least, that they share a part of the pathway. Thus, consideration of coupling between sodium and water flow, as discussed above with respect to the short-circuit studies, naturally leads to speculation on the pathways for sodium and water across the tissue. Unfortunately, the operator is capable of measuring only total transport across the tissue, which is the sum of all the movements through the various possible pathways. This immediately leads to difficulties of interpretation of data. For example, Visscher's hypothesis originally proposed two pathways for fluid transport across the intestine. A zero net transport of water indicates that the flows in the two channels were equal, but in the opposite direction. Thus, even if it were possible, in the short-circuit experiment, to adjust net water transport to zero by the use of hydrostatic pressure or osmotic gradients, we cannot exclude the possibility that net sodium transport is due to entrainment of this ion in one of the fluid streams.

The possibility of multiple pathways across the intestine and other epithelia has now become an important consideration. Kedem and Katchalsky (1963) have published a theoretical treatment of transport through parallel pathways. From the experimental point of view, both functional and morphological studies have been applied to identify pathways. Evidence of solvent drag effects have been taken to indicate that water and its affected solutes pass through common aqueous channels (Andersen and Ussing, 1957). A correlation of morphological changes with transport phenomena has been used to anatomically identify certain pathways (Diamond and Tormey, 1966a, b). This review will necessarily be brief and leave many questions unanswered, since this aspect of intestinal transport has come into focus only in recent years.

10.9. THE ACTIVE TRANSPORT PATHWAY

The experimental criteria discussed above consistently indicated that the sodium ion is actively transported across the small intestine. Sodium is transported against the prevailing electrochemical potential gradient, the observed flux ratio is higher than that calculated from the electrochemical potential gradient and sodium exhibits net transport under short-circuit conditions.

A question on the validity of this conclusion arises because water is also transported simultaneously. Although these criteria do not exclude the possibility of entrainment of sodium in an actively pumped stream of fluid, Schultz and Curran (1968) have reviewed a great deal of evidence indicating that the opposite situation is more likely to be the real state of affairs, viz., that water transfer is dependent on sodium transfer. Furthermore, it is conceptually easier to accept active transport of sodium than an active water pump. Biochemical mechanisms for active sodium transport have been proposed (Skou, 1967). It has also been indicated, by a physical model, how water transport may follow active solute flow (Curran and McIntosh, 1962). Consequently, for the purposes of this review, it will be assumed that sodium is actively transported and that water flow is dependent on solute transport.

It is clear, from purely anatomical considerations, that any pathway leading from intestinal lumen to blood is necessarily complex. A substance must cross many morphological barriers. The important question is which of these barriers is actually rate-determining. It has been generally assumed that the mucosal cell layer with the basement membrane is the only barrier worth considering. Unfortunately, there are few experimental studies to support this point of view. Removal of the epithelial cells, by a gentle scraping of the mucosa, generally results in a sharp increase in the permeability of the intestine. Munck and Schultz (1969) noted that the flux of radioactive lysine increased ten-fold when the mucosal cell layer was removed from rabbit ileum. Edmonds (1967a, b) established that the mucosal cell layer is the site of the transmural potential difference across the colon. No significant potential difference was detected across the submucosal and serosal layers of tissue. However, the contribution of the serosal layers to the total diffusional resistance of the intestine may be influenced by the type of tissue preparation. When blood vessels are perfused, glucose added to the mucosal solution rapidly appears in the perfusate (Parsons and Prichard, 1968). On the other hand, when using everted segments of intestine without perfusion of the blood vessels, the movement of the sugar on the serosal side is much slower (Clarkson and Cross, 1961).

To allow coupling to cellular metabolism, it is reasonable to suppose that the pathway for actively transported ions must include the epithelial cell. One of the first models of this type of pathway was proposed by Ussing (1960). In this model the frog skin is regarded as equivalent to a layer of epithelial cells. Sodium enters the cell from the outside (mucosal) solution flowing down its potential energy gradient into the interior of the cell. An active sodium pump then extrudes this ion out of the cell to the serosal side. The pump may function as a sodium–potassium exchange pump—forcing potassium into the cell as sodium is extruded. The impermeability of the mucosal membrane of the cell to potassium prevents net transport of potassium across the tissue. Many attempts have been made to see if this model may explain active sodium transport across other epithelia, including the intestine.

This model requires that the electrochemical potential of sodium is lower inside the cell than the potential in the solution bathing the mucosal surface. Available experimental evidence supports this requirement. Wright (1966), using intracellular micro-electrodes, observed that the potential difference across the mucosal facing membrane of the tortoise intestinal cells was 8.6 mV and across the serosal facing membrane, 21 mV. The cell interior was negative with respect to the bathing solutions. Gilles-Baillien and Schoffeniels (1967) reported that the cell interior was approximately 20 to 25 mV negative with respect to the bathing solution. The sodium concentration inside the cell has been reported in the range from 50 to 70 mM (Bosačková and Crane, 1965a; Schultz *et al.*, 1966; and Gilles-Baillien and Schoffeniels, 1967). These results indicate that there is a favorable gradient, both electrical and chemical, for sodium entry into the cell, and are therefore consistent with the Ussing model.

The serosal facing membrane must be the main site of active sodium transport in order to achieve low intracellular sodium concentrations and, at the same time, cause net transport across the tissue in the mucosal to serosal direction. Studies on the action of the cardiac glycosides, ouabain, are compatible with this conclusion. This glycoside inhibits sodium transport only when added to the serosal solution (Schultz and Zalusky, 1964). Ouabain is impermeant to frog intestinal epithelium (Csaky and Hara, 1965) and poorly permeant to guinea-pig epithelium (Forth and Rummel, 1967). Csaky and Hara (1965) have reported that, when ^{3}H-labeled-ouabain is present at inhibitory concentrations in the serosal solution, the concentration of this glycoside in the water of the "mucosal cell scrapings" was probably too low to inhibit the Na^+-K^+ activated ATP enzyme. Such evidence has been interpreted (see Schultz and Curran, 1968) to indicate that ouabain is inhibiting sodium transport by acting at the serosal facing membrane.

This "Ussing-type" model of the intestinal cell indicates that the intracellular sodium concentration is the result of a steady-state situation. The rate of passive flow of sodium into the cell is balanced by active transport to the serosal side. The rate of entry into the cell should be determined by the electrochemical gradient and the permeability of the cell membrane to sodium. An agent capable of increasing the permeability to sodium of the mucosal facing membrane should cause increased entry of sodium into the cell and, as a result of increased intracellular sodium, the active pump should extrude more sodium to the serosal side. The overall results should be an increased net transport of sodium. This conclusion was confirmed by studies on the action of low concentrations of $HgCl_2$ on the small intestine (Clarkson and Cross, 1961).

Not all the sodium flows across the mucosal facing membrane by passive diffusion. A part of the sodium flow is coupled to the flow of certain hexose sugars and amino acids (Crane, 1968; Csaky, 1961). A specific carrier-mediated mechanism has been proposed to explain the coupling between sodium and alanine flows across the epithelial surface of rabbit small intestine (Curran *et al.*, 1967). Sodium and the amino acid combine with the carrier to form a tertiary complex at the outer surface of the mucosal cell membrane. The diffusion of this complex through the cell membrane is the rate-determining step. Both sodium and alanine are released at the inner surface of the membrane. The energy for the flow derives from the sodium potential energy gradient and therefore ultimately from the active sodium pump. Specificity to alanine and certain other amino acids is due to the properties of the carrier. The number of different carrier systems in existence is still under study. Presumably at least one other type of carrier exists for coupling of sodium and sugar transport. There is some evidence to indicate that the flow of other solutes—phenylglucosides (Alvarado and Monreal, 1967; Playoust and Isselbacher, 1964), pyrimidines (Csaky, 1963) and bile salts (Holt, 1964)—may be coupled to sodium flow. If this proves to be the case the sodium pump may be the ultimate source of energy for many active transport processes across the intestine.

After extrusion from the mucosal cells, sodium probably enters the lateral spaces between the cells; the evidence comes from studies on other epithelia. Diamond and Tormey (1966a, b) have shown, in preparations of gall bladder, that when the cells are not transporting sodium chloride solution, spaces between the cells are small. However, when transport is initiated, these cellular spaces expand below the tight junctions as if fluid were entering. Inhibition of sodium transport by ouabain causes a contraction of these spaces. Similar studies on intestinal epithelium have not been reported. However, the generally similar morphological arrangement of cells in epithelia would suggest Diamond's theory to be a general mechanism.

The presence of the submucosal compartment may explain the close coupling between sodium and water flow across the intestine. Parsons and Wingate (1961) reported that the isolated rat intestine transported water against its activity gradient. Later Curran and McIntosh (1962) described a series membrane model capable of transporting water against its activity gradient. Extrapolating from the physical model to the intestine, Curran (1965) has suggested that the subepithelial spaces may be regarded as bounded by two membranes of different reflection coefficients. The transport of sodium across the first membrane (i.e. the cell membranes of the mucosal cells) gives rise to an osmotic pressure difference, causing fluid movement into the submucosal spaces. A hydrostatic pressure head will build up in these spaces, forcing fluid through the more porous serosal barrier. This pressure head is probably also responsible for the enlargement of the lateral spaces between the cells.

To summarize, what might be termed the "active transport pathway" consists of a series of barriers. The first barrier is the mucosal membrane of the epithelial cell. Sodium flow across this membrane is the rate-determining step for sodium transport; sodium flows down the potential energy gradient into the cell, and at least a part of the sodium flow is coupled with flows of sugars, amino acids, and possibly other non-electrolytes. The serosal and lateral membranes of the epithelial cells constitute the second barrier across which sodium is actively transported. Sodium then enters the subepithelial spaces, including the lateral spaces below the "tight junction" of the epithelial cells. This second compartment plays a critical role in the coupling of water flow to sodium flow. Sodium, water, and other solutes move from the submucosal compartment to the blood vessels and lymphatics. Lee (1961) has claimed that under *in vitro* conditions as much as 80% of absorbed water (and presumably sodium) enters the lymphatics. The mechanism of transport from the submucosal compartment is not known, but is probably passive, involving diffusional and bulk flow processes.

The other alkali metal cations probably do not cross the intestine by way of the active transport pathway. They cannot replace sodium in its ability to couple with sugar and amino acid flow across the mucosal membrane (Bosačková and Crane, 1965b). As reviewed earlier, by all the accepted criteria, the other alkali metal cations are not actively transported across the intestine.

10.10. PATHWAYS FOR PASSIVE TRANSPORT

In common with the proximal tubular epithelium of the kidney, and in contrast to frog skin and toad bladder, the intestinal epithelium possesses a high passive permeability (for a review, see Clarkson, 1967). The electrical resistance is low—approximately 50 ohm cm^2, as compared to the resistance of frog skin and toad bladder, of 1500 to 500 ohm cm^2. The sodium flux ratio, which according to Kedem and Essig (1965) is a measure of membrane resistance to sodium flux, is approximately 10 to 20 times lower than the corresponding figure with frog skin (Curran and Solomon, 1957; Ussing and Zerahn, 1951).

In principle, passive transport of ions could take place either through or between the epithelial cells or both. The generally accepted view that all cell membranes allow some passive flow of ions, and the electron-microscopic evidence that epithelial cells are closely attached to each other by "tight junctions" (Farquar and Palade, 1963), support the idea that passive transport of ions, as well as active transport, takes place through the epithelial cells. However, a significant body of evidence has now appeared in the literature, which is difficult to explain on the premise that movement through the epithelial cell is the rate-determining step in the passive flow of alkali metal ions across the intestine. In fact, in several experiments discussed below, the passive flows of sodium and potassium exhibit characteristics indicating an extracellular shunt pathway.

Studies on the isolated rabbit ileum by Schultz and Zalusky (1964) indicate that the serosal to mucosal unidirectional transmural flux of sodium is by simple passive diffusion. These authors derived an equation relating the serosal to mucosal flux, Φ_{sm}, to the transmural electrical potential difference ($\Psi_s - \Psi_m$) for cases where the sodium concentrations in the bathing solution were identical, viz.

$$\Phi_{sm} = {}_o\Phi_{sm} \exp\left[F(\Psi_s - \Psi_m)/RT\right]^{\frac{1}{2}}$$

where ${}_o\Phi_{sm}$ is the unidirectional transmural flux under short-circuit conditions. By applying a current across the intestine, it was possible to set ($\Psi_s - \Psi_m$) at any desired value. Measurement of Φ_{sm} using ^{24}Na isotope revealed complete agreement with this equation over values of ($\Psi_s - \Psi_m$) ranging from -30 to $+50$ mV.

A recent thermodynamic analysis of isotope flows by Kedem and Essig (1965) indicates that equations of the type derived by Schultz and Zalusky assume not only a process of passive diffusion, but that the passive flow takes place through pathways separate and distinct from active transport pathways. Thus, it seems unlikely that the serosal to mucosal flux passes through the mucosal cell, because if this were the case, the passive flux would be entering the intracellular sodium pool which is strongly influenced by active sodium transport.

This conclusion is supported by Schultz and Zalusky's (1964) data on the effects of inhibitors on the transmural fluxes. The net transport of sodium under short-circuit conditions was completely abolished by addition of 2,4-dinitrophenol or ouabain to the bathing solutions. In the case of inhibition by ouabain, it is known that the intracellular sodium concentration is greatly increased. Nevertheless, treatment with ouabain or 2,4-dinitrophenol affected only the mucosal to serosal flux. The ^{24}Na–sodium flux from serosal to mucosal solutions was unaffected.

Edmonds and Nielson (1968) concluded that at least two distinct pathways exist for sodium transport across the rat colon. They measured the transmural fluxes of $^{24}Na^+$ and the intracellular sodium concentrations. Assuming that sodium crossed the mucosal facing membrane of the colon epithelial cell by passive diffusion, and applying Ussing's flux ratio equation (p. 489), it was possible to calculate the unidirectional fluxes of sodium across this membrane. The results of these calculations indicated that the unidirectional fluxes across the mucosal facing cell membrane were far too low to account for the magnitude of the transmural fluxes across the tissue. Thus, it is necessary to postulate an additional pathway across the colon. Edmonds and Nielson (1968) suggested that this second pathway may be extracellular or through other cell types.*

The characteristics of potassium transport across the small intestine are difficult to explain on the premise that movement occurs only through the epithelial cell. The electrochemical potential of potassium is higher inside the cell than in the bathing solution by at least 40 mV (Schultz and Curran, 1968). Consequently, potassium must be actively pumped into the cell. However, there is no evidence of active potassium transfer across the tissue (Gilman *et al.*, 1962; Clarkson and Rothstein, 1960; Clarkson, 1967). One explanation is that the "potassium pumps" are so distributed around the epithelial cell that the pumps on the mucosal side exactly counteract the pumps situated on the serosal aspect of the cell (Schultz and Curran, 1968). However, these facts would be equally well explained by postulating that potassium crosses the intestinal epithelium by "by-passing" the epithelial cells. As in the case of the experiments of Edmonds and Nielson, one has to consider extracellular channels or the presence of a small number of cells having unusually high permeability to potassium. More detailed studies on the site of action of the cardiac glycoside, ouabain, might help decide between the explanations; for example, ouabain added to the serosal side not only inhibits ion transport but causes Na^{+} concentrations inside the cell to approach levels in the bathing solutions (Schultz *et al.*, 1966). If Schultz and Curran's explanation is correct, this would mean that ouabain is able to inhibit the potassium pumps situated on both the mucosal and serosal facing membranes. However, as was previously discussed (p. 493), present evidence suggests ouabain acts only on the serosal facing membrane, but unfortunately the evidence is not completely conclusive. The possibility that ouabain enters the epithelial cell has not been excluded (Csaky and Hara, 1965), and Forth and Rummel have shown that the local distribution of ouabain in the intestinal tissue is not the same if the glycoside is applied to different sides of the intestinal wall.

Studies on the influence of electrical and chemical driving forces on

*For additional discussion of this topic see also Chapter 3, pp. 202 and 203 (Eds.).

the net flows of sodium, potassium and chloride across isolated rat ileum support the conclusion that the passive transport pathway exhibits all the functional characteristics of an extracellular shunt. The data indicated that sodium and potassium passed through aqueous pores, whose diameters were large compared to the hydrated sizes of the monovalent ions. The ionic composition in the pores was equal to the mean value of the ionic concentration of the ions in the mucosal and serosal solutions. The ionic permeabilitics of the ileum to sodium, potassium and chloride were proportional to the ionic mobilities in free solution. The effects of ion flow on water transport in the absence of osmotic pressure gradients could be interpreted in terms of transport through aqueous extracellular channels.

The flows of Na^+ and Cl^- ions quantitatively account for the quantity of electrical current that is passed across the isolated ileum (Clarkson, 1967). If these ions pass through aqueous extracellular channels, it follows that the activation energy of the tissue conductance should correspond to the activation energy for free diffusion of these ions in aqueous solution. This has been shown to be the case for isolated rabbit ileum (Schultz and Zalusky, 1964) and for isolated rat colon mucosa (Edmonds and Nielson, 1968).

The possibility of extracellular channels allowing passive diffusion of iron and of certain alkali metal cations has been discussed recently by Forth *et al.* (1968) and by Pfleger *et al.* (1967) respectively.

The evidence reviewed above is derived mainly from kinetic studies, and alternative interpretations are possible. All that may be said is that the passive transport pathways possess the functional characteristics of an extracellular shunt. It is conceivable that a small number of cells, highly permeable to monovalent ions, may account for the observations. The definition of an extracellular shunt soon becomes a matter of semantics.

Unfortunately, there is no direct evidence on the anatomical location of these pathways. However, amongst the epithelia so far studied, the intestine is probably unique in its high rate of turnover of epithelial cells. In most mammals, the half-time turnover is only a few hours. This process of exfoliation may account for the extracellular channels. The cells produced in the crypts of Lieberkuhn progress in an orderly fashion to the tips of the villi where they exfoliate. Any given row of cells surrounding the base of a villus is moving over a steadily decreasing surface area as the cells progress along the villus. Some cells must move more rapidly, others more slowly, if the cells are to remain on the villus surface.

This process will require continual breaking of the junctions between cells and may lead to the appearance of transient, intercellular channels. The exfoliation process at the villus tip must also result in breaking intercellular linkages.

Evidence on the mechanism of extrusion of epithelial cells is reviewed and discussed in Chapter 1, "The Structural Basis of Intestinal Absorption". Studies to date do not indicate the presence of any visible gaps between the cells, but such gaps may be transient and difficult to observe by present techniques. For example, Curran and Solomon (1957) concluded from studies on the diffusion of mannitol across the rat ileum that the largest pores would have a radius of no more than 36 Å. It seems likely that such pores would be extracellular since Lindemann and Solomon (1962) calculated that the pore radius of the mucosal surface of the epithelial cell was only 4 Å.

ACKNOWLEDGEMENTS

This study was supported in part under contract with the U.S. Atomic Energy Commission at the University of Rochester Atomic Energy Project and has been assigned Report No. UR–49–1197.

REFERENCES

ALVARADO, F. and MONREAL, J. (1967) Sodium-dependent active transport of phenylglucosides in the chicken small intestine. *Comp. Biochem. Physiol.* **20:** 471–488.

ANDERSEN, B. and USSING, H. H. (1957) Solvent drag on non-electrolytes during osmotic flow through isolated toad skin and its response to antidiuretic hormone. *Acta Physiol. Scand.* **39:** 228–239.

AULSEBROOK, K. A. (1961) Effect of vasopressin on sodium transfer by rat colon *in vitro*. *Endocrinology* **68:** 1065–1067.

AULSEBROOK, K. A. (1965) Intestinal transport of glucose and sodium: changes in alloxan diabetes and effects of insulin. *Experientia* **21:** 346–347.

BARRY, R. J. C., SMYTH, D. H. and WRIGHT, E. M. (1965) Short-circuit current and solute transfer by rat jejunum. *J. Physiol.* **181:** 410–431.

BLICKENSTAFF, D. D. (1954) Increase in intestinal absorption of water from isosmotic saline following pitressin administration. *Am. J. Physiol.* **179:** 471–472.

BOSAČKOVÁ, J. and CRANE, R. K. (1965a) Studies on the mechanism of intestinal absorption of sugars. IX. Intracellular sodium concentrations and active sugar transport by hamster small intestine *in vitro*. *Biochim. Biophys. Acta* **102:** 436–441.

BOSAČKOVÁ, J. and CRANE, R. K. (1965b) Studies on the mechanism of intestinal absorption of sugars. VIII. Cation inhibition of active sugar transport and ^{22}Na influx into hamster small intestine *in vitro*. *Biochim. Biophys. Acta* **102:** 423–425.

CANAVAN, D. A. and LOVE, A. H. G. (1969) The effects of insulin on intestinal absorption *in vitro*. *J. Physiol.* **200:** 129–130.

CLARKSON, T. W. (1967) The transport of salt and water across the isolated rat ileum. *J. Gen. Physiol.* **50**: 695–727.

CLARKSON, T. W. and CROSS, A. (1961) *Studies of the Action of Mercuric Chloride on Intestinal Absorption.* University of Rochester AEP Report No. 588.

CLARKSON, T. W., CROSS, A. C. and TOOLE, S. R. (1961) Electrical potentials across the isolated small intestine of the rat. *Am. J. Physiol.* **200**: 1233–1235.

CLARKSON, T. W. and ROTHSTEIN, A. (1960) Transport of monovalent cations by the isolated small intestine of the rat. *Am. J. Physiol.* **199**: 898–906.

CLARKSON, T. W. and TOOLE, S. R. (1964) Measurement of short-circuit current and ion-transport across the ileum. *Am. J. Physiol.* **206**: 658–668.

CRANE, R. K. (1968) Absorption of sugars, pp. 1323–1351. In: *Handbook of Physiology,* sect. 6, vol. 7, CODE, C. F. and HEIDEL, W. (Eds.). Am. Physiol. Soc., Washington, D.C.

CSAKY, T. Z. (1961) Significance of sodium ions in active intestinal transport of non-electrolytes. *Am. J. Physiol.* **201**: 999–1001.

CSAKY, T. Z. (1963) A possible link between active transport of electrolytes and non-electrolytes. *Fedn. Proc.* **27**: 3–7 (Part 1).

CSAKY, T. Z. and HARA, Y. (1965) Inhibition of active intestinal sugar transport by digitalis. *Am. J. Physiol.* **209**: 467–472.

CURRAN, P. F. (1960) Na_2Cl and water transport by rat ileum *in vitro. J. Gen. Physiol.* **43**: 1137–1148.

CURRAN, P. F. (1965) Ion transport in intestine and its coupling to other transport processes. *Fedn. Proc.* **24**: 993–999.

CURRAN, P. F., HERRERA, F. C. and FLANNIGAN, W. J. (1963) The effect of Ca and anti-diuretic hormone on Na transport across frog skin. II. Sites and mechanisms of action. *J. Gen. Physiol.* **46**: 1011–1127.

CURRAN, P. F. and MCINTOSH, J. R. (1962) A model system for biological water transport. *Nature* **193**: 347–348.

CURRAN, P. F., SCHULTZ, S. G., CHEZ, R. A. and FUISZ, R. F. (1967) Kinetic relations of the Na^+ –amino acid interaction at the mucosal border of the intestine. *J. Gen. Physiol.* **50**: 1261–1286.

CURRAN, P. F. and SCHWARTZ, G. F. (1960) Na, Cl and water transport by rat colon. *J. Gen. Physiol.* **43**: 555–570.

CURRAN, P. F. and SOLOMON, A. K. (1957) Ion and water fluxes in the ileum of rats. *J. Gen. Physiol.* **41**: 143–168.

CURRAN, P. F., WEBSTER, E. W. and HOVSEPIAN, J. A. (1960) The effect of X-irradiation on sodium and water transport in rat ileum. *Radiation Res.* **13**: 369–380.

DAVIDSON, S. and PASSMORE, R. (1966) *Human Nutrition and Dietetics.* E. and S. Livingstone, Ltd., Edinburgh and London.

DAWSON, A. M. and ISSELBACHER, K. J. (1960) Studies on lipid metabolism of the small intestine with observations on the role of bile salts. *J. Clin. Invest.* **39**: 730–740.

DEMPSEY, E. F., CARROLL, E. L., ALBRIGHT, F. and HENNEMAN, P. H. (1958) A study of factors determining electrolyte excretion. *Metabolism* **7**: 108–118.

DIAMOND, J. M. and TORMEY, J. M. (1966a) Role of long extracellular channels in fluid transport across epithelia. *Nature* (*Lond.*) **210**: 817.

DIAMOND, J. M. and TORMEY, J. M. (1966b) Studies on the structural basis of water transport across epithelial membranes. *Fedn. Proc.* **25**: 1458.

DOMBRADI, G. A., KRIZSA, F. and JANSCO, T. (1960) Die Kinetik der intestinalen Wasserresorption der Ratte unter dem Einfluss von AOH. *Acta Physiol. Acad. Sci. Hung.* **17**: 301–308.

EDMONDS, C. J. (1967a) Transport of potassium by the rat colon of normal and sodium-depleted rats. *J. Physiol.* **193**: 603–617.

EDMONDS, C. J. (1967b) The gradient of electrical potential difference and of sodium and potassium of the gut contents along the caecum and colon of normal and sodium-depleted rats. *J. Physiol.* **193:** 571–588.

EDMONDS, C. J. and NIELSON, O. F. (1968) Transmembrane electrical potential differences and ionic composition of mucosal cells of rat colon. *Acta Physiol. Scand.* **72:** 338–349.

FARQUAR, M. G. and PALADE, G. E. (1963) Junctional complexes in various epithelia. *J. Cell. Biol.* **17:** 375–412.

FINKELSTEIN, R. A. P., ATTHASAMPUNNA, P., CHALASAMAYA, M. and CHARUNMETHEE, P. (1966) Pathogenesis of experimental cholera; biological activities of purified procholeragen A. *J. Immunol.* **96:** 440–449.

FISHER, R. B. (1955) The absorption of water and of some small solute molecules from the isolated small intestine of the rat. *J. Physiol.* (*Lond.*) **130:** 655–664.

FORDTRAN, J. S. (1968) Absorption of water, electrolyte and sugars for the human gut. In: *Handbook of Physiology,* sect. 6, vol. 3, CODE, E. F. and HEIDEL, W. (Eds.). Am. Physiol. Soc., Washington, D.C.

FORDTRAN, J. S. and LOCKLEAR, T. W. (1966) Ionic constituents and osmolality of gastric and small intestine fluids after eating. *Am. J. Dig. Dis.* **11:** 503–521.

FORDTRAN, J. S., RECTOR, F. C. JR. and CARTER, N. W. (1968) Mechanism of sodium absorption in the human small intestine. *J. Clin. Invest.* **47:** 884–900.

FORTH, W., LEOPOLD, G. and RUMMEL, W. (1968) Eisendurchtritt von der Mucosa zur Serosaseite und umgekehrt an isolierten Eisenarmen und normalen Segmenten von Jejunum und Ileum. *Arch. Pharmak. exp. Path.* **261**: 434–440.

FORTH, W. and RUMMEL, W. (1967) Wirkung von Herzglykosiden auf Calcium-, Matrium-, Wasser-, und Glukose-transport am isolierten Dünndarm. *Helv. Physiol. Acta* **25:** 8–23.

FORTH, W., RUMMEL, W. and BALDAUF, J. (1966) Wasser- und Electrolytbewegung am Dünndarm und Dickdarm unter dem Einfluss von Laxantien, ein Beitrag zur Klarung ihres Wirkungsmechanismus. *Arch. Pharmak. exp. Path.* **254:** 18–32.

FORTH, W., RUMMEL, W. and GLASNER, H. (1964) Zur resorptionshemmenden Wirkung von Gallensäuren. *Arch. Pharmak. exp. Path.* **247:** 382–383.

FORTH, W., RUMMEL, W. and GLASNER, H. (1966) Zur resorptionshemmenden Wirkung von Gallensäuren. *Arch. Pharmak. exp. Path.* **254:** 364–368.

GILLES-BAILLIEN, M. and SCHOFFENIELS, E. (1967) Bioelectric potentials in the intestinal epithelium of the Greek tortoise. *Comp. Biochem. Physiol.* **23:** 95–104.

GILMAN, A., KOELLE, E. and RICHIE, J. M. (1962) Transport of potassium ions in the rat's intestine. *Nature* (*Lond.*) **197:** 1210–1211.

GRADY, G. F., MODOFF, M. A., DUHAMEL, R. C., MOORE, E. W. and CHALMERS, T. C. (1967) Sodium transport by the human ileum *in vitro* and its response to cholera enterotoxin. *Gasteroenterology* **53:** 737–744.

GREEN, K. and MATTY, A. J. (1966) Effect of vasopressin on ion transport across intestinal epithelia. *Life Sci.* **5:** 205–209 (Part I).

GUANSON, J. M. and STANBURY, S. W. (1965) Congenital chloridorrhoea and so-called congenital alkalosis with diarrhoea. *Gut* **6:** 29–37.

HAKIM, A. A. and LIFSON, N. (1969) Effects of pressure on water and solute transport by dog intestinal mucosa *in vitro*. *Am. J. Physiol.* **216:** 276–284.

HOLDSWORTH, C. D. and DAWSON, A. M. (1964) The absorption of mucosaccharides in man. *Clin. Sci.* **27:** 371–379.

HOLT, P. R. (1964) Intestinal absorption of bile salts in the rat. *Am. J. Physiol.* **207:** 1–7.

HOSHIKO, T. and LINDLEY, B. D. (1964) The relationship of Ussing's flux ratio equation to the thermodynamic description of membrane permeability. *Biochim. Biophys. Acta* **79:** 301–317.

HOSHIKO, T. and USSING, H. H. (1960) The kinetics of ^{24}Na flux across amphibian skin and bladder. *Acta Physiol. Scand.* **49:** 74–81.

INGRAHAM, R. C., PETERS, H. C. and VISSCHER, M. B. (1938) On the movement of materials across living membranes against concentration gradients. *J. Phys. Chem.* **42:** 141–150.

INGRAHAM, R. C. and VISSCHER, M. B. (1936) The production of chloride-free solutions by the action of the intestinal epithelium. *Am. J. Physiol.* **114:** 676–680.

INGRAHAM, R. C. and VISSCHER, M. B. (1938) Further studies on epithelial absorption with the performance of osmotic wash. *Am. J. Physiol.* **121:** 771–785.

KEDEM, D. and ESSIG, A. (1965) Isotope flows and flux ratios in biological membranes. *J. Gen. Physiol.* **48:** 1047–1070.

KEDEM, O. and KATCHALSKY, A. (1961) A physical interpretation of the phenomenological coefficients of membrane permeability. *J. Gen. Physiol.* **45:** 143–179.

KEDEM, O. and KATCHALSKY, A. (1963) Thermodynamic analysis of the permeability of biological membranes to non-electrolytes. *Biochim. Biophys. Acta* **27:** 229–246.

LEAF, A., ANDERSON, J. and PAGE, L. B. (1958) Active sodium transport by the isolated toad bladder. *J. Gen. Physiol.* **41:** 657–668.

LEE, J. S. (1961) Flows and pressures in lymphatic and blood vessels of intestine in water absorption. *Am. J. Physiol.* **200:** 979–983.

LEVITAN, R. and INGELFINGER, F. J. (1965) Effect of D-aldosterone on salt and water absorption from the intact human colon. *J. Clin. Invest.* **44:** 801–808.

LEVITAN, R. and MAUER, I. (1966) The influence of pitressin administration on salt and water absorption from the human colon. *Clin. Res.* **14:** 301 (Abstr.).

LINDEMANN, B. and SOLOMON, A. K. (1962) Permeability of luminal surface of intestinal mucosal cells, *J. Gen. Physiol.* **45:** 801–810.

MALAWER, S. J., EWTON, M. F., FORDTRAN, J. S. and INGELFINGER, F. J. (1965) Interrelation between jejunal absorption of sodium, glucose and water in man. *J. Clin. Invest.* **44:** 1072–1073 (Abstr.).

MCHARDY, G. J. R. and PARSONS, D. S. (1957) The absorption of water and salt from the small intestine of the rat. *Quart. J. Exp. Physiol.* **42:** 33–48.

MCKENNEY, J. R. (1968) Electrolyte transport and voltage measurements in a preparation of the irradiated rat ileum, pp. 206–214. In: *Gastrointestinal Radiation Injury,* SULLIVAN, M. F. (Ed.). Excerpta Medica Foundation, Reidel, Dordrecht, Netherlands.

MEARES, P. and USSING, H. H. (1959) The fluxes of sodium and chloride ions across a cation-exchange resin membrane. Part 7. Effect of a concentration-gradient. *Trans. Farad Soc.* **55:** 147–155.

MEKHJIAN, H. S., PHILLIPS, S. F. and HOFMAN, A. T. (1968) Conjugated bile salts block water and electrolyte transport by the human colon. *Gasteroenterology* **54:** 1256 (Abstr.).

MUNCK, B. G. and SCHULTZ, S. G. (1969) Lysine transport across isolated rabbit ileum. *J. Gen. Physiol.* **53:** 157–182.

OGILVIE, J. T., MCINTOSH, J. R. and CURRAN, P. T. (1963) Volume flow in series membrane system. *Biochim. Biophys. Acta* **66:** 441–444.

PARSONS, D. S. (1956) The absorption of bicarbonate–saline solutions by the small intestine and colon of the white rat. *Quart. J. Exp. Physiol.* **41:** 410–420.

PARSONS, D. S. and PATERSON, C. R. (1965) Fluid and solute transport across rat colonic mucosa. *Quart. J. Exp. Physiol.* **50:** 220–231.

PARSONS, D. S. and PATERSON, C. R. (1966) Movements of fluid and glucose in an everted sac preparation of rat colonic mucosa. *Biochim. Biophys. Acta* **49:** 173.

PARSONS, D. S. and PRICHARD, J. S. (1968) A preparation of perfused small intestine for the study of absorption in amphibians. *J. Physiol.* **198:** 405–434.

PARSONS, D. S. and WINGATE, D. C. (1961) The effect of osmotic gradients on fluid transfer across intestine *in vitro. Biochim. Biophys. Acta* **46:** 170–183.

PASSOW, H., ROTHSTEIN, A. and CLARKSON, T. W. (1961) The general pharmacology of heavy metals. *Pharm. Rev.* **13:** 185–224.

PFLEGER, K., FORTH, W. and RUMMEL, W. (1967) Vergleichende Untersuchungen zur Resorption von Alkaliionen durch den Dünndarm. p. 191. In: *Radioisotope in der Gastroenterologie,* F. K. Schattauer-Verlag, Stuttgart.

PHILLIPS, S. F. and CODE, C. F. (1966) Sorption of potassium in the small and large intestine. *Am. J. Physiol.* **211:** 607–613.

PLAYOUST, M. R. and ISSELBACHER, K. J. (1964) Studies on the transport and metabolism of conjugated bile salts by intestinal mucosa. *J. Clin. Invest.* **43:** 467–476.

QUASTLER, H. (1956) The nature of intestinal radiation death. *Radiation Res.* **4:** 303–320.

ROSENBERG, T. (1954) The concept and definition of active transport. *Symp. Soc. Exp. Biol.* **8:** 27–41.

RUMMEL, W. and STUPP, H. F. (1962) The influence of diuretics on the absorption of salts, glucose and water from isolated small intestine of the rat. *Experientia* **18:** 303–309.

SACHER, D. B., TAYLOR, J. O., SAHA, J. R. and PHILLIPS, R. A. (1969) Intestinal transmural electrical potential and its response to glucose in acute and convalescent cholera. *Gasteroenterology* **50:** 512–521.

SCHEDL, H. P. and CLIFTON, J. A. (1963) Solute and water absorption by the human small intestine. *Nature* **199:** 1264–1267.

SCHULTZ, S. G. and CURRAN, P. F. (1968) Intestinal absorption of sodium chloride and water, pp. 1245–1275. In: *Handbook of Physiology,* sect. 6, vol. 3. CODE, C. F. and HEIDEL, W. (Eds.). Am. Physiol. Soc., Washington, D.C.

SCHULTZ, S. G., FUISZ, R. E. and CURRAN, P. F. (1966) Amino acid and sugar transport in rabbit ileum. *J. Gen. Physiol.* **49:** 849–866.

SCHULTZ, S. G. and ZALUSKY, R. (1964) Ion transport in isolated rabbit ileum. *J. Gen. Physiol.* **47:** 567–584.

SKOU, J. C. (1967) The enzymic basis for active transport of sodium and potassium. *Protoplasma* **63:** 303–308.

SLADEN, G. E. and DAWSON, A. M. (1968) Effect of bicarbonate on sodium absorption by the human jejunum. *Nature* **218:** 267–268.

SMYTH, P. H. and TAYLOR, C. B. (1957) Transfer of water and solutes by an *in vitro* intestinal preparation. *J. Physiol.* **136:** 632–648.

SOERGEL, K. H., WHALEN, G. E., HARRIS, J. A. and GREENEN, J. E. (1968) Effect of antidiuretic hormone on human small intestinal water and solute transport. *J. Clin. Invest.* **47:** 1071–1082.

SOLS, A., VIDAL, S. and LARROLDS, L. (1948) The effects of insulin on intestinal glucose absorption in alloxan diabetic rats. *Nature* (*Lond.*) **161**: 932–933, Part 2.

SULLIVAN, M. F. (1968) Sodium, water and ^{12}B absorption in irradiated rats, pp. 218–227. In: *Gastrointestinal Radiation Injury,* SULLIVAN, M. F. (Ed.). Excerpta Medica Foundation, Reidel, Dordrecht, Netherlands.

SUMERS, R. W. and SCHEDL, H. P. (1968) Effects of toxicity and glucose on intestinal sodium and water absorption. *Scand. J. Gastroenter.* **3:** 376–382.

USSING, H. H. (1949) The distinction by means of tracers between active transport and diffusion. *Acta Physiol. Scand.* **19:** 43–56.

USSING, H. H. (1960) The frog skin potential. *J. Gen. Physiol.* **43:** 135–147 (Suppl.).

USSING, H. H. (1963) *Transport of Electrolytes and Water across Epithelia.* Harvey Lecture. London Academic Press Inc., Ltd.

USSING, H. H. and WINDHAGER, E. E. (1966) Nature of shunt pathway and active sodium transport path through frog skin epithelium. *Acta Physiol. Scand.* **61:** 484–504.

USSING, H. H. and ZERAHN, K. (1951) Active transport of sodium as a source of electric current in the short-circuited isolated frog skin. *Acta Physiol. Scand.* **23:** 110–127.

VISSCHER, M. B. and ROEPKE, R. R. (1945) Osmotic and electrolyte concentration relationships during absorption of salt solutions from ileal segments. *Am. J. Physiol.* **144:** 468–476.

VISSCHER, M. B., ROEPKE, R. R. and LIFSON, N. (1945) Osmotic and electrolyte concentration relationships during the absorption of autogenous serum from ileal segments. *Am. J. Physiol.* **144:** 457–463.

WELCH, C. S., WAKEFIELD, E. G. and ADAMS, M. (1936) Function of the large intestine of man in absorption and excretion: a study of a subject with an ileostomy stoma and an isolated colon. *Arch. Internal Med.* **48:** 1095–1110.

WILSON, T. H. (1954) Concentration gradients of lactate, hydrogen and some other ions across the intestine *in vitro*. *Biochem. J.* **56:** 521–527.

WILSON, T. H. (1956) Fluid movement across the wall of the small intestine *in vitro*. *Am. J. Physiol.* **187:** 244–246.

WILSON, T. H. (1962) *Intestinal Absorption*. W. B. Saunders, Philadelphia.

WILSON, T. H. and WISEMAN, G. (1954) The use of sacs of everted small intestine for the study of the transference of substances from the mucosal to the serosal surface. *J. Physiol.* (*Lond.*) **123:** 116–125.

WRIGHT, E. M. (1966) The origin of the glucose-dependent increase in the potential difference across the tortoise small intestine. *J. Physiol.* (*Lond.*) **185:** 486–500.

WRONG, O. and METCALFE-GIBSON, A. (1965) The electrolyte content of feces. *Proc. Roy. Soc. Med.* **58:** 1007–1009.

CHAPTER 11

GASTROINTESTINAL ABSORPTION OF ALKALINE EARTH IONS

Alexander D. Kenny

Columbia, Missouri, U.S.A.

11.1. INTRODUCTION

Any review of the gastrointestinal absorption of the alkaline earth ions will naturally concern itself mainly with Ca for obvious reasons.

First, the ion plays a key role in biological systems, including man. Calcium is essential for the integrity of cell membranes and is necessary for maintaining normal function in muscle, nerve, and secretory organs. It is no wonder, then, that the Ca level in the plasma, and hence in extracellular fluid, is kept within very narrow limits. The major physiological control systems concerned with Ca homeostasis involve three hormonal messengers, parathyroid hormone, calcitonin, and cholecalciferol,* and three target organs, gut, bone, and kidney. Within recent years, the contribution of the gut to Ca homeostasis has been receiving greater emphasis.

Secondly, most of the research in this area has been concerned with the absorption of Ca rather than Mg and the less physiologically important alkaline earth ions, strontium, barium, radium and beryllium.

Lastly, the major thrusts forward, such as the recent developments in vitamin D metabolism research, the mechanisms of alkaline earth ion transport across the gut, and the phenomenon of adaptation, are concerned mainly with Ca absorption.

The review will include first an examination of the more recent data and concepts concerning Ca transport, followed by a discussion of the

*Recent developments in the biochemistry and pharmacology of cholecalciferol (vitamin D_3) have indicated the possibility that the vitamin is synthesized and released by a specific tissue, the skin, and is carried to its target organs, gut, bone and kidney, by the blood. It is within this framework that cholecalciferol can be classified as a hormone.

influence of growth, reproduction, and Ca deprivation. Next the pharmacological aspects of Ca transport—that is the effects of cholecalciferol, the hormones, and other agents—will be described. Finally, the remaining alkaline earth ions will be analyzed for their points of difference, both quantitative and qualitative, from the way in which Ca is handled by the gut.

The author is indebted to recent excellent reviews on this topic, particularly those by Wasserman (1968), Wasserman and Taylor (1969), Wasserman *et al.* (1969), DeLuca (1969a), and Kimberg (1969).

11.2. CALCIUM TRANSPORT

11.2.1. TECHNIQUES

Of the many *in vivo* and *in vitro* techniques which have been used in studies of gut absorption in general (Berger, 1960, 1963; Levin, 1967), most have been applied to an examination of Ca absorption. *In vivo* methods include the balance technique, perfusion of both acute and chronic preparations of isolated loops, and injection into ligated loops. The most popular *in vitro* preparation is the everted gut sac of Wilson and Wiseman (1954). Other *in vitro* approaches have included intestinal slices and isolated villi.

The techniques available for clinical studies in man are more limited (Duthie, 1967). That technique most widely used in studies of Ca absorption has been the balance method.

A brief description of these techniques and their application to studies of Ca absorption in specific species follows. Where appropriate, mention is made of the relative advantages and disadvantages. No effort has been made to cite the original application. In fact, recent rather than classical references have been cited.

11.2.1.1. *Experimental techniques in animals: in vivo*

(a) *Balance method in animals.* The balance approach is the classical method for studying Ca absorption. In its simplest form the total fecal output is subtracted from the total dietary intake to give the quantity of Ca absorbed, which may then be expressed as a percentage of the dietary intake. In order to minimize collection errors it is necessary to collect specimens over several days and use an unabsorbed marker, such as chromium sesquioxide, in the diet to mark the beginning and the end of the collection period. The balance technique has been used by Henry and Kon (1953) and Benson *et al.* (1969) in the rat, Gershoff *et al.* (1958) in the dog, and Hurwitz and Griminger (1960) in the laying hen. Marcus and Lengemann (1962a) used ^{91}Y as a marker in rats.

However, this simple approach fails to correct for the contribution of the endogenous component of fecal Ca. The existence of this component was early recognized by pioneer studies of Albright and his associates, in man (Bauer *et al.*, 1929), who found fecal losses of 300 mg/day on a Ca intake of around 100 mg/day. In the mid-50s this problem was tackled with the aid of intravenously administered ^{45}Ca and the endogenous fecal loss of Ca was demonstrated and quantitated under normal dietary conditions in cattle (Comar *et al.*, 1953; Visek *et al.*, 1953), rats (Hansard and Crowder, 1957; Hansard and Plumlee, 1954), and man (Bronner and Harris, 1956). More recent studies in rats have also attempted to quantitate the endogenous fecal Ca and to make appropriate corrections (Shah and Draper, 1966; Sammon *et al.*, 1970).

This does not mean that studies failing to take this endogenous loss into consideration necessarily lead to false conclusions. In Table 1 data taken from Hansard and Plumlee (1954) and Sammon *et al.* (1970) have been assembled to indicate the differences in the values for percent Ca absorbed both by the simpler and by the more precise approaches. It is obvious that the classical approach (apparent absorption) gives lower values than those corrected for endogenous fecal loss (true absorption). However, conclusions concerning the relative effects of dietary Ca level on the percent absorbed would be the same based on either set of data.

TABLE 1. CALCIUM BALANCE DATA IN RATS ON VARIOUS CALCIUM INTAKES

Dietary Ca (%)	Ca intake v_i (mg/day)	Ca absorbed v_a (mg/day)	Endogenous fecal loss v_f (mg/day)	Ca absorption Apparent[(a)] (%)	True[(b)] (%)
Data from Hansard and Plumlee (1954)					
0.01	0.8	0.78	0.78	—	98
0.3	24.0	20.6	8.4	65	86
0.5	45.0	28.4	24.3	46	63
1.0	102.0	47.9	64.3	37	47
Data from Sammon *et al.* (1970)					
0.05	7.3	6.6	0.3	86	90
0.5	72.8	44.5	5.1	54	61
1.4	205.0	75.9	11.1	32	37

[(a)] $(v_i - v_F)\,100/v_i$.

[(b)] $(v_i - v_F + v_f)\,100/v_i$ or $v_a \times 100/v_i$, where v_F = total fecal Ca.

The estimate of endogenous fecal Ca is not a constant value but varies with the dietary level: the higher the dietary intake the greater the endogenous loss (Table 1 and Bronner, 1969; Bronner and Aubert, 1965; Sammon *et al.,* 1970). The question can be asked whether or not the determination of endogenous fecal Ca is a *sine qua non* of acceptable work in Ca-absorption studies using the balance approach. We cannot be certain of the answer until more is known about the physiology of the endogenous loss. For example, it is still unclear to what extent the endogenous Ca, secreted into the intestine, is subject to partial reabsorption (Bronner, 1964).

The balance method has one major advantage: it is the most physiological. Its drawbacks, in addition to the problem of endogenous fecal loss already described, lie in its tedium, lack of precision in marking fecal collections, and its inability to contribute to mechanism or site of absorption studies.

(b) *Isolated loop: perfusion in chronic preparation.* The chronically prepared isolated loop (Thiry–Vella fistula) has been used mainly in larger animals such as the dog (Cramer, 1963, 1964, 1965, 1968; Cramer and Dueck, 1962; Cramer and Haqq, 1963; Cramer *et al.,* 1969) and the sheep (Care and van't Klooster, 1965; Phillipson and Storry, 1965; Scott, 1965).

Solutions of varying but known composition are perfused through the loop at a volume rate estimated to be physiological (Care and van't Klooster used 180 ml/hr in 2–3-year-old sheep). However, the perfusate may be diluted by intestinal secretions or concentrated by fluid absorption; either phenomenon will introduce an error in interpretation. This artifact may be controlled, as was done by Care and van't Klooster (1965), by the addition to the perfusate of a material such as polyethylene glycol which is not absorbed and can be measured readily by a turbidimetric method (Hyden, 1955).

One drawback of the Thiry–Vella loop is that disuse atrophy can occur as a consequence of the loop being isolated from the normally functioning gastrointestinal tract. This problem can be minimized by the use of re-entrant cannulae which permit the flow of food through the loops except when isolated during an experiment (Phillipson and Storry, 1965).

The chronically isolated loop preparation, although less physiological than the balance technique, is certainly more precise quantitatively. Certain kinetic aspects can be studied such as unidirectional flow and saturation kinetics. It can answer questions concerning sites of absorption and the direct influence of pharmacological agents at these sites. It cannot readily be used to isolate the active and passive components and hence the mechanisms underlying absorption.

(c) *Isolated loop: perfusion in acute preparation.* Perfusion of the isolated loop in an acute preparation has had more limited application. Its use in studies of Ca absorption has been restricted to the smaller animals, particularly the rat (Dumont *et al.*, 1960; Krawitt, 1967; Krawitt and Schedl, 1968; and Wasserman *et al.*, 1961) and the chicken (Holdsworth, 1965). With this method an isolated segment of the small intestine is canulated at both ends under anesthesia. The segment is perfused at a constant rate with (Holdsworth, 1965; Krawitt, 1967; Krawitt and Schedl, 1968) or without (Wasserman *et al.*, 1961) recirculation of the fluid. The advantages of the acute perfusion technique are similar to those of the chronic preparation. In addition, the problem of disuse atrophy is eliminated.

(d) *Isolated loop: injection into ligated segment.* This is probably the most widely used *in vivo* technique in smaller animals, especially in rats (Pento, 1970; Waldron-Edward *et al.*, 1966; Wasserman, 1962; Wasserman and Comar, 1961; Wasserman *et al.*, 1966; Winter *et al.*, 1969, 1970) and in chickens (Corradino and Wasserman, 1970; Coates *et al.*, 1961; Coates and Holdsworth, 1961; Ebel *et al.*, 1969; Gershoff and Hegsted, 1956; Harmeyer and DeLuca, 1969; Hurwitz *et al.*, 1967; Neville and Holdsworth, 1969; Sallis and Holdsworth, 1962a; Wasserman *et al.*, 1969; Wasserman and Kallfelz, 1962; Wasserman *et al.*, 1966; Webling and Holdsworth, 1965). The animal is anesthetized and a segment of the intestine exposed and ligated at both ends following the injection of a ^{45}Ca (or ^{47}Ca) solution. In studies involving the proximal duodenum the bile duct is also ligated. The laparotomy is closed and the animals allowed to recover from anesthesia. At the end of a certain period (usually 1 hr) the animal is bled and the segment of duct removed. The plasma ^{45}Ca, total gut ^{45}Ca, or the ^{45}Ca remaining in the gut contents and/or washings can be used as indices of Ca absorption. The technique is simple and relatively physiological. It can be used directly for studies of unidirectional fluxes. The active and passive components of Ca absorption can be determined indirectly by the use of flux ratios at varying luminal Ca concentrations (Wasserman and Kallfelz, 1962). It can also be used to identify sites of absorption. A somewhat similar technique has been used in dogs (Schedl *et al.*, 1968).

11.2.1.2. *Experimental techniques in animals: in vitro*

(a) *Everted gut sac.* The everted gut sac was first described by Wilson and Wiseman (1954) in studies of glucose and methionine absorption by rat and hamster intestine. A short segment (2–3 cm) of the intestine is removed, everted, and ligated at both ends following the introduction of a small volume (0.5 ml) of a buffer solution containing ^{40}Ca and ^{45}Ca with or without glucose. The everted sac is placed in a 25-ml Erlenmeyer flask containing a larger volume (3 ml) of the buffer solution. After incubation at 37°C for 1–3 hours with shaking, the final ^{45}Ca concentration ratios (inside/outside I/O; or serosal/mucosal, S/M) are determined.

The development of the everted gut sac preparation gave a great impetus to research in gut absorption in general. It enabled active transport to be examined directly and to be demonstrated more conclusively. The influence of environment, metabolic inhibitors, and pharmacological agents can be studied removed from neural and humoral factors (Table 2).

Since its first applications to Ca absorption by Schachter and Rosen (1959) and by Rasmussen (1959) the technique has contributed greatly to our understanding of several facets of mineral absorption, especially Ca and the other alkaline earths. Although Schachter and Rosen (1959) used the technique in both rats and rabbits its subsequent applications to studies of Ca absorption have been almost exclusively in rats (Avioli *et al.*, 1969 a, b; Blunt *et al.*, 1968a; Dowdle *et al.*, 1960; Finkelstein and Schachter, 1962; Gruson *et al.*, 1970; Harrison and Harrison, 1969; Kessner and Epstein, 1966; Kimberg *et al.*, 1961; Lifshitz *et al.*, 1967 a, b, 1969; Martin and DeLuca, 1969a; Noble and Matty, 1967; Rasmussen,

TABLE 2. EVERTED GUT SAC OF THE RABBIT: EFFECT OF METABOLIC INHIBITORS ON ACTIVE TRANSPORT OF CALCIUM[a]

Inhibitor	Concentration (mM)	Serosal/mucosal ratio	
		Control	Inhibitor
Nitrogen (anaerobiosis)	—	3.7	0.8
5°C	—	4.8	1.0
Sodium fluoride	2.0	5.2	1.0
Sodium cyanide	0.5	4.6	1.1
Sodium azide	3.0	6.0	1.1
Sodium iodoacetate	0.3	5.0	1.6
Mercuric chloride	1.0	4.6	1.1
Sodium malonate	20.0	5.0	2.5
2,4-dinitrophenol	0.05	7.2	1.2
Magnesium chloride	1.0	4.6	2.0
Strontium chloride	1.0	4.3	5.5
Barium chloride	1.0	4.5	4.6

[a] From Schachter and Rosen (1959).

1959; Schachter *et al.*, 1960a, 1966, 1970; Urban and Schedl, 1969, 1970; Wasserman, 1960; Wasserman and Taylor, 1963a; Williams *et al.*, 1961, 1962). The technique has been modified by Harrison and Harrison (1965 and 1970) to study passive transport by incubating at 5° or 22°C and under other conditions (anaerobiosis or metabolic inhibitors) which inhibit active transport. Hurwitz *et al.* (1967), Holdsworth (1965), and Sallis and Holdsworth (1962a) have used the gut sac preparation in chickens. A disadvantage of the technique is that it cannot answer such questions as to where the *bulk* of the Ca is absorbed in the gastrointestinal tract.

The everted gut sac as described above represents the most popular *in vitro* preparation. Other similar preparations have been described for special purposes. Morehead and Kessner (1969) used an open-ended gut sac of the rat similar to that described by Parsons and Paterson (1965). Schachter (1963) and Wasserman and Taylor (1969) adapted the preparation described by Crane and Wilson (1958) for Ca-absorption studies. This technique, whereby a segment of the everted gut is ligated at one end, and at the other end tied to a cannula suspended in a test tube, permits serial sampling and can be modified to facilitate the measurement of bioelectric phenomena.

(b) *Other in vitro techniques.* These include the use of rat intestinal slices (Batt and Schachter, 1969; Martin and DeLuca, 1969b; Schachter *et al.*, 1960b) and rat isolated villi (Rasmussen *et al.*, 1963) for tissue uptake studies, and a modification of the Ussing and Zerahn (1951) technique for measuring transmural unidirectional fluxes and electrical potentials (Helbock *et al.*, 1966; Martin and DeLuca, 1969; Walling and Rothman, 1969).

11.2.1.3. *Clinical techniques in man*

(a) *Balance method.* The balance method has been unquestionably the most widely used approach in studies of Ca absorption in man. The early history and the experimental details associated with balance studies in man have been adequately reviewed by Malm (1958). As in animal studies (see pp. 508–510) the balance method, when used for estimating Ca absorption, can lead to erroneous conclusions unless the endogenous component of fecal Ca is allowed for. Blau *et al.* (1954) and Bronner and Harris (1956) were the first to demonstrate this phenomenon in man. Its physiological significance has been discussed by Bronner (1964).

(b) *Other in vivo techniques.* During the past decade there have appeared several reports of a simpler method of determining relative Ca absorption in humans using a single oral dose of radiocalcium and monitoring the plasma level of radioisotope (Avioli *et al.*, 1965; Caniggia *et al.*, 1963; Curtis *et al.*, 1967; Jaworski *et al.*, 1963; Rose *et al.*, 1965; Samachson, 1963; Spencer *et al.*, 1964a and 1969). More recently, Birge *et al.* (1969) have developed a model of Ca absorption which enabled them to subject the data obtained with this technique to kinetic analysis. The method involved a single oral administration of ^{47}Ca followed by monitoring the plasma ^{47}Ca level over the next 8 hr. One to two weeks later an intravenous dose of ^{47}Ca was administered and similarly monitored. Kinetic analysis and comparison of the plasma ^{47}Ca responses to the two routes within the context of their model enabled the authors to make physiological interpretation of the data both in the normal and diseased individual.

Wensel *et al.* (1969) have used a different approach to the study of Ca absorption in the human gut. The small intestine was directly intubated and perfused using a triple-lumen polyvinyl tube. The perfusate (10 ml/min) emerged from the proximal lumen and was continuously sampled via the second and third lumens located 10 and 60 cm respectively and distally below the point of infusion. Polyethylene glycol (see pp. 510–511) was used to measure water movement.

11.2.2. MECHANISMS OF CALCIUM ABSORPTION

In this section it is intended to point out the various possible mechanisms which have been proposed as contributing to the absorption of Ca from the intestine. Some of the mechanisms, such as active transport, are well substantiated. Others, such as the existence and contribution of a Ca-activated adenosinetriphosphatase (CaATPase), are more controversial. It is not intended to take a stand at this point on the importance of a particular mechanism; this will depend on the circumstances (species, intestinal site, age, physiological and pharmacological factors) and will be discussed in later sections. But it is hoped that a brief description of the individual mechanisms will serve as an introduction to the terminology, the techniques used in the study of a certain mechanism, and to the evidence for the existence of that mechanism.

In considering the mechanisms of transport of Ca from the intestinal lumen to plasma it should be remembered that the barrier through which Ca has to cross is not a simple, unicellular, anatomical membrane, but may consist of several layers of tissues. *In vivo*, blood vessels are found close to the basement membrane so that the ion being transported must pass at least through the epithelial cells, basement membrane, lamina propria, and the vascular endothelium. Certain *in vitro* preparations, such as the everted gut sac, exaggerate this barrier by requiring the ion to be translocated through additional layers of tissue (muscularis mucosa, submucosa, circular and longitudinal muscle, and the serosa). Experiments in which the mucosal layer is stripped off and studied as such *in vitro* have been described (Berger, 1963; Crane and Mandelstam, 1960); the technique has not been applied to Ca transport studies.

It is possible that, from kinetic and functional aspects, the barrier might under certain circumstances take the form of a simple unicellular layer, the other layers not being rate-limiting. It is usually assumed that the epithelial cells of the mucosal membrane are rate-limiting and therefore form the barrier of most interest in Ca transport studies. It is in this tissue layer that drugs, active in controlling Ca transport such as vitamin D or its metabolites, are thought to act. Although this concept is reasonable in the light of current knowledge, there is little direct evidence in its support. There is even less evidence to allow conclusions as to where, in what is presumably a polarized unit, certain mechanisms are located in the epithelial cell. We do know that the cell is polarized anatomically (microvillar surface *versus* basal surface without microvilli) and therefore assume that certain functions such as active transport are polarized. A discussion of the cellular and subcellular structures and their possible relationship to Ca transport may be found elsewhere (Wasserman and Taylor, 1969).

11.2.2.1. *Active transport*

(a) *Active transport: theoretical aspects.* Active transport in simplest terms is defined as movement against an electrochemical gradient, a process which requires work or energy input. This gradient consists of two components, electrical and chemical. The electrical part is the potential difference across the barrier or membrane and could either enhance or oppose cation transport depending upon which side of the barrier is electrically negative. The chemical component is the chemical concentration, or more correctly the *activity*, gradient existing across the barrier. These two components are related to each other according to the Nernst equation:

$$E = \frac{RT}{nF} \mathrm{In} \frac{a_1}{a_2}$$

TABLE 3. TRANSMURAL POTENTIAL DIFFERENCES IN SMALL INTESTINES OF VARIOUS SPECIES *in vivo* AND *in vitro*

Species	Site	Technique	Potential difference [a] mean or range	Investigators
Rat	Duodenum	*In vitro* (Ussing) [b]	**+3.0 to +4.5**	Helbock *et al.* (1966)
Rat	Duodenum	*In vitro* (Ussing) [b]	+1.3	Martin and DeLuca (1969b)
Rat	Duodenum	*In vitro* (Ussing) [b]	+5.2	Walling and Rothman (1969)
Rat	Duodenum	*In vivo* ligated loop	+8.1	Wasserman *et al.* (1961)
Rat	Duodenum	*In vitro* everted sac	+4.9	Noble and Matty (1967)
Rat	Jejunum	*In vitro* everted sac	+9.5	Noble and Matty (1967)
Rat	Ileum	*In vitro* everted sac	+4.4	Noble and Matty (1967)
Rat	Colon	*In vitro* everted sac	+7.2	Harrison and Harrison (1969)
Rabbit	Duodenum	*In vitro* membrane	+3.0	Wasserman and Taylor (1969)
Chicken	Duodenum	*In vivo* ligated loop	+6.1	Wasserman and Kallfelz (1962)
Sheep	Duodenum	*In vivo* Thiry–Vella loop	+14.0	Scott (1965)
Sheep	Upper jejunum	*In vivo* Thiry–Vella loop	+13.0	Scott (1965)
Sheep	Lower jejunum	*In vivo* Thiry–Vella loop	**+7.5**	Scott (1965)
Sheep	Ileum	*In vivo* Thiry–Vella loop	**+7.6**	Scott (1965)

[a] + sign indicates that the serosa is positive with respect to mucosa.
[b] Short-circuit apparatus of Ussing and Zerahn (1951).

where E = potential difference; R = gas constant; T = absolute temperature; n = valence of ion; F = Faraday; a_1 and a_2 are the *activities** (concentrations) of the ion on either side of the barrier. The *in vivo* potential difference between the intestinal lumen and the blood is normally positive with respect to the lumen and is between 5 and 40 mV depending upon the site and species (Scott, 1965; Wilson, 1962). This means that with no active transport one would anticipate the ratio of the *activities* (blood/lumen) of a cation to be less than 1.0 under steady state conditions. A qualitatively and quantitatively similar potential difference exists *in vitro*. Table 3 summarizes some *in vitro* and *in vivo* bioelectric data taken from the Ca transport literature (Harrison and Harrison, 1969; Helbock *et al.*, 1966; Martin and DeLuca, 1969b; Noble and Matty, 1967; Scott, 1965; Walling and Rothman, 1969; Wasserman and Kallfelz, 1962; Wasserman and Taylor, 1969; Wasserman *et al.*, 1961). All these reports indicate that the serosa is positive with respect to the mucosa, a situation which opposes cation transport. Martin and DeLuca (1969b) calculate from their observed potential difference (1.3 mV) that a flux ratio (mucosal to serosal/serosal to mucosal) of not more than 0.9 would be expected in the absence of active transport; Walling and Rothman (1969) suggested a value of 0.68. These values are consistent with the observation that, under conditions which inhibit active transport (anaerobiosis or metabolic inhibitors), the serosal/mucosal ratios often drop to values of 0.7 to 0.9 (Schachter and Rosen, 1959; Wasserman, 1960) (Table 2).

As a first approximation the electrical component is usually ignored and the total Ca concentration is normally equated with the *activity*. Under these circumstances an equilibrium concentration ratio (serosal mucosal) of 1.0 is assumed to represent no active transport; values significantly greater than 1.0 indicate an energy-dependent transport system or, more colloquially, a Ca pump.

A more precise approach to the problem of demonstrating active transport is to use flux ratio analysis (Koefoed-Johnsen and Ussing, 1960; Ussing, 1949), an approach which has had considerable application in studies of Ca transport by the gut (Dumont *et al.*, 1960; Helbock *et al.*, 1966; Krawitt and Schedl, 1968; Noble and Matty, 1967; Walling and Rothman, 1969; Wasserman and Taylor, 1969). One advantage of this approach is that it is applicable to both the *in vitro* and *in vivo* situation. This method involves a comparison between the *observed* flux ratios (lumen to plasma/plasma to lumen) and the *theoretical* flux

*The thermodynamic term, *activity*, is synonymous with the *ionic* Ca concentration, but may be equal to, or less than, the total Ca concentration.

ratios calculated from the known chemical and electrical gradients (ignoring solvent drag) as described by Koefoed-Johnsen and Ussing (1960). If the observed ratio equals the theoretical flux ratio, then only passive transport is involved. If the observed is significantly larger than the theoretical then active transport is partly or wholly involved.

(b) *Active transport: experimental aspects.* In 1959 the existence of a Ca pump in the intestine was first demonstrated *in vitro* by Schachter and Rosen (1959) in both the rat and the rabbit. The evidence was clear-cut (Table 2). First the concentration ratio (serosal/mucosal) was always greater than 1.0 (3.7–7.2) in the absence of metabolic inhibitors. In the presence of the latter the ratio was reduced towards 1.0 or below. This initial demonstration of active Ca transport has been amply confirmed in rats using: (1) the everted gut sac technique (Blunt *et al.*, 1968a; Dowdle *et al.*, 1960; Finkelstein and Schachter, 1962; Gruson *et al.*, 1970; Harrison and Harrison, 1969; Kessner and Epstein, 1966; Kimberg *et al.*, 1961; Lifshitz *et al.*, 1969; Martin and DeLuca, 1969a; Noble and Matty, 1967; Pento, 1970; Pento and Kenny, 1970; Rasmussen, 1959; Schachter *et al.*, 1960a, 1966, 1970; Urban and Schedl, 1969, 1970; Wasserman, 1960; Wasserman and Taylor, 1963a); (2) an open everted gut sac preparation (Morehead and Kessner, 1969); and (3) the Ussing and Zerahn (1951) method (Walling and Rothman, 1969). Active transport of Ca has been shown by Schachter and his colleagues to be present also in the intestine of the rabbit, guinea pig and mouse (Schachter, 1963), as well as the hamster (Schachter, 1963; Schachter *et al.*, 1970).

The *in vivo* evidence for active transport in the rat has been well summarized by Wasserman and Taylor (1969). The positive evidence is largely that reported by Wasserman *et al.* (1969) and by Krawitt and Schedl (1968). These groups used an acute *in vivo* perfusion technique (see pp. 520 and 521), measured unidirectional fluxes in all segments of the small intestine, and determined the observed flux ratios. Wasserman *et al.* (1961), from a knowledge of the luminal and plasma Ca *Activities* and the potential difference, calculated the theoretical flux ratios and compared them with the observed values. Over a luminal Ca concentration range of 0.3–1.97 mM the *observed* flux ratio values were approximately ten-fold the *theoretical* ratios, which was interpreted as evidence for active transport. Krawitt and Schedl (1968) made no bioelectric measurements but found that, even when the perfusion fluid Ca concentration (0.4 or 0.85 mM) was kept below the plasma ionic Ca level (1 mM or above), there was still a net flux of Ca from the lumen to the plasma. In view of the fact that the plasma is always electrically positive with respect to the lumen (Table 3) and that the concentration ratio (lumen/plasma) was kept below 1.0, Krawitt and Schedl can claim that this net flux was observed in the face of an opposing electrochemical gradient, or in other words that active transport was involved.

The negative evidence in the rat is represented by the work of Helbock *et al.* (1966) and of Dumont *et al.* (1960). The work of the former group is impressive. They used several approaches including the Ussing short-circuit apparatus. Although they demonstrated active Na transport in a 400-g male rat duodenum, they were unable to find any evidence for active transport of Ca in the same preparation. The negative findings of Dumont *et al.* (1960) in 300–400-g male rats also cannot be ignored, although the intestinal segment (mainly ileal) used is not considered the best for demonstrating active transport of Ca (Kimberg *et al.*, 1961). Both these studies (Helbock *et al.*, 1966; Dumont *et al.*, 1960) used heavy rats. The age of the rats cannot be estimated with any degree of accuracy from weight data alone—they could have been any age after 6 months—but it is possible that very old rats were used and that the active transport mechanism had degenerated. Schachter *et al.* (1960a) found that active transport, as determined with the *in vitro* gut sac technique, decreased with age, but they still observed significant active transport in 400–500-g male rats over 12 months of age. Walling and Rothman (1969) reported similar findings. However, more recently Schachter *et al.* (1970) used a Ca-specific electrode in conjunction with the everted duodenal sac preparation and found no evidence of active transport in rats over 500 g. In view of the overwhelming *in vitro* evidence and of the existence of positive *in vivo* evidence, and in spite of the two reports to the contrary, the author feels that the existence of an active process for the transport of Ca in the rat's upper small intestine can be accepted as an established fact.

The existence of active transport of Ca in chicken intestine is less certain. Hurwitz *et al.* (1967) were unable to demonstrate it *in vitro* in any part of the small intestine under normal circumstances; only in a low Na medium did the ileum indicate an energy-dependent system. Norman and his associates on the other hand have reported finding it in the ileum (Adams *et al.*, 1969). Wasserman and Kallfelz (1962) used an *in vivo* acute perfusion technique and found, at luminal Ca concentrations of 5.2 mM and less, flux ratios (lumen to plasma/plasma to lumen) which were always greater than the theoretical flux ratios calculated with the equation of Ussing (1949). These data were interpreted as indicating an active process. The presence of an active transport mechanism for

Ca in the sheep is still controversial (Care and van't Klooster, 1965; Phillipson and Storry, 1965; Scott, 1965). The data of Wensel *et al.* (1969) would suggest the presence of an active transport system in the human proximal small intestine.

(c) *Active transport: saturation kinetics.* Wasserman and Taylor (1969) and Walling and Rothman (1969) have pleaded a case for the existence of an active transport system which becomes saturated at intestinal

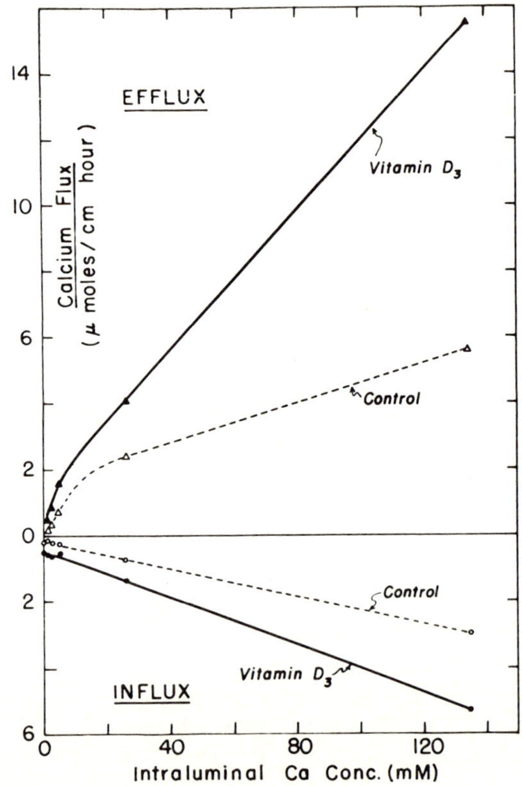

FIG. 1. Effect of vitamin D_3 and intraluminal Ca concentration on the unidirectional fluxes of Ca across the chick duodenum. Radiocalcium (^{47}Ca) was placed in the ligated duodenum for 10 min for efflux (lumen to plasma) determinations. Net flux was determined from ^{40}Ca movement; influx (plasma to lumen) was derived by difference. Note change in slope of efflux at low intraluminal Ca concentrations as active transport system became saturated. There was no evidence of a further change in slope, indicating that the passive transport system did not become saturated. The control chicks were vitamin D-deficient; the treated birds received vitamin D_3 (500 i.u. orally) 24 hr before the experiment. (From Wasserman and Kallfelz, 1962.)

luminal concentrations of around 3–5 mM Ca. Wasserman's case is based largely on his earlier work (Wasserman and Kallfelz, 1962) using an *in vivo* preparation (injection into an isolated loop) in the chicken. There appears to be no question that, as the intraluminal concentration of Ca is increased, the efflux (lumen to plasma) changes rather abruptly from a faster to a slower flux around 5 mM (Fig. 1). This was interpreted as indicating that one process had become saturated and that this process was active transport. The latter conclusion is based on the fact that at the lower luminal Ca concentrations (1.3–5.2 mM) the observed flux ratios (lumen to plasma/plasma to lumen) were always greater than the theoretical flux ratios which would pertain in the absence of an active process. The authors note that the point where one process becomes saturated (around 5 mM) is also the point at which the electrochemical gradient becomes theoretically zero. In other words, at luminal Ca concentrations greatly above 5 mM, transport would occur passively by a downhill process. However, no saturation of the downhill process was observed even with intraluminal Ca concentrations as high as 135 mM. Walling and Rothman (1969) have confirmed these findings in the rat duodenum: active transport became saturated at 3 mM whereas passive transport did not become saturated with Ca concentrations up to 12.5 mM. In humans Wensel *et al.* (1969) found no evidence of saturation in the proximal small intestine but the highest luminal Ca concentration used was only around 4 mM.

11.2.2.2. *Passive transport*

The transport of an ion across a membrane is considered completely passive if its movements can be explained entirely and quantitatively in terms of physical forces such as chemical (concentration or *activity*) gradient, electrical gradient, solvent drag, or any combination of these forces. It is to be expected as a first approximation that the concentration or *activity* ratio (serosal/mucosal) will equal unity or less at equilibrium, or approach unity with time in a non-equilibrium situation. A more precise approach is that of measuring flux ratios as discussed above (pp. 515–518).

The mechanism or mechanisms of passive transport of Ca across the gut are unknown. Two major possibilities exist: simple diffusion or facilitated (carrier-mediated) diffusion. Functionally these would express themselves as either a non-saturable or a saturable system respectively. Using the balance approach in rats Bronner and his associates (Bronner, 1969; Bronner and Aubert, 1965; Sammon *et al.*, 1970) found that, as the Ca intake (v_i) was increased, the true Ca absorption (v_a) tended to plateau (Table 1*); they suggested the mathematical relationship: $v_a = 84.0\ (1 - e^{-0.011 v_i})$. These data can be interpreted as indicating that the "downhill" transport system becomes saturated as v_i is increased. In contradiction acute *in vivo* preparations have failed to show any saturation of the Ca efflux (lumen to plasma) with intraluminal concentrations as high as 25 mM in the rat (Dumont *et al.*, 1960) or 135 mM in the chicken (Wasserman and Kallfelz, 1962). On the other hand, chronic *in vivo* preparations (Thiry–Vella loop) exhibited saturation at 12.5 mM in the dog (Cramer and Dueck, 1962) and around 40 mM in the sheep (Care and van't Klooster, 1965). Whether these different findings (saturable in dog and sheep; non-saturable in rat and chicken) have their origins in the differences between the species or in the difference between the preparations (acute *versus* chronic) is uncertain.

11.2.2.3. *Sites of absorption*

In a discussion of the sites of absorption of Ca in the gut several aspects require consideration. These include: (1) the existence of active transport and its importance relative to passive transport in the particular segment; (2) the time of passage through the segment; (3) the Ca concentration of the gut contents which obviously changes as it passes down the intestine; (4) the chemical state of the Ca as it is influenced by changes in pH and the addition of secretory products (e.g. bile); and finally (5) where the bulk of the Ca is absorbed which is a composite of the preceding factors. Much is known about the existence and location of active transport, particularly in the rat. There is some knowledge about where the bulk of the Ca is absorbed. Little information exists with regard to the other parameters.

(a) *Sites of absorption: rodents.* Active transport of Ca has been studied in all major segments of the gut in the rat from duodenum to the colon (Harrison and Harrison, 1969; Kimberg *et al.*, 1961; Krawitt and Schedl, 1968; Schachter *et al.*, 1960a, 1966; Urban and Schedl, 1969; Wasserman, 1960). It is exhibited by the duodenum to the greatest extent and decreases as the distance from the pylorus increases (Kimberg *et al.*, 1961). These findings are in accord with those of Waldron-Edward *et al.* (1966) who observed absorption in all segments but to the greatest extent in the proximal areas; these studies utilizing the *in vivo* ligated

*Here and subsequently the terminology of Aubert *et al.* (1963) is used to denote: v_i, Ca intake; v_a, true Ca absorption; v_f, endogenous fecal Ca; v_F, total fecal Ca; v_o, bone resorption; and α, fractional absorption (v_a/v_i).

loop techniques did not differentiate between active and passive transport. Some authors find little or no active transport in the jejunum and ileum in rats on a normal diet (Kimberg *et al.*, 1961; Schachter, 1963; Schachter *et al.*, 1960a, 1966; Williams *et al.*, 1961, 1962), but were able to demonstrate it in all segments of the small intestine in Ca-deprived rats (Kimberg *et al.*, 1961). Others have been able to demonstrate its existence under normal conditions in all segments of the small intestine (Krawitt and Schedl, 1968; Wasserman, 1960) as well as in the colon (Harrison and Harrison, 1969). The latter observation is interesting in the light of the finding of Kimberg *et al.* (1961) that active transport begins to increase again in the distal ileal region as the contents approach the colon.

A similar situation exists in the rabbit, mouse, and guinea pig; transport decreases as the distance from the pylorus increases (Schachter, 1963; Schachter and Rosen, 1959). Among the rodents studied to date, the hamster and the newborn rat are exceptions; active transport is greatest in the ileum in the hamster (Schachter *et al.*, 1970) and is more evenly distributed in the newborn rat (Batt and Schachter, 1969).

(b) *Sites of absorption: dogs.* Cramer (1965), using Thiry–Vella loops in dogs, found that the greatest rate of Ca absorption was in the duodenum (0.35 mg Ca/cm). The rates in the jejunum and ileum (0.2 mg Ca/cm) were only 57% of the duodenal rate. However, when other factors, such as length of segment and the amount of dietary Ca found in the segment, are considered, the *bulk* of the Ca is estimated to be absorbed in the ileum. These experiments were not designed to determine the role of active transport.

(c) *Sites of absorption: sheep.* The sheep appears to be different from other mammalian species in that secretion of Ca into the gut (plasma to lumen flux) often outweighs the translocation from the gut (lumen to plasma flux). Phillipson and Storry (1965) could not demonstrate net absorption in either the duodenum or the ileum using Thiry–Vella loops with re-entrant cannulae (see pp. 518–521). Net absorption did occur in the upper jejunum and the middle of the small intestine even at intraluminal Ca concentrations as low as 1.9 mM. In those areas of the intestine where they could not find net absorption (duodenum and lower ileum) the highest Ca concentration used was 10.5 mM. Care and van't Klooster (1965), on the other hand, found net absorption of Ca in the ileum at intraluminal Ca concentrations of 10 mM and above; in agreement with Phillipson and Storry (1965) they observed a net secretion at levels below 10 mM.

(d) *Sites of absorption: chickens.* Active transport has been demonstrated in both the duodenum (Wasserman and Kallfelz, 1962) and the ileum (Adams *et al.*, 1969). There is disagreement on the most effective site of Ca absorption in the chicken. Wasserman (1962) and Harmeyer and DeLuca (1969) found the duodenum to have the highest rate of absorption. Others (Holdsworth, 1965; Hurwitz and Bar, 1965, 1966a; Sallis and Holdsworth, 1962a; Webling and Holdsworth, 1965) are not in accord with this observation.

(e) *Sites of absorption: humans.* Two reports in this area have appeared recently (Birge *et al.*, 1969; Wensel *et al.*, 1969) using two different techniques (see pp. 513–514). Both studies found that in normal human subjects Ca absorption occurred at a much greater rate in the proximal small intestine.

11.2.2.4. *Calcium-binding protein (CaBP)*

Earlier evidence (Taylor and Wasserman, 1965; Wasserman and Taylor, 1963b) led Wasserman and his associates to report the existence of a protein in chicken intestinal tissue which preferentially bound Ca (Wasserman and Taylor, 1966) and which was increased by vitamin D treatment. Subsequently, Ca-binding protein (CaBP) from chick intestine has been purified (Wasserman *et al.*, 1968; Wasserman and Taylor, 1969); its chemical properties are summarized in Table 4. It binds to Ca about 100 times more strongly than does citrate (1:1 complex). CaBP has been shown to be present in the gut and kidney (Taylor and Wasserman, 1967) and in the shell gland (Corradino *et al.*, 1968) of the chicken, all sites of Ca transport. It has not been found in muscle, liver, blood, or bone (Wasserman and Taylor, 1969). Intestinal tissue of the rat (Kallfelz *et al.*, 1967), dog and monkey (Taylor *et al.*, 1968) and calf (Wasserman and Taylor, 1969) contains CaBP as well as the chicken, indicating that its species distribution is fairly wide. Taylor and Wasserman (1970a) used an immunofluorescent technique to demonstrate that CaBP was

TABLE 4. CHEMICAL PROPERTIES OF CALCIUM–BINDING PROTEIN (CaBP)[a]

Molecular weight	25,000–28,000
Sedimentation coefficient (S_{20})	2.96 S
Formation constants:	
Ca	2.6×10^5 M^{-1}
Sr	3.9×10^4 M^{-1}
Ba	5.8×10^3 M^{-1}
Binding capacity	1 mole Ca/mole protein

[a] From Wasserman *et al.* (1968).

located in the goblet cells and the microvillar area of the intestinal epithelial cells. Although most of the work concerning CaBP has originated from the laboratory of its discovery it is important to note that its existence has been confirmed by others in the chicken (Hamilton and Holdsworth, 1969; Harmeyer and DeLuca, 1969; MacGregor *et al.*, 1970) and in the rat (Avioli *et al.*, 1969a; Harmeyer and DeLuca, 1969; Pento and Kenny, unpublished; Schachter *et al.*, 1967).

Its physiological importance is based on the findings that wherever or whenever Ca transport in the gut is modified, the level of CaBP is changed in the same direction. This observation applied to: (1) its location in the gut* (duodenum>jejunum>ileum; Taylor and Wasserman, 1967); (2) its response to dietary Ca intake (Morrissey and Wasserman, 1970; Taylor and Wasserman, 1969; Wasserman and Taylor, 1968, 1969); (3) its response to vitamin D (Ebel *et al.*, 1969; Wasserman and

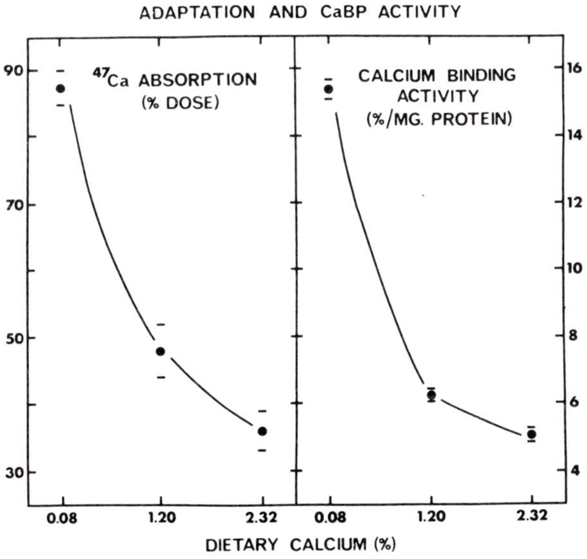

FIG. 2. Comparison of Ca absorptive capacity and CaBP content of the duodenum in chicks adapted to varying levels of dietary Ca. Radiocalcium (^{47}Ca) absorption was determined with the ligated loop technique and CaBP activity was determined by the Chelex resin method. (From Taylor and Wasserman, 1969.)

*Schachter *et al.* (1967 and 1970) report an exception to this correlation in the hamster; whereas the CaBP levels are highest in the duodenum the active transport mechanism is optimal in the ileum.

Taylor, 1966, 1968); (4) its response to actinomycin D (Corradino and Wasserman, 1968); (5) its relationship to age and egg-laying (Wasserman and Taylor, 1968, 1969); and (6) its relationship to uremia (Avioli *et al.*, 1969a) and to strontium toxicity (Corradino and Wasserman, 1970). The correlation between the binding affinity of CaBP for the alkaline earths (Ca > Sr > Ba > Mg) and the relative absorption of these ions is also impressive (Taylor and Wasserman, 1969). Figure 2 presents data taken from Wasserman *et al.* (1969), indicating the response of CaBP to dietary Ca intake and its relationship to Ca absorption.

All the above correlations may be coincidental and may not represent a causative relationship. At least two criticisms may be aimed at the concept. A minor one concerns the inefficiency of the binding process,

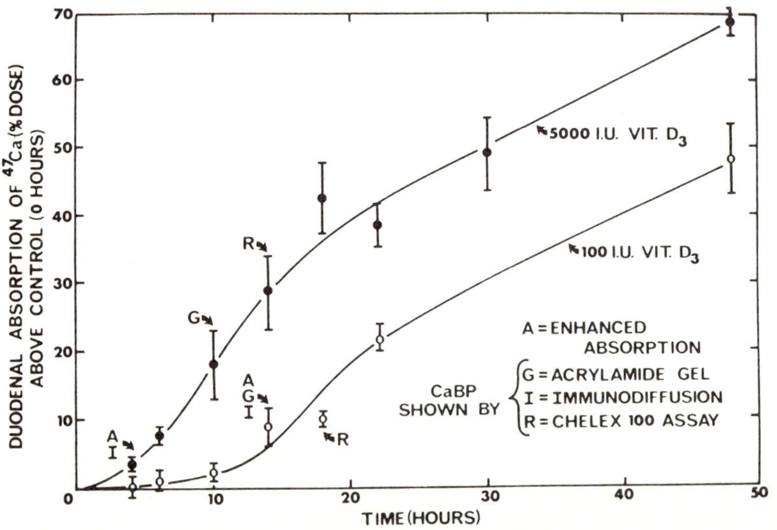

FIG. 3. Effect of vitamin D_3 at 0–48 hr after dosing and at doses of 10^2 and 5×10^3 i.u. on duodenal absorption of ^{47}Ca by rachitic chicks and the correlation of absorption with the appearance of CaBP as indicated by the Chelex resin assay, acrylamide gel electrophoresis, and immunodiffusion techniques. Absorption of ^{47}Ca was measured from a ligated duodenal loop by determining the ^{47}Ca remaining in the loop after 30 min and subtracting from the initial dose. Time after dosing at which the first *significant* increase in absorptive capacity at either 10^2 or 5×10^3 i.u. of vitamin D_3 was seen is indicated by A. Times after dosing at which CaBP was first detected and the method used are indicated by G (acrylamide gel electrophoresis), I (immunodiffusion), and R (Chelex 100 Ca-binding assay). Each point represents the group mean of five or six chicks ± standard error of the mean. Note the *simultaneous* appearance of A and I at first point. (From Ebel *et al.*, 1969.)

that is only one mole of Ca (40 parts) binds to each mole (25,000 parts) of CaBP. The major criticism is the time relationship between enhancement of Ca absorption and of CaBP levels following administration of vitamin D or its active metabolite, 25-hydroxycholecalciferol (25-(OH)-D_3). If increased CaBP levels cause enhanced absorption of Ca, then the former should be detectable before or at least simultaneously with the latter. DeLuca and his associates claim that they have never been able to observe this; enhanced Ca absorption is always detectable *before* an increase in CaBP levels (DeLuca, 1969b; Harmeyer and DeLuca, 1969), a phenomenon which also existed in the earlier work from Wasserman's laboratory (Wasserman and Taylor, 1966). Wasserman and coworkers have responded to this criticism by suggesting that the difficulty in satisfying this criterion is due to a lack of sensitivity in detecting CaBP. Recently, using more sensitive methods for detecting CaBP (immunodiffusion and gel electrophoresis rather than chelation with Chelex-100), they have been able to show an increase in CaBP levels occurring simultaneously with the enhanced Ca absorption in the chick duodenum following administration of vitamin D_3 (Ebel *et al.*, 1969; Wasserman *et al.*, 1969; Wasserman and Taylor, 1969). The data of Ebel *et al.* (1969) are presented in Fig. 3. There the matter rests at the time of writing; Harmeyer and DeLuca (1969) suggest that "CaBP therefore cannot serve as an unequivocal parameter of calcium transport", while Ebel *et al.* (1969) propose that their work "provides considerable support for the hypothesis that CaBP plays a role in calcium transport, although the nature of this role is uncertain".

11.2.2.5. *Calcium-dependent adenosine triphosphatase* (*CaATPase*)

A strong case exists for the association of certain ATPases with the phenomenon of cation transport across membranes (Skou, 1965). The association between Na-K transport and a particular Mg-dependent, Na-K-activated, ouabain-sensitive ATPase (transport-ATPase) has been delineated to the greatest extent. There have been fewer endeavors to link Ca transport with a Ca-dependent, ouabain-insensitive ATPase and much of the work has been limited to erythrocytes and skeletal muscle (Rothstein, 1968; Schatzmann, 1970; Wasserman and Kallfelz, 1970).

Attempts to link gut transport of Ca to a CaATPase have been reported from three laboratories. The first reports came from DeLuca and his associates (DeLuca, 1969b, c; Martin *et al.*, 1969; Melancon, 1970; Melancon and DeLuca, 1970) who claimed that a CaATPase was present in the proximal small intestine of both the chicken and the rat, and that the levels of intestinal CaATPase were increased by administration of vitamin D_3. These findings have been confirmed in the chicken in a preliminary report from Rasmussen's laboratory (Nagode *et al.*, 1970). However, Wasserman's group has failed to show any effects on intestinal CaATPase levels in the chicken following treatments (vitamin D, low Ca diet) which increased Ca absorption, CaBP levels, and certain other enzymatic activities (Taylor and Wasserman, 1970b). The evidence marshalled by Melancon and DeLuca (1970) in support of a role for CaATPase in gut transport of Ca in the chicken is impressive. The enzyme was located in the mucosal brush border and the time-course of the increase in Ca absorption and CaATPase levels following vitamin D_3 was similar. The latter finding is in sharp contrast to the experience of DeLuca's group with the time-course of CaBP levels (DeLuca, 1969b; Harmeyer and DeLuca, 1969). An earlier study by Spirichev and Blazhevich (1966) had found that hypervitaminosis D led to inhibition of rat intestinal CaATPase.

11.2.2.6. *Physiological aspects of mechanisms*

The information to hand is too meager to make any general conclusions about the physiological aspects of the mechanisms discussed above. In spite of this, a brief commentary follows concerning two major physiological points: (1) the relative contributions of active and passive transport; and (2) the relative contributions of the various segments of the small intestine to the overall absorption of Ca. Only one species, the rat, has been studied in any depth. In this species the active transport mechanism decreases as the distance from the pylorus increases (Kimberg *et al.*, 1961), whereas the Ca concentration of the gut contents increases (Sernka and Borle, 1969). It is obvious that "downhill" transport must play a greater role as the contents pass down the gut. If to this we add the observation that the *bulk* of the Ca is absorbed in the lower rather than the upper small intestine due to differences in transit times (Cramer, 1965; Cramer and Copp, 1959; Lengemann, 1963; Marcus and Lengemann, 1962a, b), then we must conclude that under *normal* dietary conditions active transport probably plays a minor role in Ca absorption. Table 5 presents data taken from Marcus and Lengemann (1962a, b) showing estimated transit times and relative contributions of the segments to the bulk Ca absorption in the rat. In addition the observation that in the rat duodenum the active transport mechanism may become saturated at 3 mM Ca further minimizes the contribution of the "uphill" process.

TABLE 5. TRANSPORT RATE AND CALCIUM ABSORPTION IN THE RAT GASTROINTESTINAL TRACT

Segment	Transport rate[a] (cm/hr)		Transit[a] half-time (min)		Calcium absorbed[b] % of total absorbed in all segments	
	Solid[c]	Liquid[d]	Solid[c]	Liquid[d]	Solid[c]	Liquid[d]
Stomach	—	—	60	36	0	0
Duodenum (21 cm)	220	210	6	6	8	15
Jejunum, upper (21 cm)	73	70	18	18		
Jejunum, lower (21 cm)	18	55	72	24	4	23
Ileum (21 cm)	13	11	102	120	88	62

[a] Determined using ^{91}Y; from Marcus and Lengemann (1962a).
[b] From Marcus and Lengemann (1962b).
[c] Solid diet given in form of single 10-min meal of ground diet (2 g).
[d] Liquid diet, 1 ml given by gavage.

The situation might be different in a period of Ca deprivation. First it is known that the rat adapts to this stress by increasing the efficiency of its active transport system in all segments of the small intestine (Kimberg *et al.*, 1961; Wasserman, 1960). Secondly, under conditions of Ca deprivation the Ca concentration of the gut contents would probably remain below the level (3–5 mM) at which the active transport process becomes saturated. Support for this contention may be found in the work of Sernka and Borle (1969) who determined the gut content of the ultrafilterable Ca in rats on a "tolerable Ca" diet. No analytical data were reported for this diet but it was estimated to contain 0.15% Ca, a level which approaches one-tenth that of normal commercial laboratory chows (1.2% Ca) and therefore can be considered a low Ca diet. The ultrafilterable Ca increased from a value of 0.19 mM in the duodenum to a maximum of 1.1 mM in the ileum, levels significantly lower than the active transport saturation point. It is conceivable that Ca deprivation switches the active transport system from a minor to a major role.

11.2.3. GROWTH AND CALCIUM ABSORPTION

11.2.3.1. *Experimental animals*

Only two experimental species, the rat and the bovine species, have been studied in any depth.

(a) *Rats.* It has been known for decades that the efficiency of Ca absorption, expressed as per cent of the Ca intake, decreases with increasing age. These early observations were arrived at using the balance method of approach and culminated in the classical studies of Henry and Kon (1947, 1953) in the rat (Table 6). Two major developments have occurred since the early 1950s which have allowed the phenomenon to be studied more precisely and in greater depth. One development was the recognition of, and the ability to determine, the endogenous component of fecal Ca; the other was the development of the everted gut sac technique (see pp. 515–518) and its application to studies of Ca absorption. Using the balance method coupled with radiocalcium techniques for determining the endogenous component of fecal Ca, Hansard and Crowder (1957) and Lemaire (1967) have confirmed the observation of Henry and Kon (1947, 1953) that the per cent of Ca absorbed decreases with age (Table 6). Others have found that the per cent Ca absorbed increases with age (Draper, 1963; Hironaka *et al.*, 1960). More will be said concerning the second development later.

TABLE 6. GROWTH AND CALCIUM ABSORPTION IN RATS

Age (months)	Ca intake v_i (mg/day)	Ca absorbed v_a (mg/day)	Ca absorption	
			Apparent[a] (%)	True[b] (%)
Data from Henry and Kon (1953)				
1	16.4	—	95	—
3	26.0	—	92	—
6	24.7	—	53	—
9	26.7	—	21	—
12	28.4	—	16	—
15	30.3	—	15	—
18	32.2	—	14	—
24	29.6	—	10	—
Data from Hansard and Crowder (1957)				
1	28	27	93	98
3	42	24	40	57
6	65	30	28	46
11–17	80	33	22	41
24	85	20	—	24
Data from Lemaire (1967)				
4	57.0	37.8	59	62
10	68.4	31.0	35	41

[a] $(v_i - v_F)\,100/v_i$.
[b] $(v_i - v_F + v_f)\,100/v_i$ or $v_a \times 100/v_i$, where v_F = total fecal Ca.

Before discussing further the effects of age or growth on Ca absorption it would be well to sound a note of caution concerning the interpretation of the data. Absorption may be expressed in at least two ways: (1) the efficiency of absorption or in other words either the fraction (α) or the *per cent* absorbed of the intake as determined by the balance method with or without correction for the endogenous component of fecal Ca; or (2) the absolute amount absorbed (mg/day) or the v_a in the terminology of Aubert *et al.* (1963). The former is more common; neither is ideal. At a given age both are influenced by the Ca concentration in the diet and in fact have opposite relationships to the dietary Ca level. As the latter is increased the absolute intake (v_a) increases, but the per cent absorbed decreases (Table 1 and Bronner, 1969). The question to be resolved is what parameters should be used in order to make comparisons of Ca absorption at different ages? As mentioned above, the data of Hansard and Crowder (1957) suggest that Ca absorption decreases with increasing age if per cent absorption is used as the criterion (Table 6). No such conclusion can be drawn from the consideration of the v_a data, the values being 27, 24, 30, 33, and 20 mg/day, respectively, with increasing age (Table 6). On the other hand Lemaire (1967) found a decrease in both per cent absorbed and v_a with age, but he studied only two age groups (4 and 10 months). The commonly accepted fact that Ca absorption decreases with advancing age has been based in the past largely on the criterion of per cent absorption rather than absolute intake.

Within the past decade the everted gut sac technique has given information with respect to the active transport component of Ca absorption and its relationship with age, supplying a third criterion of the efficiency of Ca absorption. In some respects this measurement is ideal but its physiological importance is not known with certainty (see p. 524). The

TABLE 7. EFFECT OF AGE ON ACTIVE TRANSPORT OF CALCIUM IN RATS[a]

Age (months)	Weight (g)	Serosal/mucosal ratio [b] (mean ± SE)
1–1½	50–90	4.8 ± 0.36
2–4	150–250	3.7 ± 0.25[c]
> 12	400–500	1.9 ± 0.30[d]

[a] From Schachter *et al.* (1960a).
[b] Everted duodenal sac technique.
[c] Significantly different from 1–1½ months ($p < 0.025$).
[d] Significantly different from 1–1½ months and 2–4 months ($p < 0.001$).
SE: Standard error of the mean.

first observation that active transport in rats declines as age increases was made by Schachter *et al.* (1960a); the data are presented in Table 7. Confirmatory evidence exists in the reports of Finkelstein and Schachter (1962), Schachter *et al.* (1970) and Walling and Rothman (1969).

(b) *Bovine*. Hansard *et al.* (1954) found in cattle that the per cent Ca absorbed decreased with advancing age, being 95 % at 1 month and declining to a value of 23 % at 12–16 years.

11.2.3.2. *Man*

The picture concerning the effects of age on Ca absorption in man is less clear. Bronner (1964) has summarized much of the data available to him prior to 1964; there have been little or no data accumulated since that time. There appears to be no obvious correlation between age and per cent Ca absorption in man even though Bronner (1964) assembled data in subjects from 11 to 72 years of age. First it should be pointed out that these data are composite, having been assembled from reports not one of which studied a wide range of ages. Secondly, the experience with experimental animals indicates that the large decline in per cent absorption occurs between birth and puberty (Table 6), an age range not included by Bronner (1964) in his summary.

11.2.4. ADAPTATION TO CALCIUM DEPRIVATION

11.2.4.1. *Experimental animals*

Mammals adapt to Ca deprivation by a more efficient absorption of Ca (defined as Ca absorbed as a per cent of the intake) and thereby remain in positive balance (Kenny, 1960). This phenomenon had been well documented by the late 1950s in rats (Hansard and Plumlee, 1954; Henry and Kon, 1953; Nicolaysen, 1943 and 1956; Rottensten, 1938) and in dogs (Gershoff *et al.,* 1958). In adapted dogs Gershoff *et al.* (1958) were unable to observe a negative Ca balance even on a diet containing only 0.034 % Ca. Adapted rats also remain in satisfactory balance on 0.04 % and 0.1 % Ca diets (Nicolaysen, 1956).

The maintenance of a positive balance in the face of Ca deprivation is not necessarily indicative of increased efficiency of absorption. Other factors such as decreases in the endogenous loss of Ca in the urine and feces also contribute to this phenomenon. The problem is identifying whether or not there has been an increase in the efficiency of absorption. Put another way, the question is deciding which parameter or parameters can be accepted as representing efficiency of absorption. Balance data coupled with radiocalcium techniques can generate the two parameters: per cent absorbed and absolute amount absorbed (v_a) per day. Neither is satisfactory as discussed previously on pp. 530–532. For example, Hansard and Plumlee (1954), Bronner and Aubert (1965) and Sammon *et al.* (1970) have studied the effects of different levels of dietary Ca, ranging from 0.01% to 1.5% Ca, on various parameters generated by the balance approach. Some of the relevant data have been presented earlier in Table 1 and indicate that as the dietary Ca level is decreased the per cent absorption increases while the absolute amount absorbed (v_a) decreases. Others have shown a similar relationship between per cent absorption and dietary Ca levels both in rats (Benson *et al.*, 1969) and in laying hens (Hurwitz and Bar, 1966b, 1969). However, Shah and Draper (1966) studied three levels of dietary Ca (0.3, 0.6 and 1.2% Ca) and found the relationship to hold only at the two higher levels. Are we to conclude then on the basis of the per cent absorption data that an endogenous adaptation had occurred with a concomitant increase in the efficiency of Ca absorption? Surely such data could be interpreted in exogenous and less mysterious terms. Perhaps, as the Ca intake is increased from a low to a high level, the only events occurring are the following in roughly the order listed: (1) active transport playing a major role (see pp. 528–529); (2) active transport becoming saturated (see pp. 520–521); (3) "downhill" transport playing a major role (see pp. 528–529); and (4) "downhill" transport becoming saturated (see pp. 521–522). These events could occur with no endogenous change in the transport systems themselves. From these considerations we can only claim that balance data *per se* are confirmatory but not conclusive evidence of increased efficiency of absorption. We know from other studies that the systems themselves can undergo endogenous changes; for example, active transport decreases with age, and vitamin D enhances "downhill" transport (see p. 548). Do endogenous changes occur in the phenomenon of adaptation or is this phenomenon explicable completely in terms of the relative roles of "uphill" and "downhill" transport and their saturation kinetics?

The *in vitro* everted gut sac technique could be used to indicate an adaptation in the active component of Ca transport. In many respects, though, the ligated segment technique (see p. 511) is ideal as it reflects both the active and passive components, is not subject to exogenous influences of the dietary Ca level such as obviously affect per cent absorption or absolute amount (v_a), and can be used to identify the sites of increased efficiency of absorption. With these remarks in mind

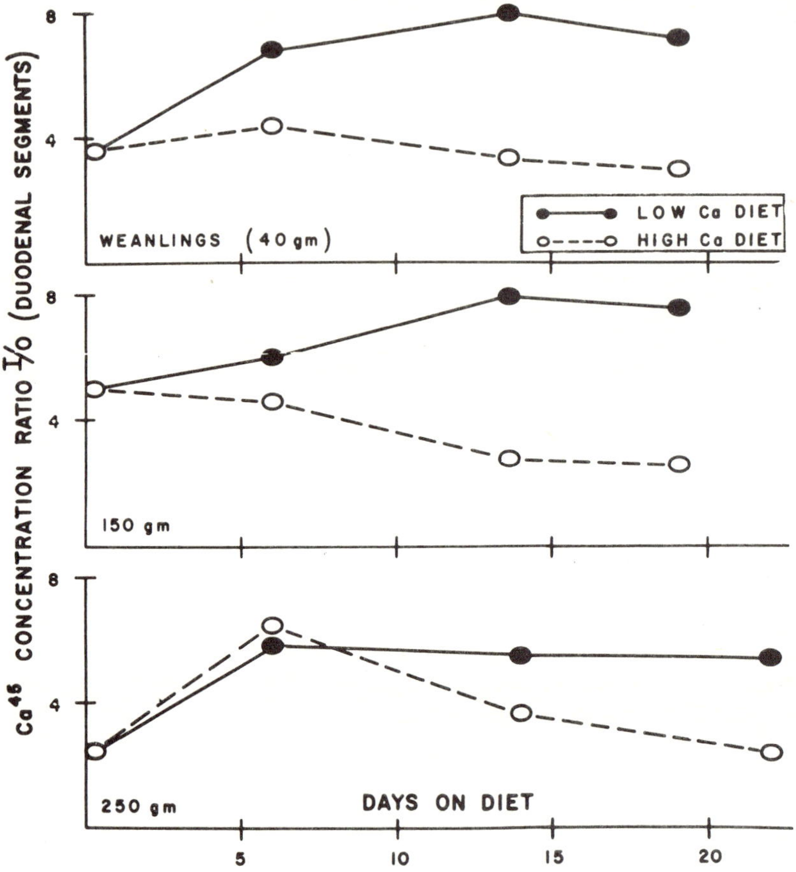

FIG. 4. Effect of age and Ca deprivation on response of the active transport system in the everted duodenal sac of the rat. The younger rats showed a more rapid adaptation to the low Ca diet; a significant response, increased I/O (serosal/mucosal) ratio, was seen within 7 days in the 40 g weanling rats. (From Kimberg *et al.*, 1961.)

let us proceed to discuss some of the more recent developments in this area, particularly those concerning the mechanisms of adaptation to Ca deprivation.

(a) *Mechanisms of adaptation: endogenous changes in the gut.* In 1960 Wasserman (1960) first demonstrated that Ca deprivation leads to an enhancement of the active transport system in rats; he used the everted gut sac preparation. This initial observation was rapidly followed by a confirmatory and more extensive report by Kimberg *et al.* (1961), from where the data presented in Fig. 4 are taken. Kimberg *et al.* (1961) reported that the increased active transport was seen in both the duodenum and the jejunum and that it was seen to a greater extent and appeared earlier (within 7 days) in younger (40 g) than in older (250 g) rats. After 14 days on a low Ca diet (0.02% Ca) the serosal/mucosal (S/M) ratios were around 8, double those obtained from rats maintained on a normal Ca diet (1.2% Ca). These initial observations have been adequately confirmed by others who have measured various parameters associated with Ca absorption: (1) S/M ratios in the *in vitro* everted gut sac preparation of the rat (Pento, 1970; Pento and Kenny, 1970; Schachter *et al.*, 1970; Wasserman, 1960); (2) Ca absorption *in vivo* from ligated duodenal and jejunal loops in rats (Pento, 1970; Pento and Kenny, 1970; Winter *et al.*, 1969); (3) Ca absorption *in vivo* from ligated duodenal loops in chickens (Morrissey and Wasserman, 1970; Taylor and Wasserman, 1969; Wasserman *et al.*, 1969); (4) *in vitro* Ca flux ratio measurements using the Ussing and Zerahn (1951) technique with rat duodenum (Walling and Rothman, 1969); and (5) CaBP determinations in chicken duodenum (Corradino and Wasserman, 1970; Morrissey and Wasserman, 1970; Taylor and Wasserman, 1969, 1970b; Wasserman *et al.*, 1969). No effect of Ca deprivation was seen on intestinal CaATPase in chickens (Taylor and Wasserman, 1970b). A selection of these data are summarized in Table 8.

It is therefore well established that Ca deprivation does lead to endogenous changes, such as in the active transport system, which can be interpreted unequivocally as increased efficiency of absorption. The repeated finding that active transport is enhanced by Ca deprivation (Kimberg *et al.*, 1961; Pento, 1970; Pento and Kenny, 1970; Schachter *et al.*, 1970; Walling and Rothman, 1969; Wasserman, 1960) is of great significance in view of the fact that in periods of Ca deprivation the active transport system probably plays a major role in Ca absorption (see pp. 528–529).

(b) *Mechanisms of adaptation: role of parathyroid hormone.* Another question demanding an answer is: what are the links in the pathway between dietary Ca level and increased efficiency of absorption? Over 25 years ago Nicolaysen (1943) proposed the existence of an "endogenous factor" which linked the body stores of Ca with intestinal absorption of Ca and required vitamin D for its action. He suggested that as the amount of skeletal Ca fell the endogenous factor was released, perhaps from bone itself, and transported to the gut where it increased the effi-

TABLE 8. EFFECT OF CALCIUM DEPRIVATION ON VARIOUS PARAMETERS ASSOCIATED WITH CALCIUM ABSORPTION

Species	Preparation	Days on diet	Parameter	Dietary calcium[a]		p	Investigators
				High	Low		
Rat	Everted duodenal sac	7	S/M	1.7	3.2	< 0.02	Wasserman (1960)
Rat	Everted duodenal sac	14	S/M	1.7	11.9	< 0.02	Pento (1970); Pento and Kenny (1970)
Rat	Ligated duodenal loop	14	% [b]	48.1	59.3	< 0.001	Pento (1970); Pento and Kenny (1970)
Chicken	Ligated duodenal loop	10	% [b]	48	87	< 0.001	Taylor and Wasserman (1969)
Rat	*In vitro* Ussing[c]	7	MS	17.1	29.9	< 0.001	Walling and Rothman (1969)
			SM	7.9	7.1	NS	
			MS/SM	2.16	4.21	< 0.001	
Chicken	Duodenum	10	CaBP	6.1	15.1	< 0.001	Taylor and Wasserman (1969)

p: probability level; NS: not significant ($p > 0.05$).
S/M: serosal/mucosal ratio.
MS: mucosal to serosal flux (nmoles/cm^2 and 10 min).
SM: serosal to mucosal flux (nmoles/cm^2 and 10 min).
CaBP: Calcium-binding protein (%/mg protein).

[a] The figures in this column represent the values of the parameters indicated in the preceding column under either high or low dietary Ca conditions.

[b] % absorption from ligated loop.

[c] Apparatus of Ussing and Zerahn (1951).

TABLE 9. EFFECT OF THYROPARATHYROIDECTOMY ON THE ADAPTIVE RESPONSE TO CALCIUM DEPRIVATION OF THE ACTIVE TRANSPORT SYSTEM FOR CALCIUM IN THE RAT [a]

Operation	Serum calcium [b] (mg/100 ml)		Serosal/mucosal ratio (mean ± SE)		*p*
	HCD	LCD	HCD	LCD	
Sham	6.9	7.4	2.9 ± 0.58	6.6 ± 0.22	<0.001
TPTX	4.4	3.5	2.6 ± 0.22	5.5 ± 0.36	<0.001

[a] From Kimberg *et al.* (1961).
[b] Median values given; see footnote * below.
HCD: high Ca diet (1.2% Ca).
LCD: low Ca diet (0.02% Ca).
SE: standard error of the mean.
p: probability level of significance between HCD and LCD responses.
TPTX: thyroparathyroidectomy.

ciency of Ca absorption. Nicolaysen's endogenous factor has yet to be identified. In 1960 Kenny (1960) and Dowdle *et al.* (1960) suggested independently that parathyroid hormone (PTH) might be Nicolaysen's endogenous factor. This concept was generated by the following facts: (1) Ca deprivation causes parathyroid gland hypertrophy (Greep, 1948) and presumably PTH release; and (2) Ca absorption is enhanced by PTH (see pp. 559–564). The following year Kimberg *et al.* (1961) produced evidence which did not support the involvement of PTH in the adaptive response to Ca deprivation; thyroparathyroidectomy (TPTX) did not abolish the adaptive response, as measured by increased S/M ratios in the everted duodenal sac in rats, to an 18-day Ca-deprivation period (Table 9). Three aspects of this study led our laboratory to re-investigate the problem 2 years ago. First the fact that Kimberg *et al.* (1961) had used TPTX rats and thus were studying the effects of three different types of hormones (PTH, iodinated thyroid hormones, and calcitonin), all of which are known to influence Ca metabolism in general, if not the gut absorption of Ca in particular. The second aspect was the fact that it did not appear that the food intake was controlled. The third aspect was the unusually low serum Ca levels which ranged from 6.4 to 7.4 mg/100 ml (3.2–3.7 mEq/l) in normal rats on a high Ca diet (1.2% Ca) as can be seen in Table 9 where the median values are given.*

Preliminary data from our laboratory have indicated that the conclusion reached by Kimberg *et al.* (1961) concerning the non-involvement of PTH

*In response to a recent inquiry Dr. Daniel V. Kimberg was kind enough to comment that he had no explanation for the unusually low serum Ca values.

in the adaptive response is not clear-cut. Pento (1970) and Pento and Kenny (1970) found that parathyroidectomy (PTX) did abolish the adaptive response to 7- and 14-day Ca deprivation. Both the *in vitro* everted duodenal sac preparation (7- and 14-day data) and the *in vivo* ligated loop technique (14-day data) were used in conjunction with quad-feeding.* Waite, Tracy and Kenny (unpublished observations), using the ligated loop technique, have continued these studies and have included a 21-day Ca deprivation period in addition to the 7- and 14-day periods. The 7-day data confirm the earlier observation of Pento and Kenny (1970), whereas the 21-day data were in agreement with the 18-day data of Kimberg *et al.* (1961). To our surprise the 14-day data did not confirm our earlier findings; PTX did not abolish the adaptive response. We are left with the conclusion that PTH is involved in the *early* part (7 days) of adaption but does not appear to play a role in *later* periods. However, the present author will not be satisfied with the latter conclusion until it has been demonstrated that accessory parathyroid tissue is not implicated. Such tissue is a common occurrence in rats (Casewell and Fennell, 1970; Van Dyke, 1959); 65% of the rats were found by Casewell and Fennell (1970) to contain ectopic parathyroid tissue in the thymus. Nevertheless if accessory tissue is invoked to explain the breakthrough of the adaptive response in PTX rats at longer time intervals, it is necessary to postulate that the gut response is more sensitive to PTH action than the blood Ca response; the blood Ca levels remain low in the PTX-low Ca diet group at 21 days. Such a postulate meets with little favor. But it is certain from the work of both Kenny (1962) and Casewell and Fennell (1970) that the accessory tissue, known to be present in the latter work and assumed to be present in the former, was unable to restore the blood Ca levels to normal following ablation of the regular parathyroid glands. Casewell and Fennell (1970) did find that PTX rats with accessory tissue in the cervical region were able to maintain slightly but significantly higher levels of serum Ca (7.9 mg/100 ml) than those with no accessory tissue (6.6 mg/100 ml). Kenny (1962) also found that rats subjected to the stress of Ca deprivation survived to a much higher degree if the stress were applied 7 days, rather than immediately after PTX; this could be interpreted as evidence for the gradual development of functional accessory tissue. Is it possible with the passage of time and with the constant hypocalcemic stimulus that sufficient PTH is released from accessory

*The term quad-feeding is used to describe the situation in which three groups of rats (intact-high Ca diet; intact-low Ca diet; and PTX-high Ca diet) are fed that quantity of diet consumed by the fourth group (PTX-low Ca diet) the previous day.

tissue to enhance Ca absorption without any gross effects on the blood Ca levels? This hypothesis is currently under study in our laboratory. Before leaving this topic it is interesting to note that Morehead and Kessner (1969) have found that PTX abolished the adaptive response (Ca absorption) following Mg deprivation.

(c) *Mechanisms of adaptation: other pathways.* Only one report has been concerned with pathways other than that involving the release of PTH in the adaptive response to Ca deprivation. Kimberg *et al.* (1961) found that in addition to TPTX, neither hypophysectomy nor adrenalectomy abolished the adaptive response, a finding that eliminates the pituitary and adrenal hormones from consideration as the endogenous factor.

A pathway which deserves more attention in the future is that involving calcitonin. Although calcitonin has not been shown to have any *acute* effects on Ca absorption (see pp. 564–565) there is evidence accumulating that the hormone may act *chronically* to suppress Ca absorption. If this proves to be so then shutting off calcitonin release would result in an increased efficiency of absorption. It is known from preliminary experiments in Japanese quail that Ca deprivation results in a fall in plasma calcitonin levels (Boelkins and Kenny, unpublished observation) as determined by bioassay using the Sephadex method of Kenny (1969). On the other hand, Tracy and Kenny (unpublished observations) have found that the adaptive response to 14-day Ca deprivation in rats can be rapidly shut down if a high Ca diet is reimposed before the end. Such a rapid shut off would appear to be inconsistent with a chronic response such as is claimed for the effect of calcitonin on gut Ca absorption.

11.2.4.2. *Man*

That man adapts to Ca deprivation by eventually going into zero or positive balance has been well documented (Malm, 1958; Nicolaysen *et al.*, 1953; Walker *et al.*, 1948). However, the evidence that this adaptive response is due to increased efficiency of absorption is incomplete. Malm (1958) notes in his studies that, when men were shifted from an intake of 940 mg Ca/day to a lower one of 463 mg Ca/day, the main change in the excretory loss occurred in the fecal Ca; there was no significant fall in urinary Ca. This was interpreted as indicating an increased efficiency of absorption. Malm assumed that the endogenous fecal loss (digestive juice Ca) remained relatively constant at a level of 750 mg Ca/day. These assumptions may be questioned. Estimates of endogenous fecal loss of Ca made with radiocalcium techniques subsequent to Malm's report indicate that the normal loss is considerably lower, ranging between 80 and 180 mg Ca/day, and that the loss is not necessarily constant (Bronner, 1964; Bronner and Harris, 1956; Bronner *et al.*, 1963; Heaney and Skillman, 1964). In fact Heaney and Skillman (1964) found that the endogenous fecal Ca (v_f) was positively correlated with the dietary Ca intake (v_i) as follows: $v_f = 0.0343v_i + 103$ (in terms of mg Ca/day). Nevertheless if we assume this relationship to be correct then the endogenous fecal Ca should be 135 mg Ca/day when the intake was 940 mg Ca/day and 118 mg Ca/day at the lower intake of 463 mg Ca/day. This fall in endogenous fecal Ca from 135 to 118, or 17 mg Ca/day, is insufficient to account for Malm's observed fall in total fecal Ca (v_f) from 338 to 266 mg Ca/day. These considerations do permit the conclusion from Malm's data that increased efficiency of absorption had occurred as a result of adaptation. Whether this response in humans is due to endogenous changes in the transport mechanisms or whether it is completely explicable in terms of the relative roles of the transport systems and their saturation kinetics (as discussed on pp. 532–539) is not known with certainty at this time. The fact that the adaptive response is not immediate but often takes time to develop favors the former, endogenous explanation. If adaptation in humans were due to the latter explanation, in which the response is dependent entirely on an exogenous factor (dietary Ca level), one would expect the adaptive response to be immediate.

11.2.5. ADAPTATION TO REPRODUCTIVE STATES

It is obvious that pregnancy must impose an increased demand for Ca on the mother, particularly during the third trimester when the bulk of the fetal Ca stores are being laid down. Species differ in this demand; on a body weight basis the relative demands are : rat > pig > bovine > human (Simkiss, 1967). The question is: from where does this extra Ca come—from the maternal bones, the diet, or both? If it comes from the diet and the dietary intake remains the same then an increased efficiency of absorption must be postulated. The same remarks would apply to other reproductive states demanding extra Ca, such as lactation and egg-laying. The discussion will concern itself mainly with the question whether or not increased efficiency of absorption results from a particular reproductive state.

11.2.5.1. *Adaptation to pregnancy*

In most species a mild hyperparathyroidism exists in pregnancy (Greep,

TABLE 10. EFFECT OF PREGNANCY AND LACTATION ON CALCIUM ABSORPTION IN RATS MAINTAINED ON A LOW OR HIGH CALCIUM INTAKE [(a)]

Period	Days of experiment	Ca intake v_i (mg/day)	Ca absorbed $v_i - v_F$ (mg/day)	Ca absorption $(v_i - v_F)100/v_i$ (%)
Low Ca diet study (0.22% Ca)				
Control	1–12	27	7.41	27
Pregnancy	14–34	27	8.1	30
Lactation	35–56	27	23.6	87
Post-lactation				
1st (4 days)	57–60	27	22.9	85
2nd (10 days)	61–70	27	22.6	84
3rd (8 days)	71–88	27	12.7	47
High Ca diet study (0.83% Ca)				
Control	1–17	100	7.9	8
Pregnancy	18–37	100	7.5	8
Lactation	38–62	100	39.2	39
Post-lactation				
1st (3 days)	63–65	100	33.9	34
2nd (3 days)	66–68	100	11.4	11
3rd (4 days)	69–72	100	8.0	8

[(a)]From Fournier and Susbielle (1952a, b); based on seven (low Ca diet) and five (high Ca diet) rats given 12 g food per day.

1948; Kenny, 1960). In some species PTH is thought to increase the efficiency of Ca absorption (see pp. 559–564). It is therefore not unreasonable to expect that pregnancy also will result in an increased efficiency of absorption. What then is the evidence for this postulated event, and is its occurrence widespread among the species? The rat and the bovine are the only species which have been adequately studied. Precise information in the human is particularly lacking in this area, presumably due to a natural reluctance to use radioisotopes which might endanger the development of the fetus.

In the rat the *in vivo* studies of Fournier and Susbielle (1952a, b) remain the definitive work in spite of the approach used (balance technique). No correction was made for the endogenous loss of fecal Ca (v_f); the work was done before the methods for determining this component of the total fecal Ca were fully developed. Hence estimates of the amount of Ca absorbed will necessarily be lower than the true value. With this reservation in mind the data of Fournier and Susbielle lead to a cautious conclusion that whether the rats were on a diet rich in Ca (0.83 %) or low in Ca (0.225 %) there was no significant increase in absorptive efficiency $\{(v_i - v_F)100/v_i\}$. All rats were fed a constant intake of 12 g of diet per day. Therefore, if it is assumed that there was no change in v_f,* it can be claimed that pregnancy in rats does not result in an increased efficiency of absorption of Ca (Table 10).

Opposed to this observation are the more recent findings of Schachter and his associates (Schachter *et al.*, 1960a, 1970). This group has shown, using the everted duodenal sac, that active transport is enhanced during the third week of gestation in rats (Table 11). Reconciliation of these apparently opposed findings is needed. The disagreement may have its origins in one or more of the following points. First, Schachter *et al.* (1960a, 1970) observed the increased active transport during the third week, but did not specify the day of gestation. Thus their observations could have been made anytime during the third week and may in fact have been close to the end of the third week. If this were so it is to be expected that the balance method, even though Fournier and Subielle (1952a, b) collected urinary and fecal samples daily, would not detect such a change until the beginning of the lactation period, when indeed a very marked increase in absorptive efficiency did occur (Table 10). Secondly, it is not necessarily predictable on the basis of present knowledge that a marked change in active transport will result in a marked change in absorptive efficiency. It will depend on the relative importance of the active and passive transport system as discussed in pp. 528–529. If, for example,

TABLE 11. ADAPTIVE RESPONSE TO PREGNANCY OF THE ACTIVE TRANSPORT SYSTEM FOR CALCIUM ABSORPTION IN THE RAT

Parameter	Serosal/mucosal ratio mean ± SE		*p*
	Non-pregnant	Pregnant	
^{45}Ca [(a)]	2.0 ± 0.38	4.6 ± 0.38	<0.001
Ionized ^{40}Ca [(b)]	1.4	2.0	<0.02

[(a)] From Schachter *et al.* (1960a).
[(b)] From Schachter *et al.* (1970).
SE: standard error of the mean.
p: probability level.

* This is a reasonable assumption as changes in v_f tend to correlate best with changes in either v_F (total fecal Ca) or v_i (Ca intake) as discussed by Bronner (1964). Presumably neither of these parameters changed in the study under discussion.

an increase in active transport was accompanied by a decrease in transit time in the gastrointestinal tract, the effect of the latter would negate that of the former. Thirdly, the lack of sensitivity of the balance method, particularly in the absence of endogenous fecal Ca determinations, may not allow detection of small but significant changes in efficiency of absorption.

Absorptive efficiency of Ca in bovine pregnancy has received little attention. The major definitive study is that of Plumlee (1953; quoted by Comar, 1956). Pregnancy had no significant effect on the efficiency of absorption as measured by the balance method coupled with radiocalcium techniques. However, Ramberg *et al.* (1970) found during the latter part of pregnancy that the intestinal absorption of Ca (v_a) is much more important quantitatively in meeting the demand for Ca than is resorption (v_{o-}) of the maternal bones.

The response of the human female with respect to Ca absorption during pregnancy has been studied only by the classical balance method with no correction for endogenous fecal loss. Simkiss (1967) has summarized balance data taken from the early work of Coons and Blunt (1930) and of Macy *et al.* (1930). In four of the five patients there was an increase in the extent of the positive balance and in the efficiency of absorption $\{(v_i - v_f)100/v_i\}$ as pregnancy progressed. However, it is difficult to draw this conclusion with any degree of conviction.

11.2.5.2. *Adaptation to lactation*

Whereas pregnancy imposes a mild strain of Ca metabolism lactation causes a much more severe stress often resulting in a prolonged period of negative Ca balance. As in pregnancy, species differ in this demand. However, perhaps of more importance in the case of lactation is the difference between individuals within a particular species; this difference can be as much as tenfold in cows (Kleiber and Luick, 1956). It is surprising how little information there is on the subject of adaptation to lactation with respect to intestinal absorption of Ca.

The only definitive study is in rats and again is the work of Fournier and Susbielle (1952a, b). In contrast to the response to pregnancy, rats responded to lactation by a marked increase in absorptive efficiency $\{(v_i - v_F)100/v_i\}$ whether the rats were on a diet rich in Ca (0.83%) or low in Ca (0.225%). On the low Ca diet the absorption of Ca increased from 30% of the intake during gestation to 87% during lactation; on the high Ca diet the figures were 8% and 39% respectively (Table 10). There is no evidence available to indicate whether or not this increase in the efficiency of absorption is due to endogenous changes in the active and passive transport systems. This point needs to be studied with the everted gut sac and ligated loop techniques.

Lactation in the bovine species has been studied recently with more precise methods using Ca kinetics and systems analysis (Mayer *et al.*, 1969; Ramberg *et al.*, 1970). It is possible to conclude from their data that the initial adaptive response to lactation is an increase in both Ca absorption (v_a) and efficiency of absorption $\{(v_a/v_i) \times 100\}$. In the data presented by Mayer *et al.* (1969) the efficiency rose from 22.6% during the 6 days immediately prior to parturition to 34% during the 8- to 14-day post-partum period. Later as lactation proceeds the gut response declines as bone resorption takes over to meet the increased demand.

Little information exists to permit acceptable conclusions with respect to adaptation to lactation in the human female. No studies with radio-calcium are readily available. All information is based on the classical balance approach. There does not seem to be any major adaptation in the form of increased efficiency of absorption of Ca. In many cases the total fecal Ca (v_F) exceeds the Ca intake (v_i), making it difficult to entertain the existence of increased efficiency (see table 10.3 in Simkiss, 1967). More precise work is badly needed in this area. This is a situation which calls for the application of the stable tracer, ^{48}Ca, which can be subsequently converted outside the body to the gamma-emitting ^{49}Ca, by neutron activation. The background for such an application lies in the rat bone studies of Conaway *et al.* (1971) and of Firschein and Miller (1966).

11.2.5.3. *Adaptation to avian reproduction*

Reproduction subjects the Ca metabolism of birds to an extraordinary stress. A hen with total Ca stores of 20 g can lay an egg containing 2 g of Ca a day 75% of the time. How does the laying hen adapt to this stress with respect to Ca absorption from the gut? There are two aspects of this question. The one concerns itself with the larger picture: non-laying days *versus* laying days. The other relates to the problem of adaptation within the egg-laying cycle, that is the interval between consecutive ovipositions.

Most hens immediately enter a state of negative balance at the start of egg production, in spite of a prompt increase in food, and therefore Ca, intake (Hurwitz and Griminger, 1960). Much of this negativity is accounted for by the loss in the egg of approximately 2 g Ca/day, an amount which often exceeds the total Ca absorbed (v_a). In the report of

Mueller *et al.* (1964) the v_a equalled 1.81 g Ca/day on a laying day; this value was only 3% higher than the mean value (1.76 g Ca/day) for a non-laying day. Thus it seems that the hen does not adapt to egg production by increasing its absorptive efficiency to any great extent, assuming in these studies that Ca intake remained unchanged.

Hurwitz and Bar (1969) studied the interval between ovipositions and obtained results which are not easy to reconcile with those of Mueller *et al.* (1964). Hurwitz and Bar (1969) measured absorptive efficiency in the laying hen at three different periods during the egg-laying cycle—at the time of no shell calcification, early in the calcification period, and later in the same period. The approach used was to: (1) label uniformly two diets (1.90% and 3.56% Ca, respectively) with a non-absorbable marker, ^{91}Y; (2) feed the diets for 4 days; (3) kill the hens at each of the three periods of the egg-laying cycle; and (4) calculate the degree of Ca absorption from the Ca/^{91}Y ratios in the distal intestine. The per cent absorption increased from 40 during the no-calcification period to values between 68 and 77% during the period of calcification. The overall response was relatively independent of the dietary Ca level (1.90% *versus* 3.56%). It appears from these data that the hen responds to the stress of calcification by an increase in the efficiency of Ca absorption.

How can the data of Hurwitz and Bar (1969) and of Mueller *et al.* (1964) be reconciled? Both report the same qualitative response. It is possible that the discrepancy is due to the fact that two different experimental approaches were used. More information is needed before it can be unequivocally claimed that egg-production leads to a greatly enhanced efficiency of Ca absorption by the intestine.

11.2.6. PHARMACOLOGICAL ASPECTS OF CALCIUM ABSORPTION

11.2.6.1. *Vitamin D*

(a) *Introduction.* The first recognition of a dietary factor, which could cure experimental rickets, enhance Ca absorption from the gut, and was related to exposure to sunlight, dates back to the early 1920s in the classical studies of Mellanby, McCollum, Steenbock, and Hess, and their respective associates. Fourman *et al.* (1968) and DeLuca (1967) present an excellent review of the early history of vitamin D. Subsequently two provitamins, ergosterol and 7-dehydrocholesterol, and the active forms to which they are converted by ultraviolet irradiation, vitamin D_2 and vitamin D_3, respectively, have been identified. Vitamin D has actions on the bone and kidney, but its main physiological and pharmacological actions are on Ca absorption by the intestine.

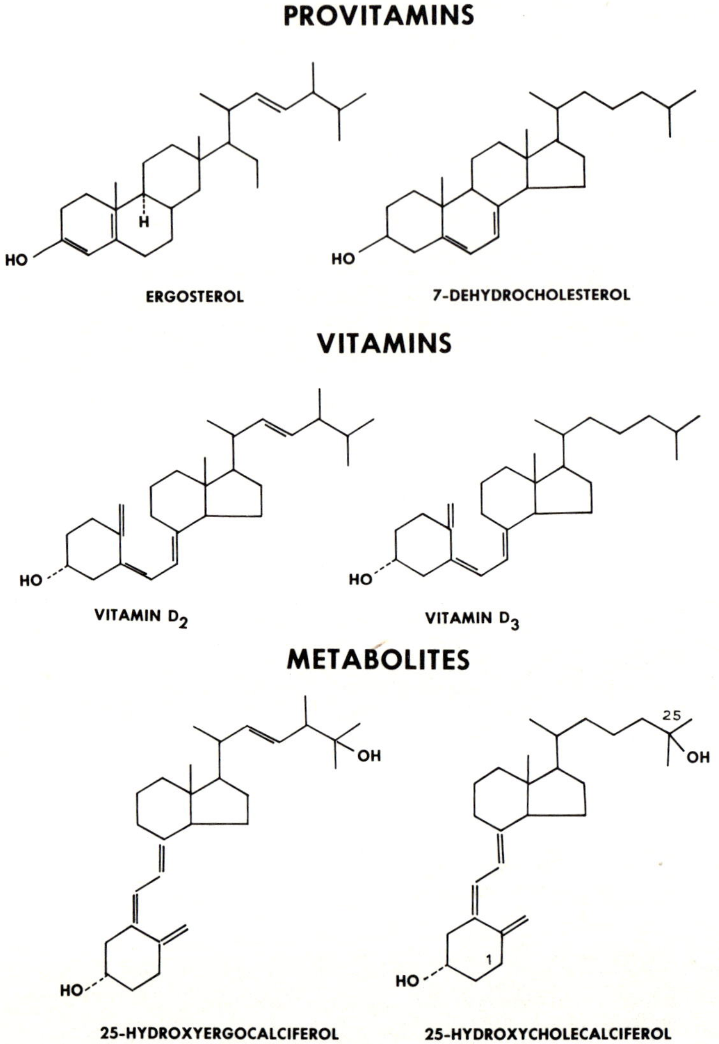

FIG. 5. Chemical structures of the provitamins (ergosterol, 7-dehydrocholesterol), vitamins (D_2 and D_3), and the active metabolites (25-hydroxyergocalciferol, 25-hydroxycholecalciferol). At present 1α,25-dihydroxycholecalciferol (1,25-$(OH)_2$-D_3) is considered to be the most active metabolite (for reference see K. Ewe, in: *Erg. inn. Med. u. Kinderhlkd.* **33:** 231, Springer, Berlin–Heidelberg–New York, 1972). The hydroxylation of 25-(OH)-D_3 to 1,25-$(OH)_2$-D_3 takes place in the kidneys (Frázer, D. R. and Kodicek, E. (1970) *Nature* **228:** 764; Gray *et al.* (1971) *Science* **172:** 1232). An important synthetic product appears to be 1α-hydroxycholecalciferol. See also author's addendum on p. 581 (Eds.).

TABLE 12. VITAMIN D TERMINOLOGY

Generic name	Source	Vitamins	Provitamins	Metabolites [a]
Vitamin D	Plants	Vitamin D_2 (Ergocalciferol) (Calciferol)	Ergosterol (Provitamin D_2)	25-Hydroxyergocal-ciferol (25-(OH)-D_2)
	Animals	Vitamin D_3 (Cholecalciferol)	7-Dehydro-cholesterol (Provitamin D_3)	25-Hydroxycholecal-ciferol (25-(OH)-D_3)

Synonyms in parentheses.
[a]Other metabolites have been indentified; these are the major active metabolites at time of writing. Cf. p. 546.

The vitamin D terminology needs some explanation. Vitamin D itself is generic, there being no particular molecule associated with the term. A compilation of the terms for the provitamins, the vitamins and their active metabolites, and the respective synonyms, is presented in Table 12. Their chemical structures are given in Fig. 5.

This is not the place to launch into a general review of the physiology and pharmacology of vitamin D. Details of its actions on bone and kidney, its therapeutic uses, its toxicity, and its dosage forms may be found elsewhere (DeLuca, 1967) and in the more comprehensive pharmacological textbooks. In the discussion which follows only recent studies on its mechanism of action on the gut and its conversion to more active metabolites will be emphasized.

(b) *Mechanism of vitamin D action.* That vitamin D is an essential factor for the optimal absorption of Ca from the gut had been solidly documented by the early 1950s when Nicolaysen and his associates reviewed the material (Nicolaysen and Eeg-Larsen, 1953; Nicolaysen *et al.*, 1953). Most of the early work was done with the classical balance approach and therefore could not supply answers to the mechanism of the essentiality of vitamin D for optimal Ca absorption. Was the action of vitamin D due to decreased excretion of endogenous fecal Ca or was it due to increased efficiency of absorption? If the latter, did it enhance active transport, passive transport, or both?

By the mid-1950s it was possible to conclude that vitamin D enhances the efficiency of absorption (Carlsson, 1954; Conrad and Hansard, 1957; Gershoff and Hegsted, 1956; Underwood *et al.*, 1951). As the vitamin will cause this effect in the absence of any change in Ca intake, we may further conclude that the increased efficiency must be due to an endogenous change in the transport systems, assuming that the vitamin has no effect on transit time. Questions to be answered are: (1) In which segment or segments of the intestine does vitamin D act? (2) Does vitamin D enhance active transport, passive transport, or both? (3) How does it influence the transport mechanisms? and (4) Which parameters play the most important role in the overall effect of the vitamin on Ca absorption? These questions will be discussed one by one.

(i) *Sites of vitamin D action:* in vivo *studies.* Vitamin D has been shown to enhance Ca absorption in all segments of the small intestine of the chicken using the *in vivo* ligated loop (Hurwitz *et al.*, 1967; Wasserman, 1962; Webling and Holdsworth, 1965). Others have reported similar findings in the duodenum (Hamilton and Holdsworth, 1969; Sallis and Holdsworth, 1962a) and in the ileum (Holdsworth, 1965; Neville and Holdsworth, 1969; Sallis and Holdsworth, 1962a) of the chicken, and in the duodenum of the rat (Urban and Schedl, 1969). The observation that the rat ileum does not respond to vitamin D (Urban and Schedl, 1969) is not in accord with the *in vivo* experiments of Harrison and Harrison (1951), nor with *in vitro* experiments described below.

(ii) *Sites of vitamin D action:* in vitro *studies.* The action of vitamin D on the intestinal transport of Ca has been much more extensively studied *in vitro*, particularly in the rat and the chicken. All segments of the rat small intestine respond to vitamin D as measured by the *in vitro* everted gut sac technique (Harrison and Harrison, 1960, 1965, 1966; Schachter *et al.*, 1961). Others have also shown *in vitro* that specific segments of the rat small intestine respond; these segments include the duodenum (Avioli *et al.*, 1969a; Blunt *et al.*, 1968a; Czarnowska-Misztal *et al.*, 1966; DeLuca, 1969b; Dowdle *et al.*, 1960; Harrison and Harrison, 1970; Kessner and Epstein, 1965; Kimberg *et al.*, 1961; Lifshitz *et al.*, 1967a, b; Martin and DeLuca, 1969a; Morii *et al.*, 1967; Schachter *et al.*, 1970; Urban and Schedl, 1969, 1970; Williams *et al.*, 1961; Zull *et al.*, 1965, 1966), the jejunum (Harrison and Harrison, 1970), and the ileum (Kimberg *et al.*, 1961). In addition, Harrison and Harrison (1969) have shown that the rat colon responds to vitamin D. A similar situation exists in the hamster and the chicken; all segments of the small intestine respond to the vitamin using *in vitro* techniques (Hurwitz *et al.*, 1967; Schachter *et al.*, 1970).

(iii) *Vitamin D and active transport.* It has been frequently demonstrated that vitamin D enhances active transport in the rat duodenum as measured by the *in vitro* gut sac technique (Avioli *et al.*, 1969a; Blunt *et al.*, 1968a; Czarnowska-Misztal *et al.*, 1966; DeLuca, 1969a; Dowdle *et al.*, 1960; Harrison and Harrison, 1966, 1969; Kessner and Epstein, 1965; Kimberg *et al.*, 1961; Lifshitz *et al.*, 1967a, b; Martin and DeLuca, 1969a; Morii *et al.*, 1967; Schachter *et al.*, 1961, 1970; Urban and Schedl, 1969, 1970; Williams *et al.*, 1961, 1962; Zull *et al.*, 1965 and 1966). The question to be resolved is whether or not this response represents a primary effect of the vitamin. This will be discussed below in this section (pp. 551–556).

(iv) *Vitamin D and passive transport.* There is a considerable body of evidence to support the concept that vitamin D enhances passive transport by increasing permeability of the mucosal cells to Ca. Two main approaches have been made: (1) the use of *in vitro* techniques under conditions (anaerobiosis, cold, and metabolic inhibitors) in which active transport is presumably inhibited; and (2) *in vivo* experiments using the flux ratio approach.

Harrison and his associates have used the former approach. In their first reports they demonstrated that vitamin D enhanced the mucosal to serosal transport in everted loops prepared from all segments of the rat intestine (Harrison and Harrison, 1960 and 1963a). This enhanced transport was seen in the presence of potassium cyanide, under anaerobiosis, and at both 5°C and 25°C incubation temperatures (Table 13). Subsequent work from the same laboratory has confirmed these findings and contributed additional observations (Harrison and Harrison, 1965, 1966, 1969, 1970; Hurwitz *et al.*, 1967). These include: (1) demonstration of the vitamin D response in the rat in the presence of *N*-ethyl maleimide which blocks active transport of Ca, Na and associated water movements (Harrison and Harrison, 1965, 1966); (2) absence of the response in rat intestinal preparations stripped of their mucosal epithelium (Harrison and Harrison, 1965); (3) presence of the response in rat colon (Harrison and Harrison, 1969); and (4) presence of the response in the chicken intestine (Hurwitz *et al.*, 1967).

The use of the flux ratio approach to demonstrate an effect of vitamin D on passive transport of Ca in both the chicken and the rat is largely attributable to Wasserman and his associates (Wasserman and Kallfelz, 1962); the data are presented in Fig. 1. The efflux (lumen to plasma) was measured by ^{47}Ca disappearance from the loop over a short time period of 10 min. The net Ca flux was determined from ^{40}Ca disappearance. The influx (plasma to lumen) was not specifically measured; it was derived

TABLE 13. EFFECT OF VITAMIN D ON PASSIVE PERMEABILITY IN ALL SEGMENTS OF THE RAT SMALL INTESTINE [a]

Conditions			Passive permeability [b]					
			Segment					
Gas phase	Temp. (°C)	Inhibitor (0.5 mM)	Proximal 1/6		Middle 3/6		Terminal 2/6	
			−D	+D	−D	+D	−D	+D
O_2	37	—	0.163	0.519	0.100	0.230	0.157	0.280
N_2	37		0.186	0.464	0.153	0.285	0.173	0.338
O_2	25		0.147	0.403	0.096	0.138	0.080	0.163
O_2	5	—	0.099	0.155	0.072	0.095	—	—
O_2	37	KCN	0.136	0.600	0.105	0.269	0.122	0.274

[a] From Harrison and Harrison (1963a).

[b] Data represent diffusion rate constants (k) in $(\text{min})^{-1}$; ^{45}Ca was placed on mucosal side of everted segment and rate of transfer to serosal side was determined, total Ca being equal on both sides. All effects of vitamin D are significant.

−D: vitamin-D-deficient rats.

+D: vitamin-D-deficient rats treated with vitamin D.

TABLE 14. EFFECT OF VITAMIN D ON CALCIUM ABSORPTION IN THE CHICKEN DUODENUM: FLUX RATIO METHOD[a]

Infused Ca (mM)	Efflux, lumen to plasma (μmoles/cm/hr)		Influx, plasma to lumen (μmoles/cm/hr)		Flux ratio (Efflux/Influx)			
					Observed[b]		Theoretical[c]	
	−D	+D	−D	+D	−D	+D	−D	+D
1.3	0.22	0.47	0.14	0.53	1.6	0.9	0.5	0.5
2.7	0.37	0.82	0.19	0.60	1.9	1.4	1.1	1.0
5.2	0.72	1.54	0.24	0.52	3.0	3.0	1.7	1.6
26	2.43	4.08	0.71	1.40	3.4	2.9	9.1	7.0
135	5.6	15.5	3.0	5.3	2.4	2.9	41.2	43.2

[a] From Wasserman and Kallfelz (1962); ^{47}Ca placed in ligated duodenum for 10 min for efflux determination; net flux was determined from ^{40}Ca movement; influx was derived by difference.

[b] Vitamin D treatment had no significant effect on observed flux ratios.

[c] Calculated from diffusion equation of Ussing (1949); the fact that the observed exceeded the theoretical flux ratios at 1.3 and 2.7 mM infused Ca was interpreted as evidence for active transport.

−D: vitamin-D-deficient chicks.

+D: vitamin-D-deficient chicks treated with vitamin D (500 i.u. orally) 24 hr prior to experiment.

from the difference between the efflux and the net flux. The most important observation was that vitamin D had no effect on the flux ratio (efflux/influx) over a range of intraluminal Ca concentrations between 1.3 and 135 mM (Table 14). Secondly the vitamin increased the individual fluxes, notably the influx (plasma to lumen). This latter point was confirmed in a subsequent publication with actual measurement of the influx (intravenous injection of ^{47}Ca) rather than by deriving it from the efflux and net flux data (Wasserman, 1963). More recently Wasserman *et al.* (1966) have measured flux ratios in the chick ileum and rat duodenum and have come to a similar conclusion: that vitamin D enhances Ca transport by increasing bi-directional permeability.

(v) *Vitamin D and calcium uptake.* There is a considerable body of evidence to indicate that a specific step in the translocation of Ca from lumen to plasma involves the uptake and concentration of Ca in mucosal tissue. This uptake phenomenon was first studied by Schachter *et al.* (1960b and 1961) *in vitro*, using slices of rat intestine; the technique was also used by Avioli (1969). Subsequent studies have employed different approaches; these include: (1) *in vitro* incubation of the everted gut sac with radiocalcium followed by analysis of either the whole tissue (Holdsworth, 1965; Martin and DeLuca, 1969a), mucosal scrapings (Holdsworth, 1965; Schachter *et al.*, 1966, 1970; Wasserman, 1963; Wasserman and Taylor, 1969), or muscle layer (Holdsworth, 1965; Schachter *et al.*, 1966, 1970); (2) *in vitro* incubation of isolated intestinal loops, either with radiocalcium (Sallis and Holdsworth, 1962a, b) or with stable Ca (Urban and Schedl, 1969), followed by analysis of the whole tissue; and (3) *in vitro* incubation of a sheet of intestinal tissue in an apparatus which permitted exposure of only the mucosal side to the fluid containing radiocalcium (Martin and DeLuca, 1969b). Different conclusions have been drawn by different groups depending upon the approach used. Some claim that this uptake phenomenon is partially energy-dependent (Martin and DeLuca, 1969b; Rasmussen *et al.*, 1963; Schachter *et al.*, 1960b, 1961). However, the energy-dependence of the uptake step has not been emphasized in more recent publications from Schachter's group (Schachter *et al.*, 1966, 1970) in which mucosal scrapings rather than whole tissue were analyzed. Figure 6 is taken from the work of Schachter *et al.* (1966) and diagrammatically represents their later

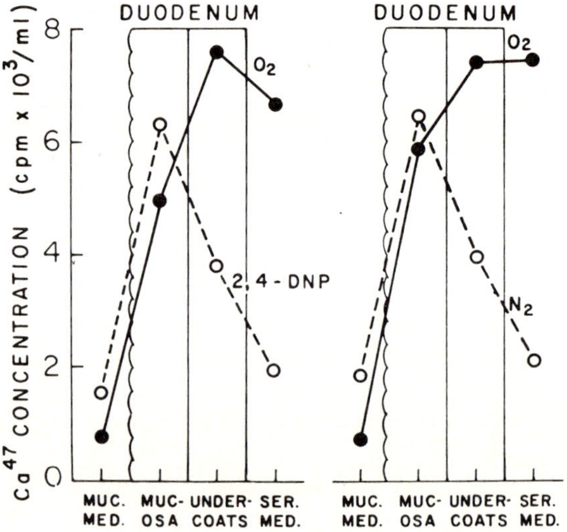

FIG. 6. Effects of incubation under N_2 or with 2,4-dinitrophenol (DNP) on ^{47}Ca gradients across duodenal sacs prepared from six 80- to 90-g rats. Half the sacs were incubated under O_2 and the remainder under N_2 for 2 hr at 37°C. Duodenal sacs were also prepared from each of twelve rats and were incubated in the presence or absence of 1 mM DNP for 2 hr at 37°C under O_2. Net movement of ^{47}Ca to the serosal surface was observed only under O_2 or in the absence of DNP. (From Schachter *et al.*, 1966.)

findings. Other investigators, who also separated mucosal epithelial uptake from whole tissue uptake, support the concept that Ca uptake by mucosal epithelium, although apparently "uphill" in terms of *total* Ca concentration, is not energy-dependent (Holdsworth, 1965; Wasserman, 1963 and 1968; Wasserman and Taylor, 1969).

Two questions immediately present themselves. Does vitamin D influence this uptake of Ca by the mucosal epithelium? and What is the chemical state of the Ca taken up by the mucosa? Most investigators agree that vitamin D enhances Ca uptake by intestinal tissue (Holdsworth, 1965; Martin and DeLuca, 1969b; Schachter *et al.*, 1960b, 1961, 1970; Wasserman, 1963, 1968; Wasserman and Taylor, 1969). These include those who isolated, and measured uptake in, mucosal epithelium following incubation of the whole tissue with radiocalcium. Only in those studies in which isolated mucosal cells were isolated first and then incubated with radiocalcium was there no effect of vitamin D on Ca uptake (Holdsworth, 1965; Rasmussen *et al.*, 1963).

With respect to the second question it is obvious that the Ca taken up by the mucosal epithelium cannot be in the ionic form. First, such concentrations would be deleterious to the integrity of the cell. Secondly, if this Ca were ionic it would have to be transported against the gradient and therefore would require energy but, as discussed above, the consensus of opinion is that the uptake process is not dependent upon energy. It may be assumed then that most of this Ca pool is chemically bound, perhaps to CaBP, which itself is increased as a result of vitamin D action (see p. 554).

(vi) *Vitamin D and protein synthesis.* That protein synthesis is a vital step in the mechanism of action of vitamin D on the intestine has been demonstrated with the aid of actinomycin D. One of the main pharmacodynamic actions of actinomycin D is to inhibit protein synthesis by preventing DNA-directed m-RNA synthesis in the nucleus. It has been repeatedly shown that this agent will inhibit the action of vitamin D on Ca absorption by the intestine of both the rat (DeLuca, 1969b; Harrison and Harrison, 1966; Moriuchi *et al.*, 1970; Schachter and Kowarski, 1965; Zull *et al.*, 1965, 1966) and the chicken (Bosmann and Chen, 1966; Corradino and Wasserman, 1968; Norman, 1965, 1966a; Norman *et al.*, 1969). Such observations only support the hypothesis that vitamin D stimulates protein synthesis in the mucosal epithelial cells as a prerequisite to enhancing Ca absorption; they by no means prove it.

However, these findings did lead to further studies aimed at proving that vitamin D or its active metabolites have a primary action on the nucleus of the intestinal mucosal cells. First it was shown that vitamin D enhanced the incorporation of ^{3}H-orotic acid into the nuclear RNA of intestinal mucosa of the rat (DeLuca, 1969b; Lawson *et al.*, 1969c; Norman, 1966a, b; Stohs *et al.*, 1967) and that actinomycin D inhibited this incorporation (Stohs *et al.*, 1967). Secondly it was observed that in both rats and chickens the nucleus of the intestinal mucosal cell is a major intracellular site of accumulation of vitamin D and its metabolites following administration of a *physiological* dose (10 i.u.) of ^{3}H-labeled vitamin D (DeLuca, 1969b; Haussler *et al.*, 1968; Haussler and Norman, 1967; Norman *et al.*, 1969; Stohs and DeLuca, 1967). Disagreement exists as to whether the nuclear accumulation is primarily on the nuclear membrane as claimed by DeLuca and his associates, or primarily on the nuclear chromatin as maintained by Norman's group. A third observation which supports the nuclear action of vitamin D is that the vitamin stimulates the template activity of chromatin prepared from rat intestinal nuclei (DeLuca, 1969b; Hallick and DeLuca, 1969). The template activity was measured by determining the incorporation of ATP into acid insoluble RNA in the presence of the chromatin and an RNA polymerase preparation from *E. coli*.

(vii) *Vitamin D and calcium binding protein* (*CaBP*). It is well established that vitamin D stimulates the formation of CaBP in the intestine of the chicken (Corradino and Wasserman, 1968, 1970; Ebel *et al.*, 1969; Harmeyer and DeLuca, 1969; MacGregor *et al.*, 1970; Taylor and Wasserman, 1967, 1969; Wasserman *et al.*, 1969; Wasserman and Taylor, 1966, 1968, 1969), of the rat (Avioli *et al.*, 1969a; Harmeyer and DeLuca, 1969; Kallfelz *et al.*, 1967), and of the dog (Taylor *et al.*, 1968). The chicken data of Ebel *et al.* (1969) are presented in Fig. 3. Actinomycin D and cycloheximide inhibit its formation in chicken intestine (Corradino and Wasserman, 1968; Wasserman and Taylor, 1969), making it a candidate for the end product of vitamin D's action on protein synthesis. The objections to this concept have been discussed above (pp. 524–527) and rest mainly on the time relationship between the administration of vitamin D and the relative appearances of the Ca-absorption response and the CaBP response.

(viii) *Vitamin D and calcium-dependent adenosine triphosphatase* (*CaATPase*). The evidence for and against the hypothesis that a CaATPase is an important endproduct of vitamin D's actions on protein synthesis in the intestine has been reviewed on pp. 527–528; nothing will be added here.

(ix) *Vitamin D and adenosine 3′,5′-cyclic monophosphate* (*CAMP*). Recently there have appeared two reports linking Ca absorption by the intestine with the second messenger system. Neville and Holdsworth (1969) noted that vitamin D increased adenyl cyclase activity in the intestine of the chicken. They further reported that the dibutyryl derivative of CAMP (DB-CAMP) increased Ca transport both *in vivo* from ligated ileal loops and *in vitro* using everted ileal sacs. In the latter experiments DB-CAMP was added *in vitro* and caused the effect only in sacs removed from rachitic chicks. Neville and Holdsworth suggested that CAMP is the second messenger through which vitamin D acts. Harrison and Harrison (1970) studied the effects of DB-CAMP on Ca absorption in a different species, the rat, and came to somewhat different conclusions. They were able to demonstrate an enhancement of passive transport of Ca by the rat duodenum but, in contrast to the experience of Neville and Holdsworth (1969) in the chicken, they observed this effect only in

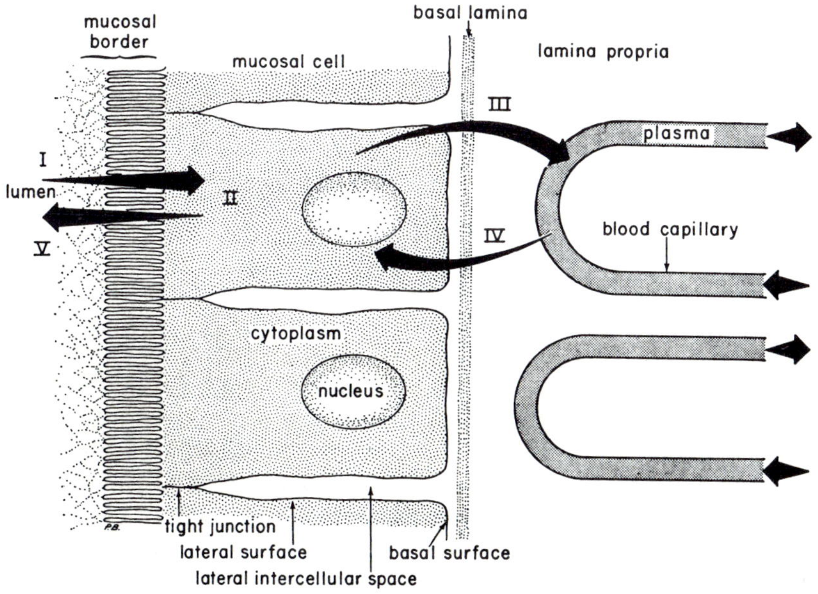

FIG. 7. Schematic representation of the stages in the transport of Ca across an intestinal epithelial cell taken from Wasserman (1968).

the vitamin D replete animal. No effect of DB-CAMP was seen in the jejunum. Harrison and Harrison (1970) concluded that CAMP's effect is dependent upon a vitamin D-induced factor and suggested that these observations may have more relevance to the mechanism of parathyroid hormone's action on Ca absorption.

(x) *Summary of vitamin D mechanism.* The following discussion presents a summary of the action of vitamin D on Ca absorption by the intestine. It represents the opinion of the author at the time of writing. It is a simplification of the problem and ignores certain discrepant findings, some of which have been reviewed above in Section 11.2.6.1 on pp. 548–555. For more extensive reviews of this subject the reader is referred to those of DeLuca (1969b), Wasserman (1968), Wasserman *et al.* (1969), and Wasserman and Taylor (1969). A schematic representation of the steps involved in Ca transport is presented in Fig. 7 taken from Wasserman (1968).

Vitamin D through its active metabolite or metabolites has the following actions on the gut in facilitating the translocation of Ca from intestinal lumen to plasma: (1) the vitamin acts primarily on the nucleus of the mucosal epithelial cells to stimulate protein synthesis which results in increased levels of a protein or proteins involved in either passive (CaBP) or active (CaATPase) transport, or both; (2) the vitamin increases *directly* the bidirectional permeability of mucosal epithelial cells in all segments of the small intestine by a passive process not requiring energy (steps I and II in Fig. 7); and (3) this increase in permeability *indirectly* increases the unidirectionally oriented (lumen to plasma) and the presumably basally located (basement membrane rather than luminal side) active transport system (step III in Fig. 7).

(c) *Active metabolites of vitamin D.** In 1956 Kodicek, using ^{14}C-ergocalciferol of low specific activity prepared biosynthetically, first demonstrated that vitamin D_2 was metabolized by the rat to break down products. He was unable to associate biological activity with any of these metabolites. This field remained relatively dormant until the late 1960s when DeLuca and his associates made a breakthrough of great importance: they discovered that a metabolite of vitamin D_3, 25-hydroxycholecalciferol (25-(OH)-D_3, was even more active than the parent vitamin, which in the light of this discovery is now considered relatively inactive (DeLuca, 1969a, b, c, d). The first step in this development was the synthesis of ^{14}C- and ^{3}H-labeled vitamins of high specific

*See also p. 546.

activity; these included: 1,2-^{3}H-vitamin D_3 with 26,000 dpm/i.u. (Neville and DeLuca, 1966); randomly labeled ^{14}C-vitamin D_2 with 30,000 dpm/i.u. (Imrie *et al.*, 1967); and 22,23-^{3}H-vitamin D_4 with 100,000 dpm/i.u. (DeLuca *et al.*, 1968). The next step was the demonstration that a major metabolite, more polar than vitamin D_3 and termed peak IV, was found in rat blood and intestine but not in liver (Lund and DeLuca, 1966). This metabolite was identified as 25-(OH)-D_3 (Blunt *et al.*, 1968b; Ponchon and DeLuca, 1969a) and shown to enhance Ca transport in the everted gut sac of the rat (Avioli *et al.*, 1969a; Blunt *et al.*, 1968a; Morii *et al.*, 1967). The conversion of vitamin D_3 to 25-(OH)-D_3 has been demonstrated in the human (Avioli, 1969; Avioli *et al.*, 1967a, b, 1968a, b; Mawer *et al.*, 1969), the pig (Blunt *et al.*, 1968b), the rat (Cousins *et al.*, 1970; Horsting and DeLuca, 1969; Morii *et al.*, 1967; Ponchon and DeLuca, 1969a, b; Ponchon *et al.*, 1969; Stohs and DeLuca, 1967), and the chicken (Drescher *et al.*, 1969; Haussler *et al.*, 1970; Lawson *et al.*, 1969a, b; Stohs and DeLuca, 1967).

Of extreme interest from both the physiological and pharmacological points of view are the reports of Blunt *et al.* (1968a) and of Olson and DeLuca (1969). The former found that the response of the rat intestine with respect to Ca absorption occurred much more rapidly after intravenous administration of 25-(OH)-D_3 (within 2–3 hr) than after the administration of vitamin D_3 by the same route (8–10 hr). The relevant data taken from Blunt *et al.* (1968a) are presented in Fig. 8. Olson and

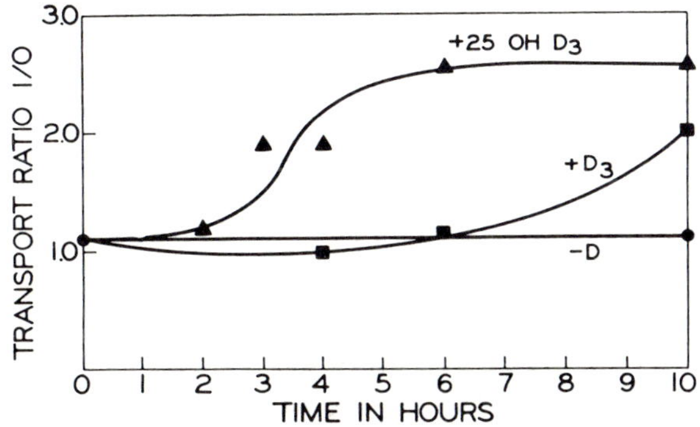

FIG. 8. Response of active transport system in everted duodenal sacs of vitamin-D-deficient (—D) rats following treatment with either vitamin D_3 (+D_3) or 25-hydroxycholecalciferol (+25-(OH)-D_3) at a dose of 0.25 mcg (10 i.u.) intravenously. The rapid response to 25-hydroxycholecalciferol is clearly seen (within 3 hr) while the response to vitamin D_3 is seen only after 8–10 hr. (From DeLuca, 1969a, and Blunt *et al.*, 1968a.)

DeLuca (1969) used an *in vivo* preparation, whereby they perfused the small intestine of the rat with the drug from the blood side and with ^{45}Ca from the luminal side. They found that a small dose of 25-(OH)-D_3 added to the blood perfusate caused a significant rise in Ca transport; no effect was seen with 1000 times greater dose (in terms of weight) of vitamin D_3. These observations, together with those concerned with *in vitro* effects on bone (Trummel *et al.*, 1969), indicate that vitamin D_3 is inactive *per se* and that its biological activity is due entirely to the fact that it is converted *in vivo* to active metabolites such as 25-(OH)-D_3.

It is well known that there are species differences in the relative responses to vitamins D_2 and D_3. Whereas in man and in the rat the two vitamins are approximately equipotent, the chicken discriminates against vitamin D_2. It has now been demonstrated in pigs that vitamin D_2 is converted to an analogous metabolite, 25-hydroxyergocalciferol (Suda *et al.*, 1969a, b). Is the relative ineffectiveness of vitamin D_2 in the chicken due to the inability of this species to convert the vitamin to its active metabolite, 25-hydroxyergocalciferol (25-(OH)-D_2)? Drescher *et al.* (1969) found that the chicken was able to effect this conversion quite readily and that the product, 25-(OH)-D_2, although equipotent with 25-(OH)-D_3 in the rat, was relatively ineffective in the chicken. The basis for this discrimination must lie elsewhere; Drescher *et al.* (1969) suggest that it may be due to a more rapid elimination of 25-(OH)-D_2 by the chicken.

The liver appears to be the major site of conversion of vitamin D_3 to its active metabolite, 25-OH-D_3 (Horsting and DeLuca, 1969; Ponchon and DeLuca, 1969b; Ponchon *et al.*, 1969); this conversion may be under feedback control (Horsting and DeLuca, 1970). Avioli and his associates have proposed that certain pathological conditions associated with depressed intestinal absorption of Ca, such as uremia and vitamin D-resistant rickets, may be due to suppression of the hepatic* conversion of inactive vitamin D to its active metabolite or metabolites (Avioli *et al.*, 1965; Avioli *et al.*, 1967b, 1968a, 1969a, b). The experimental basis for this concept is the fact that in uremic rats, in which Ca transport (everted gut sac technique) was depressed, vitamin D_3 failed to restore the response to normal, whereas 25-(OH)-D_3 was successful in this respect (Avioli *et al.*, 1969a). This concept is fascinating and its more widespread application to the variety of disorders of Ca absorption is awaited with interest.

Evidence is beginning to appear that other metabolites more polar

*Cf. p. 546. It is now clear cut that the conversion of 25-(OH)-D_3 into 1,25-$(OH)_2$-D_3 takes place in the kidneys (Eds.).

than 25-(OH)-D_3 may be of importance with respect to intestinal function (Haussler *et al.*, 1970; Lawson *et al.*, 1969a, b). Whether or not these metabolites prove to be biologically active must await further work. However, the radioactivity which preferentially accumulates in the nuclear fraction of the intestinal mucosal cells following ^{3}H-vitamin D_3 administration (see pp. 553–554) has been found to be mainly 25-(OH)-D_3 (Cousins *et al.*, 1970; Stohs and DeLuca, 1967).

11.2.6.2. *Hormones*

In the past decade the endocrine aspects of Ca absorption have been concerned largely with three hormones: parathyroid hormone, calcitonin, and the iodinated thyroid hormones. There has been much less activity in the area of the steroid hormones and the pituitary hormones associated with their synthesis and release. Essentially no research activity of any significance and relevant to this review can be found with any of the other hormones.

(a) *Parathyroid hormone* (*PTH*). Historically it had been assumed that the parathyroid glands had no direct influence on Ca absorption from the intestine (Kenny, 1960). Categorical statements to this effect were made in the review literature as late as the mid-1950s (Irving, 1957; Nicolaysen *et al.*, 1953). Today it is generally recognized that the glands do exercise some influence on Ca absorption; the only argument is over the degree and importance of this influence. Pure parathyroid hormone is not readily available. Only in two studies discussed in this section (pp. 563–564) did the investigators use a partially purified preparation (Birge *et al.*, 1969; Robinson *et al.*, 1968). In the remaining studies only very crude preparations such as the commercially available pharmaceutical product, Parathyroid Injection (100 USP units/ml), were used; in terms of units/mg protein the commercial product is only about 0.5% pure. For this and other reasons many investigators in the past have often preferred to rely on the endocrinectomy approach, using either pure parathyroidectomy (PTX) or the less satisfactory thyroparathyroidectomy (TPTX) in those species, such as the dog, where pure PTX is a more complicated surgical procedure.

The following discussion will outline the relationships between PTX, PTH, and Ca absorption followed by a review of the information concerning the mechanism of PTH's action on the gut.

(i) *Parathyroidectomy and calcium absorption.* A brief glance at the literature reveals a degree of confusion concerning the effects of PTX on Ca absorption by the small intestine. The discrepancies do not appear to have their origins either in the species or in the techniques used. For example, in the rat with the everted gut sac technique there have been reports of PTX (or TPTX) leading both to a decrease in Ca absorption (Lifshitz *et al.,* 1969; Rasmussen, 1959; Schachter, 1963) and to no effect (Gruson *et al.,* 1970; Kimberg *et al.,* 1961; Morehead and Kessner, 1969; Wasserman and Comar, 1961). Similar discrepancies exist in those studies using the balance method in the rat. Aubert *et al.* (1964), Milhaud and Moukhtar (1966), and Shah and Draper (1966) found decreased Ca absorption following PTX (or TPTX), whereas Sammon *et al.* (1970) and Clark (1969a) found no consistent effects. The *in vivo* ligated loop method in the rat has also led to discordant findings. Wasserman and Comar (1961) and Cramer *et al.* (1961) were not able to demonstrate an effect of PTX on Ca absorption. Winter *et al.* (1970) obtained different effects depending upon the dietary levels of Ca while Talmage and Elliott (1958) and Kodicek *et al.* (1964) reported a fall in Ca absorption. Cramer *et al.* (1961) studied the absorption of an oral dose of ^{45}Ca in rats and found that it was decreased by PTX. Other species have been studied less thoroughly. Nelson *et al.* (1969) claimed no effect of TPTX in the sheep using the balance technique although the data are not clear cut. On the other hand, both the dog (Cramer, 1963) and the goat (Payne and Sansom, 1966) respond to TPTX by a decrease in Ca absorption. Hypoparathyroid patients also have decreased Ca absorption relative to normal subjects (Birge *et al.,* 1969).

Is it possible to bring a semblance of order to these apparently discordant findings? The apparent chaos is not due to differences between PTX and TPTX as no correlation can be found in these terms. However, if all the rat studies mentioned above, with only five exceptions (Cramer *et al.,* 1961; Kodicek *et al.,* 1964; Sammon *et al.,* 1970; Schachter, 1963; Talmage and Elliott, 1958), are arranged in descending order of Ca content of the diet (Table 15) a pattern develops. A very sharp division takes place at about 0.65 % Ca; all studies using dietary Ca levels above this value report no significant effect of PTX on Ca absorption by the intestine. The studies below 0.65 % are not as clear cut. However if, in those studies using either the ligated loop or duodenal sac, a distinction is made between the length of time on the special diet, a pattern again develops. In adaptation studies, as discussed above on pp. 535–539, Kenny and his associates have shown that the parathyroid glands are important for adaptation at 7 days, are unimportant at 21 days, and may or may not

TABLE 15. RELATIONSHIP BETWEEN DIETARY CALCIUM LEVEL AND EFFECT OF PARATHYROIDECTOMY (PTX) OR THYROPARATHYROIDECTOMY (TPTX) ON CALCIUM ABSORPTION

Dietary Ca (%)	Technique	Parameter	Response[a] p level	Investigators
High Ca series				
2.0	*in vivo* ligated loop	% absorbed	N.S.	Wasserman and Comar (1961)
2.0	*in vitro* duodenal sac	S/M	N.S.	Wasserman and Comar (1961)
1.5	*in vitro* duodenal sac	S/M	N.S.	Pento (1970); Pento and Kenny (1970)
1.5	*in vivo* ligated loop	% absorbed	N.S.	Pento (1970); Pento and Kenny (1970)
1.2	*in vitro* duodenal sac	S/M	N.S.	Kimberg *et al.* (1961)
1.2	balance method	v_a	N.S.	Shah and Draper (1966)
0.8	balance method	α	N.S.	Clark (1969a)
0.76	*in vitro* duodenal sac	S/M	N.S.	Gruson *et al.* (1970)
0.68	*in vitro* duodenal sac	S/M	N.S.	Morehead and Kessner (1969)
Low Ca series: short-term studies*				
0.6	*in vivo* ligated loop	% absorbed	N.S.*	Winter *et al.* (1970)
0.6	*in vivo* ligated loop	% absorbed	<0.001*	Winter *et al.* (1970)
0.6	balance method	v_a or α	<0.001	Milhaud *et al.* (1966)
0.6	balance method	v_a	<0.01	Shah and Draper (1965)
0.54	*in vitro* duodenal sac	S/M	<0.025*	Lifshitz *et al.* (1969)
0.44	balance method	α	<0.001	Aubert *et al.* (1964)
0.3	balance method	v_a	<0.001	Shah and Draper (1966)
0.1	*in vivo* ligated loop	% absorbed	<0.001*	Winter *et al.* (1970)
0.01	*in vivo* ligated loop	% absorbed	<0.01*	Pento (1970); Pento and Kenny (1970)
0.01	*in vitro* duodenal sac	S/M	<0.05*	Pento (1970); Pento and Kenny (1970)
Low	*in vitro* duodenal sac	S/M	<0.001*	Rasmussen (1959)
Low Ca series: long-term studies				
0.4	*in vivo* ligated loop	% absorbed	N.S.†	Cramer *et al.* (1961)
0.2	*in vivo* ligated loop	% absorbed	N.S.†	Wasserman and Comar (1961)
0.2	*in vitro* duodenal sac	S/M	N.S.†	Wasserman and Comar (1961)
0.02	*in vitro* duodenal sac	S/M	N.S.†	Kimberg *et al.* (1961)
0.01	*in vivo* ligated loop	% absorbed	N.S.†	Waite, Tracy and Kenny (unpublished)
0.01	*in vivo* ligated loop	% absorbed	N.S.†	Waite, Tracy and Kenny (unpublished)

[a] Fall in Ca absorption following PTX on TPTX.
N.S.: not significant ($p > 0.05$). S/M: serosal/mucosal ratio.
v_a: amount absorbed. α: v_a/dietary intake (v_i).
* Rats were 2 weeks or less on diet. †Rats were 2 weeks or more on diet.

be important at 14 days (Pento, 1970; Pento and Kenny, 1970; Waite, Tracy and Kenny, unpublished observations). Hence if we divide the low Ca series into two categories, less than or greater than 2 weeks of dietary treatment (remembering that 2 weeks itself is equivocal), we find significant effects in the former* and no effects in the latter situation. At least this concept reconciles the negative data of Wasserman and Comar (1961) which have often been explained by others in terms of the acuteness of the PTX (24 hr) and who at the same time ignored the fact that a positive effect was seen by Rasmussen (1959) only 4 hr after PTX. It may be concluded from the above discussion that, in order to demonstrate an effect of PTX on Ca absorption from the rat intestine with either the ligated loop or duodenal sac, certain conditions must be met. The rats must be placed on a diet moderately or markedly low in Ca and ideally they should be on this diet about 7 days, assuming that the rats were maintained previously on a normal commercial laboratory chow which usually contains more than 1.0% Ca. Under the right conditions there appears to be no doubt that parathyroidectomy results in a suppression of Ca absorption from the intestine.

A word about the exceptions and why they were eliminated from Table 15. Cramer *et al.* (1961), Kodicek *et al.* (1964), Schachter (1963), and Talmage and Elliott (1958) did not report their dietary Ca levels.† Only the data of Sammon *et al.* (1970) cannot be fitted into the scheme; no explanation can be offered. It is obvious that in presenting this simplified scheme only the dietary Ca level has been taken into consideration.

Dietary P level is of significance too and therefore caution must be exercised in extrapolating this scheme too indiscriminately.

If the pattern presented in Table 15 is accepted there is a logical explanation for it: that the dietary Ca levels influence PTH secretion rate, such that the higher the dietary Ca level the lower will be the plasma PTH concentration. If this is so then one would expect that at high dietary Ca levels the difference between plasma PTH levels of the intact and PTX rats would be negligible, at least with respect to the gut Ca response. At low dietary Ca levels the difference is presumably great enough to be reflected in the gut response.

*The one exception is that of Winter *et al.* (1970) and they report a significant effect in one experiment and no effect in a second experiment at the same Ca level, 0·6%, where a variable response might be expected close to the cross-over point.

†In the studies of Cramer *et al.* (1961) and Schachter (1963), stock diets of unstated Ca content were used in the relevant experiments.

(ii) *Parathyroid hormone and calcium absorption.* Since Rasmussen's first demonstration of an effect of PTX on active transport of Ca in the everted duodenal sac of the rat (Rasmussen, 1959) there have been only three reports of an opposite effect of PTH. Harrison and Harrison (1969) used the commercially available impure parathyroid extract (PTE) at a subcutaneous dose of 1000 USP units/kg 5 hr before the intestines were removed for preparation of everted duodenal sacs. In TPTX rats the hormone increased the S/M ratios significantly back to control levels. However, no effect was seen in intact rats. Addition of PTE *in vitro* had no effect, confirming the former observation of Rasmussen (1959). Robinson *et al.* (1968) found highly significant increases in Ca absorption measured by the ligated loop technique in PTX rats following administration of PTH. This study is important for two reasons. First, a highly purified preparation (900 USP units/mg) of PTH was used; it was administered subcutaneously in a total dose of 600 USP units in eight divided doses over a period of 48 hr. Secondly, all segments of the small intestine were studied; all responded, but the jejunum gave the greatest response. This latter fact is interesting in view of the fact that Birge *et al.* (1969) concluded that in humans the more distal segments of the small intestine were more sensitive to controlling factors such as PTH. In an earlier study Cramer *et al.* (1961) using the balance method observed a definite enhancement of Ca absorption following a subcutaneous injection of 50 USP units/rat twice daily for 3 days. Schachter (1963) obtained equivocal results after PTE treatment. In everted gut preparations removed from hypophysectomized rats, Finkelstein and Schachter (1962) have found no response to injection of PTE at a subcutaneous dose of 30 USP units/rat given daily for 7 days prior to the experiment.

Recently there have been two reports concerning the gut response to PTH in humans. Birge *et al.* (1969) used a partially purified preparation of PTH and a kinetic approach. Although no response was seen following a 4-hr infusion of 400 USP units they did observe a two-fold increase in Ca absorption following treatment with 200 USP units in gelatin given intramuscularly twice daily over a 3-week period. In addition they found that Ca absorption was greatly enhanced in hyperparathyroid patients. Wensel *et al.* (1969) also found no effect in humans with a low dose of PTE (a single dose of 120–200 USP units) given intravenously.

It thus appears that PTH has a definite effect, opposite to that of PTX, on Ca absorption from the gut. It does not seem to be a very sensitive response and therefore its normal physiological importance may be questioned. In some preliminary studies Tracy and Kenny (unpublished observations) have found that when PTE replacement therapy is given to PTX rats the plasma Ca levels respond to lower doses than does the gut Ca-absorption response measured by the ligated loop method. However, at least in man the gut response may be of importance in pathological conditions such as hyperparathyroidism.

(iii) *Mechanism of action of parathyroid hormone on calcium absorption.* In the past the major concern of those interested in the mechanism of PTH's action on gut Ca absorption has been whether or not vitamin D is needed for the response. Toverud (1964) used the balance method and found that PTX and PTE-treatment in PTX rats caused significant responses in the face of vitamin-D-deficiency. In contrast to this observation Dowdle *et al.* (1960) and more recently Winter *et al.* (1970) using *in vitro* and *in vivo* methods respectively found no effect of PTX on Ca absorption in the vitamin-D-deficient rat. At the time of writing this matter must remain undecided.

An interesting development which may prove to have some bearing on the problem of the mechanism of action of PTH on the gut is that reported by Harrison and Harrison (1970). In an *in vitro* study of passive transport in the rat duodenum they observed that DB-CAMP, either injected *in vivo* or added *in vitro,* caused a significant increase in passive transport, but only when the rats were not vitamin-D-deficient. This finding would indicate that CAMP is not the second messenger for the vitamin. However, the authors suggest that the messenger might be involved in PTH's action on the gut. The further exploration of this hypothesis is awaited with interest.

(b) *Calcitonin.* Calcitonin has no *acute* effect on gut function with respect to Ca. The first studies were in the rat and were indirect. Hirsch and his associates observed that the hypocalcemic response to a single injection of calcitonin was not affected if the rat had been previously subjected to a low Ca diet (Hirsch *et al.,* 1964) or to complete removal of the gastrointestinal tract (Munson *et al.,* 1966); they concluded that the gut was not involved in the response. Kenny and Heiskell (1965) came to a similar conclusion after showing that fasting for 48 hr did not impair the response. Wase *et al.* (1966) found that repeated administration of calcitonin to intact rats increased the positive Ca balance significantly. Interpretation of these data is not simple. The authors claim that this response is largely due to decreased endogenous Ca excretion; a single dose of calcitonin had no effect on the absorption of an oral dose of ^{45}Ca. Other studies confirming the absence of an acute effect of calcitonin in the rat include the use of: (1) perfusion of an isolated loop of the rat *in vivo* and the determination of flux ratios (Krawitt, 1967); (2) *in vivo* ligated loops in PTX rats with and without PTH treatment (Robinson *et al.*, 1968); (3) balance method coupled with radiocalcium techniques (Milhaud and Moukhtar, 1966); and (4) everted duodenal sacs (Gruson *et al.*, 1970; Pento, 1970). Similar negative responses to acute calcitonin administration, of both avian and porcine origin, have been observed in the dog using Thiry–Vella loop preparations (Cramer *et al.*, 1969; Kraintz and Cramer, 1966).

An intriguing concept is being developed by Care and his associates: that a *chronic* response to repeated administration of calcitonin may be the suppression of Ca absorption from the intestine and that a feedback control of this response might exist between the gut and the calcitonin secreting cells of the thyroid. Prolonged administration of calcitonin in sheep causes a definite fall in Ca absorption within 2 or 3 days (Care, 1970). In addition Care (1970) and Care *et al.* (1971) have shown that a gut hormone, pancreozymin, is capable of releasing calcitonin from the perfused thyroid gland of the pig; another gut hormone, secretin, did not possess this property, indicating some specificity in this response. Care suggests that pancreozymin might be the link in the negative feedback control between Ca absorption and calcitonin secretion.

(c) *Iodinated thyroid hormones: thyroxine* (T_4) *and triiodothyronine* (T_3). Most of the earlier studies of thyroid dysfunction in man, particularly in cases of hyperthyroidism, had led to the conclusion that the iodinated thyroid hormones, T_4 and T_3, depress Ca absorption from the intestine (Fourman *et al.*, 1968). Within the past decade this relationship has received greater attention in experimental animals with very clear-cut results. The thyroid hormones definitely suppress Ca absorption from the intestine of the rat. The relevant studies include: (1) suppression of active transport in the everted duodenal sac following subcutaneous administration of either thyroid-stimulating hormone (TSH) at a dose of 1 USP unit per day for 2 weeks, or T_3 at a dose of 10 mcg per day for either 7, 14, or 28 days (Friedland *et al.*, 1965); (2) suppression of both active and passive transport in the everted duodenal, jejunal, or ileal sac following subcutaneous administration of T_4 at a dose of 1 mg/kg daily for 7 days (Noble and Matty, 1967); (3) suppression of active transport in the everted duodenal sac removed from hypophysectomized rats after subcutaneous treatment with T_4 at a dose of 10 mcg daily for 6 days (Finkelstein and Schachter, 1962); and (4) suppression of Ca absorption as measured by the balance method after addition of T_4 to the diet at a concentration of 0.008% (Forbes, 1963). The suppression was immediate (1 day) and showed no evidence of escape even after 98 days of treatment (Friedland *et al.*, 1965).

The effects of the thyroid hormones have been studied in other species. The Ca balance data of Jones *et al.* (1966) in human hypothyroid and hyperthyroid patients treated with T_3 and propylthiouracil respectively are in agreement with the rat data. Propylthiouracil given to hyperthyroid patients moved them from negative to positive balances, while T_3 treatment of hypothyroid individuals moved the balances in the opposite direction. On the other hand, in goats replacement with T_4 (1 mg/day or 5 mg/week intramuscularly in arachis oil) had no effect on Ca absorption following an oral dose of ^{45}Ca in either thyroparathyroidectomized or thyroidectomized animals (Payne and Sansom, 1966). In addition no effect was seen on the Ca balance of the goats.

(d) *Growth hormone*. Clinical experience has led to the general conclusion that administration of growth hormone in humans leads to increased Ca absorption from the intestine (Fourman *et al.*, 1968). The only studies of the relationship between growth hormone and Ca absorption in the rat have emerged from Schachter's laboratory. The first observation was that of Kimberg *et al.* (1961) who found that hypophysectomy was followed by a decrease in the active transport system in the everted duodenal sac in both Ca-depleted and Ca replete rats. The pituitary hormone responsible was identified as growth hormone in a subsequent publication (Finkelstein and Schachter, 1962). Growth hormone given subcutaneously to hypophysectomized rats at a dose of 0.5 mg daily for 7 days restored the impaired active transport system (everted duodenal sac) to 70–100% of normal. No such effect was seen with either ACTH, TSH, or the gonadotropins with the exception of prolactin. The latter finding could not be explained on the basis of contamination with growth hormone. Examination of the time course of the effect of hypophysectomy revealed that the initial response (4–5 days) was an enhancement of active transport followed by a decline which was seen at 7 days and persisted through 21 days, the last time interval studied. The fall in S/M ratios seen at 14 days is very impressive, reaching well below 50% of control levels. Equally impressive is the ability of replacement therapy with growth hormone to restore the *status quo*. These observations of Schachter's group are important and merit further and more extensive study.

(e) *Steroid hormones.*

(i) *Adrenal steroid hormones.* Recent studies of the effects of the adrenal corticosteroids have been mainly in the rat and have been concerned with the glucocorticoids rather than the mineralocorticoids. There appears to be a discrepancy in the conclusions depending upon the technique used. All *in vitro* approaches with the everted duodenal sac lead to the conclusion that the glucocorticoids (cortisone, hydrocortisone, or corticosterone) inhibit the active transport process (Finkelstein and Schachter, 1962; Harrison and Harrison, 1960; Kimberg, 1969; Williams *et al.*, 1961, 1962) and that adrenalectomy enhances the process (Kimberg *et al.*, 1961). The mineralocorticoid, desoxycorticosterone, had no effect (Finkelstein and Schachter, 1962). However, all the *in vivo* studies in this species report no effect from glucocorticoid administration whether the technique was the ligated loop (Winter *et al.*, 1969), the balance method (Williams *et al.*, 1962), or the absorption of an oral dose of ^{45}Ca (Clark and Smith, 1964). These disparate findings have yet to be explained.

Kimberg (1969) has found that the gut from the cortisone-treated rat, although depressed with respect to active transport, contains higher levels of CaBP. In addition, cortisone-treated rats have more vitamin D activity in their intestinal mucosa than the mucosa from control rats following treatment of both groups with a single dose of vitamin D_3. Kimberg (1969) is forced to the conclusion that cortisone's action on Ca absorption is independent of an interaction with vitamin D.

In the chicken, Sallis and Holdsworth (1962b) found that hydrocortisone and desoxycorticosterone inhibited Ca absorption. Avioli *et al.* (1968b) have recently proposed that in man the well-known antagonism between vitamin D and the glucocorticoids might be due to a reduction in the production of the active metabolites of the vitamin.

(ii) *Gonadal steroid hormones.* There has been very little research activity in this area within the past decade. Only negative data were reported by Finkelstein and Schachter (1962). Neither estradiol, progesterone, nor testosterone had any effect on active transport in everted duodenal sacs removed from hypophysectomized rats.

11.2.6.3. *Other pharmacological agents*

(a) *Phosphate.* It is a widely accepted maxim that addition of inorganic phosphate to the diet suppresses the absorption of Ca by the intestine, in spite of informed denials of this generalization (Bronner, 1964; Irving, 1957). This conclusion is based largely on early and extensive rat studies with the balance method in which extremes of Ca:P ratios were often used. It is unfortunate that these findings are frequently extrapolated to other species and to more moderate Ca : P ratios. It is therefore worthwhile emphasizing that by the mid-1950s it became generally recognized that, in the presence of adequate levels of dietary Ca and vitamin D, changing the Ca : P ratio over a fairly wide range had little or no effect on Ca absorption either in man (Bronner, 1964; Irving, 1957; Malm, 1953) or in other species (Bronner, 1964; Davis, 1963). More recently Spencer and her associates (Spencer *et al.*, 1965) have found that varying the Ca : P ratio from 2 : 1 through 1 : 8 by the addition of glycerophosphate to both a low Ca diet (200 mg/day intake) and a high Ca diet (1500 mg/day intake) had no consistent effects on Ca absorption in human patients except possibly to *enhance* absorption in the low Ca diet study. Similarly in rats Clark (1969b) using the balance method found that addition of P to a diet adequate in Ca *enhanced* Ca absorption.

The influence of P on Ca absorption in experimental animals has been examined with techniques other than the balance method. In the dog using the Thiry–Vella loop Cramer (1968) studied various Ca : P ratios, including the addition of no P. He found that addition of P enhanced Ca absorption but, once P was present, varying the Ca : P molar ratio from 0.5 : 2 : 1 had no effect on the Ca absorption rate. *In vitro* studies in the rat led to similar findings. Addition of P, in situations where the solubility product of calcium phosphate was not exceeded, either had no effect (Martin and DeLuca, 1969b), slightly depressed (Walling and Rothman, 1969), or greatly enhanced Ca transport (Helbock *et al.*, 1966). In the ligated loop of the chicken Wasserman (1962) found that addition of a chemically equivalent amount of P (presumably around 25 mM) in the form of either orthophosphate or glucerophosphate to the loop contents containing 25 mM Ca depressed Ca absorption. However, this inhibition can be explained on the basis of precipitation of calcium phosphate (Wasserman, 1964); Helbock *et al.* (1966) observed precipitation with concentrations of 3.0 and 10.7 mM for Ca and P respectively.

It thus appears that in situations of adequate Ca and vitamin D intake, varying the P content of the diet does not lead to a depression of Ca absorption unless levels are reached at which precipitation of calcium phosphate becomes a limiting factor. The major influence of P is to *enhance* Ca absorption when P addition is compared with the P-deficient situation.

(b) *Phytates*. Since Mellanby's first discovery in 1925 of a rachitogenic factor present in cereals, later identified as phytic acid or inositol hexaphosphoric acid, a considerable controversy has raged in nutritional circles as to its importance. There is no question, as was later shown, that phytic acid can inhibit Ca absorption from the diet (see reviews by Bronner, 1964; Davis, 1963; Fourman *et al.*, 1968; Irving, 1957). This action has in fact been applied therapeutically in man in cases of sarcoidosis and hypercalciuria (Henneman *et al.*, 1956). Its therapeutic effectiveness was not dramatic; diarrhea was the only side-effect. However, in the human adaptation occurs; the initial fall in Ca absorption following phytate ingestion is eventually overcome (Walker *et al.*, 1948).

By the mid-1950s Harris (1955) and Bronner *et al.* (1954) were led to conclude that "when the intake of unrefined cereals is relatively low and that of Ca relatively high nutritional problems due to phytate ingestion are negligible" (Bronner, 1964). The nutritional controversy has subsided and interest in phytate and Ca absorption has waned to insignificant levels.

(c) *Magnesium*. The effect of Mg on Ca absorption is not consistent and is dependent upon many factors (Wasserman and Taylor, 1969). There are reports which conclude that addition of Mg to the diet can either enhance, depress, or have no effect on Ca absorption (Alcock and MacIntyre, 1962, 1964; Clark, 1965, 1968, 1969a; Ebel and Comar, 1968; Forbes, 1963; Heaton and Parsons, 1961; Miller *et al.*, 1965a). There appear to be few points of agreement. In some laboratories Mg deficiency in the rat leads to increased transport as measured by the everted duodenal sac (Alcock and MacIntyre, 1962; Kessner and Epstein, 1966; Morehead and Kessner, 1969); this response was abolished by prior PTX (Morehead and Kessner, 1969), indicating that it might be secondary to stimulation of the parathyroid glands. In the Harrisons' laboratory no effect due to Mg deficiency was seen in the same preparation (Lifshitz *et al.*, 1967a, b). Addition of Mg to the fluid used in the everted duodenal sac has been shown either to decrease (Hendrix *et al.*, 1963; Schachter and Rosen, 1959)* or to have no effect (Kessner and Epstein, 1966; Lifshitz *et al.*, 1967a) on active transport of Ca. In the Thiry–Vella loop preparation Mg depressed Ca absorption in both the dog (Cramer and Dueck, 1962) and the sheep (Care and van't Klooster, 1965). The picture is far from clear and must await further work for clarification.

(d) *Sodium*. Controversy exists over whether or not Na is required for

*See Table 2 for Schachter and Rosen (1959) data, p. 512.

the active transport of Ca. Earlier reports (Harrison and Harrison, 1963b; Wasserman and Taylor, 1963a) indicated that Na was not required. On the other hand Martin and DeLuca (1969a) found that in the absence of Na, active transport of Ca was greatly decreased; they attributed the discrepancy between the two sets of observations to the presence of K and phosphate in the media used by the earlier workers.

(e) *Potassium*. The overall effect of K on Ca absorption also lacks clarity. Whereas K deficiency resulted in a decreased absorption of Ca *in vivo* as measured by a short-term balance technique (Cuisinier-Gleizes and Mathieu, 1969), the addition of K *in vitro* to media depressed uptake and transport of Ca (Harrison and Harrison, 1963b; Schachter *et al.*, 1960a).

(f) *Lactose*. It has been known for over 40 years that lactose, when incorporated into experimental diets, will enhance the intestinal absorption of Ca in many species. The effect of lactose in the rat is directly on the gut (Chang and Hegsted, 1964; Lengemann, 1959; Lengemann *et al.*, 1959; Wasserman, 1964; Wasserman and Comar, 1959; Wasserman and Lengemann, 1960). Other sugars (mannose, cellobiose, raffinose, D- and L-xylose, D- and L-arabinose) and polyalcohols (mannitol, sorbitol and inositol) have a similar effect; glucose and sucrose are effective *in vitro* but ineffective *in vivo* due to their rapid absorption in the upper part of the small intestine (Wasserman and Comar, 1959).

In man lactose gave only a slight enhancement of Ca absorption from the intestine (Greenwald *et al.*, 1963). On the other hand, Pansu *et al.* (1969) have recently made the interesting observation that osteoporotic patients, intolerant to lactose with respect to the hyperglycemic response to ingested lactose, show a much more dramatic response in Ca absorption.

(g) *Amino acids*. The fact that certain amino acids directly and immediately enhance the intestinal absorption of Ca in the rat was first documented by Wasserman's group (Raven *et al.*, 1960; Wasserman *et al.*, 1956, 1957a). The relative effectiveness of the amino acids is as follows: (1) highly effective, L-lysine, and L-arginine; (2) moderately effective, L-tryptophane, L-leucine, L-histidine, L-methionine, L-aspartic acid, hydroxyl-L-proline, L-glutamic acid, and DL-tyrosine; and (3) relatively ineffective, glycine, L-isoleucine, L-valine, and L-phenylalanine. In the chicken Wasserman *et al.* (1957a) found that lysine inhibited Ca absorption; Sallis and Holdsworth (1962a) found no effect of either L-lysine or L-arginine in the ligated loop preparation of the rachitic chick. The effect of lysine in man is not dramatic (Spencer and Samachson, 1963).

(h) *Hydrogen ion.* Two factors make the relationship between pH and intestinal absorption of Ca worthy of study: (1) the pH of the small intestine varies from the proximal to the distal regions; and (2) the solubilities of Ca salts generally decrease as pH rises. The pH of the rat small intestine varies from around 6.5 in the duodenum, decreases to a minimum of 6.0 in the proximal jejunum, and increases to a maximum of 7.2 in the terminal ileum (Waldron-Edward *et al.*, 1966). In the chicken the pH increases progressively from a value of 6.55 in the duodenum to a value of 7.83 in the distal region of the small intestine (Coates and Holdsworth, 1961). Earlier work reviewed by Irving (1957) had led to the conclusion that intestinal pH under normal conditions was relatively unimportant. In a study using the ligated duodenal loop of the rat, Sallis and Holdsworth (1962a) found no difference in Ca absorption from the loop whether the contents of the loop were at pH 4 or at pH 6. In the chicken Wasserman (1963) tested the effect of pH 1.8, 4.0 and 6.9 on Ca absorption from ligated duodenal loops in both normal and rachitic chicks. There was no dramatic effect of pH on absorption in the normal chick. However, there were sharp differences between the normal and the rachitic chicks at pH 4.0 and 6.9 (the rachitic absorption was suppressed relative to the normal); there was no difference between the two nutritional states at pH 1:8. In the dog, Cramer (1968) found no differences in Ca absorption rates from Thiry–Vella loops between pH 3.3, 5.2 and 7.4.

(i) *Bile and bile acids.* The chronic effects of bile and the bile acids are complicated by the fact that in the rat, and presumably in other species, bile is normally required for the optimal absorption of vitamin D (Schachter *et al.*, 1964). However, bile does have an immediate and direct effect on Ca absorption both in the rat (Lengemann and Dobbins, 1958; Schachter *et al.*, 1964; Webling and Holdsworth, 1966) and in the chicken (Coates and Holdsworth, 1961; Webling and Holdsworth, 1965, 1966). Rachitic bile was just as effective and the response was rapid, indicating that the effect was not due to the vitamin D or active metabolite content of the bile. Three observations in the rat cloud this picture. Vaughan and Filer (1960) found no positive effect of bile added to ligated duodenal and ileal sacs. Cholestyramine is an anion exchange resin which binds bile acids in the lumen and prevents their absorption; therefore its administration to rats would predictably decrease Ca absorption. However, the resin has been found both to increase Ca absorption (Briscoe and Ragan, 1963) and to have no effect (Thompson and Thompson, 1969). The positive effects of bile acids are also seen with other materials of an anionic detergent nature, such as sodium lauryl sulphate, whereas cationic (benzalkonium chloride) and neutral (polyoxyethylene sorbiton mono-oleate or Tween 80) detergents were ineffective (Webling and Holdsworth, 1965). This generalization does not necessarily hold as a cationic detergent (cetyltrimethylammonium bromide) enhances Ca absorption from ligated duodenal loops of rachitic chicks but depresses Ca absorption in normal chicks (Wasserman and Taylor, 1969).

(j) *Antibiotics.* Certain antibiotics, such as penicillin, chloramphenicol, and neomycin, have been shown to increase Ca absorption from the intestine (Heggeness, 1959; Migicovsky *et al.*, 1951; Wasserman and Lengemann, 1960). Whether or not this response is related to the fact that germ-free rats absorb Ca more efficiently (Reddy *et al.*, 1968) is not known.

11.3. MAGNESIUM TRANSPORT

The information concerning the physiological factors controlling Mg homeostasis is more meager than that concerning Ca homeostasis (Walser, 1967). It is clear that the maintenance of Mg homeostasis is a greater problem in ruminants than in non-ruminants, hypomagnesemia of pathological proportions being a more frequent event in the former (Care, 1967). It is also becoming clear that the gut plays an important role in Mg homeostasis in ruminant species. For this reason the intestinal transport of Mg in ruminants and non-ruminants will be discussed separately.

11.3.1. MAGNESIUM ABSORPTION IN NON-RUMINANTS

11.3.1.1. *Physiological aspects*

Magnesium absorption from the intestine has been studied in several non-ruminant species. These include the rat (Alcock and MacIntyre, 1962, 1964; Chutkow, 1964a, b, 1965; Heggeness, 1959; Hendrix *et al.*, 1963; Kessner and Epstein, 1966; MacIntyre and Robinson, 1969; Ross, 1961, 1962; Schachter *et al.*, 1960a), the chicken (Wasserman,

1962, 1963), the dog (Cramer *et al.*, 1969), the pig (Miller *et al.*, 1965a, b, c), the rabbit (Aikawa and David, 1969; Anast *et al.*, 1964), the guinea pig (Ross and Care, 1962) and man (Graham *et al.*, 1960). All segments of the small intestine of the rat are capable of transporting Mg (Chutkow, 1964a; Hendrix *et al.*, 1963; MacIntyre and Robinson, 1969); the ileum seems to be the major site (Chutkow, 1964a; Hendrix *et al.*, 1963; MacIntyre and Robinson, 1969). Absorption of Mg is generally at a slower rate than that of Ca (MacIntyre and Robinson, 1969). Little or no active transport appears to be involved either in the rat (Hendrix *et al.*, 1963; Schachter *et al.*, 1960a), the rabbit (Aikawa and David, 1969; Anast *et al.*, 1964), or the guinea pig (Ross and Care, 1962). The transport mechanism becomes saturated as luminal Mg concentration is increased in the rat (Ross, 1962). *In vitro* Na stimulates Mg transport in the rat (Ross, 1961). Magnesium binds to CaBP less strongly than does either Ca, Sr, or Ba (Taylor and Wasserman, 1969).

There are conflicting reports on the effect of Mg deprivation on Mg absorption. Kessner and Epstein (1966) found no effect on the S/M ratio in the everted duodenal sac of the rat, whereas in rabbits Aikawa and David (1969) report that Mg deficiency led to an increase in the passive transport of Mg. Calcium deprivation led to an increase in Mg absorption in the rat as determined by the balance technique (Alcock and MacIntyre, 1962, 1964). Addition of Ca appears to depress Mg absorption (Hendrix *et al.*, 1963). These observations led Alcock and MacIntyre (1962) and MacIntyre (1967) to suggest that Ca and Mg share a common pathway in intestinal transport, a concept which Walser (1967) feels has not yet been adequately verified.

11.3.1.2. *Pharmacological aspects*

The pharmacological aspects of Mg absorption from the intestine resemble those of Ca absorption except that Mg absorption is much less responsive to the drugs.

Recent reports from MacIntyre's laboratory have indicated that PTH in the form of a purified preparation (900 USP units/mg) increases Mg absorption from ligated duodenal, jejunal, and ileal loops of the PTX rat (MacIntyre and Robinson, 1969; MacIntyre *et al.*, 1966). The hormone (total dose, 600 USP units) was injected subcutaneously in eight divided doses over 48 hr and absorption from the loop was studied for a period of 4 hr. MacIntyre and Robinson (1969) suggest that Mg absorption is largely controlled physiologically by PTH.

Vitamin D appears to have slight effects on Mg metabolism in the intestine. The vitamin has been reported to improve the Mg balance in pigs (Miller *et al.*, 1965a) and to enhance Mg absorption from ligated duodenal loops in rachitic chicks (Wasserman, 1962).

Calcitonin has no acute effects on Mg absorption from Thiry–Vella loops in dogs (Cramer *et al.*, 1969). Growth hormone may enhance Mg absorption in man (Hanna *et al.*, 1961).

11.3.2. MAGNESIUM ABSORPTION IN RUMINANTS

11.3.2.1. *Physiological aspects*

Intestinal absorption of Mg has been investigated in both the bovine (Smith, 1959, 1962, and 1963) and the sheep (Care and Keynes, 1964; Care and van't Klooster, 1965; Care *et al.*, 1967; Field, 1961; McAleese *et al.*, 1961; Phillipson and Storry, 1965; Scott, 1965; Stewart and Moodie, 1956) but more extensively in the latter. The secretion of Mg into the intestine is considerable in ruminants, so that a defect in absorption or dietary restriction of Mg can lead to a considerable endogenous loss of Mg and to hypomagnesemic complications (Care, 1967).

Magnesium is absorbed from all segments of the upper gastrointestinal tract of the sheep with the exception of the rumen (Phillipson and Storry, 1965; Stewart and Moodie, 1956); the middle region of the small intestine is the major site of net absorption (Care, 1967; Care and van't Klooster, 1965; Field, 1961). In the young bovine the large intestine is an important site of Mg absorption; the small intestine assumes a greater role as the calf grows (Smith, 1962). The transport mechanism appears to be mostly passive in sheep (Care and van't Klooster, 1965). Saturation was observed, which led Care and van't Klooster (1965) to suggest that the mechanism was one of facilitated diffusion. Sodium was found to stimulate, and K and Ca to suppress, Mg absorption from Thiry–Vella loops of the mid-ileum (Care and van't Klooster, 1965; Care *et al.*, 1967). Magnesium deficiency enhanced Mg absorption in sheep (McAleese *et al.*, 1961).

11.3.2.2. *Pharmacological aspects*

The pharmacological aspects of Mg absorption in ruminants have received very little attention. This is somewhat surprising in view of the agricultural importance of the hypomagnesemic ruminant condition known as grass tetany, a condition which is assumed to be due to defective intestinal absorption of Mg (Care, 1967). Perhaps the explanation of this relative neglect lies in the fact that grass tetany in the bovine responds therapeutically to simple treatment with Mg (Smith, 1961).

Although the effects of PTH itself have not been investigated, Care and Keynes (1964) reported that TPTX decreased Mg absorption by the mid-ileum of the sheep. These authors also noted that triiodothyronine inhibited Mg absorption (quoted in Care, 1967).

11.4. STRONTIUM TRANSPORT

11.4.1. CONCEPT OF DISCRIMINATION

The transport of Sr across the intestinal barrier would probably have remained of academic interest only, had it not been for the toxicological problem of radioactive fallout from nuclear fissions. Stable Sr can replace Ca to a large extent and is relatively harmless. It is this ability to follow Ca that makes *radio*strontium (^{89}Sr or ^{90}Sr) a bone-seeking isotope of long biological half-life and therefore potentially toxic. It is understandable that much research effort has been applied in this area in an attempt to delineate the nuances of Sr metabolism. This effort was noticeable particularly in the 1950s at the height of the international concern over radioactive pollution. Comar and Wasserman (1964) note that between 1957 and 1961 there were over 1800 references related to Sr and Ca metabolism listed in the cumulative index of *Nuclear Science Abstracts*. An excellent review of several aspects of Sr metabolism both in man and in animals may be found in the proceedings of a recent symposium (Lenihan *et al.*, 1967). One of the consoling facets about the problem of radioactive pollution with the radionuclides of Sr is that biological processes in general discriminate against Sr in favor of Ca. Not least among these is the process of intestinal absorption. Comar and his colleagues (Comar, 1967; Comar and Wasserman, 1964; Comar *et al.*, 1957) developed a terminology to express these discriminations. First they proposed the Sr–Ca Observed Ratio (*OR*) to represent the *overall* discriminations observed in a series of discriminatory processes:

$$OR_{\text{sample/precursor}} = \frac{\text{Sr/Ca}_{\text{sample}}}{\text{Sr/Ca}_{\text{precursor}}}.$$

For example, we may represent the discrimination from the diet to the urine as follows:

$$OR_{\text{urine/diet}} = \frac{\text{Sr/Ca}_{\text{urine}}}{\text{Sr/Ca}_{\text{diet}}}.$$

Secondly, they suggested the Sr–Ca Discrimination Factor (*DF*) to represent the discrimination in a *single* physiological process:

$$DF_{\text{absorptive}} = \frac{\text{Sr transported across gut}}{\text{Ca transported across gut}}.$$

Thirdly, it follows that with several barriers in series:

$$OR = (DF_1)(DF_2)(DF_3) \ldots (DF_n).$$

11.4.2. PHYSIOLOGICAL ASPECTS

Strontium metabolism with respect to intestinal absorption has been investigated in several species. These have included studies in rats (Bruce, 1963; Comar *et al.*, 1956; Cramer and Copp, 1959; Dumont *et al.*, 1960; Gran, 1960; Greenberg, 1945; Harrison *et al.*, 1957; Hendrix *et al.*, 1963; Kawin, 1959; Kostial *et al.*, 1963, 1964, 1965, 1967; Lengemann, 1963; Lengemann and Comar, 1961; Lengemann *et al.*, 1959; MacDonald *et al.*, 1955; Marcus and Lengemann, 1962a, b; Mraz, 1962; Palmer *et al.*, 1958a, b; Paul *et al.*, 1964; Schachter, 1963; Schachter *et al.*, 1960a; Skoryna *et al.*, 1964 and 1965; Talmage and Elliott, 1958; Taylor, 1967; Volf, 1965; Waldron-Edward *et al.*, 1964, 1966, 1967; Wasserman, 1963; Wasserman and Comar, 1959, 1961; Wasserman and Lengemann, 1960; Wasserman *et al.*, 1956, 1957b, 1966), in chickens (Corradino and Wasserman, 1970; Wasserman, 1962, 1963, 1968), in man (Bedford *et al.*, 1960; Carr, 1967; Comar *et al.*, 1957; Greenwald *et al.*, 1963; Hesp and Ramsbottom, 1967; Samachson, 1963; Shimmins *et al.*, 1967; Spencer *et al.*, 1960, 1961, 1964b, 1965, 1967a), in rabbits (Kidman *et al.*, 1950) and in sheep (Jones and Mackie, 1959).

11.4.2.1. *Sites of strontium absorption*

All segments of the rat small intestine can absorb Sr (Marcus and Lengemann, 1962b; Waldron-Edward *et al.*, 1966; Wasserman, 1963; Wasserman and Comar, 1961), the most rapid rate being in the duodenum (Cramer and Copp, 1959). However, as with Ca, the ileum appears to be the major site of Sr absorption when both rates of absorption and transit times are taken into consideration (Cramer and Copp, 1959; Marcus and Lengemann, 1962a, b). A similar situation exists in the chicken (Wasserman, 1962, 1963).

11.4.2.2. *Discrimination phenomenon*

The approximate percentages of Sr absorbed by various species on

TABLE 16. STRONTIUM ABSORPTION AND DISCRIMINATION FACTORS IN VARIOUS SPECIES [a]

Species	Sr absorption (%)	Discrimination factor ($DF_{\text{absorptive}}$)
Man	25	0.7
Dog	4	—
Cow	10	0.2
Goat	5	0.25
Sheep	15	0.4
Pig	9	—
Rat	20	0.5

[a] From Comar and Wasserman (1964).

$$DF_{\text{absorptive}} = \frac{\text{Sr transported across gut}}{\text{Ca transported across gut}}.$$

normal calcium intakes are presented in Table 16 taken from Comar and Wasserman (1964). It can be seen that Sr is absorbed to the extent of only about 5–25% of the Sr intake. These values are below those of Ca, a fact which is reflected in the *DF* data which quantitatively indicate the discrimination against Sr relative to Ca. Particularly fortunate from the health point of view is the low discrimination factor of 0.2 for the cow, signifying that Ca is favored over Sr by a factor of 5. A further discrimination takes place between the plasma and the milk of the cow, making an overall discrimination, $OR_{\text{mill/diet}}$, against Sr. This indicates that the gut is by far the most effective discriminatory barrier with respect to Sr metabolism. The basis for this discrimination in the rat lies partly in the following observations: (1) Sr is absorbed to a lesser extent than Ca in the ligated duodenal and ileal loops of the rat (Wasserman and Comar, 1961); (2) unlike Ca, Sr does not appear to be actively transported from the mucosal to serosal side as determined either with the everted duodenal and ileal preparations (Wasserman, 1960; Wasserman and Comar, 1961) or with flux ratio approach in perfused segments *in vivo* (Dumont *et al.*, 1960); and (3) perhaps of more importance is the fact that Sr, unlike Ca, appears to be actively secreted into the lumen of the ileum (Wasserman, 1960). It is also of interest to note that CaBP has less affinity for Sr than for Ca (Taylor and Wasserman, 1969).

11.4.2.3. *Dietary calcium and strontium absorption*

Calcium deprivation, a stimulus for increased Ca absorption (see Table 8 and Section 11.2.4.1 above), can enhance Sr absorption, but only under certain circumstances. Corradino and Wasserman (1970) found that Ca deprivation in chickens led to enhanced absorption of Sr from ligated duodenal loops *in vivo*. No such response was seen in rats as measured by the effect on S/M ratio in everted duodenal sacs (Wasserman, 1960). Similarly in man the effect of Ca deprivation on Sr absorption is not striking (Shimmins *et al.*, 1967; Spencer *et al.*, 1967a).

Increasing the dietary Ca level has been found to decrease Sr absorption, particularly in rats (MacDonald *et al.*, 1955; Palmer *et al.*, 1958a; Wasserman *et al.*, 1957b). These findings are supported by the *in vivo* perfusion experiments of Mraz (1962), who found that addition of Ca to the perfusate decreased the absorption of Sr from isolated intestinal loops. Little effect of high Ca diet on Sr absorption has been seen in man (Shimmins *et al.*, 1967; Spencer *et al.*, 1967a).

11.4.2.4. *Growth and strontium absorption*

Strontium absorption decreases with increasing age in rats and resembles that of Ca in this respect. However, the decline is more rapid with Sr; the discrimination factor decreases with age (Gran, 1960). The discrimination factor ($DF_{\text{absorptive}}$) in the human infant is approximately 1.0, indicating no discrimination in favor of Ca (Harrison *et al.*, 1965). However, the factor decreases with increasing age; in the human adult the discrimination factor has fallen to a more favorable level of 0.42 (Comar, 1967; Spencer *et al.*, 1960). The $OR_{\text{body/diet}}$ data of Lough *et al.* (1963) also support these findings. Children in the first month of life have *OR* values of between 0.9 and 1.0; between 1 and 2 years of age the *OR* values fall close to the adult value of around 0.25.

11.4.3. STRONTIUM ABSORPTION: PHARMACOLOGICAL ASPECTS

Many of the agents which affect Ca absorption (see pp. 545–572) also influence Sr absorption and usually in the same direction. However, the pharmacological aspects of Sr absorption have not been as thoroughly studied. Few of the studies have been direct; many have used bone uptake following the placement of Sr in the gastrointestinal tract as the criterion of absorption.

11.4.3.1. *Vitamin D*

Vitamin D has been shown to increase Sr absorption from the duodenum and ileum of rats (Greenberg, 1945; Lengemann, 1963; Schachter, 1963) and from all segments of the small intestine of the chicken (Wasserman, 1962, 1963). In addition, vitamin D enhances mucosal tissue uptake of Sr in chickens (Wasserman, 1963). The indirect data of Patrick and Bacon (1957) in rats and in chickens also support these findings. In the human adult Spencer *et al.* (1967a) were unable to demonstrate an enhancement of ^{85}Sr absorption (as judged by plasma and fecal levels of the isotope) following daily administration of 50,000 i.u. of vitamin D for several weeks.

11.4.3.2. *Parathyroid hormone*

Parathyroidectomy had no effect on active transport of Sr in the everted duodenal or ileal sacs of the rat, but this was a study where no effect was seen on Ca transport either (Wasserman and Comer, 1961). In a study in which PTX did cause a reduction in absorption of Ca from ligated loops of the rat small intestine, similar effect was seen on Sr transport (Talmage and Elliott, 1958). No report could be found of the direct effect of PTH on Sr absorption in experimental animals.

The effect of PTE on ^{85}Sr absorption in man has been studied by Spencer *et al.* (1967a, b). Administration of 200 USP units/day to hypoparathyroid patients had no effect on Sr absorption. However, Ca absorption was not influenced in the same studies either.

11.4.3.3. *Other hormones*

Indirect evidence in human patients with thyroid dysfunction indicates that the iodinated thyroid hormones probably inhibit Sr absorption as they do Ca absorption (see pp. 565–566). Spencer *et al.* (1967a, b) have found depressed absorption in hyperthyroid patients relative to euthyroid and hypothyroid patients. These same authors studied the effects of the gonadal and adrenal steroid hormones on ^{85}Sr metabolism in man but found no dramatic effects on Sr absorption (Spencer *et al.*, 1967a).

11.4.3.4. *Miscellaneous agents*

Certain carbohydrates such as lactose and certain amino acids such as lysine enhance Ca absorption (see pp. 570–571). These agents also enhance Sr absorption in the rat (Taylor, 1967; Wasserman and Comar, 1959; Wasserman and Lengemann, 1960; Wasserman *et al.*, 1956). In addition, Taylor (1967) has shown that various metabolic inhibitors (phloridzin, 2,4-DNP, barbital, and oligomycin), when administered either orally or intraperitoneally, enhanced both Ca and Sr absorption from the gastrointestinal tract of the rat. The interrelationships between dietary P levels and Sr absorption have been studied in rats by several investigators (Bruce, 1963; Kostial *et al.*, 1963, 1964, 1965, 1967; MacDonald *et al.*, 1955; Palmer *et al.*, 1958b; Volf, 1965; Wasserman and Comar, 1960). In man addition of P to the diet decreased Sr absorption, whether the subjects were on a high or a low Ca diet (Spencer *et al.*, 1964b, 1965, 1967a). Ebel and Comar (1968) have studied the influence of dietary Mg levels on Sr absorption.

Attempts have been made to find a pharmacological agent which would specifically lower the discrimination factor ($DF_{\text{absorptive}}$) and thus favor Ca over Sr absorption. Among the more effective agents in this regard are the naturally occurring polyuronic acids, alginic and pectic acids and their derivatives, which function both in rats (Paul *et al.*, 1964; Skoryna *et al.*, 1964, 1965; Waldron-Edward *et al.*, 1964, 1967) and in humans (Hesp and Ramsbottom, 1965, 1967). Both pectic and alginic acids inhibit Sr absorption markedly from ligated loops of the rat intestine without any major effect on Ca absorption (Skoryna *et al.*, 1964; Waldron-Edward *et al.*, 1967).

11.5. TRANSPORT OF OTHER ALKALINE EARTHS

Information on the intestinal absorption of the other alkaline earths (Ba, Be, and Ra) is sparse. Schachter *et al.* (1960a) were the first to study Ba transport by the everted duodenal sac of the rat and found little evidence of active transport (S/M ratio of 1.2). Barium is absorbed in the ligated duodenal loops of the chicken but to a much lesser extent than Ca; vitamin D enhanced its absorption and increased its uptake by mucosal tissue (Wasserman, 1962, 1963). Barium is bound by CaBP but to a lesser extent than Ca and to a greater extent than Sr (Taylor and Wasserman, 1969; Wasserman *et al.*, 1968).

ACKNOWLEDGEMENTS

Supported in part by NIH grant AM 12184 and Dalton Research Center, University of Missouri. The author is indebted to Phyllis Strawn particularly, and to his son, Alexander L. Kenny. Their diligence in maintaining a literature retrieval system has made this review a much easier, and hopefully a more complete, task than would have been possible otherwise.

ADDENDUM

This review was completed September 1, 1970. Since that time rapid developments have occurred in some of the areas under discussion, but particularly in the area of Vitamin D metabolism. The reader is referred to Kenny and Dacke (in press) for additional information.

REFERENCES

ADAMS, T. H., WONG, R. G. and NORMAN, A. W. (1969) Vitamin D mediated calcium transport. *Fedn Proc. Fedn Am. Socs Exp. Biol.* **28**: 759. (Abstract.)

AIKAWA, J. K. and DAVID, A. P. (1969) ^{28}Mg studies in magnesium-deficient animals. *Ann. N.Y. Acad. Sci.* **162:** 744–757.

ALCOCK, N. and MACINTYRE, I. (1962) Inter-relation of calcium and magnesium absorption. *Clin. Sci.* **22:** 185–193.

ALCOCK, N. and MACINTYRE, I. (1964) Some effects of magnesium repletion on calcium metabolism in the rat. *Clin. Sci.* **26:** 219–225.

ANAST, C., KENNEDY, R., VOLK, G. and ADAMSON, L. (1964) Studies of active transport of calcium, magnesium and sulfate by the small intestine. *J. Pediat.* **65:** 1105. (Abstract.)

AUBERT, J.-P., BRONNER, F. and RICHELLE, L. J. (1963) Quantitation of calcium metabolism theory. *J. Clin. Invest.* **42:** 885–897.

AUBERT, J.-P., CHERIAN, A. G., MOUKHTAR, M. S. and MILHAUD, G. (1964) Etude du métabolisme du calcium chez le rat à l'aide de calcium 45. V. La thyroparathyroïdectomie et l'effet de la thyroxine et de la parathormone. *Biochem. Pharmac.* **13**: 31–44.

AVIOLI, L. V. (1969) Absorption and metabolism of vitamin D_3 in man. *Am. J. Clin. Nutr.* **22:** 437–446.

AVIOLI, L. V., BIRGE, S. J. and LEE, S. W. (1968b) Effects of prednisone on vitamin D metabolism in man. *J. Clin. Endocr. Metab.* **28:** 1341–1346.

AVIOLI, L. V., BIRGE, S., LEE, S. W. and SLATOPOLSKY, E. (1968a) The metabolic fate of vitamin D_3-^3H in chronic renal failure. *J. Clin. Invest.* **47:** 2239–2252.

AVIOLI, L. V., LEE, S. W., BIRGE, S. J., SLATOPOLSKY, E. and DELUCA, H. F. (1969b) The nature of the defect in intestinal calcium absorption in chronic renal disease. *J. Clin. Invest.* **48**: 4a. (Abstract.)

AVIOLI, L. V., LEE, S. W., MCDONALD, J. E., LUND, J. and DELUCA, H. F. (1967a) Metabolism of vitamin D_3–^3H in human subjects: distribution in blood, bile, feces and urine. *J. Clin. Invest.* **46:** 983–992.

AVIOLI, L. V., MCDONALD, J. E., SINGER, R. A. and HENNEMAN, P. H. (1965) A new oral isotopic test of calcium absorption. *J. Clin. Invest.* **44:** 128–139.

AVIOLI, L. V., SCOTT, S., LEE, S. W. and DELUCA, H. F. (1969a) Intestinal calcium absorption: nature of defect in chronic renal disease. *Science, N.Y.* **166:** 1154–1156.

AVIOLI, L. V., WILLIAMS, T. F., LUND, J. and DELUCA, H. F. (1967b) Metabolism of vitamin D_3-^3H in vitamin D-resistant rickets and familial hypophosphatemia. *J. Clin. Invest.* **46:** 1907–1915.

BATT, E. R. and SCHACHTER, D. (1969) Developmental pattern of some intestinal transport mechanisms in newborn rats and mice. *Am. J. Physiol.* **216:** 1064–1068.

BAUER, W., ALBRIGHT, F. and AUB, J. C. (1929) Studies of calcium and phosphorus metabolism. II. The calcium excretion of normal individuals on a low calcium diet, also data on a case of pregnancy. *J. Clin. Invest.* **7:** 75–96b.

BEDFORD, J., HARRISON, G. E., RAYMOND, W. H. A. and SUTTON, A. (1960) The metabolism of strontium in children. *Brit. Med. J.* **1:** 589–592.

BENSON, J. D., EMERY, R. S. and THOMAS, J. W. (1969) Effects of previous calcium intakes on adaptation to low and high calcium diets in rats. *J. Nutr.* **97:** 53–60.

BERGER, E. Y. (1960) Intestinal absorption and excretion, pp. 249–286. In: *Mineral Metabolism: An Advanced Treatise,* vol. 1, part A, COMAR, C. L. and BRONNER, F. (Eds.). Academic Press, New York.

BERGER, E. Y. (1963) Techniques for studying ion transfer across the alimentary tract, pp. 57–74. In: *The Transfer of Calcium and Strontium Across Biological Membranes,* WASSERMAN, R. H. (Ed.). Academic Press, New York.

BIRGE, S. J., PECK, W. A., BERMAN, M. and WHEDON, G. D. (1969) Study of calcium absorption in man: a kinetic analysis and physiologic model. *J. Clin. Invest.* **48:** 1705–1713.

BLAU, M., SPENCER, H., SWERNOV, H. and LASZLO, D. (1954) Utilization and intestinal excretion of calcium in man. *Science, N.Y.* **120:** 1029–1031.

BLUNT, J. W., DELUCA, H. F. and SCHNOES, H. K. (1968b) 25-Hydroxycholecalciferol. A biologically active metabolite of vitamin D_3. *Biochemistry, N.Y.* **7**: 3317–3322.

BLUNT, J. W., TANAKA, Y. and DELUCA, H. F. (1968a) The biological activity of 25-hydroxycholecalciferol, a metabolite of vitamin D_3. *Proc. Nat. Acad. Sci. U.S.A.* **61**: 1503–1506.

BOSMANN, H. B. and CHEN, P. S. (1966) Actinomycin D inhibition of vitamin D- and dihydrotachysterol-induced responses in the chick. *J. Nutr.* **90:** 405–415.

BRISCOE, A. M. and RAGAN, C. (1963) Enhancement of calcium absorption in man by a bile acid sequestrant. *Am. J. Clin. Nutr.* **13**: 277–284.

BRONNER, F. (1964) Dynamics and function of calcium, pp. 341–444. In: *Mineral Metabolism: An Advanced Treatise,* vol. II, part A, COMAR, C. L. and BRONNER, F. (Eds.). Academic Press, New York.

BRONNER, F. (1969) Calcium absorption. *Am. J. Clin. Nutr.* **22**: 376–380.

BRONNER, F. and AUBERT, J.-P. (1965) Bone metabolism and regulation of the blood calcium level in rats. *Am. J. Physiol.* **209:** 887–890.

BRONNER, F. and HARRIS, R. S. (1956) Absorption and metabolism of calcium in human beings, studied with calcium^{45}. *Ann. N.Y. Acad. Sci.* **64:** 314–325.

BRONNER, F., HARRIS, R. S., MELETSKOS, C. J. and BENDA, C. E. (1954) Studies in calcium metabolism. Effect of food phytates on calcium^{45} uptake in children on low-calcium breakfasts. *J. Nutr.* **54:** 523–542.

BRONNER, F., RICHELLE, L. J., SAVILLE, P. D., NICHOLAS, J. A. and COBB, J. R. (1963) Quantitation of calcium metabolism in postmenopausal osteoporosis and in scoliosis. *J. Clin. Invest.* **42:** 898–905.

BRUCE, R. S. (1963) Influence of calcium phosphate on the absorption of radioactive strontium. *Nature* (Lond.) **199:** 1107–1108.

CANIGGIA, A., GENNARI, C., BIANCHI, V. and GUIDERI, R. (1963) Intestinal absorption of ^{45}Ca in senile osteoporosis. *Acta Med. Scand.* **173:** 613–617.

CARE, A. D. (1967) Magnesium homeostasis in ruminants. *World Review of Nutrition and Dietetics* **8:** 127–142.

CARE, A. D. (1970) The effects of pancreozymin and secretin on calcitonin release. *Fedn Proc. Fedn Am. Socs. Exp. Biol.* **29**: 253. (Abstract.)

CARE, A. D., BRUCE, J. B., BOELKINS, J. N., KENNY, A. D., CONAWAY, H. H. and ANAST, C. A. (1971) The role of pancreozymin-cholecystokinin and structurally related compounds as calcitonin secretogogues. *Endocrinology* **89**: 262–271.

CARE, A. D. and KEYNES, W. M. (1964) The role of parathyroid hormones in the absorption of calcium and magnesium from the small intestine. *Proc. R. Soc. Med.* **57:** 867–868.

CARE, A. D. and VAN'T KLOOSTER, A. T. (1965) *In vivo* transport of magnesium and other cations across the wall of the gastrointestinal tract of sheep. *J. Physiol.* (Lond.) **177:** 174–191.

CARE, A. D., VOWLES, L. E., MANN, S. O. and ROSS, D. B. (1967) Factors affecting magnesium absorption in relation to the aetiology of acute hypomagnesaemia. *J. Agrie. Sci., Camb.* **68:** 195–204.

CARLSSON, A. (1954) The effect of vitamin D on the absorption of inorganic phosphate. *Acta Physiol. Scand.* **31:** 301–307.

CARR, T. E. F. (1967) An attempt to quantitate the short-term movement of strontium in the human adult, pp. 139–148. In: *Strontium Metabolism,* LENIHAN, J. M. A., LOUTIT, J. F. and MARTIN, J. H. (Eds.). Academic Press, New York.

CASEWELL, M. W. and FENNELL, R. H. (1970) Supernumerary parathyroid structures in the neck and thymus of parathyroidectomized rats and their relationship to recovery from hypocalcaemia. *Brit. J. Exp. Path.* **51:** 197–202.

CHANG, Y. O. and HEGSTED, D. M. (1964) Lactose and calcium transport in gut sacs. *J. Nutr.* **82:** 297–300.

CHUTKOW, J. G. (1964a) Sites of magnesium absorption and excretion in the intestinal tract of the rat. *J. Lab. Clin. Med.* **63:** 71–79.

CHUTKOW, J. G. (1964b) Metabolism of magnesium in the normal rat. *J. Lab. Clin. Med.* **63:** 80–99.

CHUTKOW, J. G. (1965) Studies on the metabolism of magnesium in the magnesium-deficient rat. *J. Lab. Clin. Med.* **65:** 912–926.

CLARK, I. (1965) Relation of magnesium ions to calcium and phosphate absorption. *Nature* (Lond.) **207:** 982.

CLARK, I. (1968) Effects of magnesium ions of calcium and phosphorus metabolism. *Am. J. Physiol.* **214:** 348–356.

CLARK, I. (1969a) Effects of magnesium on calcium and phosphate metabolism in parathyroidectomized rats. *Endocrinology* **85:** 1103–1113.

CLARK, I. (1969b) Metabolic interrelations of calcium, magnesium and phosphate. *Am. J. Physiol.* **217:** 871–878.

CLARK, I. and SMITH, M. R. (1964) Effects of parathyroidectomy and hydrocortisone on the intestinal absorption of calcium and phosphate. *Endocrinology* **74:** 421–428.

COATES, M. E., HARRISON, G. F. and HOLDSWORTH, E. S. (1961) The effect of a rachitogenic factor on calcium metabolism in chicks. *Brit. J. Nutr.* **15:** 149–155.

COATES, M. E. and HOLDSWORTH, E. S. (1961) Vitamin D_3 and absorption of calcium in the chick. *Brit. J. Nutr.* **15:** 131–147.

COMAR, C. L. (1956) Radiocalcium studies in pregnancy. *Ann. N.Y. Acad. Sci.* **64:** 281–298.

COMAR, C. L. (1967) Some principles of strontium metabolism: implications, applications, limitations, pp. 17–31. In: *Strontium Metabolism,* LENIHAN, J. M. A., LOUTIT, J. F. and MARTIN, J. H. (Eds.). Academic Press, New York.

COMAR, C. L., MONROE, R. A., VISEK, W. J. and HANSARD, S. L. (1953) Comparison of two isotope methods for determination of endogenous fecal calcium. *J. Nutr.* **50:** 459–467.

COMAR, C. L., RUSSELL, R. S. and WASSERMAN, R. H. (1967) Strontium–calcium movement from soil to man. *Science, N.Y.* **126:** 485–492.

COMAR, C. L. and WASSERMAN, R. H. (1964) Strontium, pp. 523–572. In: *Mineral Metabolism: An Advanced Treatise,* vol. II, part A, COMAR, C. L. and BRONNER, F. (Eds.). Academic Press, New York.

COMAR, C. L., WASSERMAN, R. H. and NOLD, M. M. (1956) Strontium–calcium discrimination in the rat. *Proc. Soc. Exp. Biol. Med.* **92:** 859–863.

COMAR, C. L., WASSERMAN, R. H., ULLBERG, S. and ANDREWS, G. A. (1957) Strontium metabolism and strontium–calcium discrimination in man. *Proc. Soc. Exp. Biol. Med.* **95:** 386–391.

CONAWAY, H. H., LEDDICOTTE, G. W. and KENNY, A. D. (1971) Neutron activation analysis of rat bone: simultaneous determination of calcium, chlorine, magnesium and sodium. *Analyt. Biochem.* **39:** 218–227.

CONRAD, H. R. and HANSARD, S. L. (1957) Effects of massive doses of vitamin D on physiological behavior of calcium in cattle. *J. Appl. Physiol.* **10:** 98–102.

COONS, C. M. and BLUNT, K. (1930) The retention of nitrogen, calcium, phosphorus, and magnesium by pregnant women. *J. Biol. Chem.* **86:** 1–16.

CORRADINO, R. A. and WASSERMAN, R. H. (1968) Actinomycin D inhibition of vitamin D_3-induced calcium-binding protein (CaBP) formation in chick duodenal mucosa. *Archs Biochem. Biophys.* **126:** 957–960.

CORRADINO, R. A. and WASSERMAN, R. H. (1970) Strontium inhibition of vitamin D_3-induced calcium-binding protein (CaBP) and calcium absorption in chick intestine. *Proc. Soc. Exp. Biol. Med.* **133:** 960–963.

CORRADINO, R. A., WASSERMAN, R. H., PUBOLS, M. H. and CHANG, S. I. (1968) Vitamin D_3 induction of a calcium-binding protein in the uterus of the laying hen. *Archs Biochem. Biophys.* **125:** 378–380.

COUSINS, R. J., DELUCA, H. F., SUDA, T., CHEN, T. and TANAKA, Y. (1970) Metabolism and subcellular location of 25-hydroxycholecalciferol in intestinal mucosa. *Biochemistry, N.Y.* **9:** 1453–1459.

CRAMER, C. F. (1963) Participation of parathyroid glands in control of calcium absorption in dogs. *Endocrinology* **72:** 192–196.

CRAMER, C. F. (1964) *In vivo* intestinal transport of calcium and water from solutions recycled through healed gut loops in dogs. *J. Nutr.* **84:** 118–124.

CRAMER, C. F. (1965) Sites of calcium absorption and the calcium concentration of gut contents in the dog. *Can. J. Physiol. Pharmac.* **43:** 75–78.

CRAMER, C. F. (1968) Effect of Ca/P ratio and pH on calcium and phosphorus absorption from dog gut loops *in vivo. Can. J. Physiol. Pharmac.* **46:** 171–173.

CRAMER, C. F. and COPP, D. H. (1959) Progress and rate of absorption of radiostrontium through intestinal tracts of rats. *Proc. Soc. Exp. Biol. Med.* **102:** 514–517.

CRAMER, C. F. and DUECK, J. (1962) *In vivo* transport of calcium from healed Thiry–Vella fistulas in dogs. *Am. J. Physiol.* **202:** 161–164.

CRAMER, C. F. and HAQQ, T. A. (1963) The effect of flow rate and osmolarity of lumen contents on calcium and water absorption from Thiry–Vella fistulas in dogs. *Can. J. Biochem. Physiol.* **41:** 127–130.

CRAMER, C. F., PARKES, C. O. and COPP, D. H. (1969) The effect of chicken and hog calcitonin on some parameters of Ca, P, and Mg metabolism in dogs. *Can. J. Physiol. Pharmac.* **47:** 181–184.

CRAMER, C. F., SUIKER, A. P. and COPP, D. H. (1961) Parathyroid influence on calcium and phosphorus absorption by the gut, pp. 158–166. In: *The Parathyroids*, GREEP, R. O. and TALMAGE, R. V. (Eds.). Charles C. Thomas, Springfield, Illinois.

CRANE, R. K. and MANDELSTAM, P. (1960) The active transport of sugars by various preparations of hamster intestine. *Biochem. Biophys. Acta* **45:** 460–476.

CRANE, R. K. and WILSON, T. H. (1958) *In vitro* method for the study of the rate of intestinal absorption of sugars. *J. Appl. Physiol.* **12:** 145–146.

CUISINIER-GLEIZES, P. and MATHIEU, H. (1969) Effet de la carence en potassium sur l'absorption intestinale du calcium chez le rat en croissance. *Revue fr. Etud. Clin. Biol.* **14:** 395–400.

CURTIS, F. K., FELLOWS, H. and RICH, C. (1967) Estimation of human calcium absorption by external radioisotope counting. *J. Lab. Clin. Med.* **69:** 1036–1041.

CZARNOWSKA-MISZTAL, E., ZULL, J. E. and DELUCA, H. F. (1966) Response to vitamin D in adrenalectomized animals. *Nature* (Lond.) **210:** 96–97.

DAVIS, G. K. (1963) Interactions of calcium with other nutrients in intestinal absorption, pp. 129–142. In: *The Transfer of Calcium and Strontium Across Biological Membranes*, WASSERMAN, R. H. (Ed.). Academic Press, New York.

DELUCA, H. F. (1967) Mechanism of action and metabolic fate of vitamin D. *Vitamins and Hormones* **25:** 315–367.

DELUCA, H. F. (1969a) 25-Hydroxycholecalciferol, the probable metabolically active form of vitamin D. *Am. J. Clin. Nutr.* **22:** 412–424.

DeLuca, H. F. (1969b) Recent advances in the metabolism and function of vitamin D. *Fedn Proc. Fedn Am. Socs Exp. Biol.* **28:** 1678–1689.

DeLuca, H. F. (1969c) Mechanism of action of 25-hydroxycholecalciferol: the active form of vitamin D. *Calcif. Tiss. Res.* **4:** 283. (Abstract.)

DeLuca, H. F. (1969d) 25-Hydroxycholecalciferol; the probable metabolically active form of vitamin D_3: its identification and subcellular site of action. *Archs Int. Med.* **124:** 442–450.

DeLuca, H. F., Weller, M., Blunt, J. W. and Neville, P. F. (1968) Synthesis, biological activity, and metabolism of 22,23-^{3}H-vitamin D_4. *Archs Biochem. Biophys.* **124:** 122–128.

Dowdle, E. B., Schachter, D. and Schenker, H. (1960) Requirement for vitamin D for the active transport of calcium by the intestine. *Am. J. Physiol.* **198:** 269–274.

Draper, H. H. (1963) The relationship of age and the intestinal absorption of calcium, pp. 97–105. In: *The Transfer of Calcium and Strontium Across Biological Membranes,* Wasserman, R. H. (Ed.). Academic Press, New York.

Drescher, D., DeLuca, H. F. and Imrie, M. H. (1969) On the site of discrimination of chicks against vitamin D_2. *Archs Biochem. Biophys.* **130:** 657–661.

Dumont, P. A., Curran, P. F. and Solomon, A. K. (1960) Calcium and strontium in rat small intestine, their fluxes and their effect on Na flux. *J. Gen. Physiol.* **43:** 1119–1136.

Duthie, H. L. (1967) Methods for studies of intestinal absorption in man. *Brit. Med. Bull.* **23:** 213–216.

Ebel, J. G. and Comar, C. L. (1968) Effect of dietary magnesium on strontium–calcium discrimination and incorporation into bone of rats. *J. Nutr.* **96:** 403–408.

Ebel, J. G., Taylor, A. N. and Wasserman, R. H. (1969) Vitamin D-induced calcium-binding protein of intestinal mucosa. Relation to vitamin D dose level and lag period. *Am. J. Clin. Nutr.* **22:** 431–436.

Field, A. C. (1961) Studies on magnesium in ruminant nutrition. 3. Distribution of ^{28}Mg in the gastrointestinal tract and tissues of sheep. *Brit. J. Nutr.* **15:** 349–359.

Finkelstein, J. D. and Schachter, D. (1962) Active transport of calcium by intestine: effects of hypophysectomy and growth hormone. *Am. J. Physiol.* **203:** 873–880.

Firschein, H. E. and Miller, O. P. (1966) Comparison of calcium-48 and carbon-14–proline as indicators of bone metabolism. *Nature* (Lond.), **212:** 1252–1253.

Forbes, R. M. (1963) Mineral utilization in the rat. I. Effects of varying dietary ratios of calcium, magnesium and phosphorus. *J. Nutr.* **80:** 321–326.

Fourman, P., Royer, P., Levell, M. J. and Morgan, D. B. (1968) *Calcium Metabolism and the Bone,* 2nd ed. Blackwell Scientific Publications, Oxford.

Fournier, P. and Susbielle, H. (1952a) Les échanges de calcium chez le rat au cours de la gestation, de la lactation et du sevrage. I. Influence d'un régime riche en calcium. *J. Physiol.* (Paris) **44:** 123–134.

Fournier, P. and Susbielle, H. (1952b) Les échanges de calcium chez le rat au cours de la gestation, de la lactation et du sevrage. II. Influence d'un régime pauvre en calcium. *J. Physiol.* (Paris) **44:** 575–590.

Friedland, J. A., Williams, G. A., Bowser, E. N., Henderson, W. J. and Hoffeins, E. (1965) Effect of hyperthyroidism on intestinal absorption of calcium in the rat. *Proc. Soc. Exp. Biol. Med.* **120:** 20–23.

Gershoff, S. N. and Hegsted, D. M. (1956) Effect of vitamin D and Ca:P ratios on chick gastrointestinal tract. *Am. J. Physiol.* **187:** 203–206.

Gershoff, S. N., Legg, M. A. and Hegsted, D. M. (1958) Adaptation to different calcium intakes in dogs. *J. Nutr.* **64:** 303–312.

Graham, L. A., Caesar, J. J. and Burgen, A. S. V. (1960) Gastrointestinal absorption and excretion of Mg^{28} in man. *Metabolism* **9:** 646–659.

Gran, F. C. (1960) *Studies on Calcium and Strontium-90 Metabolism in Rats.* Oslo University Press, Oslo.

GREENBERG, D. M. (1945) Studies in mineral metabolism with the aid of artificial radioactive isotopes. VIII. Tracer experiments with radioactive calcium and strontium on the mechanism of vitamin D action in rachitic rats. *J. Biol. Chem.* **157**: 99–104.

GREENWALD, E., SAMACHSON, J. and SPENCER, H. (1963) Effect of lactose on calcium metabolism in man. *J. Nutr.* **79**: 531–538.

GREEP, R. O. (1948) The physiology and chemistry of the parathyroid hormone, pp. 255–299. In: *The Hormones: Physiology, Chemistry and Applications,* vol. 1, PINCUS, G. and THIMANN, K. V. (Eds.). Academic Press, New York.

GRUSON, M., CERLAND, M., MIRAVET, L., PAUL, J. and HIOCO, D. (1970) Action de la calcitonine de porc sur le transfert *in vitro* du Ca 45 au niveau du duodénum de rat normal et thyroparathyroïdectomisé. *C. r. hebd. Séanc. Acad. Sci., Paris* **270**: 1014–1017.

HALLICK, R. B. and DELUCA, H. F. (1969) Vitamin D_3-stimulated template activity of chromatin from rat intestine. *Proc. Natn. Acad. Sci. U.S.A.* **63**: 528–531.

HAMILTON, J. W. and HOLDSWORTH, E. S. (1969) Calcium transport by the chick small intestine. The role of vitamin D_3, the mitochondria and binding protein. *Calcif. Tiss. Res.* **4**: 284. (Abstract.)

HANNA, S., HARRISON, M. T., MACINTYRE, I. and FRASER, R. (1961) Effects of growth hormone on calcium and magnesium metabolism. *Brit. Med. J.* **11**: 12–15.

HANSARD, S. L., COMAR, C. L. and DAVIS, G. K. (1954) Effects of age upon the physiological behavior of calcium in cattle. *Am. J. Physiol.* **177**: 383–389.

HANSARD, S. L. and CROWDER, H. M. (1957) The physiological behavior of calcium in the rat. *J. Nutr.* **62**: 325–339.

HANSARD, S. L. and PLUMLEE, M. P. (1954) Effects of dietary calcium and phosphorus levels upon the physiological behavior of calcium and phosphorus in the rat. *J. Nutr.* **54**: 17–31.

HARMEYER, J. and DELUCA, H. F. (1969) Calcium-binding protein and calcium absorption after vitamin D administration. *Archs Biochem. Biophys.* **133**: 247–254.

HARRIS, R. F. (1955) Phytic acid and its importance in human nutrition. *Nutr. Rev.* **13**: 257–259.

HARRISON, G. E., JONES, H. G. and SUTTON, A. (1957) The effects of carrier strontium on the absorption of oral doses of radioactive strontium in rats. *Brit. J. Pharmac. Chemother.* **12**: 336–339.

HARRISON, G. E., SUTTON, A., SHEPHERD, H. and WIDDOWSON, E. M. (1965) Strontium balance in breast-fed babies. *Brit. J. Nutr.* **19**: 111–117.

HARRISON, H. C. and HARRISON, H. E. (1969) Calcium transport by rat colon *in vitro. Am. J. Physiol.* **217**: 121–125.

HARRISON, H. C. and HARRISON, H. E. (1970) Dibutyryl cyclic AMP, vitamin D and intestinal permeability to calcium. *Endocrinology* **86**: 756–760.

HARRISON, H. E. and HARRISON, H. C. (1951) Studies with radiocalcium: the intestinal absorption of calcium. *J. Biol. Chem.* **188**: 83–90.

HARRISON, H. E. and HARRISON, H. C. (1960) Transfer of Ca^{45} across intestinal wall *in vitro* in relation to action of vitamin D and cortisol. *Am. J. Physiol.* **199**: 265–271.

HARRISON, H. E. and HARRISON, H. C. (1963a) Theories of vitamin D action, pp. 229–251. In: *The Transfer of Calcium and Strontium Across Biological Membranes*, WASSERMAN, R. H. (Ed.). Academic Press, New York.

HARRISON, H. E. and HARRISON, H. C. (1963b) Sodium, potassium, and intestinal transport of glucose, L-tyrosine, phosphate, and calcium. *Am. J. Physiol.* **205**: 107–111.

HARRISON, H. E. and HARRISON, H. C. (1965) Vitamin D and permeability of intestinal mucosa to calcium. *Am. J. Physiol.* **208**: 370–373.

HARRISON, H. E. and HARRISON, H. C. (1966) Actinomycin D inhibition of intestinal transport of calcium and of vitamin D action. *Proc. Soc. Exp. Biol. Med.* **121**: 312–317.

HAUSSLER, M. R., LITTLEDIKE, E. T., BOYCE, D. W. and RASMUSSEN, H. (1970) Separation of vitamin D metabolites by countercurrent distribution. *Fedn Proc. Fedn Am. Socs Exp. Biol.* **29**: 368Abs. (Abstract.)

HAUSSLER, M. R., MYRTLE, J. F. and NORMAN, A. W. (1968) The association of a metabolite of vitamin D_3 with intestinal mucosa chromatin *in vivo*. *J. Biol. Chem.* **243:** 4055–4064.

HAUSSLER, M. R. and NORMAN, A. W. (1967) The subcellular distribution of physiological doses of vitamin D_3. *Archs Biochem. Biophys.* **118:** 145–153.

HEANEY, R. P. and SKILLMAN, T. G. (1964) Secretion and excretion of calcium by the human gastrointestinal tract. *J. Lab. Clin. Med.* **64:** 29–41.

HEATON, F. W. and PARSONS, F. W. (1961) The metabolic effect of high magnesium intake. *Clin. Sci.* **21:** 273–284.

HEGGENESS, F. W. (1959) Effect of antibiotics on the gastrointestinal absorption of calcium and magnesium in the rat. *J. Nutr.* **68:** 573–582.

HELBOCK, H. J., FORTE, J. G. and SALTMAN, P. (1966) The mechanism of calcium transport by rat intestine. *Biochem. Biophys. Acta* **126:** 81–93.

HENDRIX, J. Z., ALCOCK, N. W. and ARCHIBALD, R. M. (1963) Competition between calcium, strontium, and magnesium for absorption in the isolated rat intestine. *Clin. Chem.* **9:** 734–744.

HENNEMAN, P. H., DEMPSEY, E. F., CARROLL, E. L. and ALBRIGHT, F. (1956) The cause of hypercalcuria in sarcoid and its treatment with cortisone and sodium phytate. *J. Clin. Invest.* **35:** 1229–1242.

HENRY, K. M. and KON, S. K. (1947) The effect of age and of the supply of phosphorus on the assimilation of calcium by the rat. *Biochem. J.* **41:** 169–176.

HENRY, K. M. and KON, S. K. (1953) The relationship between calcium retention and body stores of calcium in the rat: effect of age and of vitamin D. *Brit. J. Nutr.* **7:** 147–159.

HESP, R. and RAMSBOTTOM, B. (1965) Effect of sodium alginate in inhibiting uptake of radiostrontium by the human body. *Nature* (Lond.) **208:** 1341–1342.

HESP, R. and RAMSBOTTOM, B. (1967) Studies on the inhibition of radiostrontium uptake from the human gastrointestinal tract with sodium alginate, pp. 313–321. In: *Strontium Metabolism,* LENIHAN, J. M. A., LOUTIT, J. F. and MARTIN, J. H. (Eds.). Academic Press, New York.

HIRONAKA, R., DRAPER, H. H. and KASTELIC, J. (1960) Physiological aspects of aging. III. The influence of aging on calcium metabolism in rats. *J. Nutr.* **71:** 356–360.

HIRSCH, P. F., VOELKEL, E. F. and MUNSON, P. L. (1964) Thyrocalcitonin: hypocalcemic hypophosphatemic principle of the thyroid gland. *Science, N.Y.* **146:** 412–413.

HOLDSWORTH, E. S. (1965) Vitamin D_3 and calcium absorption in the chick. *Biochem. J.* **96:** 475–483.

HORSTING, M. and DELUCA, H. F. (1969) *In vitro* production of 25-hydroxycholecalciferol. *Biochem. Biophys. Res. Commun.* **36:** 251–256.

HORSTING, M. and DELUCA, H. F. (1970) Feed-back control of 25-hydroxycholecalciferol production. *Fedn Proc. Fedn Am. Socs Exp. Biol.* **29:** 542 Abs. (Abstract.)

HURWITZ, S. and BAR, A. (1965) Absorption of calcium and phosphorus along the gastro-intestinal tract of the laying fowl as influenced by dietary calcium and egg shell formation. *J. Nutr.* **86:** 433–438.

HURWITZ, S. and BAR, A. (1966a) Rate of passage of calcium-45 and yttrium-91 along the intestine, and calcium absorption in the laying fowl. *J. Nutr.* **89:** 311–316.

HURWITZ, S. and BAR, A. (1966b) Calcium depletion and repletion in laying hens. 1. Effect on calcium in various bone segments, in egg shells and in blood plasma, and on calcium balance. *Poult. Sci.* **45:** 345–352.

HURWITZ, S. and BAR, A. (1969) Intestinal calcium absorption in the laying fowl and its importance in calcium homeostasis. *Am. J. Clin. Nutr.* **22:** 391–395.

HURWITZ, S. and GRIMINGER, P. (1960) Observations on the calcium balance of laying hens. *J. Agric. Sci. Camb.* **54:** 373–377.

HURWITZ, S., HARRISON, H. C. and HARRISON, H. E. (1967) Effect of vitamin D_3 on the *in vitro* transport of calcium by the chick intestine *J. Nutr.* **91:** 319–323.

HYDÉN, S. (1955) A turbidimetric method for the determination of higher polyethylene glycols in biological materials. *Ann. Agric. Coll. Sweden* **22,** 139–145.

IMRIE, M. H., NEVILLE, P. F., SNELLGROVE, A. W. and DELUCA, H. F. (1967) Metabolism of vitamin D_2 and vitamin D_3 in the rachitic chick. *Archs Biochem. Biophys.* **120:** 525–532.

IRVING, J. T. (1957) *Calcium Metabolism,* Methuen, London.

JAWORSKI, Z. F., BROWN, E. M., FEDORUK, S. and SEITZ, H. (1963) A method for the study of calcium absorption by the human gut using a standard dose of calcium labeled with calcium^{47}. *New Engl. J. Med.* **269:** 1103–1111.

JONES, H. G. and MACKIE, W. S. (1959) The metabolism in sheep of the alkaline earth products of fission. The absorption and excretion of ^{45}Ca and ^{89}Sr by blackface wethers. *Brit. J. Nutr.* **13:** 355–362.

JONES, J. E., DESPER, P. C., SHANE, S. R. and FLINK, E. B. (1966) Magnesium metabolism in hyperthyroidism and hypothyroidism. *J. Clin. Invest.* **45:** 891–900.

KALLFELZ, F. A., TAYLOR, A. N. and WASSERMAN, R. H. (1967) Vitamin D-induced calcium-binding factor in rat intestinal mucosa. *Proc. Soc. Exp. Biol. Med.* **125:** 54–58.

KAWIN, B. (1959) Effects of stable calcium and strontium on deposition of calcium-45 and strontium-89 in bone. *Experientia* **15:** 313–314.

KENNY, A. D. (1960) Parathyroid glands and calcium metabolism, pp. 159–183. *World Review of Nutrition and Dietetics,* vol. 2, BOURNE, G. H. (Ed.). Pitman Medical Publishing Co., London.

KENNY, A. D. (1962) Survival and serum calcium levels of rats after parathyroidectomy. *Endocrinology* **70:** 715–722.

KENNY, A. D. (1969) Determination of plasma calcitonin by bioassay. *Pharmacologist* **11:** 252. (Abstract.)

KENNY, A. D. and DACKE, C. G. (in press) Parathyroid hormone and calcium metabolism. In: *World Review of Nutrition and Dietetics*, BOURNE, G. H. (Ed.). Hafner Publishing Co., New York.

KENNY, A. D. and HEISKELL, C. A. (1965) Effect of crude thyrocalcitonin on calcium and phosphorus metabolism in rats. *Proc. Soc. Exp. Biol. Med.* **120:** 269–271.

KESSNER, D. M. and EPSTEIN, F. H. (1965) Effect of renal insufficiency on gastrointestinal transport of calcium. *Am. J. Physiol.* **209:** 141–145.

KESSNER, D. M. and EPSTEIN, F. H. (1966) Effect of magnesium deficiency on gastrointestinal transfer of calcium. *Proc. Soc. Exp. Biol. Med.* **122:** 721–725.

KIDMAN, B., TUTT, M. and VAUGHAN, J. M. (1950) The retention and excretion of radioactive strontium and yttrium (Sr^{89}, Sr^{90} and Y^{90}) in the healthy rabbit. *J. Path. Bact.* **62:** 209–227.

KIMBERG, D. V. (1969) Effects of vitamin D and steroid hormones on the active transport of calcium by the intestine. *New Engl. J. Med.* **280:** 1396–1405.

KIMBERG, D. V., SCHACHTER, D. and SCHENKER, H. (1961) Active transport of calcium by intestine: effects of dietary calcium. *Am. J. Physiol.* **200:** 1256–1262.

KLEIBER, M. and LUICK, J. R. (1956) Calcium and phosphorus transfer in intact dairy cows. *Ann. N.Y. Acad. Sci.* **64:** 299–313.

KODICEK, E. (1956) Metabolic studies on vitamin D, pp. 161–172. In: *Ciba Foundation Symposium on Bone Structure and Metabolism,* WOLSTENHOLME, G. E. W. and O'CONNOR, C. M. (Eds.). Little, Brown & Co., Boston.

KODICEK, E., CRUICKSHANK, E. M., DELUCA, H. F. and RAISZ, L. G. (1964) Effects of vitamin D and parathyroidectomy on the absorption of Ca^{45} from *in vivo* loops of small intestine, p. 363. In: *Bone and Tooth,* BLACKWOOD, H. J. J. (Ed.). The Macmillan Company, New York. (Abstract.)

KOEFOED-JOHNSEN, V. and USSING, H. H. (1960) Ion transport, pp. 169–203. In: *Mineral Metabolism,* vol. 1, part A, COMAR, C. L. and BRONNER, F. (Eds.). Academic Press, New York.

KOSTIAL, K., LUTKIĆ, A., GURDEN, N., VOJVODIĆ, S. and HARRISON, G. E. (1963) The effect of dietary phosphorus on the metabolism of calcium and strontium in the rat. *Int. J. Radiat. Biol.* **6:** 431–439.

KOSTIAL, K., SIMONOVIĆ, I. and PISONIĆ, M. (1967) Effect of calcium and phosphates on gastrointestinal absorption of strontium and calcium in newborn rats. *Nature* (Lond.) **215:** 1181–1182.

KOSTIAL, K., VOJVODIĆ, S. and COMAR, C. L. (1965) Effects of dietary levels of phosphorus and calcium on the comparative behavior of strontium and calcium. *Nature* (Lond.) **208:** 1110–1111.

KOSTIAL, K., VOJVODIĆ, S., GRUDEN, N. and LUTKIĆ, A. (1964) Skeletal uptake of calcium-47 and strontium-85 as influenced by the phosphorus content of the diet, pp. 111–119. In: *Bone and Tooth,* BLACKWOOD, H. J. J. (Ed.). The Macmillan Company, New York.

KRAINTZ, L. and CRAMER, C. F. (1966) Lack of effect of thyrocalcitonin on calcium absorption from gut loops in the dog. *Program of the 48th Meeting of The Endocrine Society, Chicago,* p. 70. (Abstract.)

KRAWITT, E. L. (1967) Effect of thyrocalcitonin on duodenal calcium transport. *Proc. Soc. Exp. Biol. Med.* **125:** 1084–1086.

KRAWITT, E. L. and SCHEDL, H. P. (1968) *In vivo* calcium transport by rat small intestine. *Am. J. Physiol.* **214:** 232–236.

LAWSON, D. E. M., WILSON, P. W., BARKER, D. C. and KODICEK, E. (1969c) Isolation of chick intestinal nuclei. Effect of vitamin D_3 on nuclear metabolism. *Biochem. J.* **115:** 263–268.

LAWSON, D. E. M., WILSON, P. W. and KODICEK, E. (1969a) New vitamin D metabolite localized in intestinal cell nuclei. *Nature* (Lond.) **222:** 171–172.

LAWSON, D. E. M., WILSON, P. W. and KODICEK, E. (1969b) Metabolism of vitamin D. A new cholecalciferol metabolite, involving loss of hydrogen at C-1, in chick intestinal nuclei. *Biochem. J.* **115:** 269–277.

LEMAIRE, R. (1967) Modifications du métabolisme calcique avec l'âge. *C. r. Séanc. Soc. Biol.* **161:** 726–730.

LENGEMANN, F. W. (1959) The site of action of lactose in the enhancement of calcium utilization. *J. Nutr.* **69:** 23–27.

LENGEMANN, F. W. (1963) Over-all aspects of calcium and strontium absorption, pp. 85–96. In: *The Transfer of Calcium and Strontium Across Biological Membranes,* WASSERMAN, R. H. (Ed.). Academic Press, New York.

LENGEMANN, F. W. and COMAR, C. L. (1961) Distribution of absorbed strontium-85 and calcium-45 as influenced by lactose. *Am. J. Physiol.* **200:** 1051–1054.

LENGEMANN, F. W. and DOBBINS, J. W. (1958) The role of bile in calcium absorption. *J. Nutr.* **66:** 45–54.

LENGEMANN, F. W., WASSERMAN, R. H. and COMAR, C. L. (1959) Studies on the enhancement of radiocalcium and radiostrontium absorption by lactose in the rat. *J. Nutr.* **68:** 443–456.

LENIHAN, J. M. A., LOUTIT, J. E. and MARTIN, J. H. (1967) *Strontium Metabolism.* Academic Press, New York.

LEVIN, R. J. (1967) Techniques, terminology and parameters in intestinal absorption. *Brit. Med. Bull.* **23:** 209–212.

LIFSHITZ, F., HARRISON, H. C. and HARRISON, H. E. (1967a) Intestinal transport of calcium and phosphate in experimental magnesium deficiency. *Proc. Soc. Exp. Biol. Med.* **125:** 19–25.

LIFSHITZ, F., HARRISON, H. C. and HARRISON, H. E. (1967b) Response to vitamin D of magnesium deficient rats. *Proc. Soc. Exp. Biol. Med.* **125:** 472–476.

LIFSHITZ, F., HARRISON, H. C. and HARRISON, H. E. (1969) Influence of parathyroid function upon the *in vitro* transport of calcium and phosphate by the rat intestine. *Endocrinology* **84:** 912–917.

LOUGH, S. A., RIVERA, J. and COMAR, C. L. (1963) Retention of strontium, calcium, and phosphorus in human infants. *Proc. Soc. Exp. Biol. Med.* **112:** 631–636.

LUND, J. and DELUCA, H. F. (1966) Biologically active metabolite of vitamin D_3 from bone, liver, and blood serum. *J. Lipid Res.* **7:** 739–744.

MCALEESE, D. M., BELL, M. C. and FORBES, R. M. (1961) Magnesium-28 studies in lambs. *J. Nutr.* **74:** 505–514.

MACDONALD, N. S., SPAIN, P. C., EZMIRLIAN, F. and ROUNDS, D. E. (1955) The effects of calcium and phosphate in foods on radiostrontium accumulation. *J. Nutr.* **57:** 555–563.

MACGREGOR, R. R., HAMILTON, J. W. and COHN, D. V. (1970) The induction of calcium-binding protein biosynthesis in intestine by vitamin D_3. *Fedn Proc. Fedn Am. Socs Exp. Biol.* **29:** 368Abs. (Abstract.)

MACINTYRE, I. (1967) Magnesium metabolism. *Adv. Internal Med.* **13:** 143–154.

MACINTYRE, I., MATTHEWS, E. W. and ROBINSON, C. J. (1966) Parathyroid hormone and magnesium absorption. *J. Physiol.* (Lond.) **184:** 83P–84P.

MACINTYRE, I. and ROBINSON, C. J. (1969) Magnesium and the gut: experimental and clinical observations. *Ann. N.Y. Acad. Sci.* **162:** 865–873.

MACY, I. G., HUNSCHER, H. A., NIMS, B. and MCCOSH, S. S. (1930) Metabolism of women during the reproductive cycle. I. Calcium and phosphorus utilization in pregnancy. *J. Biol. Chem.* **86:** 17–35.

MALM, O. J. (1953) On phosphates and phosphoric acid as dietary factors in the calcium balance of man. *Scand. J. Clin. Lab. Invest.* **5:** 75–84.

MALM, O. J. (1958) *Calcium Requirement and Adaptation in Adult Men.* Oslo University Press, Oslo.

MARCUS, C. S. and LENGEMANN, F. W. (1962a) Use of radioyttrium to study food movement in the small intestine of the rat. *J. Nutr.* **76:** 179–182.

MARCUS, C. S. and LENGEMANN, F. W. (1962b) Absorption of Ca^{45} and Sr^{85} from solid and liquid food at various levels of the alimentary tract of the rat. *J. Nutr.* **77:** 155–160.

MARTIN, D. L. and DELUCA, H. F. (1969a) Influence of sodium on calcium transport by the rat small intestine. *Am. J. Physiol.* **216:** 1351–1359.

MARTIN, D. L. and DELUCA, H. F. (1969b) Calcium transport and the role of vitamin D. *Archs Biochem. Biophys.* **134:** 139–148.

MARTIN, D. L., MELANCON, M. J. and DELUCA, H. F. (1969) Vitamin D-stimulated, calcium-dependent adenosine triphosphatase from brush borders of rat small intestine. *Biochem. Biophys. Res. Commun.* **35:** 819–823.

MAWER, E. B., LUMB, G. A. and STANBURY, S. W. (1969) Long biological half-life of vitamin D_3 and its polar metabolites in human serum. *Nature* (Lond.) **222:** 482–483.

MAYER, G. P., RAMBERG, C. F. and KRONFELD, D. S. (1969) Calcium homeostasis in the cow. *Clin. Orthopaed.* **62:** 79–94.

MELANCON, M. J. (1970) Vitamin D-induced, calcium-dependent adenosine triphosphatase in chick intestinal brush borders. *Fedn Proc. Fedn Am. Socs Exp. Biol.* **29:** 268Abs. (Abstract.)

MELANCON, M. J. and DELUCA, H. F. (1970) Vitamin D stimulation of calcium-dependent adenosine triphosphatase in chick intestinal brush borders. *Biochemistry, N.Y.* **9:** 1658–1664.

MIGICOVSKY, B. B., NIELSON, A. M., GLUCK, M. and BURGESS, R. (1951) Penicillin and calcium absorption. *Archs Biochem. Biophys.* **34:** 479–480. (Abstract.)

MILHAUD, G. and MOUKHTAR, M. S. (1966) Thyrocalcitonin: effects on calcium kinetics in the rat. *Proc. Soe. Exp. Biol. Med.* **123:** 207–209.

MILHAUD, G., MOUKHTAR, M. S., CHERIAN, G. and PÉRAULT, A. M. (1966) Effet de l'administration du thyrocalcitonine sur les principaux paramètres du métabolisme de calcium du rat normal et du rat thyroparathyroïdectomisé. *C. r. hebd. Séanc. Acad. Sci. Paris* **262:** 511–514.

MILLER, E. R., ULLREY, D. E., ZUTAUT, C. L., HOEFER, J. A. and LUECKE, R. W. (1965a) Mineral balance studies with the baby pig: effects of dietary vitamin D_2 level upon calcium, phosphorus and magnesium balance. *J. Nutr.* **85**: 255–259.

MILLER, E. R., ULLREY, D. E., ZUTAUT, C. L., HOEFER, J. A. and LUECKE, R. L. (1965b) Comparisons of casein and soy proteins upon mineral balance and vitamin D_2 requirement of the baby pig. *J. Nutr.* **85**: 347–354.

MILLER, E. R., ULLREY, D. E., ZUTAUT, C. L., HOEFER, J. A. and LUECKE, R. W. (1965c) Mineral balance studies with the baby pig: effects of dietary magnesium level upon calcium, phosphorus and magnesium balance. *J. Nutr.* **86**: 209–212.

MOREHEAD, R. M. and KESSNER, D. M. (1969) Effects of Mg deficiency and parathyroidectomy on gastrointestinal Ca transport in the rat. *Am. J. Physiol.* **217**: 1608–1613.

MORII, H., LUND, J., NEVILLE, P. F. and DELUCA, H. F. (1967) Biological activity of a vitamin D metabolite. *Archs Biochem. Biophys.* **120**: 508–512.

MORIUCHI, S., WATANABE, T. and HOSOYA, N. (1970) Distribution of orally administered ^{45}Ca in rat intestinal tissues and vitamin D_3 effect. *J. Vitaminology* **16**: 58–63.

MORRISSEY, R. L. and WASSERMAN, R. H. (1970) Adaptation, calcium binding protein (CaBP) and the intestinal absorption of calcium. *Fedn Proc. Fedn Am. Socs Exp. Biol.* **29**: 847Abs. (Abstract.)

MRAZ, F. R. (1962) Intestinal absorption of Ca-45 and Sr-85 as affected by the alkaline earths and pH. *Proc. Soc. Exp. Biol. Med.* **110**: 273–275.

MUELLER, W. J., SCHRAER, R. and SCHRAER, H. (1964) Calcium metabolism and skeletal dynamics of laying pullets. *J. Nutr.* **84**: 20–26.

MUNSON, P. L., HIRSCH, P. F., TASHJIAN, A. H. and ALIAPOULIOS, M. A. (1966) Calcitonin and thyrocalcitonin; evaluation of hypocalcemic factors, pp. 467–480. In: *Methods in Drug Evaluation,* MANTEGAZZA, P. and PICCININI, F. (Eds.). North-Holland Publishing Co., Amsterdam.

NAGODE, L. A., HAUSSLER, M. R., BOYCE, D. W., PECHET, M. and RASMUSSEN, H. (1970) Vitamin D induced phosphatases in bone and intestine: inhibitions by theophylline and diphosphonates. *Fedn Proc. Fedn Am. Socs Exp. Biol.* **29**: 368Abs. (Abstract.)

NELSON, T. E., TAVERNOR, W. D., JONES, E. W. and TILLMAN, A. D. (1969) Influence of age and calcium-free diet on thyroparathyroidectomized sheep. *J. Nutr.* **97**: 359–366.

NEVILLE, E. and HOLDSWORTH, E. S. (1969) A "second messenger" for vitamin D. *Febs Letters* **2**: 313–316.

NEVILLE, P. F. and DELUCA, H. F. (1966) The synthesis of [1,2-^{3}H] vitamin D_3 and the tissue localization of a 0.25-μg (10 IU) dose per rat. *Biochemistry, N. Y.* **5**: 2201–2207.

NICOLAYSEN, R. (1943) The absorption of calcium as a function of the body saturation with calcium. *Acta Physiol. Scand.* **5**: 200–211.

NICOLAYSEN, R. (1956) Studies in calcium metabolism in rats. III. The adaption to low Ca intakes of old rats. *Acta Physiol. Scand.* **36**: 114–118.

NICOLAYSEN, R. and EEG-LARSEN, N. (1953) The biochemistry and physiology of vitamin D. *Vitamins and Hormones* **11**: 29–60.

NICOLAYSEN, R., EEG-LARSEN, N. and MALM, O. J. (1953) Physiology of calcium metabolism. *Physiol. Rev.* **33**: 424–444.

NOBLE, H. M. and MATTY, A. J. (1967) The effect of thyroxine on the movement of calcium and inorganic phosphate through the small intestine of the rat. *J. Endocr.* **37**: 111–117.

NORMAN, A. W. (1965) Actinomycin D and the response to vitamin D. *Science, N.Y.* **149**: 184–186.

NORMAN, A. W. (1966a) Actinomycin D effect on lag in vitamin D-mediated calcium absorption in the chick. *Am. J. Physiol.* **211**: 829–834.

NORMAN, A. W. (1966b) Vitamin D-mediated synthesis of rapidly labeled RNA from intestinal mucosa. *Biochem. Biophys. Res. Commun.* **23**: 335–340.

NORMAN, A. W., HAUSSLER, M. R., ADAMS, T. H., MYRTLE, J. F., ROBERTS, P. and HIBBERD, K. A. (1969) Basic studies on the mechanism of action of vitamin D. *Am. J. Clin. Nutr.* **22:** 396–411.

OLSON, E. B. and DELUCA, H. F. (1969) 25-Hydroxycholecalciferol: direct effect on calcium transport. *Science, N.Y.* **165:** 405–407.

PALMER, R. F., THOMPSON, R. C. and KORNBERG, H. A. (1958a) Effect of calcium on deposition of strontium-90 and calcium-45 in rats. *Science, N.Y.* **127:** 1505–1506.

PALMER, R. F., THOMPSON, R. C. and KORNBERG, H. A. (1958b) Factors affecting the relative deposition of strontium and calcium in the rat. *Science, N.Y.* **128:** 1505–1506.

PANSU, D., CHAPUY, M. C. and BERNARD, J. (1969) L'Absorption du calcium en présence de lactose chez des sujets ostéoporotiques intolérants ou non au lactose. *C. r. hebd. Séanc. Acad. Sci., Paris* **268:** 1310–1313.

PARSONS, D. S. and PATERSON, C. R. (1965) Fluid and solute transport across rat colonic mucosa. *Q. J. Exp. Physiol.* **50:** 220–231.

PATRICK, H. and BACON, J. A. (1957) The effect of vitamin D upon bone mineralization of Ca^{45} and Sr^{89} as chlorides and as phosphopeptides. *J. Biol. Chem.* **228:** 569–572.

PAUL, T. M., WALDRON-EDWARD, D. and SKORYNA, S. C. (1964) Studies on inhibition of intestinal absorption of radioactive strontium: II. Effects of administration of sodium alginate by orogastric intubation and feeding. *Can. Med. Ass. J.* **91:** 553–557.

PAYNE, J. M. and SANSOM, B. F. (1966) Calcium metabolism in normal and thyro-parathyroidectomized goats. *J. Physiol.* (Lond.) **184:** 433–443.

PENTO, J. T. (1970) A study of calcium transport in the small intestine of the rat. Ph.D. Thesis. University of Missouri.

PENTO, J. T. and KENNY, A. D. (1970) Mechanism of adaptation to calcium deprivation in the rat. *Program of the 52nd Meeting of The Endocrine Society, St. Louis,* p. 121. (Abstract.)

PHILLIPSON, A. T. and STORRY, J. E. (1965) The absorption of calcium and magnesium from the rumen and small intestine of the sheep. *J. Physiol.* (Lond.) **181:** 130–150.

PLUMLEE, M. P. (1953) Placental transfer of calcium in cattle and rats using radioactive $calcium^{45}$. Ph.D. Thesis. Purdue University.

PONCHON, G. and DELUCA, H. F. (1969a) Metabolites of vitamin D_3 and their biologic activity. *J. Nutr.* **99:** 157–167.

PONCHON, G. and DELUCA, H. F. (1969b) The role of the liver in the metabolism of vitamin D. *J. Clin. Invest.* **48:** 1273–1279.

PONCHON, G., KENNAN, A. L. and DELUCA, H. F. (1969) "Activation" of vitamin D by the liver. *J. Clin. Invest.* **48:** 2032–2037.

RAMBERG, C. F., PHANG, J. M. and KRONFELD, D. S. (1970) A compartmental model of calcium metabolism in cows, pp. 119–134. In: *Parturient Hypocalcemia,* ANDERSON, J. J. B. (Ed.). Academic Press, New York.

RASMUSSEN, H. (1959) The influence of parathyroid function upon the transport of calcium in isolated sacs of rat small intestine. *Endocrinology* **65:** 517–519.

RASMUSSEN, H., WALDORF, A., DZIEWIATKOWSKI, D. D. and DELUCA, H. F. (1963) Calcium exchange in isolated intestinal villi. *Biochem. Biophys. Acta* **75:** 250–256.

RAVEN, A. M., LENGEMANN, F. W. and WASSERMAN, R. H. (1960) Studies of the effect of lysine on the absorption of radiocalcium and radiostrontium by the rat. *J. Nutr.* **72:** 29–36.

REDDY, B. S., PLEASANTS, J. R. and WOSTMANN, B. S. (1968) Calcium, phosphorus and magnesium metabolism in germfree rats. *Fedn Proc. Fedn Am. Socs Exp. Biol.* **27:** 311. (Abstract.)

ROBINSON, C. J., MATTHEWS, E. W. and MACINTYRE, I. (1968) The effect of parathyroid hormone and thyrocalcitonin on the intestinal absorption of calcium and magnesium, pp. 279–282. In: *Les Tissus Calcifiés, Ve Symposium Européen, Bordeaux, France,* MILHAUD, G., OWEN, M. and BLACKWOOD, H. J. J. (Eds.). Société d'Edition d'Enseignement Supérieur, Paris.

ROSE, G. A., REED, G. W. and SMITH, A. H. (1965) Isotopic method for measurement of calcium absorption from the gastro-intestinal tract. *Brit. Med. J.* **1:** 690–692.

ROSS, D. B. (1961) Influence of sodium on the transport of magnesium across the intestinal wall of the rat *in vitro*. *Nature* (Lond.) **189:** 840–841.

ROSS, D. B. (1962) *In vitro* studies on the transport of magnesium across the intestinal wall of the rat. *J. Physiol.* (Lond.) **160:** 417–428.

ROSS, D. B. and CARE, A. D. (1962) The movement of $^{28}Mg^{2+}$ across the cell wall of guinea-pig small intestine *in vitro*. *Biochem. J.* **82:** 21p. (Abstract.)

ROTHSTEIN, A. (1968) Membrane phenomena. *A. Rev. Physiol.* **30:** 15–72.

ROTTENSTEN, K. V. (1938) The effect of body stores on the efficiency of calcium utilization. *Biochem. J.* **32:** 1285–1292.

SALLIS, J. D. and HOLDSWORTH, E. S. (1962a) Influence of vitamin D on calcium absorption in the chick. *Am. J. Physiol.* **203:** 497–505.

SALLIS, J. D. and HOLDSWORTH, E. S. (1962b) Calcium metabolism in relation to vitamin D_3 and adrenal function in the chick. *Am. J. Physiol.* **203:** 506–512.

SAMACHSON, J. (1963) Plasma values after oral ^{45}calcium and ^{85}strontium as an index of absorption. *Clin. Sci.* **25:** 17–26.

SAMMON, P. J., STACEY, R. E. and BRONNER, F. (1970) Role of parathyroid hormone in calcium homeostasis and metabolism. *Am. J. Physiol.* **218:** 479–485.

SCHACHTER, D. (1963) Vitamin D and the active transport of calcium by the small intestine, pp. 197–210. In: *The Transfer of Calcium and Strontium Across Biological Membranes*, WASSERMAN, R. H. (Ed.). Academic Press, New York.

SCHACHTER, D., DOWDLE, E. B. and SCHENKER, H. (1960a) Active transport of calcium by the small intestine of the rat. *Am. J. Physiol.* **198:** 263–268.

SCHACHTER, D., DOWDLE, E. B. and SCHENKER, H. (1960b) Accumulation of Ca^{45} by slices of the small intestine. *Am. J. Physiol.* **198:** 275–279.

SCHACHTER, D., FINKELSTEIN, J. D. and KOWARSKI, S. (1964) Metabolism of vitamin D. I. Preparation of radioactive vitamin D and its intestinal absorption in the rat. *J. Clin. Invest.* **43:** 787–796.

SCHACHTER, D., KIMBERG, D. V. and SCHENKER, H. (1961) Active transport of calcium by intestine: action and bio-assay of vitamin D. *Am. J. Physiol.* **200:** 1263–1271.

SCHACHTER, D. and KOWARSKI, S. (1965) Radioactive vitamin D: preparation, metabolism, and mechanism of action. *Bull. N.Y. Acad. Med.* **41:** 241. (Abstract.)

SCHACHTER, D., KOWARSKI, S., FINKELSTEIN, J. D. and MA, R. I. W. (1966) Tissue concentration differences during active transport of calcium by intestine. *Am. J. Physiol.* **211:** 1131–1136.

SCHACHTER, D., KOWARSKI, S. and REID, P. (1967) Molecular basis for vitamin D action in the small intestine. *J. Clin. Invest.* **46:** 1113–1114. (Abstract.)

SCHACHTER, D., KOWARSKI, S. and REID, P. (1970) Active transport of calcium by intestine: studies with a calcium activity electrode, pp. 108–123. In: *A Symposium on Calcium and Cellular Function*, CUTHBERT, A. W. (Ed.). St. Martin's Press, New York.

SCHACHTER, D. and ROSEN, S. M. (1959) Active transport of Ca^{45} by the small intestine and its dependence on vitamin D. *Am. J. Physiol.* **196:** 357–362.

SCHATZMANN, H. J. (1970) Transmembrane calcium movements in resealed human red cells, pp. 85–95. In: *A Symposium on Calcium and Cellular Function*, CUTHBERT, A. W. (Ed.). St. Martin's Press, New York.

SCHEDL, H. P., OSBALDISTON, G. W. and MILLS, I. H. (1968) Absorption, secretion, and precipitation of calcium in the small intestine of the dog. *Am. J. Physiol.* **214:** 814–819.

SCOTT, D. (1965) Factors influencing the secretion and absorption of calcium and magnesium in the small intestine of the sheep. *Quart. J. Exp. Physiol.* **50:** 312–328.

SERNKA, T. J. and BORLE, A. B. (1969) Calcium in the intestinal contents of rats on different calcium diets. *Proc. Soc. Exp. Biol. Med.* **131:** 1420–1423.

SHAH, B. G. and DRAPER, H. H. (1966) Depression of calcium absorption in parathyroidectomized rats. *Am. J. Physiol.* **211:** 963–966.
SHIMMINS, J., SMITH, D. A., NORDIN, B. E. C. and BURKINSHAW, L. (1967) A comparison between calcium-45 and strontium-85 absorption, excretion and skeletal uptake, pp. 149–159. In: *Strontium Metabolism,* LENIHAN, J. M. A., LOUTIT, J. F. and MARTIN, J. H. (Eds.). Academic Press, New York.
SIMKISS, K. (1967) *Calcium in Reproductive Physiology: A Comparative Study of Vertebrates.* Chapman & Hall, London.
SKORYNA, S. C., PAUL, T. M. and WALDRON-EDWARD, D. (1964) Studies on inhibition of intestinal absorption of radioactive strontium. I. Prevention of absorption from ligated intestinal segments. *Can. Med. Ass. J.* **91:** 285–288.
SKORYNA, S. C., PAUL, T. M. and WALDRON-EDWARD, D. (1965) Studies on inhibition of intestinal absorption of radioactive strontium. IV. Estimation of the suppressant effect of sodium alginate. *Can. Med. Ass. J.* **93:** 404–407.
SKOU, J. C. (1965) Enzymatic basis for active transport of Na+ and K+ across cell membrane. *Physiol. Rev.* **45:** 596–617.
SMITH, R. H. (1959) Absorption of magnesium in the large intestine of the calf. *Nature* (Lond.) **184:** 821–822.
SMITH, R. H. (1961) Importance of magnesium in the control of plasma calcium in the calf. *Nature* (Lond.) **191:** 181–182.
SMITH, R. H. (1962) Net exchange of certain inorganic ions and water in the alimentary tract of the milk-fed calf. *Biochem. J.* **83:** 151–163.
SMITH, R. H. (1963) Small intestine transit time and magnesium absorption in the calf. *Nature* (Lond.) **198:** 161–162.
SPENCER, H., LEWIN, I., FOWLER, J. and SAMACHSON, J. (1969) Effect of sodium fluoride on calcium absorption and balances in man. *Am. J. Clin. Nutr.* **22:** 381–390.
SPENCER, H., LEWIN, I. and SAMACHSON, J. (1967a) Effect of thyroid and parathyroid function on radiostrontium absorption. *Fedn Proc. Fedn Am. Socs Exp. Biol.* **25:** 368. (Abstract.)
SPENCER, H., LEWIN, I. and SAMACHSON, J. (1967b) Influence of dietary and hormonal factors on radiostrontium metabolism in man, pp. 111–129. In: *Strontium Metabolism,* LENIHAN, J. M. A., LOUTIT, J. F. and MARTIN, J. H. (Eds.). Academic Press, New York.
SPENCER, H., LI, M. and SAMACHSON, J. (1961) Effect of high calcium intake on strontium-85 metabolism in man. *J. Clin. Invest.* **40:** 1339–1345.
SPENCER, H., LI, M., SAMACHSON, J. and LASZLO, D. (1960) Metabolism of strontium-85 and calcium-45 in man. *Metabolism* **9:** 916–925.
SPENCER, H., MENCZEL, J., LEWIN, I. and SAMACHSON, J. (1964a) Absorption of calcium in osteoporosis. *Am. J. Med.* **37:** 223–234.
SPENCER, H., MENCZEL, J., LEWIN, I. and SAMACHSON, J. (1965) Effect of high phosphorus intake on calcium and phosphorus metabolism in man. *J. Nutr.* **86:** 125–132.
SPENCER, H., MENCZEL, J. and SAMACHSON, J. (1964b) Effect of high phosphorus intake on Sr^{85} excretions in man. *Proc. Soc. Exp. Biol. Med.* **117:** 59–63.
SPENCER, H. and SAMACHSON, J. (1963) Effect of lysine on calcium metabolism in man. *J. Nutr.* **81:** 301–306.
SPIRICHEV, V. B. and BLAZHEVICH, N. V. (1966) Inhibitory effect of vitamin D_2 on adenosinetriphosphatase activity. *Nature* (Lond.) **212:** 203–204.
STEWART, J. and MOODIE, E. W. (1956) The absorption of magnesium from the alimentary tract of sheep. *J. Comp. Path. Therap.* **66:** 10–21.
STOHS, S. J. and DELUCA, H. F. (1967) Subcellular location of vitamin D and its metabolites in intestinal mucosa after a 10-IU dose. *Biochemistry, N.Y.* **6:** 3338–3349.
STOHS, S. J., ZULL, J. E. and DELUCA, H. F. (1967) Vitamin D stimulation of [^{3}H] orotic acid incorporation into ribonucleic acid of rat intestinal mucosa. *Biochemistry, N.Y.* **6:** 1304–1310.

SUDA, T., DELUCA, H. F., SCHNOES, H. K. and BLUNT, J. W. (1969a) The isolation and identification of 25-hydroxyergocalciferol. *Biochemistry, N.Y.* **8:** 3515–3520.

SUDA, T., DELUCA, H. F., SCHNOES, H. and BLUNT, J. W. (1969b) 25-Hydroxyergocalciferol: a biologically active metabolite of vitamin D_2. *Biochem. Biophys. Res. Commun.* **35:** 182–185.

TALMAGE, R. V. and ELLIOTT, J. R. (1958) Influence of parathyroids on intestinal absorption of radiocalcium and radiostrontium. *Fedn Proc. Fedn Am. Socs Exp. Biol.* **17:** 160. (Abstract.)

TAYLOR, A. N. and WASSERMAN, R. H. (1965) A vitamin D_3-dependent factor influencing calcium binding by homogenates of chick intestinal mucosa. *Nature* (Lond.) **205:** 248–250.

TAYLOR, A. N. and WASSERMAN, R. H. (1967) A vitamin D_3-induced calcium-binding protein: partial purification, electrophoretic visualization, and tissue distribution. *Archs Biochem. Biophys.* **119:** 536–540.

TAYLOR, A. N. and WASSERMAN, R. H. (1969) Correlations between the vitamin D-induced calcium-binding protein and intestinal absorption of calcium. *Fedn Proc. Fedn Am. Socs Exp. Biol.* **28:** 1834–1838.

TAYLOR, A. N. and WASSERMAN, R. H. (1970a) Immunofluorescent localization of vitamin D-dependent calcium-binding protein. *J. Histochem. Cytochem.* **18:** 107–115.

TAYLOR, A. N. and WASSERMAN, R. H. (1970b) Vitamin D stimulation of calcium-binding protein and brush border enzyme activities. *Fedn Proc. Fedn Am. Socs Exp. Biol.* **29:** 368Abs. (Abstract.)

TAYLOR, A. N., WASSERMAN, R. H. and JOWSEY, J. (1968) A vitamin D-dependent calcium-binding protein in canine intestinal mucosa. *Fedn Proc. Fedn Am. Socs Biol.* **27:** 675. (Abstract.)

TAYLOR, D. M. (1967) The role of oxidative phosphorylation in calcium and strontium absorption from the gastro-intestinal tract, pp. 175–179. In: *Strontium Metabolism*, LENIHAN, J. M. A., LOUTIT, J. F. and MARTIN, J. H. (Eds.). Academic Press, New York.

THOMPSON, W. G. and THOMPSON, G. R. (1969) Effect of cholestyramine on the absorption of vitamin D_3 and calcium. *Gut* **10:** 717–722.

TOVERUD, S. U. (1964) Parathyroid effect on intestinal absorption of calcium and on secretion of calcium with the digestive juices in vitamin D-deficient rats. *Acta Physiol. Scand.* **62:** Suppl. 234, 1–31.

TRUMMEL, C. L., RAISZ, L. G., BLUNT, J. W. and DELUCA, H. F. (1969) 25-Hydroxycholecalciferol: stimulation of bone resorption in tissue culture. *Science, N.Y.* **163:** 1450–1451.

UNDERWOOD, E., FISCH, S. and HODGE, H. C. (1951) Metabolism of calcium in normal, rachitic and vitamin D-treated rats as evidenced by radiocalcium Ca^{45} studies. *Am. J. Physiol.* **166:** 387–393.

URBAN, E. and SCHEDL, H. P. (1969) Comparison of *in vivo* and *in vitro* effects of vitamin D on calcium transport in the rat. *Am. J. Physiol.* **217:** 126–130.

URBAN, E. and SCHEDL, H. P. (1970) Effect of vitamin D on tissue calcium of rat duodenum. *Scand. J. Gastroent.* **5:** 33–37.

USSING, H. H. (1949) The distinction by means of tracers between active transport and diffusion. The transfer of iodide across the isolated frog skin. *Acta Physiol. Scand.* **19:** 43–56.

USSING, H. H. and ZERAHN, K. (1951) Active transport of sodium as the source of electric current in the short-circuited isolated frog skin. *Acta Physiol. Scand.* **23:** 110–127.

VAN DYKE, J. H. (1959) Aberrant parathyroid tissue and the thymus: postnatal development of accessory parathyroid glands in the rat. *Anat. Rec.* **134:** 185–203.

VAUGHAN, O. W. and FILER, L. J. (1960) The enhancing action of certain carbohydrates on the intestinal absorption of calcium in the rat. *J. Nutr.* **71:** 10–14.

VISEK, W. J., MONROE, R. A., SWANSON, E. W. and COMAR, C. L. (1953) Calcium metabolism in dairy cows as studies with Ca^{45}. *J. Dairy Sci.* **36:** 373–384.
VOLF, V. (1965) Effect of phosphates, carbonates, and magnesium oxide upon the intestinal absorption of Sr-85 in rats. *Experientia* **21:** 571–572.
WALDRON-EDWARD, D., PAUL, T. M. and SKORYNA, S. C. (1964) Studies on the inhibition of intestinal absorption of radioactive strontium. III. The effect of administration of sodium alginate in food and in drinking water. *Can. Med. Ass. J.* **91:** 1006–1010.
WALDRON-EDWARD, D., PAUL, T. M. and SKORYNA, S. C. (1966) Effects of the counter ion and pH on intestinal absorption of calcium and strontium. *Proc. Soc. Exp. Biol. Med.* **123:** 532–538.
WALDRON-EDWARD, D., PAUL, T. M. and SKORYNA, S. C. (1967) Inhibition of absorption of radioactive strontium by alginic acid derivatives, pp. 329–340. In: *Strontium Metabolism,* LENIHAN, J. M. A., LOUTIT, J. F. and MARTIN, J. H. (Eds.). Academic Press, New York.
WALKER, A. R. P., FOX, F. W. and IRVING, J. T. (1948) Studies in human mineral metabolism. I. The effect of bread rich in phytate phosphorus on the metabolism of certain mineral salts with special reference to calcium. *Biochem. J.* **42:** 452–462.
WALLING, M. W. and ROTHMAN, S. S. (1969) Phosphate-independent, carrier-mediated active transport of calcium by rat intestine. *Am. J. Physiol.* **217:** 1144–1148.
WALSER, M. (1967) Magnesium metabolism. *Ergb. Physiol. Biol. Chim. Exp. Pharmakol.* **59:** 185–341.
WASE, A. W., PETERSON, A., RICKES, E. and SOLEWSKI, J. (1966) Some effects of thyrocalcitonin on the calcium metabolism of the rat. *Endocrinology* **79:** 687–691.
WASSERMAN, R. H. (1960) Metabolic basis of calcium and strontium discrimination: studies with surviving intestinal segments. *Proc. Soc. Exp. Biol. Med.* **104**: 92–95.
WASSERMAN, R. H. (1962) Studies on vitamin D_3 and the intestinal absorption of calcium and other ions in the rachitic chick. *J. Nutr.* **77**: 69–80.
WASSERMAN, R. H. (1963) Vitamin D and the absorption of calcium and strontium *in vivo,* pp. 211–228. In: *The Transfer of Calcium and Strontium Across Biological Membranes,* WASSERMAN, R. H. (Ed.). Academic Press, New York.
WASSERMAN, R. H. (1964) Lactose-stimulated intestinal absorption of calcium: a theory. *Nature* (Lond.) **201**: 997–999.
WASSERMAN, R. H. (1968) Calcium transport by the intestine: a model and comment on vitamin D action. *Calcif. Tiss. Res.* **2:** 301–313.
WASSERMAN, R. H. and COMAR, C. L. (1959) Carbohydrates and gastrointestinal absorption of radiostrontium and radiocalcium in the rat. *Proc. Soc. Exp. Biol. Med.* **101**: 314–317.
WASSERMAN, R. H. and COMAR, C. L. (1960) Effect of dietary calcium and phosphorus levels on body burdens of ingested radiostrontium. *Proc. Soc. Exp. Biol. Med.* **103:** 124–129.
WASSERMAN, R. H. and COMAR, C. L. (1961) The parathyroids and the intestinal absorption of calcium, strontium and phosphate ions in the rat. *Endocrinology* **69:** 1074–1079.
WASSERMAN, R. H., COMAR, C. L. and NOLD, M. M. (1956) The influence of amino acids and other organic compounds on the gastrointestinal absorption of $calcium^{45}$ and $strontium^{89}$ in the rat. *J. Nutr.* **59:** 371–383.
WASSERMAN, R. H., COMAR, C. L. and PAPADOPOULOU, D. (1957b) Dietary calcium levels and retention of radiostrontium in the growing rat. *Science, N.Y.* **126:** 1180–1182.
WASSERMAN, R. H., COMAR, C. L., SCHOOLEY, J. C. and LENGEMANN, F. W. (1957a) Interrelated effects of L-lysine and other dietary factors on the gastrointestinal absorption of calcium 45 in the rat and chick. *J. Nutr.* **62:** 367–376.
WASSERMAN, R. H., CORRADINO, R. A. and TAYLOR, A. N. (1968) Vitamin D-dependent calcium-binding protein: purification and some properties. *J. Biol. Chem.* **243:** 3978–3986.

WASSERMAN, R. H., CORRADINO, R. A. and TAYLOR, A. N. (1969) Binding proteins from animals with possible transport function. *J. Gen. Physiol.* **54:** 114s–137s.

WASSERMAN, R. H. and KALLFELZ, F. A. (1962) Vitamin D_3 and unidirectional calcium fluxes across the rachitic chick duodenum. *Am. J. Physiol.* **203:** 221–224.

WASSERMAN, R. H. and KALLFELZ, F. A. (1970) Transport of calcium across biological membranes, pp. 313–345. In: *Biological Calcification. Cellular and Molecular Aspects,* SCHRAER, H. (Ed.). Appleton-Century-Crofts, New York.

WASSERMAN, R. H., KALLFELZ, F. A. and COMAR, C. L. (1961) Active transport of calcium by rat duodenum *in vivo. Science, N.Y.* **133:** 883–884.

WASSERMAN, R. H. and LENGEMANN, F. W. (1960) Further observations on lactose stimulation of the gastrointestinal absorption of calcium and strontium in the rat. *J. Nutr.* **70:** 377–384.

WASSERMAN, R. H. and TAYLOR, A. N. (1963a) The non-essentiality of sodium ions for intestinal calcium transport. *Proc. Soc. Exp. Biol. Med.* **114:** 479–482.

WASSERMAN, R. H. and TAYLOR, A. N. (1963b) Vitamin D_3 inhibition of radiocalcium binding by chick intestinal homogenates. *Nature* (Lond.) **198:** 30–32.

WASSERMAN, R. H. and TAYLOR, A. N. (1966) Vitamin D_3-induced calcium-binding protein in chick intestinal mucosa. *Science, N.Y.* **152:** 791–793.

WASSERMAN, R. H. and TAYLOR, A. N. (1968) Vitamin D-dependent calcium-binding protein: response to some physiological and nutritional variables. *J. Biol. Chem.* **243:** 3987–3993.

WASSERMAN, R. H. and TAYLOR, A. N. (1969) Some aspects of the intestinal absorption of calcium with special reference to vitamin D, pp. 321–403. In: *Mineral Metabolism: An Advanced Treatise,* vol. III, COMAR, C. L. and BRONNER, F. (Eds.). Academic Press, New York.

WASSERMAN, R. H., TAYLOR, A. N. and KALLFELZ, F. A. (1966) Vitamin D and transfer of plasma calcium to intestinal lumen in chicks and rats. *Am. J. Physiol.* **211:** 419–423.

WEBLING, D. D'A. and HOLDSWORTH, E. S. (1965) The effect of bile, bile acids and detergents on calcium absorption in the chick. *Biochem. J.* **97:** 408–421.

WEBLING, D. D'A. and HOLDSWORTH, E. S. (1966) Bile salts and calcium absorption. *Biochem. J.* **100:** 652–660.

WENSEL, R. H., RICH, C., BROWN, A. C. and VOLWILER, W. (1969) Absorption of calcium measured by intubation and perfusion of the intact human small intestine. *J. Clin. Invest.* **48:** 1768–1775.

WILLIAMS, G. A., BOWSER, E. N., HENDERSON, W. J. and UZGIRIES, V. (1961) Effects of vitamin D and cortisone on intestinal absorption of calcium in the rat. *Proc. Soc. Exp. Biol. Med.* **106:** 664–666.

WILLIAMS, G. A., BOWSER, E. N., HENDERSON, W. J. and UZGIRIES, V. (1962) Calcium absorption in the rat in relation to excessive vitamin D and cortisone. *Proc. Soc. Exp. Biol. Med.* **110:** 889–892.

WILSON, T. H. (1962) *Intestinal Absorption.* Saunders, Philadelphia.

WILSON, T. H. and WISEMAN, G. (1954) The use of sacs of everted small intestine for the study of the transference of substances from the mucosal to the serosal surface. *J. Physiol.* (Lond.) **123:** 116–125.

WINTER, M., MORAVA, E. and SIMON, G. (1969) Effect of cortisone on the intestinal absorption of calcium in rats. *Med. Exp.* **19:** 52–57.

WINTER, M., MORAVA, E., SIMON, G. and SÓS, J. (1970) The role of the parathyroid glands in the absorption of calcium from the small intestine. *J. Endocr.* **47:** 65–72.

ZULL, J. E., CZARNOWSKA-MISZTAL, E. and DELUCA, H. F. (1965) Actinomycin D inhibition of vitamin D action. *Science, N.Y.* **149:** 182–184.

ZULL, J. E., CZARNOWSKA-MISZTAL, E. and DELUCA, H. F. (1966) On the relationship between vitamin D action and actinomycin-sensitive processes. *Proc. Natn. Acad. Sci., U.S.A.* **55:** 177–184.

CHAPTER 12

GASTROINTESTINAL ABSORPTION OF HEAVY METALS*

W. Forth, *Bochum*, and W. Rummel, *Homburg/Saar*

Federal Republic of Germany

INTRODUCTION

The subject of this chapter is the absorption of heavy metals of biological and toxicological interest. These metals differ from alkali metals primarily because they are not ionized at the hydrogen ion concentrations prevailing in biological media; instead, depending on their coordination numbers, they are bound to ligands. Water molecules are the simplest ligands which form aquo-ions with heavy metals. Other ligands can occupy the coordination sites, especially if the resulting complexes are thermodynamically more stable than the aquo-ions. Amino acids and polybasic hydroxy acids are the most common ligands found in biological media.

The consequences arising from these properties of the heavy metals, compared with those of the alkali and alkaline earth metals, can be illustrated by their behavior in blood plasma (Williams, 1966). The *alkali metals,* viz. sodium and potassium, are completely ionized in plasma. Of the *alkaline earth metals*, viz. calcium and magnesium, about half is ionized while the remainder is relatively loosely bound to plasma proteins and also to phosphoric and carboxylic acids. By contrast, none of the three, biologically most important, *heavy metals* (biometals) in the plasma, i.e. iron, copper and zinc, are ionized to any appreciable extent; these metals are partly bound to specific proteins (Fe to transferrin, Cu to ceruloplasmin), and partly bound unspecifically to proteins, principally albumins. It is likely that low molecular compounds of these

* Investigations by the authors' laboratory were supported by a grant of the Sonderforschungsbereich 38, "membrane research" at the University of the Saarland, Federal Republic of Germany.

metals also exist in the plasma; thus, amino acid complexes of copper (Neumann and Sass-Kortsak, 1967; Sarkar and Kruck, 1966) and iron (Prasad and Oberleas, 1971) have been identified.

Clearly this capacity of heavy metals to form coordination compounds entails a number of consequences after oral administration. Firstly, their *availability* for absorption from the intestinal lumen could be affected and secondly, the *absorption process,* i.e. the transfer across the mucosal cells, can be influenced. Accordingly, the absorption of a heavy metal is governed more by the rate of association with and dissociation from intraluminal and intracellular ligand systems than by the rate of the free diffusion of metal ions. It is very difficult to obtain information about the intracellular ligands which are significant for the transcellular movement.

Comparing the distance which a metal travels along the gastrointestinal tract to the site of absorption, the final passage across the mucosal epithelium into the blood seems to be negligible. It must, however, be remembered that this distance, along which the absorption actually takes place, is, for instance, 100,000 to 200,000 times the diameter of the bivalent iron ion.

This introductory consideration leads to the following division of this chapter. The first part deals with the *intraluminal factors* that determine mainly the *availability* of the metals for absorption, i.e. the interaction between the metals and the gut contents. In the second part the *absorption process,* i.e. *uptake into the cells* and *transfer across the cells* of the mucosal epithelium into the blood, is discussed.

In literature there is little information about the absorption of toxicologically interesting heavy metals. By contrast, numerous investigations dealing with the biometals iron, copper and zinc are available. Special attention is, therefore, paid to the last-mentioned metals and an attempt is made to draw general conclusions regarding the absorption of heavy metals.

12.1. INTRALUMINAL FACTORS INFLUENCING ABSORPTION

12.1. AVAILABILITY FOR ABSORPTION; METHODOLOGICAL CONSIDERATIONS

Intraluminal factors, e.g. concentration of hydrogen ions and food constituents, influence the solubility of the heavy metals and thereby their availability for absorption.

Evidently for the evaluation of the contradictory data in literature concerning the availability of heavy metals the precise description of the methods used is a prerequisite. Obviously, the availability will vary depending on whether a metal is administered orally or is injected directly in a tied-off gut segment.

Also the parameter chosen for assessing the availability of the metal is important. Very often the quantity retained cannot be measured directly and the absorption has to be determined by assessing the biological action of the metal in the organism. Schultze *et al.* (1934, 1936), for example, observed that copper hematoporphyrin remained inactive in the anemic animal as measured by the hemoglobin synthesis, whereas other copper compounds produced a favorable effect. However, no conclusion can be drawn regarding the absorption of copper hematoporphyrin. Probably this complex is absorbed from the gut just like iron hematoporphyrin (see pp. 632–633). *Unlike* the iron complex, which can be utilized in hemoglobin synthesis, the copper of the hematoporphyrin complex does apparently not participate in the formation of cytochrome oxidase, an enzyme which plays a key role in the synthesis of hemoglobin. Such indirect methods were commonly used before the introduction of radioisotopes.

Very often the metal content of an organ, e.g. the liver, is used as a measure of metal availability after feeding. Erroneous results may occur if different compounds of a metal, e.g. organic salts and complexes, are compared. Variations in the elimination and distribution of different compounds in the organism are responsible for differences in the organ contents and, therefore, it is not justified in this case to draw any conclusions concerning the availability of the metal for absorption.

Finally, it must be pointed out that the *metabolic utilization* of biometals varies according to the demands of the body. Metabolic utilization may be measured by repair of a deficiency-state, e.g. the increase in blood hemoglobin following administration of iron. In a deficiency-state the utilization of the biometals offered in the food, i.e. the *absorptive utilization* by the gut, is increased. This is known, not only for iron (for references see Forth *et al.*, 1968c) but also for copper (for references see Van Campen, 1971; Kirchgessner *et al.*, 1973) and for zinc (for references see Becker and Hoekstra, 1971; Kirchgessner *et al.*, 1973). Direct evidence showed that, despite the equal amounts of iron complexes transferred in intestinal segments of normal and iron-deficient rats *in vitro* (cf. Table 29; Forth *et al.*, 1965c), the absorptive utilization of oral iron *in vivo* in the gastro-intestinal tract of anemic rats is remarkably greater than that in normal animals (Forth *et al.*, 1968c). These critical considerations on methods used may help to understand why there are so many conflicting data in the literature.

12.1.2. AVAILABILITY AND CHEMICAL STATE

It is well known that the solubility of a metal in the intraluminal medium is a prerequisite for absorption from the gastrointestinal tract. For example, metallic mercury administered orally is known to produce practically no symptoms of poisoning because of its slight solubility. Systematic investigations on the absorption of metals in different chemical forms have been carried out by Chapman and Bell (1963) and Schultze *et al.* (1934, 1936) for copper, and by Roberson and Schaible (1960) for zinc. These studies show that the availability of a metal for absorption increases with the solubility of the dosage form. This holds true only for

TABLE 1. THE SOLUBILITY OF SOME HEAVY METAL SALTS IN WATER

Numbers represent the – log of the solubility product (*SP*) at 25°C. The higher the – log *SP*, the less soluble is the metal salt. Values are either means or ranges from different measurements. Sol. = soluble. Values from Sillen and Martell (1964) and from Phillips and Williams (1965)

Cations	Anions						Fe(II)-CN_6^{4-}	SCN^-
	OH^-	Cl^-	I^-	CO_3^{2-}	PO_4^{3-}	S^{2-}		
Cr^{2+}	17–20	—	—	—	—	—	—	Sol
Cr^{3+}	30	Sol	—	—	—	—	—	Sol
Mn^{2+}	13	Sol	—	10	—	11–15	13	Sol
Fe^{2+}	13–15	Sol	—	10	—	18	—	Sol
Fe^{3+}	37	Sol	Sol	—	22	27	40	Sol
Co^{2+}	14	Sol	—	13	34	20–25	15	Sol
Co^{3+}	44	—	—	—	—	—	—	—
Ni^{2+}	14–17	—	—	8	30	18–20	14	Sol
Cu^+	10	7	11	—	—	~50	—	11
Cu^{2+}	19	Sol	—	10	37	~40	15	Sol
Ag^+	8	10	14–18	11	18–20	~50	27	10–12
Zn^{2+}	16	Sol	Sol	10	32	22–26	15	Sol
Cd^{2+}	14	Sol	Sol	11–1	32	28	15	Sol
Hg^{2+}	23	18	28	16	—	47	12	19
Hg_2^{2+}	25	Sol	Sol	—	—	53	Sol	7
Tl^+	Sol	Sol	8	—	—	19–23	11	4
Tl^{3+}	45	Sol	—	—	—	—	—	4
Sn^{2+}	25	Sol	Sol	—	—	26	—	Sol
Pb^{2+}	16	5	8	13	42	29	17	5
Bi^{3+}	30	Sol	18	—	23	72–90	—	Sol
Sb^{3+}	41	Sol	—	—	—	—	—	—

metal ions fed at high concentration levels. Metal ions present at low concentration levels may be kept in solution by food constituents as was shown for zinc which is equally available for absorption in chicks as oxide, sulfate or carbonate (Pensack *et al.*, 1958; Roberson and Schaible, 1960).

Sparingly soluble metal may enter the organism even as particles. Volkheimer *et al.* (1969) showed that in the dog metallic iron particles of up to 52 mcm diameter appear in the bile, lymph and even in the cerebrospinal fluid following oral administration. However, no quantitative data are as yet available to show how much iron enters the organism by this route (persorption). It seems unlikely that the organism covers its demand for biometals in this way.

Heavy metals are ingested usually in food or as drugs in the form of salts or complexes. Salts are discussed first. In Table 1 the solubility products of some important heavy metal salts are listed.

12.1.2.1. *Heavy metal salts*

Most heavy metals readily form water-soluble *halides* (see Table 1). Exceptions are copper(I), silver(II) and mercury(II) which forms the sparingly soluble mercurous chloride calomel. Iodides are generally less soluble than chlorides. Even thallium, the chloride of which is readily soluble in water, forms an iodide that is only sparingly soluble. This also holds true for lead(II).

The *cyanides* behave similarly to the halides. Thus, the cyanides of copper(II), silver(II), mercury(II) (Hg^{2+} and $Hg_2{}^{2+}$), thallium(I), thallium(II) and lead(II) are only sparingly soluble.

Compounds of metals with the other anions listed in Table 1, i.e. hydroxide, carbonate, phosphate, sulfide and cyanoferrate, are almost without exception only sparingly soluble.

The following should be noted in respect of the importance of the nature of the individual anions as partners for heavy metal ions in the gastrointestinal tract. *Phosphate ions* are abundantly available in the food, particularly in food of plant origin. When heavy metals are given along with food, formation of sparingly soluble phosphates is, therefore, likely.

Formation of sparingly soluble *metal hydroxides* in the intestinal tract is very common. Thallium(I) is an exception, forming no hydroxide, and no aquo-ions. In biological media thallium ions behave quite like potassium ions (Mullins and Moore, 1960; Gehring and Hammond, 1964, 1967); this is discussed later (see p. 605).

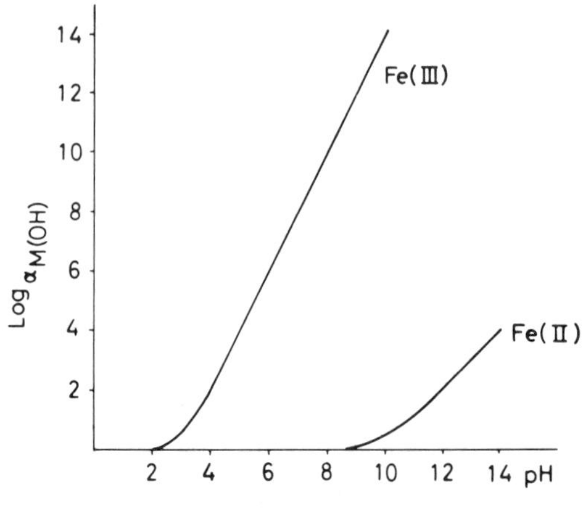

FIG. 1. Hydroxide formation of ferric and ferrous iron in solutions with increasing pH-values. The coefficient α was calculated assuming the following reactions of the metal (M) with OH-ions (OH): M(OH), $M(OH)_2$ and $M_2(OH)_2$:

$$\alpha_{M(OH)} = 1 + [OH] \times K_{M(OH)} + [OH]^2 \times K_{M(OH)_2} + \cdots .$$

(From Schubert, 1964.)

Hydroxide formation is favored by higher valency states of the metal. This relationship is brought out particularly clearly for iron by Schubert (1964) (see Fig. 1). The fact that iron(III) forms hydroxides at a pH of little more than 2 is very important; the effect on iron absorption is discussed in detail later (see pp. 618–621). The general tendency of heavy metals to form hydroxides indicates that these are precipitated with rising pH in the gut lumen, i.e. after neutralization of the acid gastric juice.

The formation of sparingly soluble *cyanoferrat*(II) compounds of heavy metals is important for the therapeutic effect in acute metal poisoning (see pp. 637–640).

Heavy metal *sulfides* are almost insoluble and are thus unsuitable for absorption. Under physiological conditions, metal sulfides are found in the lower part of the intestine, particularly in the colon in the presence of hydrogen sulfide formed by micro-organisms. The sulfides impart the characteristic color to the feces following oral heavy metal administration. Thiols, e.g. SH-containing proteins and their degradation products, may convert part of the heavy metal ions to the metallic state by reduction in the intestinal lumen. This is known to occur for silver (cf. Heubner, 1934) and bismuth (cf. Forst, 1935).

The fact that orally administered metal sulfides are absorbed to only a small extent has recently been demonstrated once again for selenium in the mouse (Henschler and Kirschner, 1969). This finding does not invalidate the view found in textbooks (Swinyard, 1970; DiPalamo, 1964) that orally taken selenium sulfide is toxic. It will probably be shown that after oral administration of such compounds the residence time in the stomach as well as the pH of the gastric juice determine how much of the more easily soluble, more readily absorbed and, hence, more toxic compounds are formed from the sparingly soluble selenium sulfide. Possibly its rate of dissolution in the stomach and the formation of toxic salts of this metal vary widely from species to species.

Excretion of heavy metals into the gut lumen. In this connection it is necessary to mention the *elimination of metals into the intestinal lumen,* which has so far not been studied systematically. Very likely, the references in the older literature to a secretion of metals into the colon are closely related to the observation of the strongly colored, sparingly soluble forms of the metals in the lower sections of the intestine (cf. Heubner, 1934). This is probably due to microbial sulfide formation and reduction to the metallic state. In a few quantitative investigations it was shown that secretion of iron and calcium in the colon plays no particular role (McGowan *et al.,* 1930; Welch *et al.,* 1936). That metals are excreted into the intestine has been shown not only for thallium (Durbin *et al.,* 1957; Lund, 1956) but also for zinc (Methfessel and Spencer, 1973b; Miller and Cragle, 1965; Miller *et al.,* 1968; Vallee, 1962), copper (Adelstein and Vallee, 1962; Van Campen, 1971; Evans, 1973), manganese and cobalt (Greenberg *et al.*, 1943).

The pathways used by heavy metals during their secretion into the gut lumen are still unknown. For some metals, e.g. copper (for references see Adelstein and Vallee, 1962; Evans, 1973; Van Campen, 1971) and cobalt and manganese (Greenberg *et al.*, 1943), the bile plays the main role, while evidently only traces of iron enter the intestine in this way (Greenberg *et al.*, 1943). This metal is mainly released into the intestinal lumen with the physiologically exfoliated mucosal cells (Crosby, 1968a). Thallium is excreted into the gut lumen with the secretions of the stomach and the intestine. Very likely the excretion of thallium by these routes is associated with the excretion of potassium (Lund, 1956).

12.1.2.2. *Heavy metal complexes*

The formation of sparingly soluble salts and hydroxides of heavy metals in the gut lumen can be prevented by compounds which form complexes. These metal complexes differ with respect to the availability of the intact compound from the simple metal salts. Because of the importance for absorption, it is necessary to say something about the principles of the formation of metal complexes and chelates with organic ligands. Details may be taken from various surveys, e.g. Catsch (1964, 1968), Dwyer and Mellor (1964), Martell and Calvin (1952, 1958) or Schubert (1964).

Stability. With respect to the availability of metals for absorption in the gut lumen the stability of the complexes is of primary importance. Chemically, a measure of the stability of metal complexes is the so-called complex formation or stability constant (K). For the formation of a simple complex [ML] between a metal [M] and a complexing agent [L] this stability constant is derived from the law of mass action:

$$K = \frac{[\mathrm{ML}]}{[\mathrm{M}] \times [\mathrm{L}]} \tag{1}$$

The brackets denote molar concentrations of the reaction partners. For simplicity the electrical charges are omitted. It is assumed that the activity equals the concentration.

TABLE 2. COMPLEXES AND CHELATES

Type	Complex or chelate	
	Coordination number 4	Coordination number 6
Monodentate (complex)	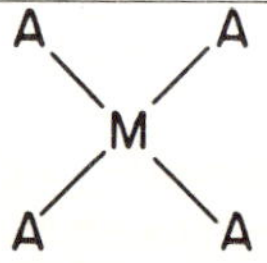	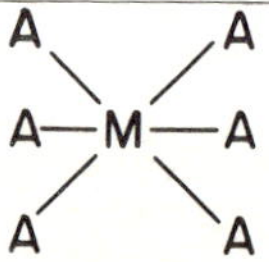
Bidentate (chelate)	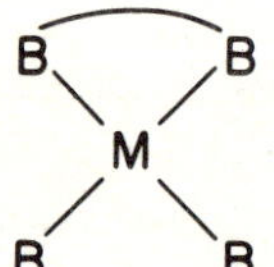 (2:1)	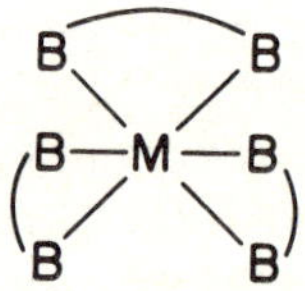 (3:1)
Tridentate (chelate)	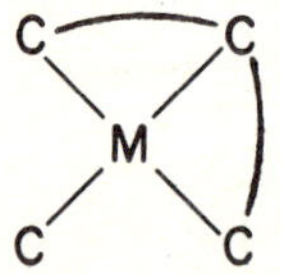 ("hetero-complex")	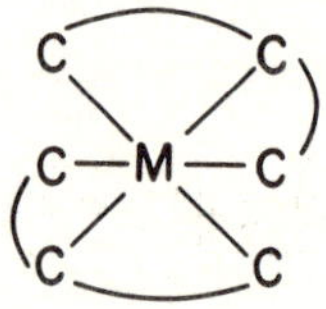 (3:1)

In general a metal can react with more than one ligand molecule of the same type. The number of the possible bonds with the ligand atoms of the molecule depends on the coordination number of the metal. Complexes formed by the participation of more than one ligand atom of one molecule are called *chelates.* According to the number of the ligand atoms of a molecule which come into contact with a metal, bidentate, tridentate, quadridentate and, in general, often, multidentate chelates are distinguished. On the basis of this nomenclature unidentate ligand molecules form only simple complexes (see Table 2).

Chelates are characterized by exceptionally high stability constants. Thermodynamically, the "chelate effect", i.e. the increase in the stability constant by formation of a multidentate chelate as compared with the stability constant of an analogue metal complex with an equivalent number of unidentate ligand molecules, can be explained by the greater positive entropy change during the formation of the chelate ring. Prerequisite for the formation of a chelate is an optimum distance between the metal and the ligand atoms of the molecule.

Chelates can be built up by a metal and only one ligand molecule (1:1-chelate) which is able to saturate all coordination sites of the metal or two ligand molecules (2:1-chelate) or even three (3:1-chelate). If the type of ligand molecules within a chelate or complex is non-uniform, then "mixed complexes" or "hetero-complexes" are the result.

It is of practical significance that a metal chelate in solution displays a degree of dissociation on dilution which is greater the more ligand molecules participate in its formation. This relation can be derived from the following equations.

If a single ligand (for the sake of simplicity ligand is used for ligand molecule) reacts with a metal of coordination number 6, then with increasing concentration of the ligand several complex types (1:1; 2:1; . . . ; 6:1) are formed until the coordination sites of the metals are filled. The reaction of the individual ligand molecules and the metals can be treated as a stepwise process. It follows that the complex formation constant can be determined for each reaction step separately.

$$K_1 = \frac{[ML]}{[M] \times [L]}; \quad K_2 = \frac{[ML_2]}{[ML] \times [L]}; \quad K_n = \frac{[ML_n]}{[ML_{n-1}] \times [L]} \tag{2}$$

The overall constant, the so-called *stability product*, is generally known as β_n, which can be calculated according to the following relationship:

$$\beta_n = K_1 \times K_2 \times \ldots \times K_n \tag{3}$$

and

$$\beta_n = \frac{[ML_n]}{[M] \times [L]^n} \tag{4}$$

From this latter formula, the complex bound fraction of iron in *tris*-acetyl-hydroxamine–Fe(III)-complex and the desferrioxamine–Fe(III)-complex can be calculated assuming that these agents are present in excess relative to iron at a concentration of 10^{-4} M.

According to formula (5) below which is a rearrangement of formula (4) the fraction of complex bound ferric iron can be calculated for acetyl-hydroxamine ($\log \beta_3 = 28$):

$$\frac{[ML_n]}{[M]} = \beta_n \times [L]^n, \tag{5}$$

$$\frac{[FeL_3]}{[Fe]} = 10^{28} \times (10^{-4})^3 = 10^{16}$$

and for desferrioxamine ($\log K = 31$):

$$\frac{[FeL]}{[Fe]} = 10^{31} \times 10^{-4} = 10^{27}.$$

This example (Schubert, 1964) shows that despite a very small difference between the stability constants of both complexes the 1:1-complex of desferrioxamine is relatively independent of dilution whereas the complex bound fraction of acetylhydroxamine is lowered remarkably by dilution.

In Table 3 a number of typical groups suitable for complex formation are summarized. In the case of acid coordinating groups one proton is replaced by a metal ion, while in the neutral groups complex formation occurs only by coordination.

As shown in Table 3, these groups, viz. carboxylic acids, hydroxy-acids, polyols, proteins, amino acids and inorganic and organic phosphates, to mention only the most important ones, occur in all biological media and particularly in food. The role that ligands of these types play is not confined to food. A complex with such compounds can also be formed in the course of transfer of the metals across the cells of the mucosal epithelium.

Kinetic stability. The *thermodynamic* stability constants provide valuable information to the chemist, but with respect to the *effective stability* of the complexes and chelates in biological media their signi-

TABLE 3. COORDINATING GROUPS OF LIGANDS (After Chenoweth, 1956)

Acid coordinating groups		Neutral coordinating groups	
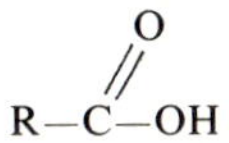	carboxyl	R—OH	alcoholic hydroxyl
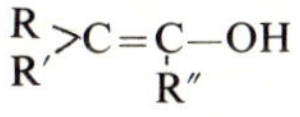	enolic hydroxyl	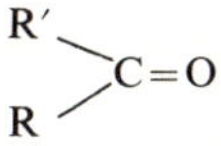	carbonyl
$R—OPO_3H_2$	primary phosphate	$R—NH_2$	primary amine
$R—OPO_3HR'$	secondary phosphate	R—NH—R′	secondary amine
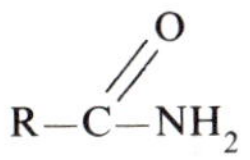	primary amido	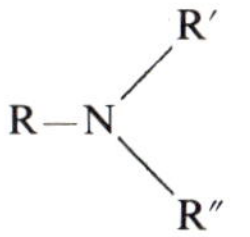	tertiary amine
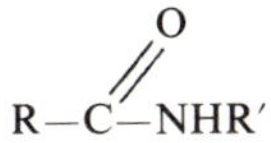	secondary amido	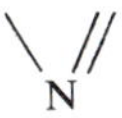	cyclic. tert. amine
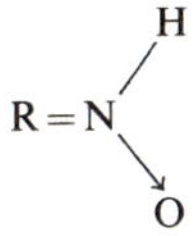	nitrone	R=N—OH	isonitroso
R—SH	thiol	R—S—R′	thio ether
$R—SO_3H$	sulfonic	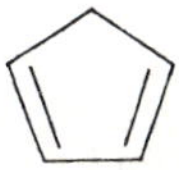	cyclopentdienyl

ficance is limited. The thermodynamic constant is by definition an equilibrium constant which is determined in a defined medium. From this constant no information can be derived as far as the velocity of association or dissociation of the complexes is concerned, especially when complex formation takes place in the presence of competing ligands or metals and oxidoreduction processes. In other words, a complex having a high thermodynamic stability constant is not necessarily inert (Schwarzenbach, 1958). There exist only a few examples of substantially inert complexes, e.g. iron–hematoporphyrin. This compound is characterized chemically by not exchanging its metal in the presence of competing ligands. However, as we shall discuss in detail later even the iron contained in this complex is released in mucosal cells by metabolic degradation of the hematoporphyrin ring (see pp. 632–633).

When assessing the stability of iron complexes in biological media one is therefore interested in kinetic rather than in thermodynamic stability. As a measure of kinetic stability the half-time of the iron exchange of complexes can be used, as shown in Table 4.

Data reproduced in Table 4 show that, despite small differences in the thermodynamic stability constants, different iron chelates reveal tremendous differences of kinetic stability as measured by their exchange of iron with transferrin as biological acceptor for iron. It is impossible to discuss in detail the factors which determine the kinetic stability of iron complexes. In addition to the thermodynamic stability and the charge of the complex, steric factors probably influence the exchange of the iron between the low molecular ligands and transferrin (Bates *et al.*, 1967a, b; Billups *et al.*, 1967). The kinetic stability of a complex can, thus, vary according to the ligand chosen for the iron exchange. Nevertheless, it is informative to use this simple method in order to assess the donor function of iron complexes in the intestinal tract especially considering that the mucosal cells possess acceptor sites for iron, as will be discussed later. In other words, the donor function of iron complexes can be investigated easily by measuring the iron uptake into the mucosal epithelium.

TABLE 4. THE KINETIC STABILITY OF SOME Fe(III)-CHELATES AS COMPARED WITH THEIR THERMODYNAMIC STABILITY CONSTANTS

The thermodynamic stability constants (log *K*) were taken from Sillen and Martell (1964). The kinetic stability was measured as the exchange time of the chelated iron with iron-free transferrin. All solutions contained 10^{-4} M/1 metal binding equivalent of transferrin and ferric chelate (ligand: Fe = 1 : 1). (From Bates *et al.*, 1967a, b)

Fe(III)-chelate of	Thermodyn. stab. constant (log *K*)	Half-time of iron exchange with iron-free transferrin
Nitrilotriacetic acid	23	3 sec
Citric acid	25	8 hr
Ethylenediamine-tetraacetic acid	25	4 days

Estimation of effective stability. As the fate of a metal complex in a biological medium usually cannot be predicted from its thermodynamic stability constant, it has been attempted to estimate the *effective* stability (Schubert, 1964; Catsch, 1964, 1968). Such computations are inevitably approximate, because generally no precise data on competing reactions with interfering ligands and metals exist.

In this connection reference is made to the formation of *polynuclear metal hydroxide complexes.* Their composition has not been fully elucidated but they are transitions to the precipitation of metal hydroxides (Schwarzenbach, 1958). The analogy between such compounds and the covalent metal hydroxides and sulfides should be mentioned, suggesting that it may be justifiable to treat both these types of compounds as complexes.

To demonstrate the extent to which the effective stability can be influenced by interfering reactions in various segments of the gastrointestinal tract, a calculation for some copper and iron complexes performed by Schubert (1964) is reproduced below. The following chelates are involved; the figures in parentheses are their thermodynamic stability constants (log *K*): Fe(III)-EDTA (25); Cu(II)-EDTA (19); Fe(III)-desferrioxamine (31); Cu(II)-desferrioxamine (14).

Theoretically the following side reactions which influence the effective stability of the complexes in the gastrointestinal tract might occur:

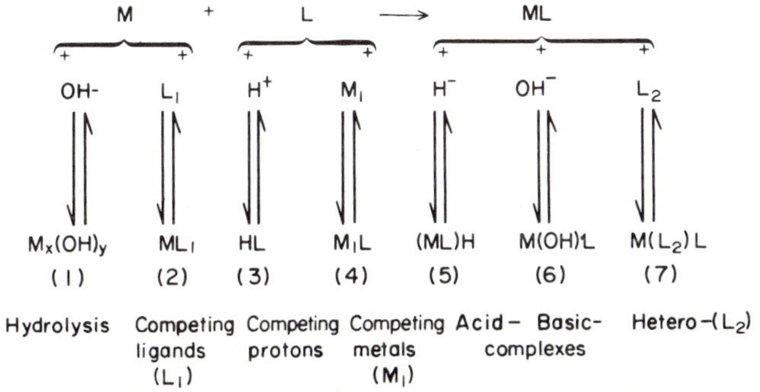

For simplicity Schubert included only reactions (1), (3), (4), (5) and (6) into the computation (see Fig. 2). Calcium was selected as the competing metal; its concentration was assumed to be 10^{-3} M.

Side reactions (1), (3), (5) and (6) predict a dependence of the effective stability of the metal complexes on the pH. As compared with the optimum, the effective stability of the chelates shown in Fig. 2 is low in the acid region. This is a consequence of the high concentration of competing

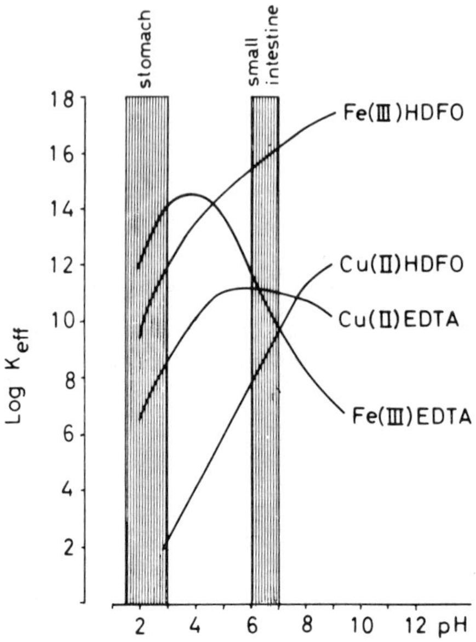

FIG. 2. Change of the effective stability of iron- and copper-chelates with concentration of H ions. Calculating the constants of effective stability (K_{eff}) the following side reactions were taken into account (cf. p. 611): side reactions 1, 3, 4 and 6. Competing metal in side reaction 4 is Ca^{2+}. EDTA = ethylenediamine-tetraacetic acid. HDFO = desferrioxamine. (From Schubert, 1964.)

hydrogen ions. The effective stability of many complexes is also low in the neutral and alkaline regions, as is the case for EDTA-chelates of iron and copper (Fig. 2). This is due mainly to the formation of both metal hydroxides and basic complexes. In contrast to EDTA-chelates the formation of such compounds is apparently of little importance in the case of desferrioxamine chelates (Fig. 2).

As Fig. 2 shows, the effective stability of metal complexes is not the same throughout the whole gastrointestinal tract. It is particularly low in the stomach, i.e. the degree of dissociation is high. However, an important finding showed that in 77% of fasted dogs and in 35% of fasted humans a pH value of 6 and more was found in the gastric juice (Kuna, 1964). The optimum effective stability is in fact restricted to a narrow pH range, as shown in Fig. 2. Considering the intraluminal conditions of the gastrointestinal tract in omniverous mammals, this applies, at most, to the short distance between the pylorus and that part of the duodenum into which the digestive secretions flow. The conditions for the existence of heavy metal complexes can be different in ruminants and in monogastric species because of different hydrogen ion concentrations in the various gastric sections.

As a rule it was assumed that food does not contain the metal and ligand in stoichiometric proportions; generally an excess of ligands is present. This ligand excess enhances the effective stability of a metal complex, as the following relationships demonstrate:

$$\frac{[ML]}{[M] \times [L]} = \alpha \times K = K_{eff} \quad (6)$$

with α as a proportionality factor symbolizing the side effects that impair the stability of the complex. Rearranging (6) to give

$$\frac{[ML]}{[M]} = K_{eff} \times [L] \quad (7)$$

reveals that the fraction of complex-bound metal, and, hence, the effective stability, increases if the ligand concentration is high, i.e. the ligand excess is high. Often the ligands in the food are substances which, like amino acids, are absorbed rapidly and, hence, the effective stability of the metal chelates decreases.

These few examples should suffice to illustrate the changes to which the effective stability of metal complexes is subjected in the gastrointestinal tract.

We can now readily identify the factors influencing the absorption of metals in the gastrointestinal tract. They are essentially the secretions of the stomach, pancreas and liver, which determine the pH in the alimentary tract, and the food *constituents* forming complexes with metals.

12.1.3. INFLUENCE OF INTRALUMINAL CONDITIONS IN DIFFERENT PARTS OF THE GASTROINTESTINAL TRACT ON AVAILABILITY

12.1.3.1. *Gastric secretion*

It is a well-established fact that metals can readily dissolve in the acid stomach medium even if presented as salts that are sparingly soluble in a neutral medium, i.e. they are converted into a well-absorbed form. This has been demonstrated for all biologically and toxicologically important heavy metals: for copper by Tompsett (1940), Eichholtz (1934a) and Van Campen (1971), for zinc by Eichholtz (1934b), for iron by Brock and Taylor (1934), Tompsett (1940), Forth *et al.* (1965a) and by Rummel (1965), for cobalt by Hendrych and Weden (1934) and by Paley and Sussman (1963), for nickel by Hendrych and Weden (1934), for manganese by Langecker (1934), for tin by Schübel (1934), for lead by Flury (1934), for thallium by Hesse (1934) and for platinum and gold by Schlossmann (1934), as well as by other authors. Even bismuth subnitrate generally held to be practically insoluble and, hence, not absorbed can be dissolved under the influence of gastric acid to a sufficient extent to occasionally cause poisoning. Aliphatic hydroxy acids (e.g. lactic acid) probably act as solubilizers (Forst, 1935; Serefis, 1934). Silver is exceptional among the metals listed here, because silver chloride is formed in the gastric juice (Heubner, 1934) which is sparingly soluble and hardly absorbed.

Conversely, the absorption of metals is reduced when proton acceptors cause the pH of the gastric juice to increase. This was shown for copper absorption in cattle and sheep by Weser and Kirchgessner (1965). However, the addition of basic components to food does not reduce copper absorption in pigs (Weser and Kirchgessner, 1965); this difference is due to the higher hydrogen ion concentration in the pig's stomach as compared to that in the rennet bag of the cattle.

The influence of gastric juice on absorption has been studied in special detail for iron. Absorption of iron in man is generally reduced when the secretion of gastric juice is restricted or entirely suppressed (Michaelides and Philis, 1959; Goldberg *et al.*, 1963; Cook *et al.*, 1964; Mailliard, 1966; Walz *et al.*, 1970) or after gastrectomy (cf. Voigt and Brüschke, 1967). Administration of hydrochloric acid restored the absorption of iron in achylous patients to normal (Cook *et al.*, 1964; Jacobs, P. *et al.*, 1964). This observation, which was confirmed in animal experiments (e.g. in rats, Whitehead and Bannerman, 1964), agrees with theoretical predictions of increased ionization and absorption of iron as the acid content of the gastric juice increases. Naturally, the acidity of the gastric juice has no effect on stable compounds such as heme. Accordingly, the absorption of hemoglobin iron is not enhanced by administering it with acid (Jacobs, P. *et al.*, 1964). In rats iron deficiency develops after gastrectomy (Rieber *et al.*, 1967).

Alcohol. Very probably the observation that alcohol promotes the absorption of iron can be explained by the enhanced production of gastric acid. Alcohol does not enhance iron absorption in achlorhydric subjects (Charlton *et al.*, 1969). However, results of investigations on the influence of alcohol iron absorption diverge (McDonald and Pechet, 1964; Tapper *et al.*, 1967, 1968).

Alcohol can influence iron absorption not only by enhancing acid secretion but also by accelerating stomach emptying, primarily, or by stimulating gastric secretion (Davenport, 1961a; Nasset, 1968). On the other hand, acute and chronic ethanol treatment has no effect on the absorption of iron from tied-off intestinal segments (Tapper *et al.*, 1968).

The significance of the intestinal transit time for iron absorption should be emphasized.* Substances like phenoxybenzamine and atropine which increase the transit time of ingested material promote the absorption of orally administered iron (Schade *et al.*, 1969).

Iron-binding constituents of gastric juice. The simple explanation that the effect of gastric juice on the absorption of iron is due solely to an acidity-induced increase of the ionized fraction has been questioned in recent years (Crosby, 1968b; Murray and Stein, 1968). Gastric juice evidently also contains substances which even after neutralization prevent the precipitation of iron (Beutler *et al.*, 1963) and this might affect the absorption of iron. Koepke and Stewart (1964) demonstrated that gastric juice of iron-deficient dogs increases iron absorption. This observation could not be confirmed in man (Jacobs, A. *et al.*, 1967; Jacobs, P. *et al.*, 1968), or in the rat (Forth and Rummel, 1968; Smith *et al.*, 1969). The recent finding by A. Jacobs and Owen (1969) that the gastric juice of anemic patients displays absorption-promoting properties in normal individuals following neutralization provides little confirmatory evidence. In these experiments the gastric juice was given together with cream of chicken soup containing strained chicken breast as the test meal. Not surprisingly, peptide fragments and amino acids are formed under these conditions which convert iron into a form suitable for absorption (Martinez-Torres and Layrisse, 1970).

An Australian group of workers (Davis and Deller, 1967; Davis *et al.*, 1966, 1967; Luke *et al.*, 1967) have detected an iron-binding factor in human gastric juice and called it gastroferrin. These authors believe it to be a protein, but this view has been challenged (Wynter and Williams, 1968; Morgan *et al.*, 1969). It is not yet clear whether gastroferrin (Davis *et al.*, 1966, 1967) and the gastric juice constituent described by Koepke and Stewart (1964) are identical; this seems unlikely, as the ability of the gastric juice to bind iron is reduced in one case and increased in the other. It has also not been established whether gastroferrin is identical with lactoferrin (eccrinosiderophilin). This iron-binding protein has been detected in the secretions of a number of exocrine glands (Schade, 1967; Masson and Heremans, 1967).

The physiological significance of the iron-binding constituent(s) of the

*See also Chapter 15, p. 824.

gastric juice is not clear. It certainly has no effect on the physiological *regulation* of iron absorption (Forth and Rummel, 1968). Whether the reduced iron-binding capacity of the gastric juice and the absence of gastroferrin in patients with hemochromatosis is important for the pathogenesis of this illness remains unsolved (Davis *et al.*, 1966; Smith *et al.*, 1969). Certainly the enhanced iron absorption—which has been described repeatedly (Block, 1958; Powell *et al.*, 1970) but which cannot be demonstrated in every case (Dreyfus and Schapira, 1964; Losowsky and Wilson, 1967)—is not the only disturbance of iron metabolism in this disease. Whether the enhanced iron absorption in hemochromatosis is merely a consequence of the simultaneous cirrhosis which also produces enhanced iron absorption (Callender and Malpass, 1963; Linscheer *et al.*, 1963) remains uncertain.

A plausible explanation for the capacity of the gastric juice to keep iron in solution after neutralization was given by Wynter and Williams (1968). These authors assume the presence of a glycoprotein in the gastric juice which forms a protective colloid and, thus, prevents iron precipitation. This interpretation was confirmed by recent investigations (Rudzki and Deller, 1973; Rudzki *et al.*, 1973).

The difference in iron-binding capacity of the gastric juice of normal and iron-deficient patients cannot be interpreted until an accurate analysis of gastric juice is available. Iron-deficiency anemia is accompanied by atrophy of the epithelia of the intestine and stomach (cf. Jacobs, A., 1969; Binder *et al.*, 1966; Cowan *et al.*, 1966a). It is, therefore, not surprising that the composition of the gastric juice differs from normal during iron-deficiency. This has been demonstrated in man (Jacobs, A. *et al.*, 1966; Stone, 1968) and in the rat (Forth and Rummel, 1968).

A factor which promotes the absorption of heme-iron in patients suffering from pernicious anemia and simultaneous iron-deficiency has recently been identified in neutralized normal gastric juice. In normal subjects or patients with simple iron-deficiency administration of this factor has no effect. It is present in normal gastric juice, but absent in patients with pernicious anemia (Waxman *et al.*, 1968).

12.1.3.2. *Pancreatic secretion*

The discussion concerning the effect of another digestive secretion on the absorption of iron, i.e. the exocrine pancreas secretion, is older than that about gastroferrin. The conditions have already been surveyed (Kavin *et al.*, 1967; Murray and Stein, 1966; Kahn, 1966; Davis and Biggs, 1967; Biggs, 1967). Originally a specific inhibitor was assumed to occur in the exocrine secretion the deficiency of which was thought to be responsible for the increased iron absorption observed in diseases of this organ. This assumption has been shown to be wrong. The decrease in the absorption of iron occasionally observed after giving pancreatic juice or extracts under experimental conditions is very probably the consequence of non-specific binding of iron to proteins, or to the alkalinity of the pancreatic juice, which reduces the ionized, i.e. absorbable, fraction of a given dosed iron by forming the sparingly soluble hydroxide. The protein is possibly lactoferrin or, as alternatively called, eccrinosiderophilin which has been identified in the secretion of exocrine glands, including the bile and the pancreas (Schade, 1967; Masson and Heremans, 1967).

Precisely the opposite effect, i.e. an increase in the availability of zinc for absorption, is ascribed to the pancreatic secretion (Strain and Pories, 1970). The function of the exocrine pancreatic secretion to neutralize the food-juice mixture leaving the stomach is of general importance for the absorption of metals. The secretion from Brunner's glands is of additional importance, neutralizing acid food. On the one hand, metals such as manganese and copper, to give two examples other than iron, form sparingly soluble poorly absorbed hydroxides following neutralization of the gastric acid. On the other hand, the decrease in the hydrogen ion concentration also favors the formation of soluble metal complexes with ligands occurring in the food (see pp. 627–637).

TABLE 5. ABSORPTION OF IRON IN THE PRESENCE OF ASCORBIC AND DEHYDROASCORBIC ACID FROM TIED-OFF JEJUNAL SEGMENTS OF RATS

Experimental conditions: fasted (16 hr) rats, Wistar (female), 200 g body weight. Tied-off jejunal segments, 13 cm length starting with the flexura duodenojejunalis (operation under ether anesthesia). Iron dose: 0.36 mcm ^{59}Fe–($FeSO_4$) in 2 ml sodium chloride solution (0.9%). Ligand: Fe = 100:1. Time: 1 hr. The absorbed amount of radioiron was measured after removal of the tied-off jejunal segments in a body counter for small animals. The values were calculated as percent of the dose. They are means from five rats ± SEM. (Forth and Lichtenberg, unpublished data)

Substance added	Amount of iron absorbed when added as			
	^{59}Fe–($FeSO_4$)		^{59}Fe–($FeCl_3$)	
	pH 2	pH 5.5	pH 2	pH 5.5
—	7.8 ±3.2	1.5[a] ±0.6	7.0 ±4.3	1.1[a] ±0.7
Ascorbic acid	18.1[a] ±6.2	3.9[a][b] ±1.2	11.8[b] ±2.4	2.6[a][b] ±1.5
Dehydroascorbic acid	17.4[b] ±4.3	5.4[a][b] ±2.4	12.4[b] ±3.3	2.3[a][b] ±0.8

[a] $p < 0.05$ as compared with the group pH 2.
[b] $p < 0.05$ as compared with the group without ligands.

Absorption of ferrous and ferric iron. Iron is a particularly impressive example of impaired absorption resulting from hydroxide formation. At pH 8 the maximum concentration of ferrous ions is 1.6×10^{-2} mole per litre, that of ferric ions is little more than $1/10^{16}$ of this value, i.e. 10^{-18} mole per litre (Charley *et al.*, 1963). This considerable difference in solubility is probably the main cause for the common observation that iron in the trivalent form is not absorbed to an appreciable extent (Starkenstein, 1934). The recommendation to use only divalent iron for therapeutic purposes dates back to Heubner (1912); it was originally motivated by the fact that the physiological form of iron in hemoglobin is ferrous.

We now know that ferrous iron and ferric iron are equally well absorbed provided that the iron is given in the ionized form (Rummel, 1965; Forth *et al.*, 1965a). Retention of ferrous and ferric iron in rats after administration (cf. Table 5) and the absorbed amounts measured 1 hr after injection of the dose in tied-off jejunal segments *in situ* are the same, provided the pH of the presented solution does not exceed 2. By contrast, if the iron solution is injected into the tied-off gut segments *in situ* at

TABLE 6. THE VALENCY STATE OF IRON IN THE LUMEN OF TIED-OFF JEJUNAL SEGMENTS OF RATS *in vivo*

Experimental conditions: fasted (16 hr) rats, Wistar (female) 200 g body weight. Normal rats (*n*): 15.8 g hemoglobin/100 ml blood (SEM = 1.2; $n = 120$); iron-deficient rats (*d*): 5.6 g hemoglobin/100 ml blood (SEM = 0.9; $n = 120$). Length of the segments: 13 cm starting with the flexura duodenojejunalis (operation under ether anesthesia). Time: 1 hr. Iron dose: 0.9 mcM in 2 ml sodium chloride solution pH 2. Fe(II) was measured spectrophotometrically by adding α,α′-dipyridyl, Fe(III) by adding 8-hydroxyquinoline-5-sulfonic acid. The values are the means of five rats ± SEM. (Forth and Lichtenberg, unpublished data)

Form of iron given	Substance added	Type of rats	Valency state of iron as *percent* of the dose					
			Fe(II)			Fe(III)		
			15	30	60	15	30	60 min
$^{59}Fe-(FeSO_4)$	—	*n*	72±6	51± 4	31±10	7±1	13±4	25±8
		d	75±8	56± 8	—	5±1	13±1	—
$^{59}Fe-(FeCl_3)$	—	*n*	34±9	22± 5	15± 6	37±4	34±6	24±5
		d	27±5	24± 6	—	37±8	26±5	—
$^{59}Fe-(FeSO_4)$	Ascorbic acid[a]	*n*	89±8	46± 8	53± 1	2±1	10±1	14±1
	Dehydro-ascorbic acid[a]	*n*	95±9	69±10	49± 6	5±1	8±2	14±3
$^{59}Fe-(FeCl_3)$	Ascorbic acid[a]	*n*	80±4	50± 8	42± 8	4±3	4±2	10±1
	Dehydro-ascorbic acid[a]	*n*	85±5	77± 4	56± 5	13±3	17±5	14±2

[a] Ligand : Fe = 30 : 1.

pH 5.5, hydroxide formation reduces the absorbed amount to one-fifth of that of the acid controls (see Table 5).

It is noteworthy that ferric iron is evidently reduced in the gut lumen of rats (Table 6). In both normal and anemic animals about one-third of a ferric iron dose is present as ferrous iron as soon as 15 min after introducing it into tied-off jejunal segments. Whether the reduction of trivalent to divalent iron after the administration of solutions of pH 5.5 has any significance with regard to the availability for absorption is doubtful because of the preferential formation of iron hydroxides in this pH region. Very likely Fe(III) hydroxide is administered in both cases. The peculiarity of the rat intestinal lumen which appears to contain reducing substances probably explains why these animals utilize oral ferrous and ferric iron equally well (Underwood, 1938; Venkatachalam *et al.*, 1956). Ascorbic acid is believed to be the main reducing agent which is excreted into the gut lumen (Conrad and Schade, 1968). There is, however, evidence that ferric iron is reduced also in tied-off segments of rats to which bile has no access (cf. Table 6).

Though the relationship between solubility and absorption of iron may

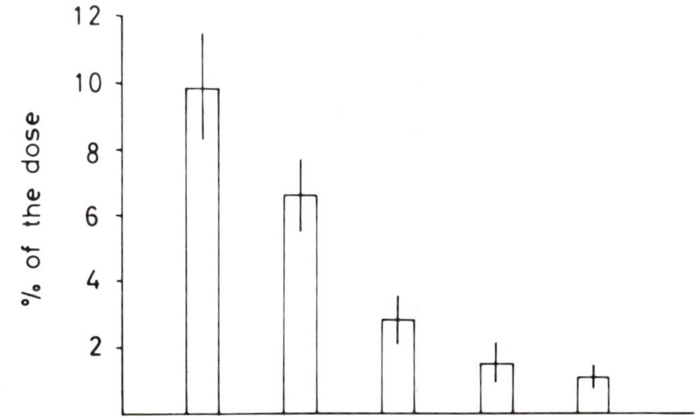

FIG. 3. Absorption of iron by rats in dependence on H^+ concentration of the applied solution. Experimental conditions: fasted rats (16 hr), Wistar (male), 220 g body weight, tied-off jejunal segments. Length: 15 cm starting from the flexura duodeno-jejunalis (operation under ether anesthesia). Iron dose: 0.36 mcM ^{59}Fe–($FeCl_3$) in 2 ml sodium chloride solution (0.9%). Time: 1 hr. The amount of the radioactive iron absorbed was measured in a body counter for small animals after removal of the tied-off segments. The columns represent means from five rats ± SEM. (Forth and Lichtenberg, unpublished data.)

seem trivial, one reason for a whole series of conflicting results—including data on the utilization of ferrous and ferric iron in man (Moore *et al.*, 1944; Hahn *et al.*, 1945) and in the dog (Hahn *et al.*, 1945)—is the fact that hydroxide is precipitated from solutions at a pH little above 2. Testing the dependence of absorption on the pH of the iron solution confirms these relationships. Such studies were carried out using tied-off rat jejunal segments *in situ* (Fig. 3). When using iron solution of pH 3.5, for example, Conrad and Schade (1968) found a substantial fraction of iron present as the hydroxide (Fig. 1), i.e. in a form unsuitable for absorption (Fig. 3).

The rules described for iron apply to all metals forming sparingly soluble hydroxides in aqueous solutions, i.e. manganese, copper, zinc and lead. The absorption of other metals such as thallium, nickel and cobalt, which do not form hydroxides in the intestinal lumen, theoretically should be independent of pH. This is indeed the case as can be demonstrated for cobalt (see Fig. 4). At pH 2 as much iron is absorbed from tied-off jejunal segments of rats *in situ* as at pH 5.5.

Figure 4 shows that the absorption of cobalt is more than twice that of iron injected into the segments at pH 2. The reason is undoubtedly the higher solubility of cobalt under the conditions prevailing in the intestinal lumen.

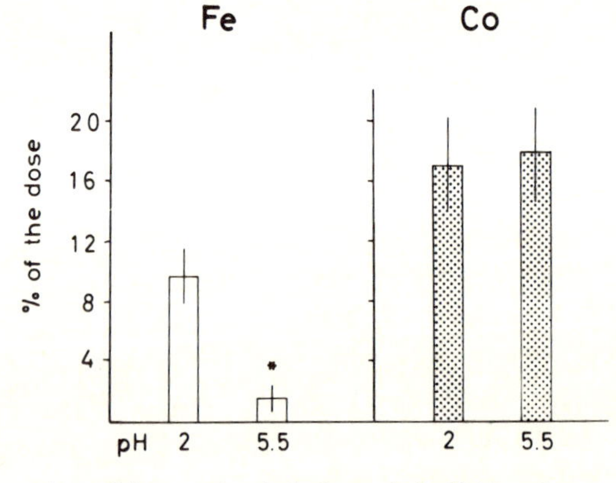

FIG. 4. Absorption of iron and cobalt from tied-off jejunal segments of rats *in vivo*. Experimental conditions: fasted rats (16 hr), Wistar (female), 250 g body weight. Length of the segments: 20 cm starting with the flexura duodenojejunalis (operation under ether anesthesia). Metal dose: 0.36 mcM as ^{59}Fe–($FeSO_4$) or ^{6}Co($CoCl_2$) in 2 ml sodium chloride solution (0.9%). The absorption of the radioactive metals was measured in a body counter for small animals after removal of the tied-off segments. Columns represent means from five rats ± SEM.* $= p < 0.01$ as compared with the controls' pH 2. (From Forth, 1966.)

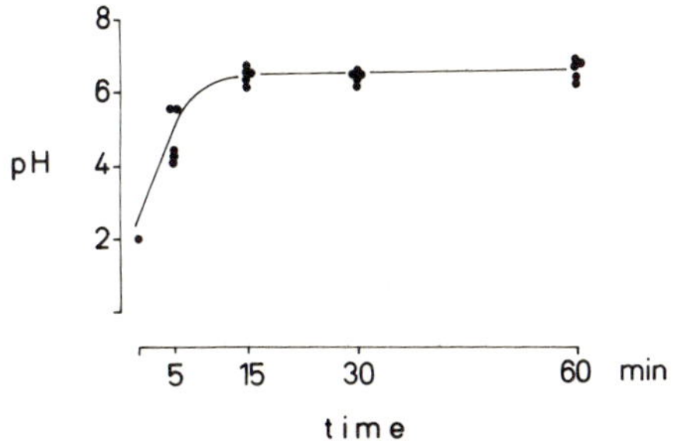

FIG. 5. Time course of intraluminal pH in the jejunum of rats. Experimental conditions: fasted rats (16 hr), Wistar (female), 220 g body weight. The experiment was started by injection of 2 ml sodium chloride solution (0.9%) of pH 2 into the tied-off jejunal segments (15 cm length). Operation under ether anesthesia. (Forth and Lichtenberg, unpublished data.)

After injection into the gut segments a solution of pH 2 is fairly quickly neutralized (Fig. 5). A pH measurement of the loop content after injection of 2 ml of pH 2 saline into a 12-cm-long segment indicated that it takes only 5 min to establish the final pH value of 6.9 which remained unchanged up to one hour. Evidently, hydroxide formation causes dissolved iron to exist for only a matter of minutes under these conditions, while the solubility of cobalt ions is unaffected by the neutralization of the loop contents. It may be added that these intraluminal pH values agree well with measurements in rats (Waldron-Edward *et al.*, 1966) and chickens (Coates and Holdsworth, 1961). In the ileum the pH rises to 7.2 in the rat and 7.8 in the chicken.

12.1.3.3. *Bile*

In contrast to the exocrine pancreatic secretion the bile increases the absorption of metals as a result of its solubilizing properties. This was demonstrated in the dog for sparingly soluble calcium and strontium compounds and also for iron phosphate. Characteristically bile did not exhibit absorption-activating properties when readily soluble iron sulfate was administered (Holdsworth, 1965; Webling and Holdsworth, 1965, 1966a, b). These authors also demonstrated that other surfactants, e.g. lauryl sulfonate, activate the absorption of metals. For sparingly soluble calcium phosphate the partition coefficient between a butanol–benzene mixture and physiological saline increases 200–400 times in the presence of bile acids and 10,000 times in the presence of lauryl sulfonate (Webling and Holdsworth, 1965). Obviously the formation of more readily soluble metal–surfactant micelles containing the metal in a form suitable for absorption may be assumed. Complex formation by bile acids may be significant and has been demonstrated for iron (Jacobs, A. and Miles, 1970) and for copper (Merkulova *et al.*, 1968; Lewis, 1973). Consequently the development of rickets after interruption of the bile flow could be explained in the same way (Holdsworth and Webling, 1971). Conrad and Schade (1968) have recently confirmed the absorption-activating effect of bile, but attribute the increase of iron absorption in rats with an open bile duct in comparison to those with a ligated one to the ascorbic acid content of the bile.

It is appropriate in this connection to return to the earlier observation of anemia in dogs caused by diverting the bile to the outside. Administration of iron restores the blood values back to normal. However, it remains open to discussion whether the iron deficiency is the only pathogenic factor involved, especially as the authors observed a normal hemoglobin content of individual erythrocytes (Syderhelm and Tammann, 1929).

12.1.4. FOOD AND ITS CONSTITUENTS

The reason why the recorded data dealing with the availability of metals for intestinal absorption are often conflicting is that the conditions during oral administration with food are confused and make evaluation difficult. Food can affect the absorption of metals by virtue of its effect on pH, its oxidoreductive activity and, above all, the capacity of some of its constituents to form metal complexes. For this reason the effect of chelates on the availability of metals for absorption from the gut lumen by citing examples in clearly defined model experiments is introduced here. Bowen (1966) compiled data about the metal content of the diet of man and the rat and the levels that produce toxic and deficiency symptoms respectively.

12.1.4.1. *Model experiments*

Theoretically there are two types of metal complexes which have a different effect on the availability of metals in the lumen of the intestine:

1. Metal complexes of high effective stability which substantially do not release their metal.
2. Metal complexes of lesser effective stability which dissociate in the gastrointestinal tract.

This classification, which was formulated for the evaluation of the absorption of complex-bound iron (Forth *et al.*, 1965b, 1968c), applies in principle to other metal complexes (Forth *et al.*, 1973).

Stable complexes of the first type are not described in detail here. Their metals are available for the organism only to the extent to which the complexes are absorbed and utilized. Transfer of intact chelates through the gut wall is discussed in detail later. All that needs to be said here is that, as theory predicts, lipoid-soluble complexes are well absorbed, water-soluble ones less well. Various factors determine the degree of metabolic utilization, e.g. the distribution in the organism, the elimination and, especially, how efficiently the organism can split the complexes and release the metal.

There are *acceptor sites* on the surface or within the mucosal cells which compete for the metals with ligands in the gut lumen. This fact is important for an understanding of the part which metal complexes, particularly those exhibiting a low effective stability, play by making metals available for absorption. The acceptor sites play an essential role in metal absorption (see pp. 640–654).

Thus, after injecting radioactive iron in the presence of a 20-fold

TABLE 7. ABSORPTION OF IRON ADMINISTERED WITH INCREASING EXCESS OF NICOTINOHYDROXAMIC ACID OR ETHYLENEDIAMINETETRAACETIC ACID IN TIED-OFF JEJUNAL SEGMENTS OF RATS *in vivo*

Experimental conditions: fasted rats (16 hr), Wistar (female), 200 g body weight. Length of the jejunal segments: 13 cm, starting from the flexura duodenojejunalis (operation under ether anesthesia). Iron dose: 0.36 mcM $^{59}Fe(FeCl_3)$ in 2 ml sodium chloride solution (0.9 %). Absorption of radioiron was measured 1 hr after the administration in a body counter for small animals after removal of the tied-off segments. In order to remove ^{59}Fe adsorbed to the surface, the segments were washed three times in 100 ml sodium chloride solution containing EDTA (10^{-2} M/l). Values are means from five rats ±SEM. (Forth and Lichtenberg, unpublished data)

Ligands	Ligand : Fe	pH	^{59}Fe transferred (cpm)	^{59}Fe transferred (%)	^{59}Fe in the intestinal tissue (cpm/g wet weight)
—	—	2.0	16,400 ± 310	11.0	43,000 ±2700
—	—	5.0	220[a] ± 38	1.5	12,800[a] ±2000
Nicotino-hydroxamic acid	20	6.0	17,300 ±2200	11.5	38,000[a][b] ±2000
	100	6.0	3950[a][b] ± 900	2.6	10,500[a] ±1050
Ethylenediamine-tetraacetic acid	20	6.0	2700[a][b] ± 600	1.8	3000[a][b] ± 650

[a] $p < 0.05$ as compared with the control group, pH 2.
[b] $p < 0.05$ as compared with the control group, pH 5.

excess of nicotinohydroxamic acid into tied-off jejunum segments, the amount of iron absorbed and the radioiron content of the tissue were the same as found after injecting free non-complex-bound iron at pH 2 (Table 7) though the solution containing the iron complex had a pH of 6. Increasing the effective stability of the Fe(III)–nicotinohydroxamate complex by using a 100-fold excess of ligand caused a fall in the amount absorbed as well as the tissue content to one-quarter of the control values (pH 2). Under these conditions, i.e. in the presence of a high excess of ligand, nicotinohydroxamic acid, which forms a medium stable complex with iron (log $\beta_3 = 12$, Bielig and Rohns, unpublished data), behaves like ethylenediaminetetraacetic acid (EDTA). The latter ligand forms a very stable complex with Fe(III) (log $K = 25$; Sillen and Martell, 1964). As little as a 20-fold excess of it reduces the tissue content of radioiron to less than one-tenth and the amount absorbed to one-sixth of that

TABLE 8. ABSORPTION OF IRON IN THE PRESENCE OF VARIOUS LIGANDS FROM TIED-OFF JEJUNAL SEGMENTS OF RATS *in vivo*

Experimental conditions: fasted rats (16 hr), Wistar (female), 200 g body weight. Length of the jejunal segments: 13 cm, starting with the flexura duodenojejunalis (operation under ether anesthesia). Iron dose: 0.36 mcM ^{59}Fe–($FeCl_3$) in 2 ml sodium chloride solution (0.9 %). Time: 1 hr. The absorption of radioiron was measured in a body counter for small animals after removal of the tied segments. Mean values from five rats ± SEM. The intestinal tissue was washed 3 times in 100 ml saline containing EDTA (10^{-2} M/l) before measuring the ^{59}Fe–activity in order to remove adsorbed radioactivity. (Forth and Lichtenberg, unpublished data)

Ligands	Ligand : Fe	pH	^{59}Fe transferred (cpm)	^{59}Fe transferred (%)	^{59}Fe in the tissue (cpm/g wet weight)
—	—	2.2	16,400 ± 310	11.0	43,000 ± 2700
—	—	5	220[a] ± 38	1.5	12,800[a] ± 200
Ascorbic acid	125	4.5	18,500[b] ±1450	12.3	43,500[a][b] ± 2600
Fructose	200	4.0	12,900[a][b] ±2800	8.6	78,000[b] ± 5500
Galactonic acid	200	4.4	17,200[b] ±2100	11.5	60,000[a][b] ± 4200
PO_4^{3-}	280	2	18,800 ± 320	12.5	47,000 ± 6500
PO_4^{3-}	280	3.4	3250[c] ± 490	2.2	26,000[c] ± 6300
PO_4^{3-} + glycine	280 550	3.4	11,500[d] ±1830	7.7	68,000[d] ±19,000
PO_4^{3-} + glutamic acid	280 550	3.4	8700[c][d] ±1400	5.8	160,000[c][d] ±13,700

[a] $p < 0.05$ as compared with the control group, pH 2.
[b] $p < 0.05$ as compared with the control group, pH 5.
[c] $p < 0.05$ as compared with the PO_4-group, pH 2.
[d] $p < 0.05$ as compared with the PO_4^{3-}-group, pH 3.4.

found with non-complex-bound iron at pH2 (Table 7).

This experiment shows that on the one hand nicotinohydroxamic acid prevents the formation of sparingly soluble iron hydroxide not suitable for absorption at pH 6. On the other hand, the Fe(III)–nicotinohydroxamate complex acts as an iron donor, because it releases its metal to the gut wall and makes it available for absorption. This donor effect takes place only if the effective stability of the complex is not too high. Incidentally it should be pointed out that by comparison with a control at pH 5 with the iron present as hydroxide, even EDTA produces increased absorption. This result clearly demonstrates to what extent the evaluation of the absorption of complex-bound metals depends on the choice of adequate controls (see Table 7).

A number of complex-forming agents present as food constituents in the intestinal lumen display a donor effect during the absorption of iron. Table 8 lists some examples and reveals that ascorbic acid, fructose, galactonic acid and amino acids, among others, may act as iron donors. Some of these ligands, particularly the amino acids, are discussed later (see pp. 699–710). Their action is discussed here only in respect of the absorption of iron phosphate by analogy with the investigations of Kroe *et al.* (1963b). Iron administered as iron phosphate in solution at pH 3–4 is poorly absorbed. Amino acids in substantial excess can compete with phosphate for binding iron and, thus, make it available for absorption. Jacobi *et al.* (1956a) were the first to describe this principle of competing iron-absorption activating and inhibiting chelators, which under alimentary conditions is of practical bearing (Martinez-Torres and Layrisse, 1970; Sayers *et al.*, 1973).

The *degree of the absorptive utilization* of alimentary biometals such as iron, copper and zinc increases appreciably in deficiency (see pp. 710–711). In other words, the varying degree of availability of complex-bound metals does not alone determine the rate of absorption. In deficiency additional factors influence the absorption. Thus, in tied-off jejunal segments of iron-deficient rats iron absorption rises to more than 4 times the value obtained with segments of normal animals (Fig. 6). Iron-deficient rats can even utilize iron if the stable Fe(III)–8-hydroxyquinolinesulfonic acid complex is given (log $\beta_3 = 35$; Sillen and Martell, 1964); the absorbed fraction is almost 20 times greater than that in nondeficient controls. It must be added that this iron complex is sparingly lipid-soluble, negatively charged, and hence, poorly absorbed (Forth *et al.*, 1965b; Rummel *et al.*, 1967). A minor change in the molecule of the ligand, viz. the removal of the polar sulfonic acid group, produces the electro-neutral, apolar and

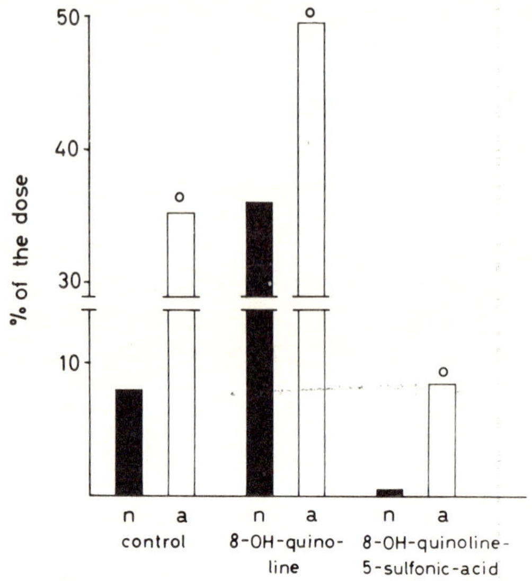

FIG. 6. Absorption of iron in the presence of 8-hydroxyquinoline and 8-hydroxy-quinoline-5-sulfonic acid in tied-off jejunal segments of normal and iron-deficient rats. Experimental conditions: fasted rats (16 hr), Wistar (female), 180–220 g body weight. Normal rats (*n*): 13.9 g hemoglobin per 100 ml blood (SEM = 1.1; $n = 30$). Iron-deficient rats (*d*): 5.8 g hemoglobin per 100 ml blood (SEM = 0.7; $n = 30$). Length of the tied-off jejunal segments: 15 cm, starting with the flexura duodeno-jejunalis (operation under ether anesthesia). Iron dose: 0.36 mcM ^{59}Fe–($FeCl_3$) in 2 ml sodium chloride solution (0.9%); pH without ligands: 2; in the presence of ligands: 3. Ligand: Fe = 10: 1. The absorption of the radioactive iron was measured by a body counter for small animals after removal of the segments. The columns represent means of five rats: $^0 = p < 0.01$ as compared with the group of normal rats. (Forth and Nell, unpublished data.)

lipid-soluble complex of Fe(III)–8-hydroxyquinoline which is, therefore, well absorbed. Normal rats absorb as much iron when this complex is presented as anemic animals do from a dose of free, non-complex-bound iron. Remarkably the absorptive utilization of iron bound in the Fe(III)–8-hydroxyquinoline complex increases in iron-deficiency (Fig. 6). The mechanism which is responsible for the absorptive utilization of stable iron chelates by the mucosal cells in deficiency studies is still unknown (see pp. 690–699). All that needs to be stated here is that in interpreting the ability of the mucosa to make use of iron of such stable complexes (Forth *et al.*, 1965b, 1968c) *hetero-complex* formation may occur between the acceptor sites of the mucosa, the administered ligand, and the co-ordination sites of the metal (see p. 606). If one accepts the formation of hetero-complexes with metals between the mucosal acceptor sites and the intraluminal ligands it appears not surprising that the size of these ligands, especially that of polynuclear-complex forming compounds, and their steric architecture may play a determining role for the availability of metals for absorption. This appears to be the correct interpretation of the findings of Terato *et al.* (1973a) rather than the assumption of the absorption of iron-complexes of molecular weights between 1500 and 9000.

In this connection it is of interest to ask up to which level of stability a metal complex may function as a metal donor in the gastrointestinal tract. Empirically, it was found that orally administered zinc complexes eliminate zinc-deficiency symptoms in chickens, i.e. that the metal of these complexes could still be utilized with thermodynamic stability constants as high as log $K = 18$ (Kratzer and Starcher, 1963; Nielsen *et al.*, 1966). In the rat the maximal stability constant compatible with absorption of iron from complexes is somewhat lower, around log $K =$ 12–14 (Forth *et al.*, 1965, 1968a). Therapeutic experience with iron complexes shows that the conditions in man are similar. The ligands used in present-day therapeutic iron preparations in this connection may be enumerated: ascorbic acid, lactic acid, malic acid, pyruvic acid, fumaric acid, glycine, fructose. Citric acid appears to be exceptional in that log K_1 for its Fe(III)-complex is stated to be 25 (Sillen and Martell, 1964). In all probability this stable complex is not present in the alimentary tract, but is transformed at least in part into the much weaker, protonated complex with a stability constant of log $K = 11–12$ (Sillen and Martell, 1964).

12.1.4.2. *Availability of heavy metals in food*

Phosphates. The phosphate content of food, especially vegetables, in general reduces the availability of heavy metals for absorption. This has been demonstrated for iron (Jacobi *et al.*, 1956a; Hegstedt *et al.*, 1949); iron and phosphate have been found to have a reciprocal influence upon their availability for absorption (Büttner and Muhler, 1959). Thus, addition of phosphate to food reduces the absorption of iron (Büttner and Muhler, 1959), and conversely iron and aluminum reduce the absorption of phosphate; rickets are a possible consequence (Deobald and Elvehejem, 1935). The absorption of zinc (Lewis *et al.*, 1957; Vohra and Kratzer, 1966; Heth *et al.*, 1966) and that of copper (Kirchgessner and Weser, 1965a) are also adversely affected by phosphate. Food contains orthophosphate, pyrophosphate and polyphosphates; these inhibit the absorption of iron both *in vivo* (Jacobi *et al.*, 1956a; Forth *et al.*, 1965b; Forth and Rummel,

1966b) and *in vitro* (Forth *et al.,* 1965c).

Among the organic phosphate compounds the *phytates* of the above-mentioned metals are particularly poorly absorbed (McCance *et al.*, 1943; Sharpe *et al.,* 1948; Savage *et al.,* 1964; Vohra *et al.,* 1965; Cowan *et al.,* 1966b). The hypothesis that the inhibition of absorption of copper and zinc by a soya bean meal is caused by its phytate content (Allred *et al.,* 1964; Davis *et al.,* 1962; O'Dell and Savage, 1960) can be extended to nickel, cobalt and manganese (Davis *et al.,* 1962). In adults (Haghshenass *et al.,* 1972) as well as in children absorption of iron from soya beans is much less than from ferrous ascorbate, especially when the soya beans have been boiled (Asworth *et al.,* 1973). In adults Layrisse *et al.* (1969) found that the availability of iron in soya beans is better than that from any other vegetable source.

It is noteworthy that phytic acid forms stable complexes particularly when five metal ions combine to one ligand molecule (Vohra *et al.,* 1965). Possibly mixed complexes, for instance, between phytate calcium and zinc are formed. In the presence of calcium the availability of zinc is reduced (Byrd and Matrone, 1965; Maddaiah *et al.*, 1964; Oberleas *et al.*, 1966a, b).

The absorption of the iron in *wheat*, *maize and bread* is less than that of simple iron sulfate (Ashworth *et al.*, 1973; Callender and Warner, 1968; Elwood *et al.*, 1968; Hussain *et al.*, 1965); these authors do not give an explanation. Possibly here, too, the reduced availability of iron is caused by the phosphate content of these foods. The same is true for *milk* (Josephs, 1958; Schulz and Smith, 1958), but this statement seems to be contradicted by the observation that *powdered milk* apparently has the opposite effect, i.e. enhances the availability of iron for absorption (Gorten *et al.,* 1963). There is no explanation for this difference. Possibly in milk powder the phosphate to protein ratio is displaced in favor of the latter and/or the proteins in powdered milk are denatured and, therefore, bind iron more strongly. They may then exercise a protective effect and prevent the formation of sparingly soluble phosphates.

Organic *nucleoside phosphates* are additional possible complexing agents for metals (Goucher and Tayler, 1964; Neuberg and Mandl, 1949), but nothing is as yet known about their significance in food in this respect.

Plant material. Speaking generally, iron is not present in a form very favorable for absorption in a diet of *vegetal origin* (Layrisse *et al.,* 1969). The oxalic acid content (e.g. in spinach) contributes to this effect along with the high phosphate content. However, plants also contain substances which promote the absorption of metals. Mills (1954, 1956, 1958, 1961) demonstrated that *meadow grass* contains copper bound in neutral or anionic complexes; these appear to be of special significance for the availability of copper for absorption. Analogous complexes of zinc and manganese appear to occur (Bremner, 1970). Copper-deficient rats absorb the metal administered in this form better than simple copper sulfate. Davis (1966) reports the similar observation that the extracted juice of grasses during certain stages of growth promotes the absorption of divalent cations, among them zinc.

Sugars. The ascorbic acid content of *fruit juices* is not solely responsible for their enhancing effect on the absorption of iron from food (Elwood *et al.,* 1968; Callender and Warner, 1968; Schulz and Smith, 1958). The effect of reducing agents will be discussed in detail at the end of this chapter (see pp. 634–635). Possible chelating agents which may enhance the availability of dietary iron are polybasic hydroxy acids such as citric acid and malic acid. The same absorption-activating effect of organic acids has also been observed for copper (Grassmann and Kirchgessner, 1969). The *sugar,* particularly the *fructose,* contained in fruit juices may contribute to their favorable effect on the absorption of iron. Complex formation with iron has been demonstrated for a number of sugars (Brodan *et al.*, 1967; Charley *et al.*, 1963, 1969; Davis and Deller, 1966; Pollack *et al.*, 1964; Saltman *et al.*, 1962; Stitt *et al.*, 1962). According to Pollack *et al.* (1964) the increase of iron absorption in the presence of fructose may be attributed to a metabolic effect by this sugar. The intermediate products formed, mainly lactic and pyruvic acids, can form complexes with iron and, thus, facilitate its transcellular passage. However, when given to rats orally with iron, these metabolites, as well as fructose, increase iron absorption (Pollack *et al.,* 1964). It is, therefore, very probable that the ligands prevent the formation of sparingly soluble, poorly absorbed forms of iron, e.g. hydroxides and phosphates, and in this way increase the availability of iron for absorption. Since in aged ferric fructose preparations Fe(II) and gluconate were detected, Bates *et al.* (1972) discuss the possibility that in addition to the effect by chelation fructose may provide a "reducing" environment generating and maintaining iron in the ferrous state. *Sorbitol* probably acts in the same way (Herndon *et al.,* 1958). A high sugar content, particularly fructose, in the diet is thought to be the cause of the excessive absorption of iron observed in Bantus, which, ultimately, produces alimentary hypersiderosis (Bothwell, 1969).

Fats. Little is known about the effect of *fats* on the absorption of metals. A high fat content in the diet reduces the absorption of iron in man (Brodan *et al.*, 1968). Fatty acids may exhibit complexing activity for metals—for example, the iron complex of dihydroxidimethylbutyrolactone which is probably of high molecular weight and, hence, poorly absorbed (Forth *et al.*, 1964). It is logical to conclude, by analogy with the conditions prevailing during calcium absorption, that fatty acids also form sparingly soluble compounds with heavy metals and for this reason reduce the availability of these metals for absorption.

Proteins, peptides and amino acids. The effect of proteins on metal absorption is described as either positive or negative. Egg protein retards the absorption of iron (Elwood *et al.*, 1968; Chodos *et al.*, 1957; Moore and Dubach, 1951); it is not known whether the effect is related to its conalbumin content. Conalbumin forms a stable complex with iron (Schade and Caroline, 1944), which *in vitro* drastically reduces the transfer of iron in jejunal segments of normal and anemic rats (Rummel, 1965). Egg yolk also contains a ligand, phosvitin, which forms a stable complex with iron (Greengard *et al.*, 1964).

The protein contained in the food depressed copper absorption in sheep where protection from toxic copper effects was investigated (McPhersons and Hemingway, 1965). In chicken fed a diet with additional copper (0.1 %) the copper content of the liver is reduced by dietary proteins (Kirchgessner *et al.*, 1970). Also, in man, the availability of cobalt for absorption in the alimentary tract is reduced by proteins (Paley and Sussman, 1963).

The effect of food proteins on the uptake of copper from the intestine may vary with the origin of the proteins (Suttle and Mills, 1966). Raw meat reduces the availability of copper for absorption but loses its effect after cooking (Moore, 1964).

An absorption-enhancing action of proteins in man is reported for lead (Milev *et al.*, 1970) and for iron (Klavins *et al.*, 1962; Brodan *et al.*, 1968; Layrisse *et al.*, 1968; Martinez-Torres and Layrisse, 1970; Moore and Dubach, 1951). In chicken fed a normal diet without any additional copper an increase in the protein content of the food was followed by an increase in the copper content of the liver (Kirchgessner *et al.*, 1970). This means that proteins in food may increase the availability of copper for absorption in low copper diets whereas in high copper diets proteins show the contrary effect (Kirchgessner *et al.*, 1970).

This ambivalent effect of proteins on copper uptake from the intestine may be due to different types of copper complexes formed in the food depending on the ratio of its copper and protein content. This, however, implies the assumption that these complexes make copper available for absorption to different degrees. With regard to the enhancing effect of protein in food on metal absorption one has to bear in mind also the effect on growth of an adequate protein and caloric nourishment which is followed by an increased uptake of biometals as for instance iron (Enwonwu *et al.*, 1972). This effect which may be involved in all longterm feeding experiments must be discerned clearly from the intraluminal effect of proteins on the availability of metals for absorption.

The differential effect of proteins on the absorption of metals could also be attributed to the different degree of hydrolysis in different experiments. On the basis of information available about the influence of polypeptides, oligopeptides and amino acids on the absorption of metals the following can be stated. After copper depletion the rats make better use of copper presented as mono-, oligo- or polymeric amino acids complexes in the food than of simple copper sulfate. The availability of copper decreases as the degree of polymerization increases (Kirchgessner *et al.*, 1967). This conclusion is based on the measurement of the copper content of rat livers. Under the same experimental conditions slightly more copper was available from complexes with L-amino acids than from complexes with the corresponding D-isomers (Kirchgessner *et al.*, 1967; Kirchgessner and Grassmann, 1970). These authors, therefore, discuss the possibility of a connection of the transport system for amino acids of the mucosal cells with the absorption of the intact copper–amino acid complex. While this may be true the possibility that the amino acid isomers form complexes which release copper to the mucosal epithelium differently must still be considered. The arguments in favor of this possibility are discussed below (see pp. 704–707).

Amino acids enhance the absorption not only of copper but also of zinc. Cysteine and histidine have been investigated most intensely (Nielsen *et al.*, 1966, 1967). However, histidine is said to become effective only after decarboxylation to histamine because it only partially eliminates the symptoms of zinc deficiency, while histamine can do so completely (Nielsen *et al.*, 1967). Concerning the effect of histidine on the absorption of zinc see pp. 704–707.

The effect of amino acids on the absorption of iron has been investigated in detail (Jacobi *et al.*, 1956a; Kroe *et al.*, 1963a, b). Among the investigated amino acids histidine proved to be particularly effective (Kroe *et al.*, 1963a, b, 1966; Van Campen and Gross, 1969).

A comparison of the effect of histidine on copper and iron absorption respectively indicates that despite the higher stability constant of the copper–histidine complex (Sillen and Martell, 1964) the effect on iron absorption seems to be greater. Histidine increases the absorption of copper 1.3 times by comparison with simple inorganic copper (Kirchgessner and Grassmann, 1970), while the absorption of iron is increased by about 30 times (Van Campen and Gross, 1969). However, such a comparison is not valid because the experimental conditions in the two cases were not comparable. In the iron experiments both groups of workers presented the metal to the controls in a particularly poorly absorbed form, i.e. as inorganic iron salt at pH 7 (Van Campen and Gross, 1969) and as iron phosphate at pH 3 (Kroe *et al.*, 1963b) respectively. These compounds were injected into tied-off jejunal segments *in vivo,* while the copper experiments were conducted by feeding, i.e. the metal passed through the stomach. In the experiments aimed at studying the absorption of iron, histidine was presented in a 20,000–100,000-fold excess; in the copper experiments the 1:1- and the 2:1-histidine–copper complexes were used.

Hemoglobin. It is certain today that hemoglobin iron is absorbed from food and utilized (Callender *et al.*, 1957; Conrad *et al.*, 1966; Goldberg *et al.*, 1963; Turnbull *et al.*, 1962; Walsh *et al.*, 1955). After administration of 5 mg of iron in man the same or a higher amount was absorbed from hemoglobin iron rather than simple ferrous sulfate (Turnbull *et al.*, 1962). In the rat, however, with similar doses per kilogram of body weight only one-fifth as much hemoglobin iron is found to be absorbed as after administration of ferrous sulfate (Weintraub *et al.*, 1965).

The peculiar observation that hemoglobin iron can be utilized better than heme iron can be explained by the tendency of the latter to form poorly absorbed *polymers* (Conrad *et al.*, 1966a). The heme iron complex is in part absorbed intact (Brown *et al.*, 1966, 1968). Chelating agents fail to decrease the absorption of hemoglobin iron (Bannerman and Malpass, 1965; Hallberg and Sölvell, 1964; Hwang and Brown, 1963, 1965; Turnbull *et al.*, 1962). The bulk of hemoglobin iron is released from the complex in epithelial cells of the mucosa (Brown *et al.*, 1966; Weintraub *et al.*, 1968a, b). This reaction which involves the splitting of the heme-ring is catalyzed enzymatically by xanthine oxidase in mucosal cells (Awai and Brown, 1969; Dawson *et al.*, 1970). This oxidase forms the hydrogen peroxide necessary for splitting the α-methene bridge in heme (Lemberg *et al.*, 1939, 1941a, b). The appearance of heme iron in the non-heme fraction within the mucosal cells agrees with the observation that ferrous sulfate administered orally or intravenously also inhibits the absorption of heme iron (Conrad *et al.*, 1966).

There is evidence that the ability of the mucosa cells to split heme is *species* dependent. In rats heme appears to be split only to a small extent (Weintraub *et al.*, 1965a), and the same seems to be true in sheep (Georgi, 1964).

In *iron-deficiency* the absorption of hemoglobin iron is increased (Conrad *et al.*, 1966; Weintraub *et al.*, 1965a; Turnbull *et al.*, 1962; Callender *et al.*, 1957; Wheby *et al.*, 1970); an explanation is not yet available. The increased uptake of heme-bound iron by the epithelial cells of the mucosa could be due to the formation of a hetero-complex between the iron acceptor sites in the mucosa and the iron coordination sites freed by the removal of globin. No reliable data are available concerning the activity of xanthine oxidase in the mucosa of normal and iron-deficient animals (Awai and Brown, 1969; Dawson *et al.*, 1970).

Metal–metal interactions. So far the discussion has been restricted to the influence of ligands present in the food on the availability of metals for intestinal absorption. Undoubtedly the availability of metals is also influenced by *competing metals*. The reduction in the availability of zinc by calcium, due probably to the formation of sparingly soluble mixed complexes with phosphates, has already been mentioned (p. 628). Kirchgessner *et al.* also achieved the reverse effect, i.e. an increase of the availability of iron, cobalt, manganese, zinc, and molybdenum, by the addition of copper to the food (Kirchgessner *et al.*, 1963; Kirchgessner and Weser, 1963, 1965a). These authors interpret the result as a consequence either of blocking by copper of ligands which withhold the metals mentioned from absorption, or by displacement of the metals from non-absorbed complexes in food. This interpretation has been supported by *in vitro* experiments, in which it was demonstrated that the dialyzability of the metals from protein-containing solutions can be increased by adding copper (Kirchgessner and Weser, 1963, 1965a). The increase in zinc retention by a large dose of calcium in the food and the converse increase in calcium retention brought about by addition of zinc does not, however, appear to be due solely to a competitive intraluminal displacement of the metals from complexes in food. A diminished excretion accompanies the increased retention of the two metals (Kirchgessner, 1965).

Here, metal–metal interactions due to growth-increasing or metabolic effects as for instance the well-known interrelationship of copper (ceruloplasmin = ferrioxidase) and iron or of molybdenum (xanthineoxidase) on iron (for ref. see Seelig, 1972) must remain out of consideration.

12.1.4.3. *Influence of reducing constituents in food*

The iron reducing power of food has repeatedly been demonstrated (Bergheim and Kirch, 1949; Kirch *et al.*, 1947; Süllman, 1931; Tompsett, 1940). Reduction of ferric to ferrous iron is favored by the acid gastric medium. Depending on the nature of the food, 75–98% of the trivalent (ferric) iron added to food is reduced to the divalent (ferrous) form. Fruit juice, tomato juice and vegetables which contain a high content of ascorbic acid have a reducing effect. Bread, meat and eggs and especially egg yolk are less active in this respect. The reducing activity of proteins is enhanced by peptic digestion (Kirch *et al.*, 1947), and attributable to their content of glutathione and cysteine.

For a long time the role of reducing agents during iron absorption formed the center of interest, because it was assumed that iron could be absorbed only in the divalent form (see pp. 618–621). The capacity of *ascorbic acid* to form complexes with iron probably contributes to the absorption-enhancing effect of this compound in addition to its reducing activity (Conrad and Schade, 1968; Jacobi *et al.*, 1956b; Höglund and Reitzenstein, 1969b; Hopping and Ruliffson, 1966; Ruskin and Merril, 1949). The same double role of simultaneously being complexing and reducing agent must be assumed for cysteine and glutathione (Jacobi *et al.*, 1956b).

The formation of a complex between ascorbic acid and iron can be deduced from the following experiment. Increasing the effective stability of the ascorbic acid–iron complex by increasing the excess of ligand (ascorbic acid: Fe = 280:1) leads to diminished iron absorption (Forth *et al.*, 1968b). Characteristically, the effect can only be shown in iron-deficient rats in which iron is absorbed very rapidly only under these conditions and the rate of release of iron from the complex limits the rate of absorption.

Dehydroascorbic acid, the oxidation product of ascorbic acid, displays the same effect as the latter (see Table 5). It may be noted that dehydroascorbic acid also has a reducing activity; on the basis of the percentage of bivalent iron in the intestinal lumen its action does not differ from that of ascorbic acid (see Table 6).

Reducing agents can influence the absorption of iron also by promoting the release of complex-bound iron. It must be remembered that, in general, complexes with ferric iron are more stable than those containing divalent (ferrous) iron (Sillen and Martell, 1964). Complexing agents protect metals from the effect of oxidoreduction reactions only to a limited extent and a number of different factors determine whether or not iron can be reduced when inside a complex. In addition to the stability of the complex, steric factors are probably decisive (Martell and Calvin, 1958; Dwyer and Mellor, 1964). A labilization of stable Fe(III)-complexes by reducing agents is well known. For instance, it plays a role in the liberation of iron from ferritin (cf. Bielig and Bayer, 1955; Mazur *et al.*, 1955, 1958). A similar mechanism is made use of in the determination of transferrin-bound iron in the plasma which becomes dissociated by reduction with ascorbic acid (Schade and Caroline, 1946; Schade *et al.*, 1954). It is possible, therefore, that reducing agents such as ascorbic acid act in the intestinal lumen by labilizing stable complexes which normally release their iron either only to a small extent or not at all and, thus, make this iron available for absorption (Forth *et al.*, 1968c).

Little is yet known about the effect of ascorbic acid on the absorption of other heavy metals. As several studies have shown, up to a threefold excess of *ascorbic acid* has no effect on the absorption of *cobalt*. Ascorbic acid reduces the absorption of *copper* (Van Campen and Gross, 1968; Hill and Starcher, 1965; Carlton and Henderson, 1965; Hunt and Carlton, 1965). On purely theoretical grounds the cause could be, firstly, the formation of a stable, poorly absorbed complex of copper with ascorbic acid, dehydroascorbic acid or another oxidation product of ascorbic acid. Alternatively, under certain conditions, e.g. in the presence of a large excess of ascorbic acid, reduction of bivalent (cupric) to monovalent (cuprous) copper could lead to the formation of sparingly soluble and, hence, poorly absorbed cuprous chloride.

12.1.4.4. *Influence of drugs*

Drugs, e.g. antibiotics added to animal food, can act as ligands for metals in the same way as do food constituents.

This is not the appropriate place for separately listing all the drugs which may form complexes with metals. In any case the only drugs of practical significance with regard to metal absorption are those which are administered therapeutically over a prolonged period. Pyrazolones and salicylic acid derivatives, especially para-aminosalicylic acid used in the treatment of tuberculosis, may be mentioned here. Other tuberculostatics such as thiosemicarbazones also form complexes with metals. Among chemotherapeutic agents 8-hydroxyquinoline and its derivatives are well-known complexing agents. Such compounds are used to treat intestinal infections, and their ability to form heavy metal complexes is related to their chemotherapeutic action (cf. Albert, 1965). Details of the effect of 8-hydroxyquinoline derivatives on the absorption of heavy metals are discussed later (see pp. 695–698). In this connection it is probably not out of place to mention the sulfonamides, especially those which are taken permanently to reduce the blood sugar level. The same is true of the biguanides which have a blood-sugar-depressing effect. Reference is also appropriate to the property of the B-group vitamins (thiamine, riboflavin, nicotinic acid derivatives) to form complexes with heavy metals. Systematic investigations about the effect of drugs on heavy metal absorption are not, as yet, available. Cholestyramine, a high molecular quaternary ammonium anion exchange resin which is used therapeutically for the removal of bile acids from the intestine, binds especially anionic drugs and, thus, delays their absorption in rats (cf. Gallo *et al.*, 1965). Surprisingly, however, cholestyramine impairs also the absorption of neutral drugs, e.g. digitoxin (Caldwell and Greenberger, 1971), vitamin B_{12} and even $FeSO_4$ (Thomas *et al.*, 1971, 1972b). In iron-deficient rats cholestyramine inhibits even the absorption of hemoglobin iron (Thomas *et al.*, 1971). This effect of cholestyramine may be the cause of the anemia observed in connection with long-term treatment in man (Kniffin *et al.*, 1970).

The manner in which antibiotics affect the metal balance in the organism is a problem that needs to be studied under therapeutic conditions in human and in veterinary medicine. The property of most antibiotics to form metal chelates leads not only to these drugs being converted into poorly absorbed compounds in the gut lumen (see Chapter 5 of this book, p. 307), but also to impaired absorption of biologically important heavy metals. This fact is well known for the *tetracyclines* (Albert and Rees, 1956) and for *penicillins* and their degradation-product *penicilloic acid,* for *cycloserine, streptomycine, kanamycine* and *novobiocin. Chloramphenicol* is an exception in apparently having only slightly developed chelate-forming properties (Niebergall *et al.*, 1966; Cressmann *et al.*, 1966; Yamabe, 1967). The complexes which the above antibiotics form with copper, nickel, cobalt and zinc are particularly stable.

A distinction must be made between this intraluminal effect of antibiotics on the availability of metals for absorption and the increase in retention of trace elements by antibiotics. The latter effect is due essentially to accelerated growth of the animals and the consequent increase in demand (Kirchgessner, 1961; Kirchgessner and Weser, 1965b). Tetracyclines and cycloheximide which inhibit the protein synthesis are known to inhibit the transfer of ferrous iron across the mucosal epithelium of rats *in vitro* and *in vivo* (Greenberger, 1973; Greenberger and Ruppert, 1966a, b; Greenberger *et al.*, 1967; Yeh and Shils, 1966; see also p. 681). Penicillin and chloramphenicol proved to be without effect on the iron absorption from tied-off intestinal segments of rats *in vivo* (Greenberger *et al.*, 1967).

12.1.4.5. *Influence of microorganisms*

For the sake of completeness it is necessary to mention the *microorganisms* of the intestinal flora. Their effect on the availability of metals for absorption by virtue of the formation of sparingly soluble sulfides has already been mentioned (see p. 604). Starting from this premise, it is reasonable to assume that in the lower intestine, i.e. the cecum and colon, only a small proportion of the metals present in the gut contents are present in a form suitable for absorption. No systematic investigations on interactions between metal absorption and enterophytes appear to have been published. That microorganisms can induce metal retention is suggested by experiments of Reddy *et al.* (1965), who found less copper and iron in the bodies of rats brought up under germ-free conditions than in normally reared rats. The manganese content of the two groups was the same.

12.1.5. AVAILABILITY FOR ABSORPTION WITH PARTICULAR REFERENCE TO THERAPEUTICS AND INTOXICATION

A long time ago heavy metals were used extensively in therapeutics. A very few heavy metals kept some significance as metalo-organic compounds in the treatment of tropic diseases, as for instance antimony, bismuth and arsenic. Mercury-containing organic compounds are considered today as obsolete diuretics. We shall therefore confine the discussion to the therapeutic *substitution* of heavy metals in cases of deficiency which can be dealt with very briefly here. For the few metals, especially iron, and possibly zinc, for which deficiency states in man are known, the intestinal mucosa apparently is able to absorb the metals from the diet according to the whole body's requirements. It is unknown in which form zinc should be given to deficient subjects. Therapeutic experience with iron shows that a normal diet with added Fe(II)-salts or, for better tolerance, weak iron complexes (see p. 629) supported by fruit juice (acid medium, polybasic hydroxy-acid ligands, ascorbic acid as reducing agent) brings optimum results. The basic principle has long been established. Fifty years ago the treatment of chlorosis in Russia and Germany consisted in giving the patients sour milk into which rusty nails had

TABLE 9. DECREASE OF METAL AVAILABILITY PRODUCED BY SOME RECOMMENDED ADDITIVES TO GASTRIC LAVAGE FLUID USED IN ACUTE METAL POISONING
(Taken from Moeschlin, 1972; Dreisbach, 1966; Wirth *et al.*, 1967; Deichmann and Gerarde, 1969)

Additives:	Milk and/or egg white	"Antidotum metallorum" (H_2S)	NaI (1%)	$NaHCO_3$ (5%)	Na_2SO_4	Ferricyanoferrat(II)	NaCl
Metal:	Zn, Cu, Fe, Cr, Hg, Ag	Cu, As, HG, Bi, Cd	Tl	Fe	Pb	Cu, Tl	Ag
Resulting compounds:	Albuminates	Sulfides	TlI	Fe-hydroxide	$PbSO_4$	Cyanoferrat(II)-complexes	$AgCl_2$
Remarks:	For first aid only; must be removed by vomiting, gastric lavage or laxative (Na_2SO_4)	Obsolete; produces H_2S intoxication		Should be added in any case when chelating of metals is desired	Lead-phosphate is less soluble than the sulfate	Life saving in experiments with animals	—

previously been placed. In Westphalia it was usual to spike apples with nails and, after some time, to use the iron-enriched fruit for therapeutic purposes! This usage probably explains the 1744 "Stahltinktur mit Borsdorffer Apfelsaffte" dispensary formulation mentioned by Turk (1940). The range of ligands used for present-day therapeutic preparations is similar to that in these old-time remedies and comprises ascorbic acid, hydroxy acids, fructose and amino acids such as glycine.

The laws determining metal availability in the gastrointestinal tract have a number of consequences that need to be considered in the treatment of cases of acute *metal poisoning*. Table 9 lists the antidotes and most important additives to gastric wash-outs in present use.

These additives cause the formation of sparingly soluble metal compounds which either can be removed by gastric lavage or else can leave the intestine with the feces without causing substantial harm. Removal of sparingly soluble precipitates by inducing vomiting or gastric wash-out should certainly not be omitted if it is technically feasible and if there are no contraindications. This is true especially if milk or egg albumin is used to form sparingly soluble *albuminates*. Experience has shown that such compounds may break up again and absorption may then take place during passage along the intestine and may even, under certain circumstances, be favored by protein hydrolysates.

Transformation of metals into sparingly soluble *sulfides* is a well-established measure which is therapeutically dangerous because of the risk of hydrogen sulfide poisoning. Buchheim (1878) mentioned the efficacy of precipitated iron sulfide in the treatment of poisoning by mercury, copper, and lead, i.e. precisely by those metals the sulfides of which have a greater solubility product than iron sulfide (Table 1). In place of the not entirely innocuous "antidotum metallorum", a concentrated stabilized solution of hydrogen sulfide K_2S (potassium sulfide) has been used as an alternative (Catsch, 1964, 1968).

Peculiarly enough, adding *bicarbonate* to gastric lavage fluid for neutralizing the gastric acid and converting the metal into sparingly soluble hydroxide is recommended only in iron poisoning; the same measure would appear to be suitable for other heavy metals which also form sparingly soluble hydroxides. The often desired formation of poorly absorbed metal complexes is also more difficult to obtain in an acid medium than after neutralization of the gastric acid.

It is not clear why *sodium-sulfate* lavages are used in the treatment of lead poisoning. Lead-phosphate ($= \log SP \sim 42$) has a lower solubility product than lead sulfate ($= \log SP \sim 8$) (Sillen and Martell, 1964). The addition of phosphate should be useful, at least on theoretical grounds, in the case of a number of other heavy metals.

Similar considerations apply to the use of *potassiumferrocyanide*. This compound should always be employed in conjunction with bicarbonate in order to prevent cyanide formation in the stomach. If it is allowed to deduce therapeutic suggestions from animal tests then the cyanoferrate (II)-complex which has given good results in removing radioactive cesium from the organism (Nigrovic and Catsch, 1965), or thallium poisoning (Dvorak, 1970, 1971), because of its small solubility product (see Table 1), should also be suitable for removing silver compound.

Complexing agents are added to gastric lavage fluid in acute metal poisoning for the purpose of forming poorly absorbed complexes. Simultaneous intravenous administration of complexing agents is recommended in order to eliminate by the kidneys the fraction of the metal which has been absorbed. At the present time *desferrioxamine B* (deferoxamine, see p. 702) is used orally as well as intravenously against acute iron poisoning (Moeschlin and Schnider, 1964). Neutralization of the gastric acid seems to be a prerequisite for the chelating of iron by deferoxamine as well as for measures inducing the formation of sparingly soluble iron hydroxide.

Diethylenetriaminepentaacetic acid (DTPA, cf. Table 33 and p. 701) and D-*penicillamine* are employed to prevent the absorption of copper in, for example, Wilson's disease. (DTPA: O'Reilly and Bank, 1964; D-penicillamine: Catsch, 1964, 1968).

Polyaminepolycarbonic acids (see pp. 699–702) have given good results especially for preventing absorption of metals which occur as radioactive fission products (Catsch, 1964, 1968; Schubert, 1955).

Acid polysaccharides (polyuronic acids) have recently been recommended for preventing the intestinal absorption of metals (Tanaka and Skoryna, 1969; Skoryna *et al.*, 1972); wide experience with such compounds has not yet been recorded.

12.2. MUCOSAL TRANSFER OF HEAVY METALS

This section deals with the mechanisms of metal transfer from the lumen across the mucosal epithelial cells into the blood, i.e. the actual absorption process. The first question is whether a transport system comparable to that responsible for the transport of sodium exists for heavy metals. This question is particularly relevant for metals where intestinal absorption is adapted to the needs of the organism, i.e. for iron, copper and zinc. Such transfer systems may be discussed for all essential heavy metals for which the supply of the organism is warranted by intestinal absorption. From the reviews of Schwarz (1970, 1973) and Kirchgessner (1972) those metals which must be regarded as essential at present may be taken. For the remaining heavy metals, for which an adaptation of absorption to the demand has not been detected, the following discussion is restricted to the question whether these metals—due to their chemical similarities with biologically important heavy metals, e.g. iron–share the same transfer system.

12.2.1. SITES OF ABSORPTION

Systematic investigations concerning the sites of absorption of heavy metals in the gastrointestinal tract are very sparsely referred to in the literature. Assessing the available data is made difficult by the fact that the experimental conditions in the various investigations often cannot be compared. The method of *in situ tied-off intestinal segments* is useful for determining regions in which a metal is preferentially absorbed. Clearly, results obtained in this manner for a given length of intestine and a given exposure period to the metals cannot always be extrapolated to physiological conditions after oral administration. In the rat under physiological conditions the transit time of ingested material through the ileum is for instance 20 times longer than that through the jejunum (Dupuis and Fournier, 1963; Lengemann, 1963). This fact needs to be considered in assessing the capacity of the two intestinal segments for absorption. Also, one must remember that experiments with tied-off segments *in situ* are necessarily short-term tests, the results of which cannot be extrapolated quantitatively to events after oral administration with free intestinal passage.

In vitro investigations on intestinal segments have often been used to study differences of absorptive activity. Our own experience shows that careful interpretation of results obtained *in vitro* leads on principle to the same conclusions as experiments with tied-off segments *in vivo*. However, the artificial conditions of *in vitro* experiments entail the risk of misinterpreting the results. *In vitro* the discharge from the mucosa is slowed down by the absence of perfusion with blood. In order to characterize this difference between the results obtained *in vitro* and *in vivo* the ratio between the radioiron content of intestinal tissue and the amount of radioiron transferred across the gut wall is shown in Table 10. This ratio

TABLE 10. TRANSFER AND TISSUE CONTENT OF ^{59}Fe PRESENTED AS $FeSO_4$ AND $FeCl_3$ TOGETHER WITH 8-HYDROXYQUINOLINE TO JEJUNAL SEGMENTS OF RATS *in vitro* AND *in vivo*

Experimental conditions: fasted rats (16 hr), Wistar (female), 180–220 g body weight. *In vivo*: tied-off jejunal segments: length 12 cm, starting from the flexura duodenojejunalis (operation under ether anesthesia). Time: 1 hr; means from five rats. *In vitro*: method according to Fisher and Parsons (1949) modified by Rummel and Stupp (1960); length 8 cm, starting from the flexura duodenojejunalis; two segments of each rat; Time: 2 hr, temp. 37°C. In order to remove adsorbed iron from the surface the segments were washed three times in 100 ml saline containing EDTA (10^{-2} M/l) (after data from Rummel *et al.*, 1967)

Method	Metal	Amount administered (mcM)	Ligand	Ligand : Fe	Amount transferred (percent of the dose)	Amount in the tissue (percent of the dose)	Amount in tissue / Amount transferred
in vivo	^{59}Fe-($FeSO_4$)	0.36	—	—	10.8	29.6	2.7
in vitro	^{59}Fe-($FeSO_4$)	0.50	—	—	0.13	3.2	25
in vivo	^{59}Fe-($FeCl_3$)	0.36	8-OH-quinoline	10:1	37.6	39.0	1
in vitro	^{59}Fe-($FeCl_3$)	0.50	8-OH-quinoline	100:1	0.24	8.6	36

is almost 10 times greater in the *in vitro* experiments than in the *in vivo*. In other words, *in vitro* relatively more iron remains in the mucosa than in the living organism and, conversely, *in vivo* more iron is discharged from the mucosa into the organism than is transferred to the serosal fluid *in vitro*. When radioiron is presented as the Fe(III)–8-hydroxyquinoline complex the ratio of tissue content of ^{59}Fe to the transferred amount *in vitro* is more than 30 times that observed *in vivo*. When extrapolating from *in vitro* results to the *in vivo* absorption metals, not only the transfer rate, but also the tissue content, should be considered. The latter is particularly significant in assessing the absorption of complex-bound metals. Here, the amount which can be found in tissue may be used as a measure of the metal-donor effect of the complex or of the absorption of the intact complex and, hence, its penetration into the mucosal epithelium, e.g. as for Fe(III)–8-hydroxyquinoline.

The relationship between the tissue-bound fraction and the amount of substance transferred into intestinal segments *in vitro* is quite generally significant in assessing absorption. Differences similar to those for the various iron compounds are found when testing the absorption of cardiac glycosides (Forth *et al.*, 1969) and barbiturates (Kakemi *et al.*, 1969).

A further difference between *in vivo* and *in vitro* results is attributed to oxidation of the metal investigated in the perfusion fluid *in vitro* due to saturation with oxygen and, hence, conversion of the metal into sparingly soluble and poorly absorbed hydroxides. Different metals are oxidized to a different extent. In contrast to iron, cobalt is unaffected, because the oxygen-saturated perfusion solution cannot oxidize cobalt(II) to cobalt (III). The formation of sparingly soluble metal compounds can be monitored by the fall of the metal concentration in the incubation fluid during an experiment (Forth and Rummel, 1965; Forth *et al.*, 1965c; Forth, 1966). In addition to metal hydroxides, sparingly soluble phosphates can also be formed in the incubation fluid. In general, the occasional differences in literature between the results obtained in *in vitro* and *in vivo* experiments can be explained by such methodological differences.

In the following discussion dealing with the site of the preferential absorption, only the metal ions and aquo-ions will be considered. The question of the absorption of metal complexes from the different intestinal regions will be dealt with in connection with the transfer of chelates through the gut wall (see pp. 690–710), as far as any information is available.

If the results obtained with tied-off intestinal segments are accepted as valid, the absorptive activity of the different sections of the gastrointestinal tract of the rat for iron, molybdenum and zinc decreases in the following order: duodenum–terminal ileum–lower ileum–stomach (Van Campen and Mitchell, 1965). For copper the sequence is: stomach–duodenum–lower jejunum–terminal ileum. The conclusion can be drawn that the stomach can be significant as the site for absorption of copper and possibly also of other metals. To these results obtained in rats should be added the results obtained in man with respect to the capacity of the stomach for copper absorption (Cartwright *et al.*, 1954; Bearn and Kunkel, 1955). From the rapid absorption of copper after oral administration these authors concluded that it is absorbed from the stomach. Lead is considered to be present in the stomach in a form suitable for absorption (Tompsett, 1940); however, this remains to be confirmed. The investigations by Van Campen and Mitchell (1965) on rats demonstrated appreciable absorption from the stomach for iron and molybdenum but not for zinc, the absorption of which amounted to only 0.5% of the dose. This was confirmed by Methfessel and Spencer (1966, 1973a) in the same species. In these experiments the absorption of zinc from the stomach was equal to that from the colon and amounted to about 1–2% of the dose.

There are probably *species differences* in the absorption of metals from the stomach. According to Miller and Cragle (1965) living bovines absorb up to 35% of the daily dose of zinc from the abomasum. In chickens the amount of zinc absorbed from the proventriculus reaches 67% of the given dose (Miller and Jensen, 1966). However, in these studies on cattle and chickens the zinc was administered in the food. The metal may therefore have been present in a form more suitable for absorption than the simple zinc salts used in the rat experiments (Van Campen and Mitchell, 1965; Methfessel and Spencer, 1966). Methfessel and Spencer (1966, 1973a) confirmed that zinc is absorbed mainly from the duodenum (Van Campen and Mitchell, 1965).

Intensive investigations concerning the site of preferential absorption in the gastrointestinal tract have been made for iron. Here the initial *in vitro* results, according to which the *duodenum* and the *upper jejunum* are the main sites of absorption (Brown and Justus, 1958; Dowdle *et al.*, 1960; Forth, 1963; Forth and Rummel, 1965), were confirmed in man and other animals *in vivo* (Duthie, 1964; Wheby, 1966; Hemmati, 1968). It is clearly shown that, especially during iron deficiency, the proximal sections of the duodenum display a high absorptive activity (Fig. 7). Neither in the stomach nor in the ileum can an increase in the absorptive activity for iron be observed for anemic rats under the conditions used in these experiments. Figure 7 shows that in this condition the region in

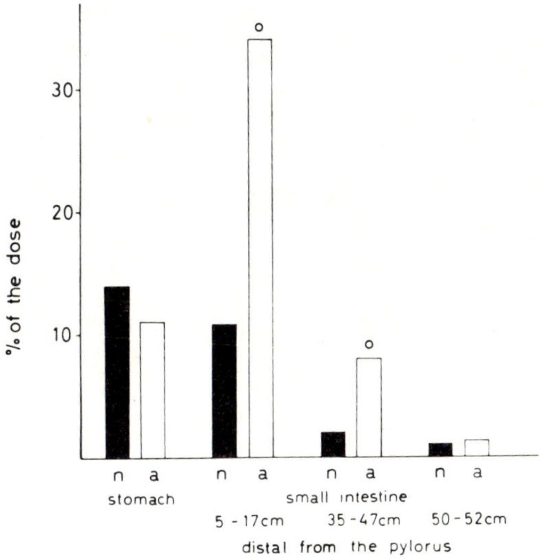

FIG. 7. Absorption of iron from tied-off segments of the gastrointestinal tract of normal and iron-deficient rats *in vivo*. Experimental conditions: fasted rats (16 hr), Wistar (female), 180–200 g body weight. Normal rats (*n*): 14.5 g hemoglobin per 100 ml blood (SEM = ± 1.2; $n = 25$). Iron-deficient rats (*d*): 6.5 g hemoglobin per 100 ml blood (SEM = ± 0.9; $n = 25$). Iron dose: 0.36 mcM ^{59}Fe–($FeCl_3$) in 2 ml sodium chloride solution (0.9%) pH 2 (operation in ether anesthesia). Time: 1 hr. The columns represent means from five rats; SEM = 20% of the mean. o = $p < 0.01$ as compared with the group of normal rats. The absorption of the radioactive iron was measured in a body counter for small animals after removal of the tied-off segments. (From Forth and Rummel, 1968.)

which iron is absorbed more efficiently during deficiency evidently extends distally to the ileum. Wack and Wyatt (1959) had previously made this observation. In iron deficiency iron can be absorbed to an appreciable extent even from the colon (Chernelch *et al.*, 1970; Terato *et al.*, 1973b).

The increase in absorptive activity of the upper jejunum in iron deficiency is not limited to iron. A similar enhancement has been demonstrated for chemically related metals, e.g. cobalt and nickel. Also zinc and manganese are absorbed at a more rapid rate in iron deficiency, but not copper (see Table 11). Enhanced absorption of these metals occurs despite the prophylactic addition of cobalt, nickel, copper, zinc and manganese to an iron-deficient diet (Forth and Andres, 1969; Forth, 1970). These findings are discussed later (see pp. 669–677).

Experiments with rat intestinal segments *in vitro* show that the amount transferred and the content of the metals in Table 11, except for manga-

TABLE 11. TRANSFER AND TISSUE CONTENT OF IRON, COBALT, NICKEL, MANGANESE, COPPER AND ZINC IN JEJUNAL AND ILEAL EVERTED SACS OF NORMAL AND IRON-DEFICIENT RATS

Experimental conditions: fasted rats (16 hr), Wistar (female), 160–190 g body weight. Normal rats (*n*): 14.6 g hemoglobin per 100 ml blood (SEM = ± 1.5; $n = 80$); iron-deficient rats (*d*): 5.6 g hemoglobin per 100 ml blood (SEM = ± 1.7; $n = 80$). Metal concentration on both sides of the everted sacs: 5×10^{-6} M/l; radioactive metals were added on the mucosal side only (50,000 cpm/ml). Mucosal fluid: 10 ml Tyrode solution. Serosal fluid: 0.5 ml Tyrode solution at the beginning of the experiment. At the end: jejunal segments 0.55 ml (SEM = ± 0.05; $n = 120$), ileal segments 0.49 ml (SEM = ± 0.04; $n = 80$). Length of the jejunal segments: 3.5 cm, starting from the flexura duodenojejunalis; two segments of each rat. Length of the ileal segments: 3.5 cm, starting 5 cm proximal of the valvula ileocoecalis; two segments of each rat. In order to remove adsorbed metals from the surface, the tissue was washed three times in 100 ml saline containing EDTA (10^{-2} M/l). Time: 2 hr; temp. 37°C. The values are means of four to twenty-five experiments, ± SEM. (From Forth, 1966)

Metal		Radioactivity in the serosal fluid (cpm/ml)		Radioactivity in the tissue (cpm/segment)	
		jejunal segments	ileal segments	jejunal segments	ileal segments
^{59}Fe–($FeSO_4$)	*n*	2000 ± 300	400[(a)] ± 10	32,000 ± 3000	8000[(b)] ± 1500
	d	16,000[(b)] ± 1500	2000[(a)(b)] ± 300	74,000[(b)] ± 6000	12,000[(b)] ± 200
^{58}Co–($CoCl_2$)	*n*	19,000 ± 1500	7000[(a)] ± 400	14,000 ± 300	10,000 ± 1600
	d	57,000[(b)] ± 3100	—	43,000[(b)] ± 500	—
^{63}Ni–($NiSO_4$)	*n*	10,000 ± 1200	6000[(d)] ± 1400	2000 ± 200	2000 ± 500
	d	42,000[(b)] ± 1100	13,000[(a)(b)] ± 3000	5000 ± 400	3000[(a)] ± 500
^{54}Mn–($MnCl_2$)	*n*	3000 ± 200	3000 ± 400	17,000 ± 1200	7000 ± 400
	d	9000[(b)] ± 1000	7000[(b)] ± 600	46,000[(b)] ± 500	15,000[(a)(b)] ± 1200
^{64}Cu–($CuSO_4$)	*n*	900 ± 300	—	22,000 ± 3000	—
	d	800 ± 150	—	17,000[(b)] ± 3000	—
^{65}Zn–($ZnCl_2$)	*n*	140 ± 60	—	11,000 ± 2000	—
	d	260[(b)] ± 90	—	20,000 ± 5000	—

[(a)] $p < 0.05$ as compared with jejunal segments.
[(b)] $p < 0.05$ as compared with the segments of normal rats.

TABLE 12. ABSORPTION OF SOME HEAVY METALS IN TIED-OFF JEJUNAL AND ILEAL SEGMENTS OF RATS *in vivo*

Experimental conditions: fasted rats (16 hr), Wistar (female), 180–220 g body weight. Metal dose: 10 nM in 2 ml saline, pH 2; in this concentration these heavy metals did not influence the "uphill" transport of glucose in everted jejunal segments *in vitro*. Length of the tied-off segments (operation under ether anesthesia): 15 cm, starting with the flexura duodenojejunalis (jejunal segments) and 3 cm proximal to the valvula ileocoecalis (ileal segments). Absorption of the radioactive metals was measured in a body counter for small animals after removing the tied-off loops. Means of five to fifteen rats ± SEM. (From Leopold *et al.*, 1968)

Segments		Metals										
		^{51}Cr ($CrCl_3$)	^{54}Mn ($MnCl_2$)	^{59}Fe ($FeSO_4$)	^{60}Co ($CoCl_2$)	^{64}Cu ($CuSO_4$)	^{65}Zn ($ZnCl_2$)	^{203}Hg ($HgCl_2$)	^{204}Tl (Tl^2SO_4)	^{113}Sn ($SnCl_2$)	^{210}Pb (Pb-acetate)	^{125}Sb ($SbCl_3$)
Jejunum:	absorption fraction in percent of the dose	5.1 ±0.5	1.8 ±0.2	10.8 ±1.8	20.8 ±5.0	14.9 ±4.0	6.9 ±1.0	0.7 ±0.07	81.4 ±2.3	0.5 ±0.1	6.9 ±0.6	7.4 ±0.8
	relative absorption ratio ($^{54}Mn = 1$)	3	1	6	11	8	4	0.4	45	0.3	4	4
Ileum:	absorption fraction in percent of the dose	7.3 ±1.5	1.0[a] ±0.1	1.2[a] ±0.4	4.1[a] ±0.4	7.4[a] ±1.4	8.4 ±1.2	0.5 ±0.03	64.4[a] ±2.4	0.4 ±0.2	6.2 ±0.7	2.3[a] ±1.6
	relative absorption ratio ($^{54}Mn = 1$)	7	1	1	4	7	8	0.5	64	0.3	6	2

[a] $p < 0.05$ as compared with jejunal segments.

nese, are higher in the upper jejunum than in the ileum. In these experiments the absorption of zinc and copper in ileum segments was not investigated.

In Table 12 the results of a systematic study of the absorption of various metals in the upper jejunum performed in tied-off segments *in situ* are recorded. The absorbed amounts have been listed in Table 12 as percent fractions of the dose given. The fractional absorption in the upper jejunum is higher than that in the ileum for iron, the closely related cobalt, for copper, antimony, thallium and manganese. For zinc, mercury, tin and lead, approximately the same fractional absorptions are found in the two sections. For chromium the fraction absorbed in the ileum is greater than in the jejunum.

For zinc these results confirm the findings of Van Campen and Mitchell (1965) and those of Methfessel and Spencer (1966).

As far as copper is concerned, the results obtained *in vivo* are precisely the reverse of the *in vitro* findings (Crampton *et al.*, 1964, 1965a, b). As these authors used hamster segments this discrepancy could be due to a species difference. However, this is not so, because in isolated rat ileum segments *in vitro* (method of Fisher and Parsons, 1949) the rate of ^{64}Cu transfer and the tissue content were also higher (Forth and Nell, unpublished data) than in jejunal segments. The reason for the discrepancy in the absorptive activity for copper measured *in vitro* and *in vivo* is not known.

Comparisons of the absorption in the upper jejunum and in the lower ileum must take into account the differential *surface area* of the mucosa in the two sections. Fisher and Parsons (1950) estimated the surface area of the upper jejunum to be about twice that of the lower ileum. This ratio agrees with recent measurements, although there is not agreement concerning the absolute magnitude of the surface area (see Chapter 1, p. 57 and Chapter 4, pp. 275). This means that the percentage absorption values of Table 12 cannot rank as the true absorptive activities of the whole mucosal epithelium of the two sections. In order to obtain a better comparison of the absorptive activities of these two sections of the intestine, Table 12 includes the *relative absorption rates* obtained by dividing the fractional absorption rates by that for manganese. This metal was chosen because its rate of absorption from the ileum is precisely half that from the jejunum. In other words, the relative absorption rate represents the rate over similar mucosal surface areas. On this basis the relative absorption rates for manganese, copper, mercury and tin are approximately the same in the jejunum and ileum. The relative absorption rates over similar surface

TABLE 13. TISSUE CONTENT OF SOME HEAVY METALS PRESENTED TO JEJUNAL AND ILEAL TIED-OFF SEGMENTS OF RATS *in vivo*
Experimental condition: cf. Table 12. In order to remove adsorbed metals from the surface the tissue was washed three times in 100 ml saline containing EDTA (10^{-2} M/l). Means of five to fifteen rats ± SEM. (From Leopold *et al.*, 1968)

Segments		Metals										
		^{51}Cr ($CrCl_3$)	^{54}Mn ($MnCl_2$)	^{59}Fe ($FeCl_3$)	^{60}Co ($CoCl_2$)	^{64}Cu ($CuSO_4$)	^{65}Zn ($ZnCl_2$)	^{203}Hg ($HgCl_2$)	^{204}Tl (Tl_2SO_4)	^{113}Sn ($SnCl_2$)	^{210}Pb (Pb-acetate)	^{125}Sb ($SbCl_3$)
Jejunum:	metal content (% of the dose)	4.5 ±1.8	1.8 ±0.7	31 ±3.5	12.1 ±2.1	11.9 ±3.1	27.9 ±3.2	18.3 ±3.0	17.0 ±2.1	27.1 ±3.4	21.2 ±6.8	24.1 ±3.1
	wet weight	1.3 ±0.1	1.3 ±0.1	1.3 ±0.1	1.2 ±0.2	1.3 ±0.2	1.3 ±0.2	1.4 ±0.1	1.4 ±0.1	1.3 ±0.1	1.1 ±0.1	1.1 ±0.1
Ileum:	metal content (% of the dose)	5.2 ±1.3	1.0[a] ±0.3	8.6[a] ±2.3	4.0[a] ±1.5	5.3[a] ±2.3	17.7[a] ±2.1	8.2[a] ±1.2	26.9[a] ±3.2	11.0[a] ±2.3	15.7 ±5.2	7.4[a] ±3.8
	wet weight	1.5 ±0.4	1.3 ±0.1	1.4 ±0.2	1.3 ±0.1	1.3 ±0.1	1.3 ±0.1	1.3 ±0.1	1.5 ±0.1	1.5 ±0.1	1.2 ±0.1	1.3 ±0.1

[a] $p < 0.05$ as compared with jejunal segments.

areas for chromium, zinc, lead and thallium are greater in the ileum than in the jejunum; the reverse holds true for iron, cobalt and antimony.

The determination of the metal *content* of the intestinal tissue was included in the investigations (Table 13). This is a measure of the amount of the administered metal still available for discharge into the blood in the intestinal mucosa 1 hr after administration. The assessment of these data is based on the assumption that most of the metal found in intestinal tissue is present in the mucosa. It has been established reliably for ^{59}Fe that at least 80% of the radioactivity measured in intestinal tissue is present in the mucosal epithelium (Manis and Schachter, 1964; Brown and Rother, 1963a, b; Forth, 1966).

The iron and cobalt content of the gut tissue corresponds to the amounts transferred (Table 13). Almost 6 times more iron is found in the jejunum than in the ileum and almost 5 times more cobalt. Even when the different surface areas of the mucosa in the two sections are taken into account the upper jejunum still possesses a higher absorptive activity for these metals.

The copper, zinc, mercury and tin content of the upper jejunum was twice as great as that of the lower ileum, i.e. it matched the surface area ratio of these two sections. The lead and chromium content of the jejunal tissue was about the same as that of the ileum while the thallium content of the ileal segment was higher than that of the jejunal segments. In view of the smaller area of the ileal mucosa the amount of lead, chromium and thallium taken up into the tissue per unit area was greater in the ileum than in the jejunum.

The differences between the absorption of *chromium* from ileum and jejunum respectively become clear when the investigations are made *in vitro,* especially when cationic chromium Cr(III) is presented to the mucosal side of the segments (see Table 14). In this case the amount of Cr(III) transferred in the ileum is 13 times that in the jejunum. The difference is reduced to 6 times when anionic chromate is presented to the mucosal side. Similar relationships for this metal were found for the tissue content of ^{51}Cr following administration of Cr(III) or chromate in jejunum and ileum segments. To underline the difference between the jejunum and ileum obtained during testing of transfer and content of chromium, Table 14 includes the data for iron and cobalt.

Under certain conditions the varying absorption of Cr(III) and chromate can also be demonstrated in man (Donaldson and Barreras, 1965, 1966). Its cause is unknown. Apparently, chromium penetrates into the mucosal cells more easily as anionic chromate than as cationic Cr^{3+}. The data on

TABLE 14. TRANSFER AND TISSUE CONTENT OF ^{51}Cr PRESENTED AS CATIONIC AND ANIONIC CHROMIUM IN EVERTED JEJUNAL AND ILEAL SACS OF RATS

Experimental conditions: fasted rats (16 hr), Wistar (female), 180–220 g body weight. Method according to Wilson and Wiseman (1954). Concentration of metals administered at the mucosal side: 5×10^{-6} M/l (50,000 cpm/ml). Mucosal fluid: 10 ml Tyrode solution; serosal fluid: 0.7 ml Tyrode solution at the beginning of the experiment; at the end: jejunal segment: 0.88 ml (SEM = $\pm$ 0.06; $n = 32$); ileal segment: 0.76 ml (SEM = $\pm$ 0.04; $n = 32$). Jejunal segments: 6 cm; starting with the flexura duodenojejunalis. Ileal segments: 6 cm, starting 3 cm proximal to the valvula ileocoecalis. Time: 2 hr; temp. 37°C. In order to remove adsorbed metals from the surface the tissue was washed three times in 100 ml saline containing EDTA (10^{-2} M/l). Means of eight experiments $\pm$ SEM. (After Leopold *et al.*, 1968)

Metal	Transfer		Tissue content	
	Jejunal segment (cpm/ml)	Ileal segment	Jejunal segment (cpm/segment)	Ileal segment
^{51}Cr–($CrCl_3$)	7700 ± 1100	18,600[a] ± 2500	2100 ± 200	6200[a] ± 1000
^{51}Cr–(Na_2CrO_4)	11,000 ± 2100	24,300[a] ± 1100	28,000[b] ± 3500	38,500[b] ± 7000
^{59}Fe–($FeSO_4$)	2200 ± 400	500[a] ± 100	32,000 ± 4000	8000[a] ± 3000
^{60}Co–($CoCl_2$)	19,000 ± 4000	7000[a] ± 1000	14,000 ± 1000	10,000[a] ± 2000

[a] $p < 0.05$ as compared with jejunal segments.
[b] $p < 0.05$ as compared with the $CrCl_3$ group.

the tissue content obtained following application of both forms of the metal *in vitro* to rat intestine segments (see Table 14) confirm this view. However, it seems doubtful whether the observed differences between Cr(III) and anionic chromate *in vivo* on oral administration are significant for absorption, because anionic chromate was reduced to cationic Cr(III) in the stomach (Donaldson and Barreras, 1965, 1966).

It should be pointed out here that the mechanisms of transfer of heavy metals in the jejunum and ileum may differ, e.g. there appear to be differences in the transfer processes for iron in jejunum and ileum (see p. 717).

The results summarized in Table 12 provide information not only about the site of preferential absorption but also about the extent of absorption of the various metals. When arranging the metals in the order of their rate of absorption, expressed as a percentage of the dose, the following sequence is found for the jejunum: thallium, cobalt, copper, iron, antimony, lead, zinc, chromium, manganese, mercury and tin. In the ileum the order is thallium, zinc, copper, chromium, lead, cobalt, antimony, iron, manganese, and tin.

Table 15 lists these metals in the order of their *retention* measured in the rat: thallium, lead, iron, zinc, antimony, chromium, cobalt, manganese, mercury, tin. Copper (^{64}Cu isotope) has too short a half-life for such measurements and was not included in these investigations.

In these experiments the first measurements were performed in a whole body counter for small animals 6 days after giving the labeled metals by stomach tube. At this time the unabsorbed portion of the metals had been excreted in the feces (Forth *et al.,* 1965b).

Thallium again heads the list (cf. Table 15; retention in percent of the dose). At the opposite end of the series appear two metals shown to be poorly absorbed in the tied-off intestinal segments: manganese and tin. In the middle there are two noteworthy exceptions to the general convergence of the series: cobalt and lead.

The low retention of cobalt is unexpected in view of the amount absorbed from tied-off jejunal segments. The amount excreted between the 6th and 10th days (Table 15) is too low to explain this discrepancy. It must be remembered that the first cobalt retention measurement was not performed until 6 days after administration. Excretion of the absorbed metal proceeds very quickly. In the rat the half-time for the first rapid phase of cobalt elimination after intravenous injection is about 24 hr (Forth, 1970). Because this phase of elimination was not considered in the measurement of retention (Table 15) the calculation of absorption of the basis of the retention values must lead to an underestimation.

TABLE 15. RETENTION OF HEAVY METALS BY RATS AFTER ORAL ADMINISTRATION

Experimental conditions: fasted rats (16 hr), Wistar (female), 220–250 g body weight. Metal dose: 10 nM in 2 ml sodium chloride solution (0.9%), pH 2. Three hours after the administration of the metals by a stomach tube the rats were fed again. Retention of the radioactive metals was measured in a body counter for small animals. Mean of ten rats ± SEM. (From Leopold *et al.*, 1968)

Days after administration	Metals									
	^{51}Cr ($CrCl_3$)	^{54}Mn ($MnCl_2$)	^{59}Fe ($FeCl_3$)	^{60}Co ($CoCl_2$)	^{65}Zn ($ZnCl_2$)	^{203}Hg ($HgCl_2$)	^{204}Tl (Tl_2SO_4)	^{113}Sn ($SnCl_2$)	^{210}Pb (Pb-acetate)	^{125}Sb ($SbCl_3$)
6th: retention % of the dose	4.6 ±1.1	2.7 ±0.3	23.4 ±3.2	3.4 ±0.5	19.5 ±3.0	1.5 ±0.2	28.7 ±0.8	0.12 ±0.02	29.4 ±3.2	6.1 ±1.1
retention in relation to Sn = 1	38	22	195	28	162	12	239	1	244	51
10th: retention % of the dose	0.8 ±0.2	2.1 ±0.3	24.3 ±4.0	2.2 ±0.4	17.3 ±2.6	1.7 ±0.3	13.7 ±0.5	0.08 ±0.04	28.7 ±3.0	6.7 ±1.3
excretion between the 6th and 10th days after the application in % of the 6th day values	82	11	not measurable	35	11	not measurable	52		not measurable	

The relatively high lead content of the animals following oral administration is surprising in view of the slow absorption from tied-off jejunal and ileal segments (Table 12). This discrepancy can only be explained by assuming that lead is apparently present in the stomach in a form favorable for absorption.

The large differences between the absorption and retention rates of individual metals will not be discussed further here; they are probably due to similar reasons as have been discussed for cobalt and lead. Summarizing the essential results of this discussion about the preferential sites of heavy metal absorption in the gastrointestinal tract, the first point to make is that they have not yet been finally elucidated. The reasons are, that there have been few systematic studies of the problem and that methodological difficulties may explain the partly conflicting results. Assessing the absorptive activity of different sections of the intestine is difficult because the data can only approximately be related to the absorbing surface. An additional complication is introduced by the different residence time in different gut sections.

Some metals are probably absorbed in the stomach; this has been demonstrated for copper and iron and is very likely for lead. Taking into account the absorptive activity and the transit time, the ileum does not only equal but actually is superior to the jejunum in terms of chromium, manganese, zinc, thallium, mercury, tin and lead absorption. The jejunum is the site of preferential absorption of antimony and, in particular, of the transition metals of group 8, i.e. iron, cobalt and nickel. Residence time is longest in the colon. However, this segment is assumed generally not to play a major role in absorption of heavy metals, mostly due to the low availability of metals and absorption in this region (see p. 604). With respect to the findings with iron in iron deficiency, it is worth while assessing the true role of the colon in man and animals after administering heavy metals locally, especially those heavy metals the absorption of which increases with the increased demand of the organism.

12.2.2. TRANSFER OF IRON

Much more is known about the transfer process of sodium (for references see Schultz and Curran, 1968) and of nutrients such as sugars (for references see Crane, 1968) and amino acids (for references see Wiseman, 1968) across the mucosal cells than about that of biologically and toxicologically significant heavy metals. Methodological difficulties are probably the explanation. Performing investigations over the concentration range in which biometals occur in the food (Bowen, 1966) requires much more analytical work than studying the absorption of sodium.

In recent years the commercial availability of radioisotopes, allowing metal transfer to be studied *in vitro* under clearly defined conditions, has widened our knowledge. However, difficulties remain in determining total iron, cobalt and zinc in mucosal tissue. Further progress is needed to provide information about the turnover rates of metals in the different cell compartments; this is prerequisite in order to gain an insight into the specific transport processes.

As with other absorption processes, there are two possible theoretical transfer mechanisms for moving heavy metals across the intestinal epithelium: *diffusion* and *transport depending on metabolism.*

Free *diffusion* as a transfer mechanism across the mucosal cells can be neglected for most metals because their capacity to form coordination compounds in biological media leads to reactions with all types of ligands. Univalent thallium, which, like the alkali metals, exists as a free ion, is probably one of the few heavy metals which can diffuse freely even in biological media. Its mode of transfer across mucosal cells is still unknown. Possibly due to its physicochemical properties this metal is absorbed like potassium since there are indications that not only algae but also erythrocytes (Gehring and Hammond, 1964) and muscle cells (Mullins and Moore, 1960; Rusznyak *et al.*, 1968) accumulate thallium like potassium, while the renal tubular cells appear to secrete thallium (Lund, 1956; Gehring and Hammond, 1967).

The fact that heavy metals are as a rule bound to ligands in biological media leads to two alternative mechanisms of transfer by diffusions: (a) the metals penetrate across the mucosal epithelium as complex chelates (see p. 690); (b) following the uptake into mucosal epithelial cells, the metals are converted into a form suitable for diffusion to the blood side.

Proteins, partly in membrane and partly in solution, represent potential ligands in the mucosal cells; low molecular weight ligands, e.g. amino acids, polybasic carboxylic acids, nucleotides, are also available. A carrier of this type could play a role in specific transcellular transport, because ubiquitous reactions of the heavy metals with cell constituents which retard the transfer from the luminal to the basal pole of the cell could be avoided. Furthermore, catalysis by heavy metals which may interfere with the cellular metabolism during the transfer cell can also be prohibited. Possibly heavy metals leave the mucosal cells on the basal pole in the form of chelates such as citrate complexes. In analogy iron is apparently transported in plants in the form of carboxylic acid complexes, i.e. mainly complexes with citric and malonic acids (Palmer *et al.*, 1963; Brown and Tiffin, 1965; Tiffin, 1966a, b).

As far as we know, no data concerning the form in which metals leave the mucosal cells on the blood side are available because of immense methodological difficulties. Furthermore, in the living animal with intact intestinal blood supply binding of metals to either specific or non-specific plasma proteins interferes. In the non-blood-perfused intestinal segments *in vitro*, in which interference from plasma proteins can be excluded by rinsing the blood vessels, analytical difficulties interfere with the measurement of the small quantities of metal and ligand present. In the absorbate of rat jejunal segments *in vitro* iron is bound to transferrin and/or to a transferrin-like protein (see p. 679). The form, however, in which iron is released from the mucosal cells to the serosal side is still unknown.

Metals may be presumed, on chemical grounds, to form complexes with low-molecular-weight ligands within mucosal cells. Brown and Rother (1963a, b), for example, concluded from their results that iron is bound to amino acids in the particle-free fraction of a mucosal cell homogenate. However, this finding has been criticized on methodological grounds (Charlton *et al.*, 1965; Manis and Schachter, 1965). Amino acids as ligands must also be considered in connection with copper, especially as the existence of such complexes in the plasma has been demonstrated (Sarkar and Kruck, 1966). In this connection it should be pointed out that the possibility of metals leaving the mucosal cells in the form of amino acid complexes does not necessarily mean that they enter the cells in the same form (see p. 704).

Obviously, heavy metals, especially iron, do not cross the mucosal epithelium in a free ionized state but in a chelated state. Such a transfer mechanism can be considered as analogous to the carrier-mediated metabolically independent transfer process of glucose through erythrocyte membranes (Wilbrandt and Rosenberg, 1961).

The possibility of "active" transport system has often been suggested for the physiologically essential heavy metals. Adaptation of the organism to the needs as demonstrated for iron, copper and zinc (see p. 710) suggests that the mucosal cells of the intestine possess special transport systems for these metals. It could be expected that such systems would transport not only the biometals, but also toxic metals because of their chemical similarity to the biometals.

These preliminary considerations may be summarized by asking whether heavy metals are transported *actively* across mucosal epithelium.

The criteria indicating the presence of an active transport system are: (a) dependence on metabolism, (b) preferential transport from the mucosal to the serosal side, (c) limited capacity, (d) specificity.

These criteria are not conventional in terms of the definition of "active" transport as transport against an electrochemical gradient as formulated for alkali metals by Ussing (1960).* The following considerations may therefore be added. It makes little sense to speak of transport against an electrochemical gradient in the case of heavy metals, because the prerequisites for defining a gradient are not fulfilled.

A heavy metal, unlike sodium, does not remain in the same form during the course of an absorption experiment. Hydroxides or sparingly soluble phosphates are formed, there may be a change of valence and chemical reactions may occur with ubiquitous ligands as well as with the transport system. Secondly, we do not know the form in which a metal leaves the mucosal cell to enter the blood. It is improbable that heavy metals leave the basal pole of the mucosal cells cross the basal membrane and the capillary wall and enter the blood as ions. Instead, more probably they penetrate as a complex with a ligand or else undergo reactions with mobile and immobile ligands en route.

The literature data do not allow the criteria outlined above to be checked for all physiologically interesting heavy metals. Most of the information available deals with iron. In respect of the transfer of copper and zinc the data available allow conclusion to be drawn by analogy.

12.2.2.1. *Theoretical and methodological considerations*

As a rule isolated, non-blood-perfused gut segments are used to study the transfer of substances across the mucosal epithelium *in vitro*. The transfer of iron can easily be investigated in rats made iron-deficient by administering a low iron diet and by repeated bleeding (Kaufman *et al.*, 1966; Mendel *et al.*, 1963; Forth and Andres, 1969) or by injecting phenylhydrazine (Mendel *et al.*, 1963; Chirasiri and Isak, 1966). For investigations on the transfer of iron *radioisotopes* are commonly used. A few preliminary remarks about assessing the results obtained are appropiate.

During transfer of isotope-labeled iron in isolated gut segments *in vitro* two phases may be distinguished (Manis and Schachter, 1962;

*The reader is referred to Chapter 2, pp. 100–111 and Chapter 10, pp. 488–495 (Eds.).

Forth and Rummel, 1965, 1966). The time course of iron absorption *in vivo* is quite different.

In vitro, the first step, i.e. uptake of iron into the mucosal cells, is followed after some delay by discharge to the serosal side. This delay in transfer is essentially a consequence of the lack of blood perfusion *in vitro* (see p. 641). In this case the labeled iron travels from the basal cell pole to the serosal side of the whole gut wall with the stream of absorbed fluid. *In vivo,* in the perfused gut, the iron released from the mucosal cell enters the blood capillary directly.

The amount of iron taken up into mucosal cells may differ from that transferred across the cells (see p. 641) in isolated gut segments *in vitro.* A comparison of these two amounts in gut segments of normal and iron-deficient rats (Table 16) shows that in deficient rats the ^{59}Fe content of the tissue is about 1.7 times that of normal segments, while the amount transferred increases tenfold. *In vivo,* only after 10 min twice as much iron is transferred across the mucosal epithelium in iron-deficient animals than in normal ones, while the tissue content in the same experiment is 4 times greater. In contrast, 50 min later no difference can be observed between normal and iron-deficient rats in the ^{59}Fe tissue content (see Table 16). This means that in iron-deficient rats ^{59}Fe is rapidly released

TABLE 16. TRANSFER AND TISSUE CONTENT OF ^{59}Fe PRESENTED AS $FeSO_4$ IN JEJUNAL SEGMENTS OF NORMAL AND IRON-DEFICIENT RATS *in vivo* AND *in vitro*

Experimental conditions: fasted rats (16 hr), Wistar (male), 180–220 g body weight. Normal rats (*n*): 14.3 g hemoglobin per 100 ml blood (SEM = ± 0.8; *n* = 20). Iron-deficient rats (*d*): 4.5 g hemoglobin per 100 ml blood (SEM = ± 1.2; *n* = 20). Experiments *in vivo* (operation under ether anesthesia): tied-off jejunal segments, length 12 cm, starting with the flexura duodenojejunalis; time: 1 hr; mean of five rats. Experiments *in vitro*: method according to Fisher and Parsons (1949) modified by Rummel and Stupp (1960); two segments of each rat, length 8 cm, starting with the flexura duodenojejunalis; time 2 hr; temp. 37°C. In order to remove adsorbed iron from the surface the segments were washed three times in 100 ml saline containing EDTA (10^{-2} M/l) (Forth, unpublished data)

Method		^{59}Fe–(FeSO$_4$) administered (mcM)	Time (min)	^{59}Fe transferred (% of the dose)	Tissue content of ^{59}Fe (% of the dose)	Amount in tissue / Amount transferred
In vitro:	*n*	0.01	10	4.6	12.6	2.8
	n	0.01	60	10.6	33.8	3.2
	d	0.01	10	8.4	57.8	6.5
	d	0.01	60	58.9	29.6	0.5
In vitro:	*n*	0.25	120	0.05	1.5	30.0
	d	0.25	120	0.55	2.5	4.5

into the blood from the mucosal cells. This interpretation is confirmed by comparing the amounts of ^{59}Fe transferred: 1 hr after administration in iron-deficient rats the amount of ^{59}Fe transferred across the mucosal epithelium is 5 times greater than in normal animals (Table 16). Two hours after administration of ^{59}Fe the tissue content of iron-deficient rats is even lower than that of normal animals (Forth and Hübers, unpublished data).

These results indicate that on principle the transfer of iron across the gut wall *in vitro* proceeds in the same ways as in blood-perfused gut segments *in vivo*. Obviously the transfer *in vitro* takes place much more slowly than *in vivo*.

When using radioisotopes to study the transfer of metals across the gut wall the following difficulty must be considered. During the transfer of radioisotopes through the gut wall, they are mixed with their non-radioactive isotopes contained in different cellular pools: the specific activity of the isotope given decreases during the passage.

When investigating the absorption of isotope-labeled iron present in the physiological concentration of 10^{-5} to 10^{-6} M, the chemical determination of iron in the absorbate by conventional methods is still unreliable. Modern methods of analysis, e.g. atomic absorption, spectrophotometrically may detect metals in the concentrations in which they occur in food. At present investigators use higher iron concentrations which allow a chemical determination under *in vitro* conditions in order to confirm results obtained with tracers. Table 17 lists the results of such an experiment, in which iron was determined by the method of Schade *et al.* (1954). The experiments were carried out on isolated rat jejunal segments *in vitro* by the method of Fisher and Parsons (1949).

A decrease of about two-thirds of the iron content of mucosal tissue of iron-deficient rats was followed by a replenishment of the mucosal cells and a threefold increase of the specific activity of iron in mucosal tissue of iron-deficient rats when iron was presented to the mucosal side. Consequently, the amount of iron appearing in the absorbate under these conditions is increased also threefold as compared with the iron-deficient control segments (Table 17). In contrast to the results obtained with normal segments, the specific activity of iron in the fluid absorbed is higher than that in mucosal tissue. This indicates that the intracellular distribution of iron taken up by the mucosal cells must be different under these conditions. The iron appearing on the serosal side derives from a particular intracellular compartment. In tracer experiments, particularly those involving isolated segments, the total amount of iron appearing in the serosal side of normal segments is the same whether iron is supplied

TABLE 17. APPEARANCE OF IRON IN THE ABSORBATE AND TISSUE CONTENT OF IRON IN JEJUNAL SEGMENTS OF NORMAL AND IRON-DEFICIENT RATS *in vitro*

Experimental conditions: fasted rats (16 hr), Wistar (female), 180–220 g body weight. Normal rats (*n*): 15.6 g hemoglobin per 100 ml blood (SEM = ± 1.0; *n* = 18); iron-deficient rats (*d*): 5.4 g hemoglobin per 100 ml blood (SEM = ± 1.2; *n* = 18). Method according to Fisher and Parsons (1949) modified by Rummel and Stupp (1960). Jejunal segments: length 8 cm, starting with the flexura duodenojejunalis; two segments of each rat. Time 2 hr; temp. 37°C. Chemical determination of iron according to Schade *et al.* (1954). The jejunal segments made blood free by perfusion of 30 ml ice-cold saline. In order to remove any hemoglobin the ice-cold acidified (0.5 ml 0.1M HCl) absorbates were shaken with ice-cold methylethylketon (Teale, 1959). This procedure was repeated three times and the ketonic supernatant was discarded. (Forth, unpublished data)

Concentration of iron added to the perfusion fluid (nM/ml)		Absorbate (ml)	Iron in the absorbate		Iron in the mucosal tissue	
			(nM/ml)	specific activity (cpm/ml and nM Fe)	(nM/100 mg w.w.)	specific activity (cpm per 100 mg w.w. and nM Fe)
—	*n*	1.7 ± 0.14	8.6 ± 0.9	—	37.4 ± 10.8	—
	d	1.9 ± 0.09	3.6 ± 0.2	—	12.5[a] ± 7.2	—
250[c]	*n*	1.6 ± 0.06	8.8 ± 0.5	660 ± 170	39.2 ± 10.8	1220 ± 280
	d	1.7 ± 0.1	11.6[a][b] ± 1.4	5100[a] ± 400	41.0[b] ± 5.9	3780[a] ± 200

[a] $p < 0.05$ as compared with the normal controls.
[b] $p < 0.05$ as compared with the group without addition of iron.
[c] Specific activity of the perfusion fluid: 7650 cpm per ml and nM Fe.

on the luminal side or not; in other words only tracer amounts of iron are transferred from the lumen to the serosal side. Hence, nearly all iron appearing on the serosal side under these conditions derives from the cellular iron pool.

Table 17 shows that the results of absorption studies using radioisotopes must be corrected in several ways in order to allow quantitative conclusions.

12.2.2.2. *Metabolic dependence of transfer*

The view that transfer of iron across the mucosal cell occurs by simple diffusion was rejected by Hahn *et al.* (1943). Jacobi *et al.* (1956b) proved experimentally that the transfer of iron depends on a "chemical process". Brown and Justus (1958) demonstrated the dependence of iron absorption on metabolic processes, a result confirmed subsequently by numerous authors (Dowdle *et al.*, 1960; Manis and Schachter, 1962a; Helbock and Saltman, 1967; Pearson and Reich, 1965; Rummel and Forth, 1968).

Manis and Schachter (1962a) observed that in everted duodenal sacs prepared from normal rats, the transfer of iron is more sensitive to oxygen withdrawal than is the mucosal iron content. The effects of O_2-deprivation differ significantly in segments according to their location in the small intestine. In segments, prepared from the first 3.5 cm below the pylorus, the mucosal iron content and the transfer to the serosal side are diminished under N_2. In segments prepared from the region extending 20 cm below the pylorus, however, the opposite is true for mucosal iron transfer which is increased under anaerobic conditions. The mucosal iron content is decreased as it is in the first part of the duodenum (Manis and Schachter, 1962a). Therefore, iron transfer does not appear to depend on respiration under all conditions.

With regard to the differences of iron absorption in different sections of the small intestine it is interesting to compare segments from two regions of the jejunum which show several differences (Forth and Rummel, 1965; Rummel and Stupp, 1960). The influence of the O_2-concentration in the incubation fluid on iron transfer across these two segments from *normal* rats differs considerably (Fig. 8), while no difference exists with regard to glucose transfer. The transport of glucose in both segments decreases linearly with decreasing O_2-concentration in the incubation fluid. Iron transfer remains unchanged in segments beginning 13 cm below the pylorus whereas in segments beginning 20 cm below the pylorus it increases with decreasing O_2-concentration (Fig. 8). The latter result agrees with observations of Manis and Schachter (1962a).

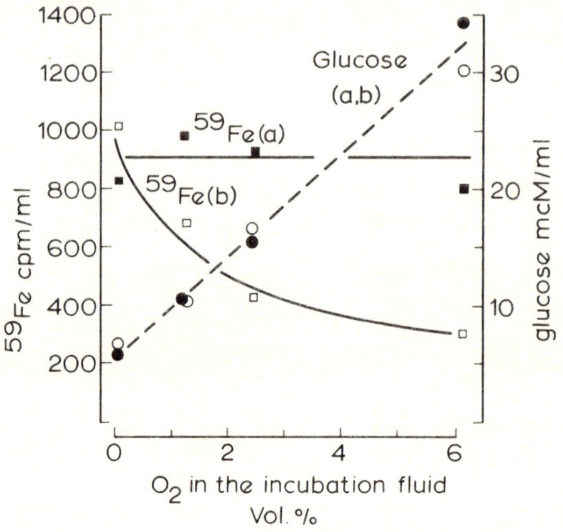

FIG. 8. Transfer of iron and glucose across the intestinal wall of jejunal segments of rats *in vitro* as a function of the oxygen concentration of the incubation fluid. Experimental conditions: fasted rats (16 hr), Wistar (female), 200 g body weight. Method according to Wilson and Wiseman (1954). Length of the everted sacs: 3.5 cm; (a) 13 cm distal from the pylorus; (b) 20 cm distal from the pylorus. The everted sacs (filled with 0.5 ml saline solution 0.9%) were gently shaken in Erlenmeyer flasks containing 10 ml Tyrode solution under 1.5 atmosphere pressure of a gas mixture of 5% CO_2 and O_2 and N_2, respectively, in variable proportions. Half an hour before starting the experiment, the Tyrode solution was equilibrated with the gas mixture. The calculated O_2 concentration in the incubation fluid is shown on the abscissa in vol.%. Iron concentration on both sides of the sacs: 10^{-5} M $FeSO_4$. ^{59}Fe was added on the mucosal side only. Glucose concentration in the Tyrode solution: 12×10^{-2} M/l. Time: 2 hr; temp. 37°C. Each point represents the mean of weight of twenty experiments; SEM for glucose-values less than 2%, for ^{59}Fe activity less than 15%. *Right ordinate:* glucose concentration, mcM/ml, in the serosal fluid. ● = segment (a) ○ = segment (b) No statistically significant difference between (a) and (b). *Left ordinate:* ^{59}Fe activity in cpm/ml in the serosal fluid. ■ = segment (a); □ = segment (b). At 1.2 vol.% O_2 the value of segment (b) was statistically significantly different ($p < 0.01$) from the value at 2.4 vol.% O_2. (From Rummel and Forth, 1968.)

Table 18 summarizes the results obtained, and includes also figures for the chemically related cobalt. The following comments apply to a jejunum segment localized 15–10 cm below the pylorus. In segments from *normal* animals under nitrogen, 2.5 times more iron and 1.3 times more cobalt are transported to the serosal side than under oxygen. In segments of iron-deficient animals the enhanced transfer of iron and cobalt transfer persists under nitrogen. Thus, in a condition which the transport of

TABLE 18. TRANSFER AND TISSUE CONTENT OF ^{59}Fe AND ^{58}Co PRESENTED AS $FeSO_4$ AND $CoCl_2$ IN JEJUNAL SEGMENTS OF NORMAL AND IRON-DEFICIENT RATS *in vitro*

Experimental conditions: fasted rats (16 hr), Wistar (female), 180–200 g body weight. Normal rats (*n*): 13.8 g hemoglobin per 100 ml blood (SEM = ± 0.7; $n = 25$). Iron-deficient rats (*d*): 6.5 g hemoglobin per 100 ml blood (SEM = ± 0.8; $n = 25$). Method according to Wilson and Wiseman (1954). Jejunal segments, 5 cm length, starting 15 cm distal of the pylorus (two segments of each rat). Metal concentration at both sides of the everted sacs: 5 nM/ml. Radioactive metals were added at the mucosal side only (22,000 cpm/ml). Mucosal fluid: 10 ml Tyrode solution, glucose concentration 15 mcM/ml. Serosal fluid: 0.5 ml Tyrode solutions. Gas: 5% CO_2 and 95% O_2 or N_2. Time: 2 hr; temp. 37°C. Mean of three to twelve experiments ± SEM. (After Forth, 1967; Forth and Rummel, 1968)

Incubation medium	Metal	Concentration of radioactive metal in the serosal fluid (cpM/ml)		Glucose concentration in the serosal fluid (cpM/ml)		Creatinin concentration in the serosal fluid (mg%)	
		n	*d*	*n*	*d*	*n*	*d*
Tyrode solution O_2	^{59}Fe–($FeSO_4$)	640 ± 60	7050[a] ± 560	39.5 ± 1.4	37.5 ± 1.3	14.4 ± 3.4	9.8 ± 2.4
	^{58}Co–($CoCl_2$)	8350 ± 590	25,000[a] ± 1500	—	—	—	—
Tyrode solution N_2	^{59}Fe–($FeSO_4$)	1580[b] ± 63	8300[a] ± 820	7.2[b] ± 0.2	6.8[b] ± 0.07	71.2[b] ± 3.1	65[b] ± 2.3
	^{58}Co–($CoCl_2$)	11,000[b] ± 440	21,000[a] ± 1850	—	—	—	—
Tyrode solution without glucose O_2	^{59}Fe–($FeSO_4$)	—	340[b] ± 70	—	3.0[b] ± 0.6	—	—
Tyrode solution + DNP 10^{-3} m O_2	^{59}Fe–($FeSO_4$)	—	392[b] ± 90	—	8.9[b] ± 1.0	—	—

[a] $p < 0.05$ as compared with the normal controls (*n*).
[b] $p < 0.05$ as compared with the O_2 control.

glucose completely ceases, the enhanced transfer of iron remains unaffected. Withdrawal of glucose or the presence of dinitrophenol, on the other hand, depresses iron transfer to values similar to those found in depleted segments. Therefore, in iron-deficient segments a metabolic step of the anaerobic glycolysis appears to be required for the activation of iron transfer.

12.2.2.3. *Preferential direction of transfer*

In segments from iron-deficient rats iron is preferentially transferred

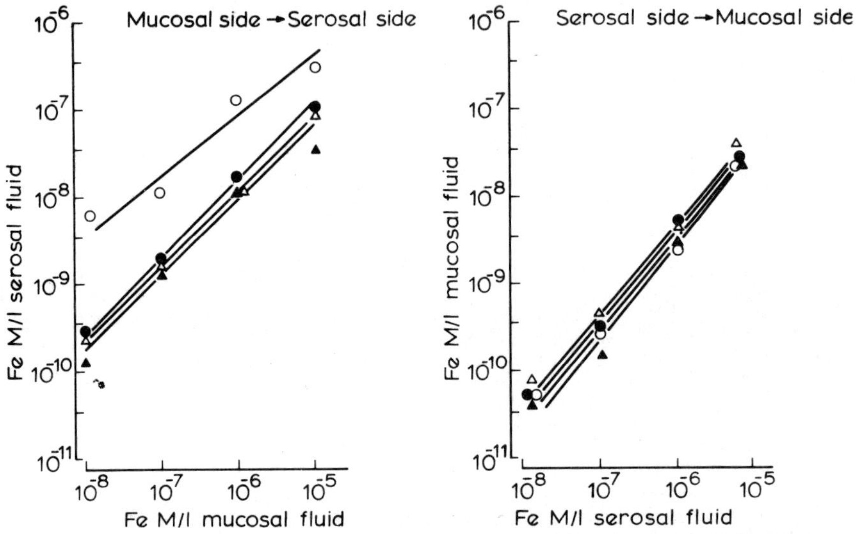

FIG. 9. Dependence of iron transfer across everted intestine sacs on concentration in normal and iron-deficient rats. Experimental conditions: fasted rats (16 hr), Wistar (female), 160–190 g body weight. Normal rats (black symbols): 14 g hemoglobin per 100 ml blood (SEM = ± 1.4; $n = 60$). Iron-deficient rats (open symbols): 5.4 g hemoglobin per 100 ml blood (SEM = ± 0.9; $n = 60$). Method according to Wilson and Wiseman (1954). Length of the segments: 5 cm. Jejunal segments (circles), starting with the flexura duodenojejunalis. Ileal segments (triangles) starting with the valvula ileocoecalis. Mucosal fluid: 12 ml Tyrode solution; serosal fluid: 0.7 ml Tyrode solution at the beginning of the experiment; at the end 0.85 ml (SEM = ± 0.09; $n = 64$) for jejunal segments and 0.72 ml (SEM = ± 0.05; $n = 64$) for ileal segments. Each point represents the mean of four experiments. *Left:* transfer of ^{59}Fe–($FeCl_3$) administered together with citric acid (ligand : Fe = 10 : 1) at the mucosal side. The difference between the jejunal segments of normal and iron-deficient rats is statistically significant ($p < 0.01$), *Right:* transfer of ^{59}Fe–($FeCl_3$) administered together with citric acid (ligand : Fe = 10 : 1) at the serosal side. No statistically significant difference between the different groups. (From Forth *et al.*, 1968a.)

from the mucosal to the serosal side: the transfer increases only in one direction, from the mucosal to the serosal side (Fig. 9). This increase was observed only in segments from the upper jejunum, known to be one of the most active sites of absorption (see p. 644), but not in the ileum.

In addition it is interesting to note that the amount of iron (calculated from the concentration shown in Fig. 6) transferred in the reverse direction, i.e. from the serosal to the mucosal side, is higher in segments of both normal and iron-deficient animals for jejunum as well as for ileum (see also Helbock and Saltman, 1967). The observation of a higher appearance rate on the mucosal side following the administration on the serosal side is not restricted to iron. This peculiarity is also described for other heavy metals (Sahagian *et al.*, 1967) and other substances, e.g. cardiac glycosides (Lauterbach, 1969; Forth and Rummel, 1969). The conclusions deduced from this anisotropy of the gut wall is in the first instance that the pathway which a substance takes from the mucosal to the serosal side is not necessarily the same as that taken in the opposite direction. From the mucosal side a substance contacts the luminal membrane of the mucosal cells, which is enlarged many times by the microvilli, and reacts with it to be transferred subsequently across the epithelium. The route in the opposite direction follows the blood and lymph vessels and ends in the intercellular spaces between mucosal cells. The passage to the mucosal side could then occur paracellularly, if the optically dense junctions of the terminal bars of the mucosal epithelium were in fact not as tight as they are generally assumed to be. Indications that this route could be open for the passage of substances through the mucosal epithelium have been discussed elsewhere in this book (Chapter 3, p. 203, and Chapter 10, pp. 496–497).

In iron-deficiency not only the transfer of ^{59}Fe from the mucosal to the serosal side is increased but also the tissue ^{59}Fe content is higher when radioactive iron is presented to the mucosal side, but not when ^{59}Fe is presented to the serosal side (Forth *et al.*, 1969).

12.2.2.4. *Limited capacity of the transfer system*

Investigations on iron absorption in man (Hahn *et al.*, 1951; Bonnet *et al.*, 1960) and in animals (Smith and Pannacciulli, 1958; Beutler *et al.*, 1962; Forrester *et al.*, 1962; Gitlin and Cruchaud, 1962; Wheby *et al.*, 1964; Thomson and Valberg, 1971; Thomson *et al.*, 1971b) demonstrated that the percentage absorption decreases as the quantity administered increases. Analogous results were obtained *in vitro* with jejunum segments of normal and iron-deficient rats. As the iron dose increases, the fraction taken up into the mucosal tissue and transferred across the gut wall to the serosal side decreases (Forth and Rummel, 1965, 1966).

Table 19 gives the results of such an experiment on isolated jejunal segments from iron-deficient rats. The table shows that iron transfer as measured by the ^{59}Fe concentration ratio on the serosal and mucosal sides (S/M) decreases as the dose increases. Also, as the iron dose increases the tissue content of ^{59}Fe decreases. A comparison of the mucosal ^{59}Fe activity in 1 g tissue (w.w.) with the ^{59}Fe activity in 1 ml of the fluid presented shows that iron is accumulated in the tissue. At the lowest concentration presented to the mucosal side the accumulation ratio of ^{59}Fe amounts to almost 13. This ratio falls with increasing iron concentration; at the highest concentration it is just above 2 (see Table 19).

The capacity of the system responsible for iron transfer across the mucosal cell is limited, as has already been shown by the results given in Table 17. In isolated jejunal segments of normal rats *in vitro* (Fisher and Parsons method) the release of iron into the absorbate during 2 hr perfusion by an iron-containing fluid is just as high as in segments perfused by an iron-free fluid. Under these artificial conditions the iron

TABLE 19. DEPENDENCE ON IRON CONCENTRATION OF TRANSFER AND TISSUE CONTENT OF ^{59}Fe PRESENTED AS $FeSO_4$ IN JEJUNAL EVERTED SACS OF IRON-DEFICIENT RATS

Experimental conditions: fasted rats (16 hr), Wistar (female), 210 g body weight. 5.6 g hemoglobin per 100 ml blood (SEM = ± 0.9; $n = 20$). Method according to Wilson and Wiseman (1954). Length of the jejunal segments: 3.5 cm, starting with the flexura duodenojejunalis (two segments of each rat). At the beginning of the experiment, mucosal fluid: 25 ml Tyrode solution; serosal fluid: 0.5 ml Tyrode solution; at the end: 0.55 ml (SEM = ± 0.04; $n = 25$). The different $FeSO_4$ concentrations were labeled with ^{59}Fe: 50,000 cpm/ml. Time: 2 hr, temp. 37°C. Means of four experiments ± SEM in order to remove adsorbed iron from the surface the segments were washed three times in 100 ml saline containing EDTA (10^{-2} M). (From Forth and Rummel, 1966a)

Quantity measured	Iron concentration in the mucosal fluid (nM/ml)		
	0.01	1.0	10.0
^{59}Fe in 1 ml serosal fluid in cpm × 10^3	40 ± 5	36.5 ± 1.4	8.7 ± 1.3
S/M[a]	0.8	0.7	0.17
^{59}Fe in the tissue of the segments in cpm × 10^3	95 ± 7.5	65 ± 4.7	18 ± 1.5
^{59}Fe accumulation by mucosal tissue[b]	12.7	9	2.4

[a] Calculated by dividing cpm/ml serosal fluid by cpm/ml mucosal fluid.

[b] cpm/g tissue wet weight divided by cpm/ml mucosal fluid. The mucosal tissue amounts to 50% of the wet weight of the entire segment and contains 80% of the ^{59}Fe-activity.

transfer is very small as compared with the content of iron in mucosal cells. Segments of iron-deficient rats, however, to which iron was presented at the mucosal side release 3 times as much iron into the absorbate as the control segments of normal animals. The limited capacity of the transfer system can be demonstrated also by the following experiments. In rats following an initial saturation of the transfer system by oral administration of iron, iron transfer was investigated in isolated segments *in vitro* (Forth *et al.*, 1963; Forth and Rummel, 1965). The time required for the transfer to recover its initial rate, i.e. the rate observed before saturating by an oral iron dose, amounts to 5 hr in normal animals. This period is roughly equal to that found by Wheby *et al.* (1964) *in vivo* with rats given repeated iron doses at regular intervals. As shown by Manis and Schachter (1964) preloading of rats with 4 mg iron orally 3 hr before segments are excised depresses the transfer of iron *in vitro* by about 90%.

In iron-deficient rats the preloaded iron-transfer system of the mucosa is emptied more rapidly; this has been shown by investigations on tied-off jejunal segments (see p. 658). By giving iron orally before an *in vitro* experiment the enhanced ^{59}Fe transfer of iron-deficiency can be reduced to values found in jejunal segments of normal rats (Rummel, 1965). The regulatory effect of the limited capacity of the iron transfer system is evident.

For higher doses of iron (100–2500 mg/kg) the amount absorbed increases as a linear fraction of the dose: this has been demonstrated in normal rats (Wheby *et al.*, 1964), in normal mice (Gitlin and Cruchaud, 1962) and in normal dogs (Moore, E. W. *et al.*, 1964). In a lower dose range, however, these authors obtained a non-linear relationship between dose and absorption rate. When the data were plotted as a Lineweaver and Burk diagram, a linear relationship resulted. This evidence alone does not justify the conclusion that an enzymatic step located within the mucosal cells determines the absorption of iron. It appears, however, that for the lower dose range a rate-limiting process, e.g. a carrier system with limited capacity, determines the transfer from the intestinal lumen to the blood. The process determining the rate of transfer in the higher dose range apparently has an unlimited capacity. Such behavior indicates a passive process, such as diffusion. For chemical reasons *free* diffusion, however, can be excluded because of the chemical properties of iron and of the constituents of mucosal cells. In the low, i.e. physiological, dose ranges the transfer of iron across mucosal cells appears to be determined mainly by specific binding sites of limited capacity while in the higher, i.e. toxic, dose range unspecific binding sites of a nearly unlimited capacity determine the absorption rate.

Other authors have described a linear relationship between the logarithm of the dose of iron administered and the logarithm of the amount absorbed (Beutler *et al.*, 1962; Bonnet *et al.*, 1960; Höglund and Reitzenstein, 1969b; Smith and Pannacciulli, 1958). However, since the dose range in these experiments extended over a range of 6–7 orders of magnitude and reached doses of 1000 mg in man and 10 mg in mice, and since the shape of the curves in the low range was determined by two points only, the disagreement between these observations and the data discussed above becomes insignificant.

Wheby *et al.* (1964) showed for the early rapid phase of iron absorption between 10 and 35 min after injection into tied-off segments: (a) that it is not the uptake of iron from the intestinal lumen into mucosal cells but the extrusion of iron out of the cells into the blood which is the step limiting the absorption rate, and (b) that for the transfer of iron from the mucosa into the blood, the process becomes saturated with doses in the range of 5 to 10 mcg in normal and of 50 to 100 mcg in iron-deficient rats.

Time course of absorption. The onset of iron absorption is very rapid as Stewart and Gambino (1961) showed in normal dogs. Data for the kinetics of the initial, very rapid phase have been obtained in blood per-

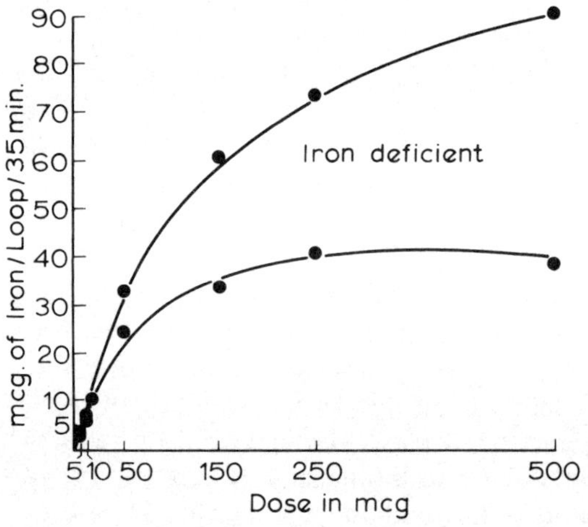

FIG. 10. Rate of mucosal uptake of iron from lumen and rate of mucosal transfer from duodenal segments into the body after single doses of varying amounts of labeled iron. *Upper curve:* mucosal uptake, i.e. the radioiron content of the washed duodenal segment plus the radioiron content of the carcass. *Lower curve:* mucosal transfer, i.e. radioiron content of the carcass. Iron-deficiency produced by repeated bleeding and feeding of an iron-reduced diet, $n=4$–7. (From Wheby *et al.*, 1964.)

fused preparations *in vitro* (Forth, 1968) and *in situ* (Pollack, 1968); in both cases the ^{59}Fe-activity in the venous outflow of the perfused segment has been measured. One minute after injecting radioiron into jejunal segments of rats *in vitro* ^{59}Fe can be detected in the portal outflow (Forth 1968).

In man (mild iron-deficiency anemia) the absorption rate within 30 min after an oral dose of 40 mg iron reached maximal values ranging between 15 and 20 mcg Fe per kg per 10 min (Hallberg and Sölvell, 1960). In the body of iron-deficient rats radioiron could be detected within 15 sec after injection into a tied-off duodenal segment. Up to 2.5% of a 2.5 mcg dose was transferred across the mucosa in 26 sec (Wheby *et al.*, 1964).

The time dependence of the absorption rate is shown in Fig. 10. The rate of mucosal transfer may differ by a factor of more than 10 during the first 35 min depending upon body iron stores (Wheby *et al.*, 1964).

When iron was administered by stomach tube to rats with normal iron stores, a proportionality was found to exist between the amount of iron taken up into the mucosal tissue and the amount transferred into the body. The release of iron from the mucosal cells into the body decreased simultaneously with the content of iron in the mucosal cells of the proximal part of the small intestine. The half-time of release was 6–9 hr (Forth and Rummel, 1966b).

Within 2 hr after administration, iron-deficient rats had absorbed 75% of the total fraction absorbed after 8 days. Consequently, two phases of absorption must be distinguished: (1) a *rapid phase* lasting up to 2 hr during which between 60 and 80% of total absorption occurs and (2) a *slow phase* extending over the subsequent 10 to 12 hr during which absorption is completed (Brown, 1963; Hallberg and Sölvell, 1960; Wheby and Crosby, 1963).

Iron absorption is usually investigated during the initial rapid phase because the absorption process underlying this rapid phase adapts rapidly to the demands of the organism in iron-deficiency. The rapid phase of iron absorption can easily be studied in jejunal segments of rats.

12.2.2.5. *Specificity of the transfer system*

The iron-transfer system of the mucosal cells of the duodenum and jejunum is highly specific for iron, as shown by investigations *in vitro* and *in vivo*.

The first observation of enhanced absorption of iron as well as of chemically related metals, e.g. cobalt and manganese, in iron-deficiency

TABLE 20. ABSORPTION OF METALS OTHER THAN IRON IN IRON-DEFICIENCY

	Increased absorption of	No change in absorption of	Refs.
Rats			
In vitro	Co, Ni, Mn, Zn	Cu	Forth (1966, 1970, 1971); Forth and Rummel (1971); Forth *et al.* (1966)
In vivo; tied-off segments or intragastric injection	Co, Mn, Zn	Cu, Cs, Mg, Hg, Ca	Pollack *et al.* (1965)
	Co, Mn, Zn	Cu	Forth (1966, 1970, 1971); Forth and Rummel (1971)
	Co, Mn		Diez-Ewald *et al.* (1968)
	Co		Schade *et al.* (1970a)
	Mn		Thomson *et al.* (1971c)
	Co, Mn		Thomson and Valberg (1972)
In vivo; gastric tube	Co, Mn, Zn		Forth (1966, 1970, 1971); Forth and Rummel (1971)
	Co		Thomson *et al.* (1971a)
	Cr		Hopkins and Noble (1969)
Man			
In vivo	Co		Valberg and Olatunbosun (1968); Valberg *et al.* (1969)
	Mn		Thomson *et al.* (1971c)

was published by two groups working on rats *in vivo* (Pollack *et al.*, 1965) and *in vitro* (Forth *et al.*, 1966) respectively. Their observations have been confirmed in iron-deficient animals as well as in man (see Table 20). Conversely, overloading rats with iron reduces the absorption of manganese as well as that of iron. Furthermore, it was shown that large amounts of manganese in food induce iron-deficiency (Diez-Ewald *et al.*, 1968).

Data on the absorption of iron and chemically related heavy metals obtained with the method of segments tied-off *in situ* in normal iron-deficient rats is shown in Fig. 11. The greatest increase of absorption in iron-deficiency is found with iron. The chemically related metals cobalt and manganese follow; even the less closely related zinc is absorbed more rapidly than in normal animals, while copper is not. Needless to say that the iron-deficient rats were not deficient with respect to the heavy

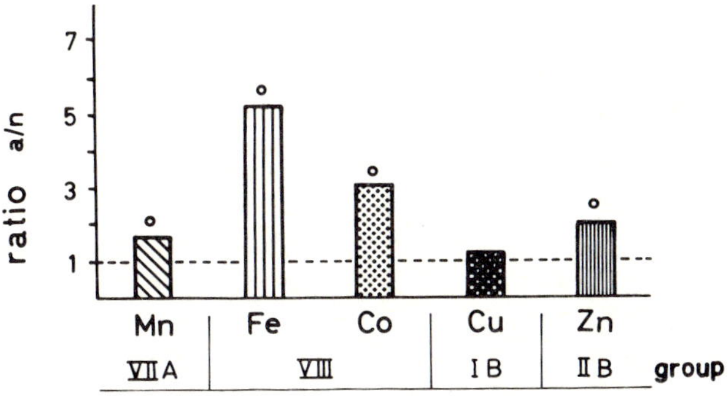

FIG. 11. The relative increase of absorption of manganese, iron, cobalt, copper and zinc in tied-off jejunal segments of iron-deficient and normal rats *in vivo*. The columns represent the amount absorbed by iron-deficient rats divided by the amount absorbed by normal rats, i.e. the ratio d/n. o indicates a statistically significant difference between the absorption in normal and that in iron-deficient rats ($p < 0.01$). The roman numbers indicate the group in the periodic system of elements. Experimental conditions: fasted rats (16 hr), Wistar (female), 160–190 g body weight. Normal rats: 14.6 g hemoglobin per 100 ml blood (SEM = $\pm$ 1.2; $n = 80$). Iron-deficient rats: 5.6 g hemoglobin per 100 ml blood (SEM = $\pm$ 0.9; $n = 80$). Length of the jejunal segments: 12 cm. starting with the flexura duodenojejunalis (operation under ether anesthesia). Metal dose: 0.36 mcM in 2 ml sodium chloride solution (0.9%), pH 2.4. (Forth, 1966, 1970; Forth and Rummel, 1971.)

metals chemically related to iron. This was proved by the retention rate of these metals injected intravenously in normal and iron-deficient rats. The diet of the iron-deficient animals contained all heavy metals tested in these experiments except for iron (Forth and Rummel, 1971).

Similar results were obtained with isolated, jejunal segments of normal and iron-deficient rats *in vitro*. Nickel was included; its transfer is also increased in iron-deficiency (Forth, 1970). The result of these and similar investigations (see Table 21 and Fig. 11) is that the transport system of the mucosa is highly specific for iron. It appears to react with chemical relatives of iron, such as cobalt, nickel and manganese, and even with zinc and chromium, but not with copper (Table 20).

When studying the uptake of heavy metals into the mucosal tissue, this preference for iron is also found (see Table 21). The investigations were made on isolated jejunal segments from normal and iron-deficient rats *in vitro* (everted sac technique). As judged by the comparison of the radioactivity per gram wet weight with that per ml of incubation fluid, all the heavy metals tested, with the exception of nickel, are accumu-

TABLE 21. UPTAKE OF SOME HEAVY METALS BY TISSUE IN EVERTED JEJUNAL SEGMENTS OF NORMAL AND IRON-DEFICIENT RATS

Experimental conditions: fasted rats (16 hr), Wistar (female), 160–190 g body weight. Normal rats: 14.6 g hemoglobin per 100 ml blood (SEM = ±1.5; $n = 80$). Iron-deficient rats: 5.6 g hemoglobin per 100 ml blood (SEM = ±1.7; $n = 80$). Method according to Wilson and Wiseman (1954). Length of the jejunal segments: 3.5 cm, starting with the flexura duodenojejunalis (two segments of each rat). At the beginning of the experiment; mucosal fluid: 10 ml Tyrode solution; serosal fluid: 0.5 ml Tyrode solution; at the end: 0.55 ml (SEM = ±0.05; $n = 120$). Metal concentration on both sides of the everted sacs: 5×10^{-6} M/l. Radioactive metals were added at the mucosal side only (50,000 cpm/ml). Time: 2 hr; temp. 37°C. Means of four to sixteen experiments ± SEM). (From Forth, 1966, 1970; Forth and Rummel, 1971)

Metal	Normal rats			Iron-deficient rats		
	Metal content of intestinal tissue			Metal content of intestinal tissue		
	cpm × 10^3 per segment	cpm × 10^3/g[a] mucosal	accumulation	cpm × 10^3 per segment	cpm × 10^3/g[a] mucosal	accumulation[b]
^{54}Mn–($MnCl_2$)	16.6±1.1	156	3.1	46[c]±5.0	306	6.1
^{59}Fe–($FeSO_4$)	18.5±2.1	174	3.5	75[c]±6.0	500	10.0
^{58}Co–($CoCl_2$)	13.5±0.8	125	2.5	43[c]±4.7	290	5.8
^{63}Ni–($NiSO_4$)	2.0±0.2	18.7	0.4	5.3[c]±0.4	35	0.7
^{64}Cu–($CuSO_4$)	22.0±3.0	206	4.1	17±2.1	114	2.3
^{65}Zn–($ZnCl_2$)	11.0±0.6	103	2.1	20[c]±2.3	134	2.7

[a] The mucosal tissue amounts to 50% of the total wet weight of the segment and contains 80% of the radioactivity.
[b] Calculated by dividing cpm/g tissue by cpm/ml mucosal fluid.
[c] $p < 0.01$ as compared with the values of normal segments.

lated. The degree of accumulation in the mucosal tissue of iron-deficient rats decreases in the order iron, manganese, cobalt, nickel, zinc.

The order of this series agrees satisfactorily with the transfer rates in the same experiment (Forth, 1970). Copper forms once again an exception: in iron-deficiency the degree of accumulation actually falls in this case. This result has a parallel in the enhanced uptake of iron and chemically related heavy metals by reticulocytes in iron-deficiency. Reticulocytes take up to a greater extent not only iron but also cobalt, manganese and zinc; again copper forms an exception (Forth *et al.*, 1968b; Forth, 1970).

If the heavy metals chemically related to iron are, at least in part, transported by the iron-transfer system these metals must *compete* with iron during absorption.

The findings of Pollack *et al.* (1965) give an indication that the absorption of manganese and cobalt is inhibited by iron. However, the differences were statistically not significant. The reason is that the concentration of the inhibiting metals could not be increased sufficiently without at the same time inducing toxic effects of heavy metals.

When lower concentration and tied-off jejunal segments of iron-deficient rats are used it is possible to detect *in vivo* a mutual inhibition of absorption between iron and cobalt, iron and manganese and even iron and zinc (Forth, 1966, 1970). The results for cobalt and manganese have meanwhile been confirmed by Schade *et al.* (1970a, b) and the group of Valberg (Thomson and Valberg, 1971, 1972; Thomson *et al.*, 1971a–c). The exceptional status of copper is also confirmed by Schade *et al.* (1970a) and Schwarz and Kirchgessner (1973). Administered in a 10-fold excess to physiological values, cobalt hinders the absorption of iron but not that of copper (Schade *et al.*, 1970a).

Table 22 shows the results of an experiment aimed at detecting the interference of some heavy metals with iron absorption. It shows that the absorption of $^{59}FeSO_4$ and $^{60}CoCl_2$ is retarded by more than 80% in the presence of a 100-fold excess of $CoCl_2$ or $FeSO_4$. With a smaller 10-fold excess the reduction of iron absorption is 70%, that for cobalt only 50%. The more severe inhibition of iron absorption is also found when the interactions between iron and zinc are investigated.

With regard to the great sensitivity of iron absorption to the influence of competing heavy metals it must be added that the inhibition of iron absorption may not be exclusively the consequence of a mutual displacement of the heavy metals at mucosal binding sites. It is quite possible that an additional toxic effect of heavy metals plays a role, particularly in

TABLE 22. MUTUAL INHIBITION OF ABSORPTION BETWEEN IRON, COBALT, MANGANESE AND ZINC IN TIED-OFF JEJUNAL SEGMENTS OF IRON-DEFICIENT RATS *in vivo*

Experimental conditions: fasted rats (16 hr), Wistar (female), 200 g body weight. 5.6 g hemoglobin per 100 ml blood (SEM = ± 0.9; $n = 35$). Jejunal segments: length 15 cm starting with the flexura duodenojejunalis (operation under ether anesthesia). Time: 1 hr. Dose of the metals labeled with radioactive tracers: 0.05 mcM in 1 ml sodium chloride solution (0.9%). The values are the means of five rats ± SEM, indicating the amount absorbed in percent of the administered dose. The radioactivity was measured in a body counter for small animals. (From Forth, 1966, 1970, 1971; Forth and Rummel, 1971)

Absorption of ^{59}Fe–($FeSO_4$) in presence of $CoCl_2$ (mcM/ml)				Absorption of ^{60}Co–($CoCl_2$) in presence of $FeSO_4$ (mcM/ml)			
—	0.05	0.5	5	—	0.05	0.5	5
38.6 ± 9	30.8 ± 10	11.7* ± 4.5	7.2* ± 1.2	60.6 ± 10.6	43.0 ± 20.4	28.9* ± 10.3	11.5* ± 2.8
Absorption of ^{59}Fe–($FeSO_4$) in presence of $MnCl_2$ (mcM/ml)				Absorption of ^{54}Mn–($MnCl_2$) in presence of $FeSO_4$ (mcM/ml)			
—			5	—			5
43.0 ± 7			25* ± 2.0	6.5 ± 2.3			3.5* ± 1.4
Absorption of ^{59}Fe–($FeSO_4$) in presence of $ZnCl_2$ (mcM/ml)				Absorption of ^{65}Zn–($ZnCl_2$) in presence of $FeSO_4$ (mcM/ml)			
—			5	—			5
42 ± 6			14.3* ± 5.3	9.5 ± 1.4			5.2* ± 2.0

*$p < 0.05$ as compared with the control experiment.

TABLE 23. THE INFLUENCE OF THE CONCENTRATION OF H^+ IONS AND OF HEAVY METALS UPON THE ABSORPTION OF FLUID AND GLUCOSE IN TIED-OFF JEJUNAL SEGMENTS OF RATS *in vivo*

Experimental conditions: fasted rats (16 hr), Wistar (female), 180–200 g body weight. Jejunal segments: length 12 cm, starting with the flexura duodenojejunalis (operation under ether anesthesia). The metals were administered in 1 ml Tyrode solution (glucose concentration: 14 mcM/ml). Time: 1 hr. Means of *n* experiments ± SEM. (From Forth, 1967; Forth and Rummel, 1971)

Metal	Concentration (mcM/ml)	pH of the fluid offered	Fluid volume in loop after 1 hr	Net transfer[b] of fluid in % of the amount offered	Glucose concentration of fluid in the loops (mcM/ml)	*n*
—	—	6	0.23 ± 0.05	—77	1.0 ± 0.02	5
—	—	2.4	0.25 ± 0.04	—75	1.4[b] ± 0.04	25
$FeSO_4$	5	2.4	0.28 ± 0.05	—72	1.6[a] ± 0.03	5
$CoCl_2$	0.05	2.4	0.32 ± 0.09	—68	1.6[a] ± 0.05	5
	0.5	2.4	0.32 ± 0.08	—68	1.6[a] ± 0.03	5
	5.0	2.4	0.56 ± 0.02	—44	2.3[a] ± 0.7	20
$MnCl_2$	5.0	2.4	0.44 ± 0.06	—56	1.4[a] ± 0.04	5
$ZnCl_2$	5.0	2.4	1.0[a] ± 0.03	±0	1.3[a] ± 0.09	5

[a] $p < 0.01$ as compared with the control experiment, pH 6.
[b] The negative values indicate a net transfer from lumen to blood.

experiments, in which a 100-fold excess of heavy metal (5 mcM/ml) was used to inhibit iron absorption. Such concentrations of the investigated heavy metals—except iron—influence the absorptive activity of the intestinal segments measured by the absorption of water and glucose. Table 23 shows that 5 mcM/ml of manganese and cobalt reduce the absorption of water by about one-third. The same concentration of zinc inhibits the absorption of water completely. One-tenth this concentration of cobalt produces no statistically significant effect on the absorption of water but inhibits the absorption of $^{59}FeSO_4$ by 70% (Table 22).

The absorption of glucose is only slightly reduced under these experimental conditions (Table 23): the inhibition is due less to the heavy metal concentration than to the enhanced hydrogen ion concentration. That glucose is less well absorbed in media of high hydrogen ion concentration is known from investigations by Iida *et al.* (1968) using intestinal segments *in vitro*.

This interaction between iron and chemically related heavy metals during absorption may entail practical consequences. It is well known that an excess of manganese in the diet may produce anemia in lambs (Hartman *et al.*, 1955), in rabbits, in pigs (Matrone *et al.*, 1959) and in rats (Diez-Ewald *et al.*, 1968). The symptoms of zinc-deficiency in pigs can be aggravated by adding iron to the diet (Hoefer *et al.*, 1960).

At first glance, the finding that cobalt inhibits the absorption of iron appears to conflict with earlier observations, which showed that cobalt can promote the absorption of iron (Wöhler and Emrich, 1956; Wöhler and Körnig, 1964). However, in these older experiments cobalt and iron were administered repeatedly for 1–2 weeks and the dose of cobalt amounted to only one-tenth of that of iron. Under these conditions the demand for iron increases because, in the presence of cobalt, the production of red blood cells is enhanced (Kato and Job, 1940). A similar effect upon the blood-forming bone marrow has been reported for copper (Eichholtz, 1934) and for manganese (Cotzias, 1962).

These are indications that the release of iron from the reticuloendothelial tissue and from the mucosa is reduced in the absence of copper (Lee *et al.*, 1968). This deficiency can be remedied by administering copper (Marston and Allen, 1967). The restitution must be ascribed, however, rather to ceruloplasmin than to copper ions (Ragan *et al.*, 1969; Roeser *et al.*, 1970).

The conclusions which can be drawn for this section are that chemically related heavy metals share—at least in part—the transfer system for iron. The sites in the mucosal cells at which these metals compete with iron have not yet been identified. Theoretically, these acceptor sites may be high molecular compounds as for instance proteins, or low molecular ligands, as for instance amino acids or carbonic acids, which can form chelates with all the heavy metals listed above. However, the acceptor sites in the mucosal cells cannot be ferritin molecules because cobalt, due to the lack of micelle formation, is not taken up by ferritin at all (Schade *et al.*, 1970b).

12.2.2.6. *Properties of the transfer system*

The facts described so far remove all doubt about the existence of a transfer system for iron in the mucosa of the upper part of small intestine. However, important questions about the properties of this system cannot be answered for the moment.

Brush borders. During the search for iron acceptor sites it was logical to think of binding sites located within the membrane, possibly by analogy with the reticulocyte membrane (Katz and Jandl, 1964; Forth *et al.*, 1967). Studies on the binding of iron by the luminal part of the cell membrane, i.e. the brush border, showed that following incubation with $^{59}FeSO_4$ at 0°C the quantity of ^{59}Fe bound to the jejunal brush borders of normal rats per mg of membrane phospholipid is 3 times as high as that in the brush borders of the ileum. Furthermore, the binding of iron to jejunal brush borders is stronger than to ileal brush borders. The jejunal brush borders released very little ^{59}Fe during eight repeated washings, while those of the ileum lost their ^{59}Fe almost completely (Hübers *et al.*, 1971a).

Unexpectedly, the amount of iron bound to jejunal brush borders of iron-deficient rats was less than that bound to brush borders of normal animals. Conversely, in iron-deficiency the ileal brush borders displayed an increased iron-binding capacity. This finding is surprising because the lower ileum is by no means a preferential site for iron absorption even in iron-deficiency (see Fig. 7). As expected, the amount of iron bound to jejunal brush borders was found to be about twice that bound to ileal brush borders (Greenberger *et al.*, 1969). It is not yet possible to assess the significance of investigations on isolated brush borders *in vitro* for the iron absorption process. Further data on these open questions are required. Thus, brush borders may lose a part of their iron-binding capacity during isolating procedure. Using a particularly mild method for separating the brush borders (a PVP-density gradient), Hübers *et al.* (1971b, c) succeeded in showing that brush borders of the jejunum of iron-deficient rats bind twice as much iron as those of normal animals.

The main reason for this result, which differs from the observations of the Greenberger group, seems to be the fact that Hübers *et al.* (1971b, c) avoided the usual edetic acid in the preparation of the brush borders.

Ferritin (references of recent literature on ferritin may be taken from Crichton, 1971, 1973). On account of the ferritin content of the mucosa, Granick (1949, 1951) ascribed to apoferritin the role of an iron acceptor. However, it is doubtful whether apoferritin is significant in the rapid phase of iron absorption which predominates in iron-deficiency. In contrast to the evidence that in normal animals ferritin is formed in the intestinal mucosa during absorption (Granick, 1946; Wöhler *et al.,* 1957), the mucosa of iron-deficient animals contains less ferritin-bound iron than that of normal animals (Brown and Rother, 1963a; Charlton *et al.,* 1963, 1965; Crosby, 1963; Manis and Schachter, 1964). This observation led Crosby (1963) to postulate that the synthesis of apoferritin is decreased in iron-deficiency. However, all the authors quoted measured only ferritin-bound iron and not ferritin protein (Brittin and Raval, 1970).

Brittin and Raval (1970) have recently published convincing evidence that as much apoferritin is formed in the mucosa in iron-deficiency as under normal conditions. They measured directly the ferritin protein content. The fact that the synthesis of ferritin protein in the mucosa takes longer in iron-deficient rats than the absorption of iron is an argument against the assumption that apoferritin could be the iron carrier across the mucosa cell (Table 24).

It may be added that the iron content of ferritin in the mucosal tissue of these animals was very low (Brittin and Raval, 1970).

Ferritin could function as an iron carrier during absorption only if the

TABLE 24. DUODENAL FERRITIN PROTEIN AND IRON ABSORPTION IN RATS *in vivo*

Experimental conditions: fasted rats (24 hr), Sprague–Dawley (male). Control rats: 406 g body weight; 5.4 g hemoglobin per 100 ml blood. Iron-deficient rats: 218 g body weight; 4.0 g hemoglobin per 100 ml blood. Iron dose: 1 mg ^{59}Fe–($FeSO_4$) administered by intra-duodenal injection in ether anesthesia. (From Brittin and Raval, 1970)

Hours after intraduodenal iron	Ferritin protein absorbed (mcg per g gut)		Iron absorption into body (% of administered dose)	
	D	*C*	*D*	*C*
0	>2.0	10.4 (1.3)	—	—
1	3.8 (0.4)	—	12.9 (0.9)	—
3	12.4 (0.5)	17.7 (1.1)	25.0 (2.4)	1.6 (0.1)
5	21.3 (0.7)	—	25.4 (2.5)	2.1 (0.5)

D = six iron-deficient rats. *C* = six control rats.
Values represent the mean, with the standard error of the mean given in brackets.

turnover of ferritin iron were rapid. This is not so. In model experiments the half-life of the exchange of ferritin iron was 4 days under optimal conditions, i.e. in the presence of reducing agents (Bielig and Bayer, 1955).

The fact that during the mucosal cell transfer of cobalt as well as of iron is enhanced in iron-deficiency is another argument against a role of ferritin. Cobalt cannot be detected in ferritin during absorption (Schade *et al.,* 1970b). An incorporation of cobalt into ferritin appears unlikely, since the metal is very resistant to oxidation under biological conditions.

Apparently, ferritin plays no other role in the mucosal cells than that elsewhere in the organism, where it acts as a depot for instantaneous excess iron. In this way it may protect cells against excessive iron concentrations and provide iron for the slow phase of absorption.

Non-ferritin proteins. Proteins other than apoferritin seem to be of increasing physiological relevance with regard to iron transfer. As already indicated, there are many reasons which justify increased attention to the possibility that mucosal cells contain proteins which function as iron carriers across the cell. Several proteins could play this role.

Thus, a glycoprotein which largely binds iron can be isolated from the intestinal mucosa of rats (Blanc, 1965, 1967; Blanc and Issliker, 1965; Delaloye *et al.,* 1966). Eccrinosiderophilin which is found in the intestinal mucosa as well as in other secretory tissues must be included here as a possible carrier agent (Masson and Heremans, 1967; Schade, 1967). Furthermore, during the last years several authors have independently found iron-binding non-ferritin proteins in mucosal cells (Charlton *et al.,* 1965; Halliday and Powell, 1973; Hübers *et al.,* 1971c, d; Pearson and Reich, 1969; Pollack *et al.,* 1972; Sheehan and Frenkel, 1972; Worwood and Jacobs, 1971a, b; Worwood *et al.,* 1971). It is not yet clear whether all these reports describe the same iron-binding constituent.

Results which appear to indicate the existence of an iron-transfer protein in mucosal cells (Hübers *et al.,* 1971b, d) may briefly be described.

In homogenized mucosal cells of both normal and iron-deficient rats two iron-binding protein fractions (fractions 1 and 2; ^{59}Fe labeled) can be isolated from particle-free supernatant by acrylamide gel electrophoresis and sephadex chromatography. The purified fraction 1 (protein 1) has some properties in common with ferritin, e.g. heat stability and electrophoretic behavior. The purified fraction 2 (protein 2), however, differs from ferritin and shows similarities with transferrin. It can be shown that protein 2 is not derived from the blood plasma by measuring the degree of contamination with plasma transferrin. Less than 0.3% of the radioiron content of protein 2 can be attributed to radioiron bound to plasma transferrin (Hübers *et al.*, 1971b; Forth *et al.*, 1972). The molecular weight of protein 2 was found to be approximately 80,000 by the sephadex method. It is heat labile and it is not precipitated by anti-ferritin. At 280 nm and 417 nm identical absorption maxima are obtained for transferrin and protein 2 (unpublished data). In iron-deficient animals the concentration of iron-binding proteins in the particle-free fraction of *jejunal* mucosal cells is increased to more than 10 times its normal value, while the total concentration of proteins in this fraction remains unchanged (Hübers, unpublished data).

Protein 2 from *ileal* mucosa, i.e. the mucosa from that part of the small intestine with the lowest activity of iron absorption—contains only 18% of the ^{59}Fe activity found in the same fraction of jejunal segments (Hübers *et al.*, 1971b).

The most striking evidence in support of the functional significance of protein 2 in iron absorption was obtained by measuring the distribution of ^{59}Fe activity on proteins 1 and 2 in the particle-free supernatant of homogenized mucosal cells of rats during absorption (Hübers *et al.*, 1971b). The correlation between the time course of the ^{59}Fe activity in the total particle-free supernatant and that bound to protein 2 from mucosal cells of iron-deficient rats is very similar. Conversely, the coincidence between protein 1 and the total ^{59}Fe activity in the particle-free supernatant normal rats is striking. Protein 2, therefore, appears to be a significant factor in the process of iron transfer across the cytoplasm of mucosal cells in the proximal small intestine and may play the part of an intracellular iron transfer protein. If this assumption is to be proved the intracellular localization of protein 2 must be demonstrated. It will be necessary to exclude the possibility of the attachment of iron-free plasma transferrin on the outside of the mucosal cells. This assumption was made by Levine and Weintraub (1969) and Levine *et al.* (1972).*

The discrimination between protein 2 and membrane-attached transferrin is difficult for methodological reasons. Quantitatively only a minor part of the content of protein 2 in the mucosal tissue can be due to plasma transferrin attached to the mucosal cells. The amount of contamination with ^{59}Fe-transferrin in the mucosal tissue is the same in homogenates of jejunum and ileum while the concentration of ^{59}Fe-labeled protein 2 in the jejunal mucosa is 5 times higher than that in the ileal mucosa.

Furthermore, protein 2 could be attached to binding sites in the brush

*The increased capacity to absorb iron in iron-deficiency can be washed out by rinsing the intestinal segments with saline (unpublished results of the Homburg-group). Protein 2, therefore, may be identical with eccrinosiderophilin.

border region of the mucosal cells. If this were so protein 2 could be identical with eccrinosiderophilin possibly derived from excretory cells of the mucosal epithelium.

When evaluating the significance of mucosal proteins for the iron absorption three other observations must be discussed.

(1) Inhibitors of protein synthesis such as cycloheximide (Greenberger, 1973; Greenberger and Ruppert, 1966a) and tetracyclines (Greenberger and Ruppert, 1966b; Greenberger *et al.*, 1967; Yeh and Shils, 1966) inhibit the absorption of iron. The inhibitory effect of tetracyclines has been shown not to be due to a decrease of iron availability due to the formation of sparingly soluble complexes (see p. 636). In this connection it is interesting that iron-deficiency itself leads to a malabsorption of iron in man and in animals which may be the result of a defective protein synthesis in the epithelial cells of the mucosa (Kimber and Weintraub, 1968). Defective protein synthesis could explain the atrophy of the mucosal epithelium of the gastrointestinal tract in iron-deficiency (see p. 616).

(2) Pretreatment of rats with phenobarbital is followed by an enhanced absorption of a single dose of iron given by gastric tube (Thomas *et al.*, 1972a). It was shown that under these conditions the ^{59}Fe content of protein 2 is increased in mucosal homogenates of duodenal segments in which the absorption of iron is enhanced (Hübers, unpublished data).

(3) The capacity of the mucosal cell to transfer iron to the blood stream is at least in part genetically controlled (Bannerman *et al.*, 1968; Edwards and Bannerman, 1970a, b; Manis, 1970, 1971; Pinkerton, 1968, 1969; Pinkerton and Bannerman, 1967; Pinkerton *et al.*, 1970). It should be added that also the hereditary microcytic anemia of mice (gen. symbol mk) is associated with an impaired iron absorption (Edwards and Hoke, 1972; Bannerman *et al.*, 1972).*

Thus in duodenal everted sacs prepared from mice with sex-linked anemia (sla) the increased iron demand consequent upon a low iron diet or upon pregnancy is not associated with an increased iron transport (Pinkerton, 1969; Manis, 1970, 1971). This defect in the transfer system is present in hemizygous males and homozygous females and appears to be restricted to iron because neither the absorption of ^{64}Cu, ^{57}Co, ^{65}Zn or fat (Bannerman *et al.*, 1968; Pinkerton *et al.*, 1970) nor the absorption of calcium, galactose or proline is diminished (Manis, 1971). Sla-mice do not show a defect of transferrin; serum iron and total iron binding capacity of serum of sla-mice show a pattern which is characteristic for iron-deficiency (Pinkerton and Bannerman, 1967). The discovery that the

*Further details may be taken from Chapter 13, pp. 771–773 (Eds.).

capacity of the iron transfer system to adapt to the demand is genetically determined is of fundamental importance. Pinkerton *et al.* (1970) wrote that "the genetically determined defect in intestinal mucosa of mice with sex-linked anemia may be due to deficiency of either an enzyme or a carrier substance necessary for normal transfer of iron from the intestinal mucosa cell to the plasma". In fact, in duodenal segments the ^{59}Fe content per mg protein 2 did not increase in sla-mice fed a low iron diet in contrast to findings in normal mice (Hübers *et al.*, 1972; Forth *et al.*, 1972). This result is in agreement with the assumption that protein 2 acts as a carrier for iron transfer across the duodenal mucosa, particularly for the transfer during the rapid phase of absorption in iron-deficiency.

12.2.3. TRANSFER OF COPPER

By the same criteria that have been applied to the transfer of iron a transport system for copper can be postulated.*

12.2.3.1. *Metabolic dependence*

The transfer of copper across the mucosal epithelium depends on the cellular metabolism. Investigations on hamster segments *in vitro* demonstrated that the transfer of ^{64}Cu is inhibited by withdrawal of oxygen or by addition of 2,4-dinitrophenol, sodium iodoacetate or sodium fluoride (Crampton *et al.*, 1964, 1965b). By contrast, the ^{64}Cu content in the intestinal tissue remains unchanged; in the presence of potassium cyanide the ^{64}Cu content of the tissue is reduced. At the same time, however, the transfer of ^{64}Cu across the gut wall increases (Crampton *et al.*, 1965b). This effect of potassium cyanide is probably due to the formation of a stable Cu-complex which can penetrate the gut wall and which does not release its copper to the mucosal binding sites. The experiments in which metabolic poisons were used are open to criticism in several respects.

(1) Unfortunately no systematic investigations have up to now been performed on intestinal segments of animals suffering from copper-deficiency (Kirchgessner *et al.*, 1973).

(2) The results obtained by Crampton *et al.* are based on a very small number of experiments, in some cases involving only two or three segments.

(3) The *in vitro* investigations were made with ileal segments, which under these conditions showed the highest transfer rate from the mucosal to the serosal side. A higher transfer rate for copper of the ileum as compared to the jejunum could not be observed in tied-off intestinal segments *in vivo* (see p. 647).

*For copper-malabsorption in man see Chapter 13, p. 770.

TABLE 25. THE INFLUENCE OF O_2 DEPRIVATION ON THE TRANSFER AND TISSUE CONTENT OF ^{64}Cu PRESENTED AS $CuCl_2$ IN EVERTED ILEAL SACS OF RATS

Experimental conditions: fasted rats (16 hr), Wistar (female), 200 g body weight. Method according to Wilson and Wiseman (1954). Length of the segments 6 cm, starting 5 cm proximal from the valvula ileocoecalis (two segments of each rat). Concentration of ^{64}Cu–($CuSO_4$): 10^{-6} M/l (20,000 cpm/ml in the mucosal fluid). At the beginning of the experiment: mucosal fluid: 12 ml Tyrode solution; serosal fluid: 0.7 ml Tyrode solution; at the end: O_2: 0.77 ml (SEM = ± 0.06; $n = 8$); N_2: 0.69 ml (SEM = ± 0.04; $n = 8$). Atmosphere: 5% CO_2 and 95% O_2 or N_2. Time: 2 hr; temp. 37°C. Means of eight experiments ± SEM. (Forth and Nell, unpublished data)

Administered at the mucosal side	Atmosphere	Conc. in serosal fluid (cpm/ml)	Tissue content (cpm/g tissue wet weight)
^{64}Cu–($CuCl_2$) (10^{-6} M/l)	O_2	1400 ± 350	16,100 ± 4380
^{64}Cu–($CuCl_2$) (10^{-6} M/l)	N_2	585[a] ± 151	3840[a] ± 530

[a] $p < 0.01$ as compared with the O_2 controls.

The findings of Crampton *et al.* (1964, 1965b) on hamster segments were confirmed in experiments on the rat intestine. By withdrawal of oxygen the transfer of copper is also reduced in this species (Table 25). These experiments were performed *in vitro* with ileal segments.

12.2.3.2. *Preferential direction*

A further argument in favor of the existence of a copper transport system is the demonstrated preferential transfer from the mucosal to the serosal side (Crampton *et al.*, 1965a, b; Schwarz *et al.*, 1973b).

12.2.3.3. *Capacity of the transfer system*

The capacity of the transport system for copper is limited. Indications to this effect have been obtained not only by *in vitro* experiments with hamster segments (Crampton *et al.*, 1965b) but also *in vivo* with mice (Gitlin *et al.*, 1960) and rats (Owen, 1964; for further references see Van Campen, 1971). In normal mice the transport system is saturated by doses above 25 mcg (Gitlin *et al.*, 1960) and in normal rats by doses greater than 100 mcg (Owen, 1964; for further references see Van Campen, 1971). When these doses are exceeded copper is absorbed at a rate directly proportional to the dose and the absorption kinetics in this dosage range can be described as a first-order reaction. The sparse results obtained in man reveal no linear relationship between dosage and absorption and, thus, suggest a copper transport system (Weber *et al.*, 1969).

12.2.3.4. *Specificity*

Whether copper transport is, like that of iron, performed by a specific system can be investigated by observing the interfering effect of other heavy metals on copper absorption. However, it is necessary to distinguish exactly between the interference of heavy metals in the gut lumen (see p. 633) and that during the actual absorption process, i.e. the transfer across the mucosal epithelium.

The decrease of copper absorption induced by a high *calcium* content of the food is due essentially to intraluminal factors. On the one hand calcium salts can reduce the solubility of copper compounds and, hence, the availability of the metal for absorption (Tompsett, 1940). On the other hand, calcium may influence copper absorption indirectly by retarding the absorption of zinc (Heth and Hoekstra, 1965), thus alleviating the interference of zinc with copper absorption (see p. 633). This mechanism is assumed to be a factor in the "meat anemia" which can be prevented by either calcium or copper supplementation (Guggenheim *et al.*, 1963; Guggenheim, 1964; Moore, T. *et al.*, 1964; for further references see Van Campen, 1971). Results concerning the calcium–copper interaction in absorption reported in the literature are, however, contradictory, mainly because of species differences (cf. Waser and Kirchgessner, 1965).

It is difficult to decide whether the interference of *molybdenum* with *copper* absorption is due to an intraluminal process or to a process occurring during the transfer across the mucosa. The inhibition of copper absorption by molybdenum initially observed in calves (Ferguson *et al.*, 1938) has meanwhile been confirmed for many other species (for references see Van Campen, 1971). Molybdenum retards the absorption of copper only in the presence of sulfate ions, as first observed in sheep by Dick (1956) who postulated that the interaction between copper and molybdenum takes place in the mucosal membranes. However, it could take place intraluminally by influencing the availability of copper by molybdenum and sulfate ions (Mills, 1961). In connection with the latter hypothesis Matrone (1970) postulates the formation of a poorly absorbed copper–molybdenum sulfide complex. The sulfides are assumed to be formed by the reducing activity of micro-organisms on sulfate in the gut lumen.

As in the case of iron, heavy metals which have been clearly shown to influence the absorption of copper are chemically related elements, i.e. *cadmium* and *zinc*. Like copper these metals possess an isoelectronic valence shell, prefer the coordination number 4 and preferentially form tetrahedral complexes. Cadmium and zinc aggravate copper-deficiency

TABLE 26. INTERFERENCE OF CHEMICALLY RELATED METALS WITH COPPER DURING ABSORPTION IN RATS AND CHICKENS *in vivo*

Rats; tied-off stomach and duodenum (operation under ether anesthesia): data were taken from Van Campen (1966); absorption was calculated by summing up the ^{64}Cu-activity in blood, heart and liver; dose of ^{64}Cu–($Cu(NO_3)_2$): 0.01 mcm. Chickens: data were taken from Starcher (1969); absorption was calculated by measuring ^{64}Cu-activity in the liver. The ratio metal:Cu can be calculated in this case only approximately, because the dose of ^{64}Cu–($CuCl_2$) administered orally varied between 0.5 and 0.016 mcm

Interfering metal	Rat			Chicken	
	Tied segments from	Interfering metal : Cu ratio	Cu absorption (% of controls)	Interfering metal : Cu ratio	Cu absorption (% of controls)
Zn	stomach	500	42[a]	—	—
Zn	duodenum	500	37[a]	30– 900	33[a]
Cd	duodenum	300	9[a]	18– 540	20[a]
Ag	duodenum	300	58	18– 540	28[a]
Hg	duodenum	300	78	10– 300	61
Mo	—	—	—	22– 660	99
Mn	—	—	—	36–1100	101

[a] $p < 0.01$ as compared with the control experiment.

symptoms in chickens (Hill *et al.*, 1963, 1964). Both heavy metals retard the absorption of copper from tied-off rat duodenal segments *in situ* (Van Campen, 1966). Zinc was also found to inhibit the absorption of copper from the stomach to the same extent as from the duodenum (Table 26).

Zinc and copper mutually affect each other's absorption (Van Campen

TABLE 27. MUTUAL INHIBITION OF COPPER AND ZINC DURING ABSORPTION IN RATS *in vivo*

Experimental conditions: tied-off duodenal segments (operation under ether anesthesia). Length of the duodenal segments: 7 cm starting with the pylorus. Dose of ^{64}Cu–($Cu(NO_3)_2$): 0.016 mcm. Dose of ^{65}Zn–($ZnCl_2$): 0.08 mcm. Absorption was calculated on the base of the disappearance of radioactivity from the tied-off segments. Means of at least eight rats. (After Van Campen, 1970)

Absorption of ^{64}Cu (% of the dose)		Absorption of ^{65}Zn (% of the dose)	
Control	50.6	Control	40.6
^{64}Cu in presence of Zn (Zn : Cu = 940)	31.5[a]	^{64}Zn in presence of Cu (Cu : Zn = 40)	28.3[a]

[a] Difference statistically significant as compared with the controls.

and Scaife, 1967; Van Campen, 1969, 1970, 1971). However, a 40-fold excess of copper over zinc (Table 27) apparently produces the same retarding effect as a 1000-fold excess of zinc over copper. The acceptor sites in the mucosa controlling the absorption appear to have a greater affinity for copper than for zinc.

Silver, which shares with copper the three above-mentioned physico-chemical properties, also intensifies copper-deficiency symptoms (Hill *et al.*, 1964). Silver shows no clear effect in tied-off rat duodenal segments (Van Campen, 1966), but an effect was produced in chickens (Starcher, 1969) (see Table 26).

Mercury is similar to copper with respect to valency and to coordination number but forms different types of complexes. It does not aggravate copper-deficiency symptoms (Hill *et al.*, 1964), nor does it reduce the absorption of copper (Table 26) in the rat. An inhibitory effect has been observed in the chicken but did not appear to be statistically significant.

The nature of the copper transport system has not yet been elucidated. Starcher (1969) found a copper binding protein in mucosal cells of the chicken intestine. This protein which has an approximate molecular weight of 10,000 may be an acceptor for copper in the mucosal cells. Cadmium, zinc and silver which all retard the absorption of copper displace copper from this protein (Starcher, 1969). Possibly, the mucosal protein binding copper is the sulfhydryl-rich protein metalothioneine (for ref. see Evans, 1973).

12.2.4. TRANSFER OF ZINC

Although zinc has recently received attention especially in veterinary as well as in human medicine, the information available is not yet sufficient to decide whether its absorption mechanism is similar to that for copper and iron (Becker and Hoekstra, 1971).

12.2.4.1. *Metabolic dependence*

As in the case of iron and copper, two processes have to be distinguished, i.e. uptake of zinc into mucosal epithelial cells and transfer to the serosal side (Pearson *et al.*, 1966; Sahagian *et al.*, 1966, 1967). The two processes apparently are influenced to a different extent by metabolic poisons. While neither group of workers observed an effect of oxygen withdrawal on the transfer of zinc in isolated rat intestine segments *in vitro* (Pearson *et al.*, 1966; Sahagian *et al.*, 1967), the amount of zinc taken up into mucosal cells appears to be reduced under anaerobic conditions. These studies were performed with normally fed rats; analogous investigations with zinc-deficient animals have yet to be carried out (Kirchgessner *et al.*, 1973).

The withdrawal of oxygen from the rat jejunum *in vitro* has no effect on the transfer of inorganic zinc in Tyrode solution. Under these conditions zinc is sparingly soluble and there is little transfer of ^{65}Zn to the serosal side. The data given in Table 28 show that the transfer of ^{65}Zn amounts to only half that of iron and to one-tenth that of copper. The transfer of ^{65}Zn is increased by a factor of about 50 after adding histidine. The tissue content of ^{65}Zn increases only 4-fold under these conditions. Withdrawal of oxygen reduces the transfer and the tissue content of ^{65}Zn (Table 28). Histidine very probably holds zinc in solution in a form suitable for absorption (see pp. 704–707).

The enhancement of the transfer of *zinc* and *cadmium* by dinitrophenol (10^{+4} M) in isolated rat jejunum segments *in vitro* described by Sahagian *et al.* (1967) was explained by assuming a *higher permeability* of the gut segments under the influence of DNP.

Similar results, i.e. a rise of the concentration of iron and of cobalt on the serosal side, could be obtained by oxygen withdrawal in everted sac preparations of the rat jejunum (Table 18). The concentration on the

TABLE 28. THE INFLUENCE OF O_2 DEPRIVATION ON TRANSFER AND TISSUE CONTENT OF ^{65}Zn PRESENTED AS $ZnCl_2$ IN PRESENCE OF HISTIDINE IN EVERTED JEJUNAL SEGMENTS OF RATS

Experimental conditions: fasted rats (16 hr), Wistar (female), 200 g body weight. Jejunal segments: length 6 cm, starting with the flexura duodenojejunalis (two segments of each rat). Mucosal fluid: 12 ml Tyrode solution; serosal fluid: 0.7 ml Tyrode solution. Atmosphere: 5% CO_2 and 95% O_2 or N_2. Volume at the end of the experiment at the serosal side: O_2, 0.9 ml (SEM = 0.04); N_2, 0.7 ml (SEM = 0.03). Concentration of ^{65}Zn–($ZnCl_2$) 10^{-6} M/l (20,000 cpm/ml) in the mucosal fluid. Time: 2 hr; temp. 37°C. Means of eight experiments ± SEM. (Forth and Nell, unpublished data)

Metal (10^{-6} M/l)	Ligand (10^{-3} M/l)	Atmosphere	Amount transferred (cpm/ml)	Tissue content (cpm/g)
^{65}Zn–($ZnCl_2$)	—	O_2	148 ± 14	22,100 ± 2400
^{65}Zn–($ZnCl_2$)	—	N_2	116 ± 16	5900[a] ± 780
^{65}Zn–($ZnCl_2$)	histidine	O_2	7700[b] ± 1050	81,500[b] ± 7200
^{65}Zn–($ZnCl_2$)	histidine	N_2	1260[a] ± 97	37,200[a] ± 5200

[a] $p < 0.01$ as compared with the O_2 controls.
[b] $p < 0.01$ as compared with the O_2 experiments without addition of histidine.

serosal side of ^{14}C-ethylenediaminetetra-acetic acid, creatinine, zinc– and manganese–EDTA complexes is also increased under these conditions (Forth, 1966).

As a rule, wherever oxygen withdrawal leads to a rise of the concentration of metals on the serosal side, the tissue content is also increased. Why this rule does not apply to copper or zinc or the zinc–histidine complex (Tables 25 and 28) is an open question.

When assessing the transfer across the gut wall it is not sufficient to rely exclusively on measurements of the concentration at the serosal side. This can be demonstrated by results obtained with the preparation of Fisher and Parsons (1949) as modified by Rummel and Stupp (1960). When the transfer of ^{59}Fe in jejunal segments of iron-deficient rats is studied under anaerobic conditions the concentration of ^{59}Fe in the absorbate rises. This is mainly the result of a reduced volume of absorbed fluid under these conditions. The amount of ^{59}Fe transferred does not differ from control values in preparation with an intact oxygen supply with a normal rate of water absorption. For creatinine a rise of the concentration on the serosal side in a N_2-atmosphere was also observed; the amount transferred, however, was even less than that in the aerobic controls (Forth and Nell, unpublished data).

12.2.4.2. *Preferential direction*

In the rat jejunum *in vitro* more zinc was found to be transferred from the mucosal to the serosal side than in the opposite direction (Sahagian *et al.*, 1967). Cadmium and mercury as well as iron (see p. 687) behave similarly while the transfer of manganese occurs at the same rate in both directions. Unfortunately, no results of comparative studies on gut segments of normal and zinc-deficient animals are at hand to resolve whether the assumed transfer operates preferentially in one direction. The intestine may possibly act as an excretory organ for zinc (Gunn *et al.*, 1962; Cotzias *et al.*, 1962; Methfessel and Spencer, 1973b).

12.2.4.3. *Capacity of the transfer system*

No data are as yet available on the effect of *concentration* upon the transfer of zinc from intestinal segment *in vitro*. In living rats absorption and retention of ^{65}Zn increases with increasing doses, but not in direct proportion to the dose (Furchner and Richmond, 1962). After a 6- to 10-fold increase in the amount of zinc added to the food the retention of ^{65}Zn increased only 3-fold. Similar results were reported by Heth and Hoekstra (1965), who observed in rats a decrease of the fractional absorption with increasing zinc content of food. Apart from differences in the extent in mice (Rubini *et al.*, 1961) and in man (Furchner and Richmond, 1962) this also occurs. However, the experiments in man were carried out in a single individual.

The dependence of the fractional absorption on dose becomes more evident when the administration of ^{65}Zn is preceded by prolonged feedings with a high zinc diet (Furchner and Richmond, 1962; Rubini *et al.*, 1961; Hoekstra, 1964; Heth and Hoekstra, 1965). A smaller effect on the percentage absorption was found by Feaster *et al.* (1954) with steers and by Ballou and Thompson (1961) with rats, when a single dose of ^{65}Zn was given simultaneously with increasing amounts of unlabeled zinc.

Zinc uptake into the tissues of different rat intestinal segments was tested *in vitro* with ^{65}Zn. Increasing concentrations of 0.004–0.08 mcg/ml give a directly proportional relationship between dose and tissue content of ^{65}Zn (Pearson *et al.*, 1966). These data do not warrant the general conclusion that the absorption of zinc is independent of the concentration presented, because the concentration range investigated was too small. The zinc content of the rat food is normally 20–40 mcg per day (Bowen, 1966). The limitation of the experiments by Pearson *et al.* (1966) to this concentration region is probably due to the low solubility of inorganic zinc salts in conventional media.

12.2.4.4. *Specificity*

Chemically related metals, e.g. copper (see p. 685) interfere with zinc absorption. A distinction must be made between intraluminal interference and interference with the actual absorption process.

The interference of *calcium* with the absorption of zinc probably occurs intraluminally (see p. 633). High concentrations of calcium-phosphate in the food severely diminish the solubility of zinc and, hence, its availability for absorption (Hoekstra, 1964; Heth *et al.*, 1966; Becker and Hoekstra, 1971).

The effect of *vitamin D* on the absorption of zinc, which a decade ago attracted considerable interest (Becker and Hoekstra, 1971), appears to have now been elucidated. Vitamin D appears to exert an indirect effect on the absorption of zinc by virtue of its well-known enhancing effect upon calcium absorption, because there is a concomital increased demand for zinc during formation of bone tissue (Becker and Hoekstra, 1966).

Cadmium aggravates zinc-deficiency symptoms in cattle (Powell *et al.*,

1964) and in turkeys (Supplee, 1961). A partial explanation may be that cadmium retards the *absorption* of zinc. Experimental evidence was obtained by Powell *et al.* (1967) with goats and calves. Cadmium also inhibits the *secretion* of zinc into the gut lumen (Gunn *et al.*, 1962; Cotzias *et al.*, 1962). *In vitro* in isolated rat jejunum segments, cadmium inhibits the uptake of zinc into the cells of the mucosal epithelium (Sahagian *et al.*, 1967). Cadmium also retards the uptake of manganese and mercury in these experiments. According to these authors and in contrast to the effect of cadmium on zinc absorption, zinc promotes the uptake of cadmium into mucosal tissue. No detailed explanation for this effect is given (Sahagian *et al.*, 1967).

Absorption of cadmium was recently investigated in sheep (Doyle *et al.*, 1972). From a diet containing 60 ppm of cadmium the animals absorb about 5% of the metal; excretion of cadmium into bile and urine is minimal.

The aggravation of zinc-deficiency symptoms in pigs led to the conclusion that iron retards the absorption of this metal (Hoefer *et al.*, 1960). More recently direct proof of this effect has been obtained in rats (Forth, 1970) (see Table 22).

Addition of copper also intensifies the symptoms of zinc-deficiency (Van Campen, 1970). As has already been mentioned, copper and zinc interfere with each other's absorption (Table 27) (Van Campen, 1969, 1970). They appear to compete for acceptor sites in the mucosa. It is possible that a protein represents the zinc acceptor site, as in the case of iron and copper. Two groups of workers succeeded in isolating proteins with appreciable zinc-binding properties from the chicken intestine (Suso and Edwards, 1969, 1971) or from the rat intestine (Van Campen, 1970; Van Campen and Kowalski, 1971). However, there is at present no evidence to show that these proteins are involved in the transfer of zinc across the mucosal epithelium.

It is too early to decide whether different proteins, or only a single one, are involved in the transfer of zinc, copper and iron.

12.3. TRANSFER OF METAL CHELATES

12.3.1. METHODOLOGICAL CONSIDERATIONS

So far only the transfer of heavy metals present as inorganic salts on the mucosal side of the intestine wall has been considered. However, under physiological conditions most heavy metals are present in the diet

TABLE 29. TRANSFER OF EDTA AND IRON IN EVERTED JEJUNAL SACS OF NORMAL AND IRON-DEFICIENT RATS

Experimental conditions: fasted rats (16 hr), Wistar (female), 180–220 g body weight. Normal rats: 14.6 g hemoglobin per 100 ml blood (SEM = ± 0.8; $n = 30$). Iron-deficient rats: 5.6 g hemoglobin per 100 ml blood (SEM = ± 1.0; $n = 30$). Method according to Wilson and Wiseman (1954). Length of the segments: 6 cm, starting with the flexura duodenojejunalis (two segments of each rat). Mucosal fluid: 12 ml Tyrode solution; serosal fluid: 0.7 ml Tyrode solution, at the end of the experiment 0.8 ml (SEM = ± 0.1; $n = 48$). Concentration of ^{59}Fe–($FeCl_3$) added to the mucosal fluid: 7 nM/ml (40,000 cpm/ml); concentration of ^{14}C–EDTA (40,000 cpm/ml) as indicated in the table by the ratio EDTA: Fe. Time: 2 hr; temp. 37°C. Means of eight experiments ± SEM. (Forth and Rummel, unpublished data)

Ratio Ligand : Fe		Concentration at the serosal side (cpm/ml)		$\frac{^{59}Fe}{^{14}C}$	Decrease of the ^{14}C and ^{59}Fe–activity at the mucosal side in % of the dose	
		^{14}C	^{59}Fe		^{14}C	^{59}Fe
—	*n*	—	730 ± 308	—	—	70
	a	—	8800$^{(a)}$ ± 400	—	—	70
1:1	*n*	10,000 ± 2000	1000 ± 220	0.1	± 0	80
	a	9600 ± 1800	7800$^{(a)}$ ± 3200	0.8	± 0	80
1000:1	*n*	12,600 ± 2100	11,000$^{(b)}$ ± 2000	0.9	± 0	± 0
	a	10,800 ± 2000	9400 ± 1200	0.9	± 0	± 0

$^{(a)}$ $p < 0.01$ as compared with segments of normal rats.
$^{(b)}$ $p < 0.01$ as compared with the experiments without EDTA.

as complexes or chelates. This fact, and the role of complexing agents in keeping the metals in a form suitable for absorption, have already been discussed (see p. 622). In the section below the actual *absorbability* of metal chelates will be discussed.

It is difficult to state to what extent metal complexes permeate the mucosa because under normal conditions, *in vivo*, a fraction of the bound metal may be liberated from the complex; the amount depends on the stability constant of the complex and on intraluminal factors such as pH and on the concentration of the competing metals and ligands. As a rule the incorporation or the metabolic utilization of heavy metals is measured during studies on metal chelate absorption and, therefore, it is necessary to make a clear distinction between that fraction which is transferred across the mucosa as intact complex and that which is transferred as heavy metal liberated from the complex. This differentiation can be made only in a few cases under favorable conditions, as shown in Table 29.

Measuring the transfer of the ^{14}C-EDTA–^{59}Fe(III)-complex in jejunal everted sac of iron-deficient rats *in vitro* yields a value of 0.8 for the $^{59}Fe/^{14}C$ ratio in the serosal fluid. This value, which approaches unity, might lead one to assume that the intact complex crosses the gut wall. Such a conclusion would be premature for several reasons: (1) An 80% drop of the ^{59}Fe activity in the incubation fluid observed during the experiments (Table 29) points to dissociation of the complex and precipitation of iron as hydroxide or phosphate. (2) Under similar conditions, in intestinal segments of *normal* rats, the $^{59}Fe/^{14}C$ ratio in the serosal fluid is only 0.1. (3) The increase of transfer across the gut wall apparently due to iron-deficiency was approximately equal in animals given EDTA–Fe(III) (ligand:Fe = 1 : 1) as in animals given $^{59}FeSO_4$. These data suggest that the complex is in fact dissociated by means of the iron transfer system. There is no reason to assume that the gut segments of iron-deficient rats are more permeable to iron EDTA than those of normal animals (Forth *et al.*, 1965; see also Table 29). The transfer rate of ^{14}C-EDTA in segments from normal and iron-deficient rats is the same.

When the effective stability of EDTA–Fe(III) is increased by increasing the excess ligand (EDTA:Fe = 1000 : 1), a value of 0.9 is found for the $^{59}Fe/^{14}C$ ratio in the absorbate of jejunal segments of both normal and iron-deficient rats (Table 29). Under these conditions the ^{59}Fe activity in the incubation fluid did not decrease. This indicates that the complex did not dissociate. The small deviation of the $^{59}Fe/^{14}C$ ratios from 1 is either due to error or the result of an exchange between ^{59}Fe and inactive iron from the gut wall.

TABLE 30. TRANSFER AND TISSUE CONTENT OF ^{59}Fe AND ^{60}Co PRESENTED AS $FeSO_4$ AND $CoCl_2$ UNDER THE INFLUENCE OF LIGANDS IN JEJUNAL SEGMENTS OF RATS *in vitro*

Experimental conditions: fasted rats (16 hr), Wistar (female), 180–200 g body weight. Method according to Fisher and Parsons (1949) modified by Rummel and Stupp (1960). Jejunal segments: length 8 cm, starting with the flexura duodenojejunalis (two segments of each rat). Metal concentration: 10^{-6} M/l (23,500 cpm/ml). Ligand:Fe = 100:1. In order to remove adsorbed metals from the surface the segments of the controls without ligand were washed three times in 100 ml sodium chloride solution (0.9 M) containing EDTA (10^{-2} M/l); for the other segments pure sodium chloride solution (0.9 %) was used. Time: 2 hr; temp. 37°C. Means of 8 experiments ± SEM. (Forth *et al.*, 1973)

Metal administered as	Ligand	Absorbate			tissue content (cpm/g wet weight)
		volume (ml)	metal conc. (cpm/ml)	metal amount (cpm/cm)	
^{59}Fe–($FeSO_4$)		2.4 ± 0.1	550 ± 57	135	30,400 ± 710
	EDTA	2.3 ± 0.2	1760[a] ± 181	440	4470[a] ± 235
	8-OH-quinoline	1.9 ± 0.2	3470[a] ± 212	750	259,000[a] ± 28,200
	8-OH-quin.-sulf.[b]	2.3 ± 0.2	153[a] ± 19	36	705[a] ± 70
^{60}Co–($CoCl_2$)	—	2.0 ± 0.1	10,000 ± 1150	2740	32,600 ± 2350
	EDTA	2.1 ± 0.1	1650[a] ± 176	450	37,770[a] ± 235
	8-OH-quinoline	2.0 ± 0.2	3060[a] ± 165	640	129,000[a] ± 22,000
	8-OH-quin.-sulf.[b]	2.2 ± 0.2	1460[a] ± 146	365	8700[a] ± 940
^{65}Zn–($ZnCl_2$)	—	2.4 ± 0.2	226 ± 35	60	19,300 ± 3280
	EDTA	2.2 ± 0.2	1760[a] ± 282	460	5400[a] ± 470
	8-OH-quinoline	1.9 ± 0.2	542[a] ± 77	106	87,000[a] ± 6100
	8-OH-quin.-sulf.[b]	2.2 ± 0.1	193 ± 99	49	25,800 ± 4800
^{64}Cu–($CuSO_4$)[c]	—	1.0 ± 0.05	14,000 ± 1200	1350	220,000 ± 19,200
	EDTA[d]	1.2 ± 0.05	740[a] ± 212	83	18,800[a] ± 2600
	8-OH-quinoline	1.0 ± 0.1	15,900 ± 1350	1630	520,000[a] ± 70,000
	8-OH-quin.-sulf.[b]	1.2 ± 0.07	320[b] ± 51	39	6800[a] ± 785

[a] $p < 0.01$ as compared with the group without ligands. [b] 8-Hydroxyquinoline-5-sulfonic acid.
[c] Ileal segments, 10 cm length, starting 5 cm proximal of the valvula ileocoecalis; two segments of each rat. [d] EDTA; Cu = 500; 1.

It thus appears to be necessary to use an excess of ligand for studying the transfer of metal complexes across the intestinal wall even when investigating complexes with a high thermodynamic stability constant, *in vitro*. Reliable information concerning the absorption of chelated metals which may differ from free metals by their availability for absorption, or by their mechanism of transfer, can be obtained only by direct measurements *in vitro* or in tied-off intestinal segments *in vivo*. Methods based on measuring retention following oral administration may provide reliable data only if the chelated metal is absorbed to a smaller extent than the free metal. When, however, the chelated metal is absorbed to a greater extent than the free metal, the distinction between enhanced availability and an increase in the transfer rate of the chelate across the mucosa is difficult, if not impossible, in the intact animal (Richmond *et al.*, 1962).

In chelates the properties of metals are masked by the ligands. The absorbability of the complex depends on its physicochemical properties, e.g. the lipid solubility and electric charge. The molecular size of most metal chelates suggests passage through the "non-porous" lipid part of the cell membrane in addition to that through the "porous" portion. A noticeable exception is the complex of *cyanocobalamin* (vitamin B_{12}) and intrinsic factor. The latter is excreted into the gastric lumen and allows the vitamin to be taken up into the mucosal cells of the ileum (Castle, 1968; see also this book, Chapter 7, p. 404).

TABLE 31. ABSORPTION OF HEAVY METAL CHELATES IN TIED-OFF JEJUNAL SEGMENTS OF RATS *in vivo*

Experimental conditions: fasted rats (16 hr), Wistar (female), 200 g body weight. Jejunal segments: length 20 cm, starting with the flexura duodenojejunalis (operation under ether anesthesia). Metal dose: 0.36 mcM in 2 ml saline solution (0.9%); without ligands, pH 2; EDTA, pH 6; quinoline-derivatives, pH 3. Ligand:Fe = 10:1. Time: 1 hr. Absorption of the radioactive metals was measured in a body counter for small animals after removal of the tied-off segment. The values are given as percent of the dose; means of five rats ± SEM. (Forth *et al.*, 1973)

Metals administered as	Without ligands	EDTA	8-Hydroxyquinoline-5-sulfonic acid	8-Hydroxyquinoline
^{59}Fe–($FeSO_4$)	10.4 ± 2.5	1.6[a] ± 0.3	0·4[a] ± 0.08	36[a] ± 1.8
^{60}Co–($CoCl_2$)	16.4 ± 1.1	1.8[a] ± 0.4	0.5[a] ± 0.09	25[a] ± 1.8
^{65}Zn–($ZnCl_2$)	13.4 ± 1.4	3.0[a] ± 1.0	3.5[a] ± 0.7	26[a] ± 0.9
^{64}Cu–($CuSO_4$)	7.5 ± 0.5	1.5[a] ± 0.2	1.1[a] ± 0.1	16[a] ± 0.9

[a] $p < 0.01$ as compared with the group without ligands.

12.3.2. Fe(III)-8-HYDROXYQUINOLINE-5-SULFONIC ACID-CHELATE

Presenting ^{59}Fe together with 8-hydroxyquinoline-5-sulfonic acid to the mucosal side of gut segments *in vitro* slows the rate of transfer of ^{59}Fe to the serosal side to approximately one-quarter of the control value (Table 30). Under these conditions the ^{59}Fe content of the mucosa is reduced to one-fortieth of the control value. In other words, the stable (log $\beta_3 = 36$), water-soluble, triple electronegative Fe(III)-chelate (see Fig. 12) penetrates the gut wall very slowly and releases practically no iron to the acceptor sites in the mucosa. Even if divalent iron is used the Fe(III)-complex appears within a few moments as indicated by the green color of the incubation fluid saturated with oxygen. From the *in vitro* observation that 8-hydroxyquinoline-5-sulfonic acid-Fe(III)-chelate penetrates the intestinal wall poorly and does not release its iron one can predict that the complex should also be poorly absorbed *in vivo*. This prediction is confirmed by the results of studies on tied-off rat jejunal segments *in situ* (Table 31) and by measurements of retention following oral administration in the rat (Table 32) as well as in man (Ewe, 1968).

TABLE 32. RETENTION OF HEAVY METALS BY RATS 6 AND 20 DAYS AFTER THEIR ADMINISTRATION AS CHELATES BY STOMACH TUBE

Experimental conditions: fasted rats (16 hr), Wistar (female), 250 g body weight. Metal dose: 0.36 mcM in 2 ml saline solution (0.9%); pH: without ligands, pH 2; EDTA, pH 6; quinoline derivatives, pH 3. Ligand:metal = 10:1. Three hours after application of the metal by stomach tube the rats were fed again. The retention of the radioactive metals was measured in a body counter for small animals. The values are given as a percent of the dose; means of ten rats ± SEM. (Forth and Nell, unpublished data)

Metal (3.6×10^{-7} M/l)	Ligand (3.6×10^{-6} M/l)	Retention after 6 days (% of dose)	Retention after 20 days (% of dose)
Fe	—	17.1 ± 2.1	15.8 ± 3.3
Fe	EDTA	$1.6^{(a)} \pm 0.2$	$1.5^{(a)} \pm 0.2$
Fe	8-OH-quinoline	$26.8^{(a)} \pm 1.7$	$24.6^{(a)} \pm 4.2$
Fe	8-OH-quin.-sulf.	$3.6^{(a)} \pm 0.8$	$3.3^{(a)} \pm 0.8$
Co	—	2.0 ± 0.2	0.7 ± 0.07
Co	EDTA	$0.23^{(a)} \pm 0.07$	$0.07^{(a)} \pm 0.004$
Co	8-OH-quinoline	$3.1^{(a)} \pm 0.2$	$1.1^{(a)} \pm 0.1$
Co	8-OH-quin.-sulf.	$0.32^{(a)} \pm 0.03$	$0.11^{(a)} \pm 0.01$
Zn	—	19.6 ± 1.8	7.9 ± 0.9
Zn	EDTA	$5.1^{(a)} \pm 0.5$	$1.9^{(a)} \pm 0.2$
Zn	8-OH-quinoline	$24.8^{(a)} \pm 2.5$	$10.9^{(a)} \pm 2.1$
Zn	8-OH-quin.-sulf.	21.3 ± 2.1	8.0 ± 1.0

$^{(a)}$ $p < 0.01$ as compared with the group without ligands.

12.3.3. Fe(III)-CHELATE-8-HYDROXYQUINOLINE

A minor change in the molecule of the complex (Fig. 12) discussed in the preceding paragraph effects a complete change of its absorbability. Removing the polar sulfonic acid group in position 5 results in 8-hydroxyquinoline-Fe(III)-chelate which has the same stability constant as the

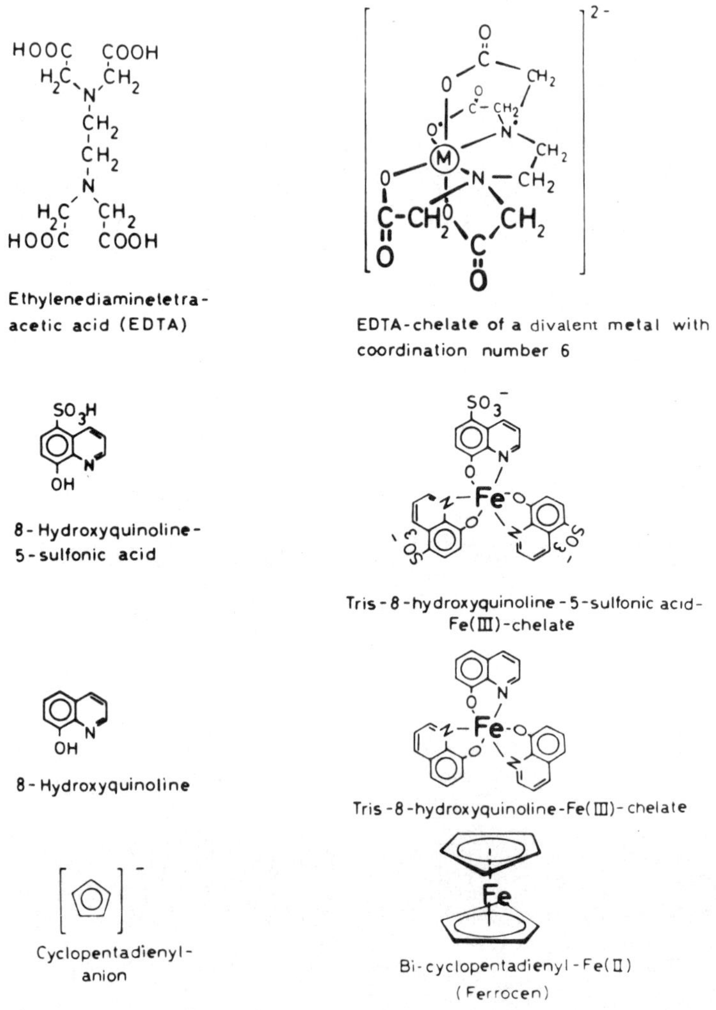

FIG. 12. For details see text.

sulfonic acid complex. However, in contrast to the latter the 8-hydroxyquinoline-Fe(III)-chelate is electroneutral and almost insoluble in water at pH 7, but highly lipid-soluble.

A trick is used for applying iron complex in aqueous solution. In acid solution (pH 2.5–3.5) the iron–hydroxyquinoline complex is water-soluble, but it is not the 3 : 1 chelate shown in Fig. 12 but probably the 2 : 1 or 1 : 1 chelate. In these compounds the free iron coordination sites are thought to be occupied by chlorine ions or water. The shift to pH 6.9–7.0 in the fluid on the mucosal side leads to the formation of the lipid-soluble 3 : 1 chelate. As predicted, this chelate penetrates the intestinal wall to a greater extent and the content of the mucosal epithelium is substantially higher than after presenting free, non-complex-bound iron (Table 30).

The green color of the intestinal segments shows that the ^{59}Fe content of the tissue is essentially due to the uptake of the intact complex. Two different penetration mechanisms can be discussed. The complex may be dissolved within the lipid part of the membrane, or may participate in an intermediate reaction with iron acceptor sites, by forming a heterocomplex. The latter assumption is supported by the observation that iron-deficient rats show enhanced absorption of iron also after administration of this complex. Heterocomplex formation between an iron compound and membrane acceptor sites has already been discussed with regard to reticulocytes: formation of a heterocomplex may be involved in the uptake of iron from transferrin by iron-binding sites in the reticulocyte membrane (Jandl and Katz, 1963; Katz and Jandl, 1964). Similarly, the membrane fraction of reticulocytes contains more 8-hydroxyquinoline-bound iron than that of mature erythrocytes (Forth *et al.*, 1967). How the iron is liberated from such a heterocomplex is unknown at present. Labilization could be due to oxidoreductive reactions of cell metabolism since reduction of trivalent to divalent is known to lead to lowered complex stability (Sillen and Martell, 1964).

According to the results obtained *in vitro* the 8-hydroxyquinoline-Fe(III)-chelate was found to be particularly well absorbed from tied-off rat jejunal segments *in situ* (Table 31) and after oral administration (Table 32). This statement also holds true in man (Ewe, 1968).

Ferrocene (dicyclopentadienyl-Fe(III); see Fig. 12), a highly lipid-soluble compound, is, like the Fe(III) complex of 8-hydroxyquinoline, well absorbed. After absorption it is initially deposited in the body fat (Goldberg and Martin, 1964). Up to 30 % of the orally administered complex is eliminated by the urine within 24 hr.

Unlike ferrocene, the Fe(III)-8-hydroxyquinoline-chelate is stored mainly in the liver and lungs of the rat. In iron-deficient rats it has been demonstrated that up to 6 days elapse before a dose of ^{59}Fe administered as the complex (0.36 mcM iron per rat) is completely utilized, i.e. incorporated into hemoglobin (Forth, 1970). Iron administered as the 8-hydroxyquinoline complex is not eliminated via the kidney as is ferrocene. It should be emphasized that both lipid-soluble chelates, i.e. ferrocene as well as the 8-hydroxyquinoline-Fe(III)-chelate, are only interesting models which have no therapeutical significance.

12.3.4. ETHYLENEDIAMINETETRAACETIC-ACID-FE-CHELATES

Ethylenediaminetetraacetic acid (EDTA) forms water-soluble complexes with iron (Fe(II)-complex, $\log K = 16$; Fe(III)-complex, $\log K = 25$; see Sillen and Martell, 1964) which, *in vitro*, penetrate the intestinal wall more rapidly than free, non-complex-bound iron (Table 30). It is unknown to what extent Fe(II) within the EDTA-complex is oxidized to Fe(III) under experimental conditions *in vitro*, i.e. perfusing intestinal segments with oxygen-saturated Tyrode solution. Simultaneously, the mucosal content of ^{59}Fe-labeled iron is presented as EDTA-Fe(II)-complex than with inorganic ^{59}Fe.

With tied-off intestinal segments of rats *in vivo*, however, less iron was absorbed when presented as EDTA-Fe(II)-complex than when free non-complex-bound iron was given (Table 31).

In order to resolve the discrepancy between the results obtained *in vitro* and *in vivo* we have to consider both the *amount* of ^{59}Fe transferred and the intestinal tissue: after presenting free non-complex-bound ^{59}Fe the sum of transferred plus stored iron, *in vitro* and *in vivo*, is nearly 4 times greater than after adding ^{59}Fe as the EDTA–Fe(II)-complex. It is, therefore, not surprising that *in vivo* less iron is absorbed from the EDTA-Fe(II)-chelate than from the same amount of metal given as free iron.

In addition EDTA–Fe is excreted in the urine to a greater extent than non-complex-bound iron: up to 40% of the amount absorbed is eliminated by the kidneys (Forth *et al.*, 1965b). This fate seems to be common to most water-soluble stable iron complexes (Forth *et al.*, 1965b; Hopping and Ruliffson, 1963; Pringle *et al.*, 1962).

12.3.5. CHELATES OF OTHER HEAVY METALS

Complexes of the ligands mentioned with zinc, copper or cobalt generally have properties similar to those of the iron complexes, and are absorbed in the same manner.

This was confirmed not only by *in vitro* experiments (Table 30), but also by experiments carried out on tied-off intestinal segments of rats *in situ* (Table 31) and by measuring retention after oral administration (Table 32). Because of the short half-life of ^{64}Cu this metal was not studied in retention tests.

For experiments with *copper* ileum segments are used. *In vitro* the EDTA–Cu-complex penetrates the gut wall less readily than the EDTA complexes of iron, cobalt and zinc (Table 30). The reason is probably that copper differs from these metals tested by having four instead of six coordination sites. Therefore, the EDTA–Cu(II)-complex may bear a negative electrical charge (Garvan, 1964). The ligand excess used in the copper experiments was 5 times greater than with the other metals. This fact, however, does not explain the smaller transfer rate.

All tested complexing agents, including 8-hydroxyquinoline, reduce the transfer of *cobalt* across the gut wall *in vitro* (Table 30), because of the high availability of inorganic cobalt for absorption. In contrast to other heavy metals cobalt is not oxidized in the perfusion fluid and its aquo-ion, unlike that of iron, does not tend to form polyhydroxides or insoluble phosphates. As a consequence, the amount of cobalt transferred across the gut wall *in vitro* is so great that no complexing agent can produce a further increase. Even ligands forming Co-complexes of low stability decrease the amount of cobalt absorbed (Kroe *et al.*, 1964).

Manganese was included in this experimental series, but results are not shown in Tables 30–32. The complexing agents displayed the same effects on isolated intestinal segments *in vitro* as were observed with iron and zinc. *In vivo,* however, none of the ligands had any effect on the absorption of manganese. This observation suggests that the excess of ligands was not large enough, so that the complexes dissociated during the passage along the gastrointestinal tract. This interpretation is supported by the thermodynamic stability constants of the other metal chelates (Sillen and Martell, 1964). Probably the dissociation is increased further by the still lower effective stability of manganese complexes in biological media. A higher absorptive utilization of the EDTA–Mn- than of the EDTA–Zn-complex was found *in vivo* in experiments with chickens (Suso and Edwards, 1968) and young turkeys (Vohra and Gonzales, 1969).

12.3.6. LIGANDS OF MEDICAL AND NUTRITIVE SIGNIFICANCE

12.3.6.1. *Polyaminopolycarbonic acids*

EDTA (see Fig. 12 and Table 33, (1)) can be regarded as the mother

TABLE 33. POLYAMINOPOLYCARBONIC ACID–Ca(II)-CHELATES

	Chemical structure	Name	Log K_1
(1)	$HOOCCH_2 \searrow NCH_2CH_2N \nearrow CH_2COOH$ $HOOCCH_2 \nearrow \qquad\qquad \searrow CH_2COOH$	Ethylenediaminetetraacetic acid (EDTA)	10.7[a]
(2)	$HOOCCH_2 \searrow N\text{–}(CH_3)_3\text{–}N \nearrow CH_2COOH$ $HOOCCH_2 \nearrow \qquad\qquad \searrow CH_2COOH$	Trimethylenediaminetetraacetic acid	7.1[a]
(3)	$HOOCCH_2 \searrow N\text{–}(CH_3)_4\text{–}N \nearrow CH_2COOH$ $HOOCCH_2 \nearrow \qquad\qquad \searrow CH_2COOH$	Tetramethylenediaminetetraacetic acid	5.0[a]
(4)	$HOOCCH_2 \searrow N\text{–}(CH_3)_5\text{–}N \nearrow CH_2COOH$ $HOOCCH_2 \nearrow \qquad\qquad \searrow CH_2COOH$	Pentamethylenediaminetetraacetic acid	4.6[a]
(5)	$HOOCCH_2 \searrow NCH_2CH_2NCH_2COOHCH_2CH_2N \nearrow CH_2COOH$ $HOOCCH_2 \nearrow \qquad\qquad \searrow CH_2COOH$	Diethylenetriaminepentaacetic acid (DTPA)	10.9[b]
(6)	$HOOCCH_2 \searrow N$ $HOOCCH_2 \nearrow$ $HOOCCH_2 \searrow N$ $HOOCCH_2 \nearrow$	1,2–Diaminocyclohexanetetraacetic acid (DCTA)	12.1[b]
(7)	$HS\text{–}(CH_2)\text{–}N \nearrow CH_2COOH$ $\qquad\qquad \searrow CH_2COOH$	Mercaptoethyliminodiacetic acid (MEIDA)	4.9[b]

[a]cf. Martell and Calvin (1952, 1958).
[b]cf. Catsch (1964, 1968).

compound of the great family of polyaminopolycarbonic acids. These ligands have been investigated extensively in view of the possibility of using them for withdrawing metals from the organism (cf. Catsch, 1964, 1968; Schubert, 1955). However, little is known about their influence on the intestinal absorption of metals. In general, these ligands are water-soluble and form complexes which are highly water-soluble. Therefore, ligands of this type may be expected to inhibit the absorption of metals which are rapidly and extensively absorbed from the intestine, e.g. iron, the absorption of which is mediated by a transfer system. The absorption of metals which are present in the gastrointestinal tract in a form which makes them unavailable for absorption and, hence, are poorly absorbed may be increased by polyaminopolycarbonic acids. Both effects can be shown with DTPA (see Table 33, (5)) in rats. DTPA reduces the absorption of iron remarkably—as does EDTA (see p. 623)—provided that the chelating agent and iron are given at nearly the same time (Nigrovic *et al.*, 1967). If, on the other hand, iron is given orally half an hour before DTPA iron absorption is increased. This result may be explained by the assumption that iron sequestered as the sparsely soluble iron hydroxide in the lower parts of the intestine may be taken up and made available for absorption by DTPA. Nigrovic *et al.* (1967) give another interpretation; they suggest iron taken up into mucosal cells could be mobilized by the subsequent dose of DTPA. It is, however, unlikely that appreciable amounts of this ligand enter the mucosal cells. Both EDTA and DTPA are absorbed only to about 5% (Foreman, 1966; Foreman and Trujillo, 1954). In rats, the absorption of the iron chelate of DTPA amounts to 3–4% of the dose. From these data it was concluded that the DTPA iron chelate is absorbed intact (Nigrovic *et al.*, 1967). Generally, the ability of polyaminopolycarbonic acids to permeate biological membranes may be increased by substituting lipophilic groups (Vlcek, 1967).

EDTA and DTPA exert toxic effects mainly in the small intestine (Weber, 1969a, b). Under the influence of DTPA the synthesis of DNA in the cells of the crypts of Lieberkühn is decreased (Weber *et al.*, 1970). In the experiments on toxic effects high ligand doses (up to 8 mM/kg) were given parenterally.

Side effects of polyaminopolycarbonic acids used as ligands for heavy metals may be predicted from the log K_1 values of the calcium chelates listed in Table 33. The relationship between structure and stability constant is exemplified by the ligands 1–4 in Table 33. The thermodynamic stability constants of the calcium chelates are known for nearly all polyaminopolycarbonic acids, whereas the constants are available only for a few of the many heavy metal chelates. With an increasing number of carbon atoms between the two nitrogen atoms the thermodynamic stability constants of the calcium chelates decrease. The relationship between structure and thermodynamic stability of heavy metal chelates is probably the same.

Replacement of one or more acetic acid groups in EDTA by hydroxy-ethyl-, propionic acid-, or methyl-phosphinic acid groups does not increase the stability constants of calcium, or heavy metal complexes.

In DTPA (Table 33, (5)) the alkylene bridge is extended by a substituted nitrogen atom. DTPA is a ligand with a remarkably high thermodynamic stability constant especially for heavy metals (Pb^{2+}, Hg^{2+}, Fe^{2+}, Fe^{3+}, Cu^{2+}, Zn^{2+}, Co^{2+}, Ce^{3+}, Y^{3+}; cf. Catsch, 1964, 1968). The stability constants of the heavy metal-DTPA-chelates are higher than those of the analogous DCTA-chelates (polyaminopolycarbonic acid with a cyclic structure, see Table 33, (6)), whereas the stability constant of the Ca(II)-DTPA-chelate is smaller than that of the Ca(II)-DCTA-chelate.

In other compounds the CH_2-groups of the alkylene bridge between the nitrogen atoms are replaced by either oxygen or thioether. Thus, higher dentate ligands with more than 6 donor atoms are formed. There are also sulfhydryl-containing compounds related chemically to the aminocarbonic-acid series; one example is given in Table 33, (7) (MEIDA).

12.3.6.2. *Sideramines*

Microorganisms of the *Streptomyces* type produce iron chelates called sideramines (Bickel *et al.*, 1960). Desferrioxamine B (Deferoxamine) is the iron-free ligand of the sideramine ferrioxamine, a metabolite of *Streptomyces pilosus* E. One mole deferoxamine binds 1M Fe^{3+}, i.e. deferoxamine can bind iron to the extent of 9.35% of its weight forming a pink water-soluble iron chelate. The thermodynamic stability constant of this chelate amounts to 10^{31} (Sillen and Martell, 1964). Other sideramines are ferrichrome (29), ferrioxamine E (32.5) and *N*-acetyl-ferrioxamine B (30.8); the numbers in brackets represent the thermodynamic stability constants (log K_1) of the iron chelates taken from Sillen and Martell (1964). In sideramines iron is bound by hydroxamic acid groups. For therapeutic purposes deferoxamine is mainly used. This compound is available either as hydrochloride or as methane-sulfonate, the water solubility of the latter being about 5 times higher than that of the former (cf. Moeschlin and Schnider, 1964). In buffer solutions of pH 6.1 deferoxamine is stable for more than 3 days whereas the compound disintegrates in acid solutions (cf. Moeschlin and Schnider, 1964). Further details of the biochemistry of desferrioxamine are given by Keberle (1964).

Deferoxamine is recommended for the treatment of secondary hemochromatosis as well as for acute iron poisoning (Moeschlin and Schnider, 1964; Wöhler, 1964). Deferoxamine is a highly specific chelator of iron. This is due to the remarkable high thermodynamic stability constant of the deferoxamine iron chelate as compared with that of chelates of this compound with other heavy metals and alkaline earth metals (see Sillen and Martell, 1964). According to its chemical properties deferoxamine decreased the oral toxicity of iron in mice provided deferoxamine is administered orally immediately after iron whereas the toxicity of other heavy metals, e.g. Cu^{2+}, Mn^{2+}, Ni^{2+}, or Zn^{2+} is not significantly influenced by deferoxamine (Tripod, 1964).

Deferoxamine is absorbed from the gastrointestinal tract to less than 15% of the dose (Tripod and Keberle, 1962). Therefore, deferoxamine is generally given parenterally for treatment of hemosiderosis. In acute iron poisoning deferoxamine must be given orally, in addition to a parenteral dose. In mice iron absorption can only be prevented if deferoxamine is given within half an hour after the iron (Tripod, 1964). Theoretically, for a child poisoned with 3–4 g ferrous sulfate at least 8 g deferoxamine must be given orally in order to trap the iron within the gastrointestinal tract. In clinical cases of iron intoxication the deferoxamine dose should be higher (by one-third) than that corresponding to the dose of iron swallowed (Moeschlin and Schnider, 1964). In rats as well as in man deferoxamine inhibits the absorption of iron provided that it is given orally either with the iron or immediately after the iron (Balcerzak *et al.*, 1966; Bannerman and Malpass, 1965; Nigrovic *et al.*, 1967); deferoxamine by no means prevents completely the absorption of iron. Because deferoxamine does react with iron ions preferentially it is not surprising that the absorption of iron bound in highly stable chelates, e.g. hemoglobin (Bannerman and Malpass, 1965; Balcerzak *et al.*, 1966), or of iron from a meal consisting mainly of pig liver (Martin *et al.*, 1967) is not impaired by deferoxamine.

The immediate source of iron removed from the organism by deferoxamine is still unknown (Brown *et al.*, 1967). Only small amounts of iron can be removed by deferoxamine from transferrin from the body stores or during absorption (Brown *et al.*, 1967; Jacobs, A. *et al.*, 1969). These observations suggest that deferoxamine takes up iron in the organism when the metal is transferred from one pool to another, e.g. during the transfer from the mucosal cells to plasma transferrin, from transferrin to the sites of hemoglobin synthesis in the bone marrow or during the mobilization of iron from the depots. During these transfer processes small but easily accessible iron pools might exist (Jacobs, A. *et al.*, 1969).

12.3.6.3. *Amino acids and the transfer of heavy metals*

It is well known that certain amino acids enhance the absorption of iron (Jacobi *et al.*, 1956; Kroe *et al.*, 1963b, 1966; Van Campen and Gross, 1969), of copper (Kirchgessner and Grassman, 1970a, b) and of zinc (Hoekstra, 1970).

Mainly L-amino acids enhance the absorption of heavy metals. The D-isomers, though possessing the same stability constants, are found to be less effective (Kirchgessner and Grassman, 1970a, b). The experiments leading to these results were carried out *in vivo* by feeding copper amino acid complexes and subsequently measuring the copper contents of the liver of rats as well as *in vitro* using everted intestinal segments of rats (Schwarz *et al.*, 1973a, b).

It is important to know whether the intact amino acid–copper complexes are absorbed or whether the amino acids make copper available for absorption from the intestinal lumen.

Experimental evidence favoring the second alternative is also available. (Forth *et al.*, 1973; Van Campen, 1973). This interpretation is not incompatible with the observation that only the L- and not the D-isomers of amino acids enhance the absorption of copper (Kirchgessner *et al.*, 1967; Kirchgessner and Grassman, 1970a, b; Kirchgessner and Weser, 1965a). If a *heterocomplex* is formed between the amino acid–copper complex and the mucosal binding sites the conformation of the amino acid–copper complex may be significant. This is particularly the case when both the metal and the ligand determine the contact with the mucosal binding sites. For steric reasons the D-isomers may be suitable for reacting with mucosal binding sites. It is well known from investigations on the exchange of complex-bound iron with transferrin that the conformation as well as the stability and the electrical charge of the iron complex is significant (Bates *et al.*, 1967a, b; Billups *et al.*, 1967).

If iron or copper is presented *in vitro* together with histidine to the mucosal side of rat jejunal segments, the transfer rate of the heavy metals increases with the concentration of L-histidine, i.e. with the excess of ligand (see Fig. 13). It is characteristic that a fairly large excess is necessary for an appreciable increase of the transfer of iron (L-histidine: Fe = 1000 :1). For copper the excess of ligand required for enhancing the

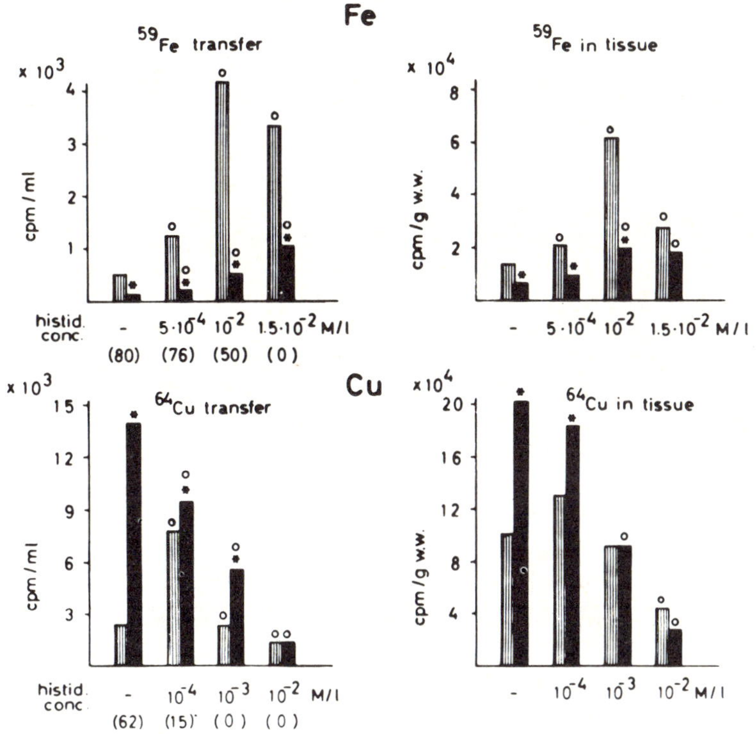

FIG. 13. Transfer and tissue content of ^{59}Fe–iron and ^{64}Cu–copper in the presence of histidine in jejunal and ileal segments of rats *in vitro*. Experimental conditions: fasted rats (16 hr), Wistar (male), 200 g body weight. Method according to Fisher and Parsons (1949) modified by Rummel and Stupp (1960). Jejunal segments (hatched columns): length: 8 cm, starting with the flexura duodenojejunalis (two segments were prepared from each rat). Ileal segments (black columns): length: 8 cm, starting with the valvula ileocoecalis (two segments were prepared from each rat). Concentration of the metals in the perfusion fluid (50 ml Tyrode solution): 10^{-6} M/l (20,000 cpm/ml). Iron: ^{59}Fe–($FeSO_4$); Copper: ^{64}Cu–($CuSO_4$). In order to remove radioactivity adsorbed to the surface, the segments were washed three times in 100 ml sodium chloride solution containing EDTA (10^{-2} M/l). Mean fluid absorption in the experiments: with jejunal segments: 2 ml (SEM = $\pm$ 0.18); with ileal segments: 1.3 ml (SEM = $\pm$ 0.09). The columns represent means from four to eight experiments; SEM did not exceed 20%. The numbers in brackets indicate the decrease of radioactivity in the perfusion fluid in percent. * = $p < 0.01$ jejunal compared with ileal segments. o = $p < 0.01$ control compared with the histidine group. (Forth *et al.*, 1973.)

transfer is lower (histidine:Cu = 100:1). The stability constant of the histidine–Cu(II)-complex is substantially greater ($\log \beta_2 = 18$) than that of the histidine–Fe(II)-complex ($\log \beta_2 = 9$). An increase in the histidine:

metal ratio beyond 1000:1 or 10,000:1, respectively, does not further increase the transfer of the metals.

The ^{64}Cu and ^{59}Fe content of the mucosal tissue is also influenced by the presence of L-histidine.

Alanine (Forth *et al.*, 1973), in agreement with the lower stability constants for its iron, copper and zinc-complexes, is less effective.

In addition to the results with jejunal segments, Fig. 13 contains data obtained with rat *ileal* segments. As mentioned previously (see p. 682), in experiments *in vitro* the transfer and the amount of copper taken up into the mucosa are greater in ileal than in jejunal segments.

L-histidine in all concentrations depresses the rate of transfer of ^{64}Cu and the amount taken up into the ileal tissue, in contrast to ^{59}Fe for which the transfer and tissue content increases steadily as the excess of L-histidine increases, reaching constant values beyond a 1000-fold excess.

In experiments with both copper and iron, the presence of L-histidine eliminates the quantitative differences between jejunum and ileum with respect to metal transfer and tissue content. The same is true for the transfer of zinc (Forth *et al.*, 1973), and this also occurs in the presence of L-alanine at high concentrations.

The data available on the transfer of metals presented to isolated gut segments *in vitro* as amino acid complexes can be interpreted by assuming that the amino acids hold the metal available in a form suitable for absorption. They also form metal complexes of low effective stability which can release their metals to acceptor sites in the mucosa.

If the stability of the amino acid–metal complexes is increased by ligand excess, these complexes (see Fig. 13) behave like stable, water-soluble metal complexes. Then an exchange with ligands within the mucosal cell takes place. Intact amino acid–metal complexes presented to the mucosal side of the intestine thus pass through the gut wall to only a very small extent, if at all. This statement does not rule out the possibility that under physiological conditions, iron, copper or zinc may leave the mucosal cells on their basal pole as amino acid complexes which were formed in the mucosal cells.

Segments of iron-deficient rats have the capacity to transport iron across the mucosal epithelium to a greater extent than do segments of normal rats, and this regardless whether L-histidine is present in a 1000-fold or even in a 10,000-fold excess. In both groups the transfer of L-histidine across the mucosal epithelium of normal and iron-deficient rats is not significantly different. In other words, in segments of iron-deficient rats iron was released—at least in part—from the L-histidine-chelate and disposed to the acceptor sites of the mucosa cells prior to the transfer across the mucosal epithelium (Forth *et al.*, 1973).

12.3.7. GENERAL CONCLUSIONS CONCERNING THE TRANSFER OF METAL CHELATES

Absorption of stable metal complexes according to the principles determining the absorption of drugs (see this book, Chapter 4, p. 254) implies that the complexes penetrate across the mucosa without reacting with the specific transport system.

Complexing agents may prevent the binding of iron to acceptor sites of mucosal cells (Forth *et al.*, 1965a, b, c; Forth and Rummel, 1966b).

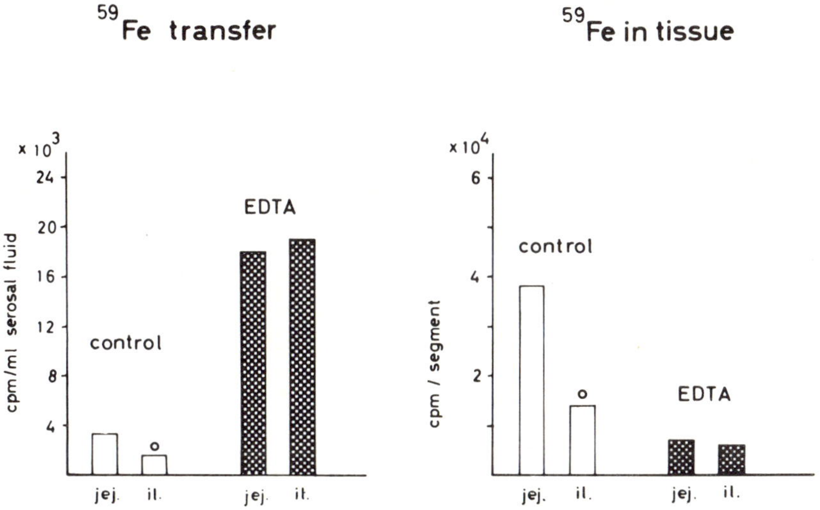

FIG. 14. Transfer and tissue content of ^{59}Fe–iron in the presence of EDTA in jejunal and ileal segments of normal rats *in vitro*. Experimental conditions: fasted rats (16 hr), Wistar (female), 180–200 g body weight. Method according to Fisher and Parsons (1949), modified by Rummel and Stupp (1960). Jejunal segments (jej.): length 8 cm, beginning with the flexura duodenojejunalis (two segments of each rat). Ileal segments (il.): length 8 cm beginning with the valvula ileocoecalis (two segments of each rat). Iron concentration in the perfusion fluid (50 ml Tyrode solution): 10^{-5} M/1 ^{59}Fe–($FeSO_4$) (100,000 cpm/ml). EDTA : Fe = 100 : 1. Time: 2 hr; temp. 37°C. In order to remove merely ^{59}Fe adsorbed by the surface, the segments were washed three times in 100 ml sodium chloride solution (0.9%) containing EDTA (10^{-2} M/1). The columns represent means of twelve (controls) and eight (EDTA) experiments. o = $p < 0.01$ jejunal compared with ileal segments. (From Forth *et al.*, 1965c.)

The difference between the *jejunal* and *ileal* segments with respect to the transfer of non-complex-bound iron through the intestinal wall as well as its accumulation in mucosal tissue disappears when complex-bound iron is administered. Figure 14 illustrates this for the EDTA–Fe(II)-complex. Other complexing agents have the same effect, e.g. citric, pyrophosphoric and nicotinehydroxamic acid, provided that a greater ligand excess is employed (Forth *et al.*, 1965c).

The characteristic difference between jejunal segments of normal and iron-deficient rats with respect to transfer of ^{59}Fe and the tissue content also disappears for complex-bound ^{59}Fe. This is illustrated for the *tris* (nicotinehydroxamato)–Fe(III)-complex in Fig. 15. Complex-bound iron,

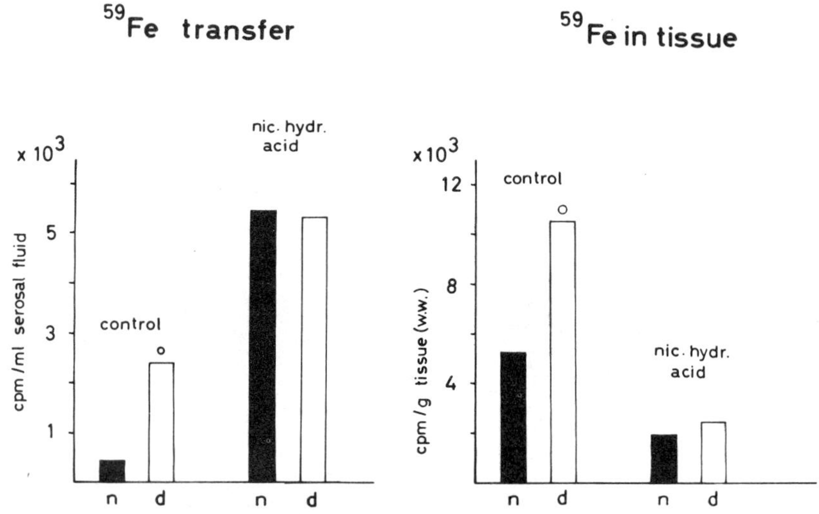

FIG. 15. Transfer and tissue content of ^{59}Fe–iron in the presence of nicotinehydroxamic acid in everted jejunal sacs of normal and iron-deficient rats. Experimental conditions: fasted rats (16 hr), Wistar (female), 160–190 g body weight. Normal rats (*n*): 14.5 g hemoglobin per 100 ml blood (SEM $= \pm 1.4$; $n = 35$). Iron-deficient rats (*d*) 6.3 g hemoglobin per 100 ml blood (SEM $= \pm 0.9$; $n = 35$). Method according to Wilson and Wiseman (1954). Jejunal segments: 6 cm beginning with the flexura duodenojejunalis. Mucosal fluid: 13 ml Tyrode solution; serosal fluid: 0.7 ml Tyrode solution at the beginning of the experiments; at the end of the experiments 0.9 (SEM $= \pm 0.008$; $n = 40$). Concentration of ^{59}Fe–($FeSO_4$): 7×10^{-6} M/1. Nicotinehydroxamic acid : Fe = 1000 : 1. Time: 2 hr; temp. 37°C. In order to remove absorbed ^{59}Fe the segments were washed three times in 100 ml sodium chloride solution (0.9%) containing EDTA 10^{-2} M/1. The columns represent means of twelve (controls) and eight (nicotinehydroxamic acid) experiments. o $= p < 0.01$ as compared with the segments of normal rats. (Forth and Rummel, unpublished data.)

thus, by-passes the transport system in the jejunal mucosa (Fig. 14 and Fig. 15).

Metal complexes like other drugs may be divided into two groups according to their physics–chemical properties which determine their absorption from the intestine:

(1) Water-soluble, polar, often negatively charged metal complexes; and

(2) Lipid-soluble, apolar, electroneutral metal complexes.

Group (1) includes the iron complexes of polybasic hydroxy-acids (Forth *et al.*, 1965a, b, c, 1968c; Rummel, 1965; Rummel *et al.*, 1967; Hopping and Ruliffson, 1963), the metal complexes of the diamino-poly-acids (Fe: Groen *et al.*, 1947; Forth and Seifen, 1961; Cleton *et al.*, 1963; Forth *et al.*, 1965a, b, c, 1968c; Rummel *et al.*, 1967; Rummel, 1965; Fe, Co, Mn and Zn; Suso and Edwards, 1968; Mn and Zn: Vohra and Gonzales, 1969; Zn: Nielson *et al.*, 1966) and the iron complexes of deferoxamine and other hydroxamic acids (Wöhler, 1964; Wöhler and Körnig, 1964; Balcerzak *et al.*, 1966; Callender, 1964; Forth *et al.*, 1965b, c; Rummel *et al.*, 1967). In general these metal complexes are poorly absorbed and the absorbed fraction is often eliminated by the kidney, at least in part. Complexing agents of group (1) are often given orally in cases of metal poisoning in order to prevent absorption (Catsch, 1964, 1968).

The metal complexes of group (2) include *ferrocene* and the metal complexes of 8-*hydroxyquinoline*. Metal complexes with quinoline derivatives readily diffuse through biological membranes. This property is a prerequisite for the antibacterial efficacy of such compounds (Albert, 1965). The absorption enhancing effect of quinolines is not limited to iron (Tables 30, 31 and 32). Thus, *bismuth–quinoline* complex preparations were used for treating angina, mainly in France.

Non-chelate metal–organic compounds are generally well absorbed because of their high lipid-solubility. Thus, tetraethyl-lead easily penetrates through biological membranes and even through intact skin. Another important example is mercury which probably is converted to *methyl* or *dimethyl-mercury* by microorganisms (for ref. see Löfroth, 1972; Experts report on methyl mercury in fish, 1971). Methyl-mercury compounds are absorbed completely from food in animals (Berglund and Berlin, 1969; Miettinen, 1969; Clarkson, 1971) and in humans (Aberg *et al.*, 1969; Miettinen, 1969) because methyl-mercury compounds increased in experimental animals by trapping these compounds intraluminally with thiol-containing resins (Clarkson *et al.*, 1971, 1973;

Clarkson and Shapiro, 1971).

The physicochemical properties determining the absorbability of a metal complex appears to be governed mainly by the ligands. Thus, the absorption of complexes of many different metals including iron, cobalt, copper and zinc with EDTA and 8-hydroxyquinoline proceeds in a similar manner *in vivo*. The nature of the metal seems to be of secondary importance for the absorbability of the complex. The differences in absorption of 8-hydroxyquinoline complexes in normal and in anemic animals (see p. 626) and differences with respect to the absorbed amount of the various quinoline–metal complexes (Table 31), however, show that the metal may also have influence.

More investigations in this field are required to determine to what extent the findings obtained here with particular ligands and a few biologically important heavy metals are representative for other heavy metal complexes. There are also important differences between different species. Thus, EDTA-bound zinc is utilized better than zinc offered as a simple inorganic salt following oral administration to chickens (Kratzer and Starcher, 1963; Koike *et al.*, 1964; Nielsen *et al.*, 1966; Hill, 1970) in contrast to rats (see Table 32). An enhanced solubility of the zinc due to complex formation probably results from peculiarities of the animal species, e.g. the acidity of the gastric juice in which the EDTA–zinc complex dissociates or a possibly exceptional avidity of the zinc-bind-sites in the chicken mucosa.

Metal chelates may be used for therapeutic substitution only if they allow the metabolic utilization of biologically important heavy metals. The ligands should only enhance the availability of biometals in the gastrointestinal tract. Very stable metal complexes are therefore usually unsuitable for substitution. Exceptions are *heme*, the iron of which is liberated in the intestinal mucosa (see p. 632), and *cyanocobalamine* (vitamin B_{12}), which is taken up into the mucosal cells of the ileum by a specific transport system (Castle, 1968; cf. Chapter 7, p. 404).

12.4. REGULATIVE FUNCTIONS OF THE INTESTINE

In deficiency states the absorption of biologically important metals such as iron (for references see Forth and Rummel, 1973), copper (for references see Van Campen, 1971; Kirchgessner *et al.*, 1973) and zinc (for references see Becker and Hoekstra, 1971; Kirchgessner *et al.*, 1973) is increased. The deficiency can be the result of a deficient *supply* of the biometals in the food or, as has been thoroughly investigated for iron, an *increased demand* due to *growth* or *sexual* functions such as menstruation or pregnancy (Smith and Schulz, 1958; Moore, 1958; Moore and Brown, 1967). The increased requirement of the young organism for copper and zinc is also satisfied by an increased rate of absorption (for references see Van Campen, 1971; Becker and Hoekstra, 1971). Though the demand for zinc and copper probably increases during pregnancy, little is known at present about possible increase of absorption.

The adaption of absorption to requirements leads to the conclusion that the *homoiostasis* of the biometals mentioned above must be regulated by special control mechanisms.

12.4.1. ABSORPTION OF IRON

Once absorbed into the organism, iron differs from other metals by its slow rate of excretion. The homoiostasis of iron metabolism is primarily warranted by the *absorption* and not by the *elimination* which is quantitatively unimportant (McCance and Widdowson, 1939; Bothwell and Finch, 1962).

A leading role in the control of absorption of iron has been assigned to almost every factor involved in iron metabolism, but usually has not been confirmed by experimental evidence. At different times iron stores and the degree of loading of the organism with iron (Bothwell *et al.*, 1958) or the rate of erythropoiesis (Bothwell *et al.*, 1958; Weintraub *et al.*, 1965b) have all been considered to play a leading role in the regulation of iron absorption. Such a role requires the assumption of humoral mediators by which the small intestine is informed about the body's requirements. *Hypophysectomy* has been shown to reduce iron absorption (Chow *et al.*, 1963), but it is by no means clear to what extent this is the result of a direct effect upon the absorption process or of an indirect effect induced by neural or hormonal stimulation of erythropoiesis (Feldman *et al.*, 1966). The following discussion will be restricted to factors which may directly affect the absorption process, while the discussion of indirect neural and hormonal influences (Schäfer, 1959) will be neglected.

The factors influencing the intestinal absorption of iron can be divided into (1) intraluminal, (2) humoral, and (3) mucosal factors. They may regulate iron absorption intraluminally (1) or by affecting the absorptive adaptation of the mucosal cells to the requirements from the blood side (2) or may be located within the mucosal cell itself (3).

12.4.1.1. *Intraluminal factors*

The influence of pH of the gastric and of the pancreatic juice has been discussed above, and no regulating function can be ascribed to these factors (see pp. 613–617).

12.4.1.2. *Humoral factors*

Erythropoietin has been thought to "inform" the absorbing cells about the iron requirements (Krantz *et al.*, 1959; Sauer *et al.*, 1969). The delayed onset of its effect on iron absorption (Reynaferye and Ramos, 1962) indicates that erythropoietin has no *direct* influence. Erythropoietin accelerates the formation of red blood cells and thus increases the demand for iron: absorption is enhanced as a *secondary* effect. As erythropoietin is synthesized in the kidneys, it is not surprising that the absorption of iron decreases following nephrectomy (Yeh and Chow, 1965; Brittin *et al.*, 1968).

It was demonstrated by Mendel (1961) that erythropoietin has no direct effect on the absorption of iron: the injection of erythropoietin does not enhance the absorption of iron if the erythropoiesis has been previously inhibited by removal of the spleen or by ^{89}Sr.

Hypoxia. Under hypoxic conditions the absorption of iron is increased (Brittin *et al.*, 1968; Greenberg *et al.*, 1960; Hathorn, 1971; Smith *et al.*, 1957; Strohmeyer *et al.*, 1964; Vasser and Taylor, 1956). The onset of the effect on the iron absorption is delayed. It was, therefore, concluded that hypoxia primarily increases erythropoiesis (Viault, 1891; Huff *et al.*, 1951). A secondary enhancement of iron absorption results from the increasing demand. This effect resembles the well-known influence of high altitudes on the absorption of iron (for references see Weintraub *et al.*, 1965b).

Independently of this indirect effect, an immediate effect of oxygen deficiency on the absorption of iron has been discussed (Brittin *et al.*, 1968; Hathorn, 1971; Mendel, 1961; Smith *et al.*, 1957; Strohmeyer *et al.*, 1964). Brittin *et al.* (1968) studied the effect of hypoxia on iron absorption in *parabiotic* rats. The parabiotic individual which was not exposed to hypoxia shows a normal oxygen saturation in blood. Therefore, the authors draw the conclusion that the increase of iron absorption in this individual must be caused by a humoral factor. In *nephrectomized* rats hypoxia enhances iron absorption without an increased erythropoiesis; the authors think that a humoral factor other than erythropoietin is involved.

The significance of the observation that a lack of oxygen in the inspired air leads to an increase in the absorption of iron is not invalidated by the findings of Prasad and Osborne (1963). These authors either clamped off the superior mesenteric artery 15 min before the administration of iron, or applied β-mercaptoethylamine (100 mg/kg), which apparently reduces the partial pressure of oxygen in tissues (Gerschman *et al.*, 1954). Under these conditions Prasad and Osborne (1963) observed a fall of iron absorption in the intraluminally perfused rat duodenum *in situ* but it must be remembered that severe ischemic damage of the tissue results after clamping off of the superior mesenteric artery for 15 min. In the rat small intestine the amino acid transport was not restored to normal for 7 days after clamping off the blood supply (Robinson *et al.*, 1965).

Dependence on blood flow. Hypoxia may be thought to influence iron absorption by modifying intestinal *blood flow*. In the isolated rat jejunum an increase of blood flow (obtained by perfusing a red cell suspension the viscosity of which was less than that of normal blood) from 9 to 20 ml/min resulted in a remarkably small variation of the absorbed amounts of iron or of cobalt. (In order to eliminate the autoregulatory influence on the vascular system papaverin, 100 ml/1, was added to the blood suspension (Forth, 1968). Unfortunately only few systematic investigations are available on the dependence of absorption (see Winne and Remischowsky, 1971; Texter *et al.*, 1971; cf. Chapter 4, p. 268).

Transferrin. The route via the *lymph* plays a quantitatively secondary role (Everett *et al.*, 1954; Moore *et al.*, 1939; Peterson and Mann, 1952; Reitzenstein *et al.*, 1960). The absorbed iron mainly enters the blood capillaries; the same is true for copper (Sternlieb *et al.*, 1967). Soon after transferrin and its role in iron metabolism had become known, a discussion about its significance for iron absorption began. This discussion is still going on. Undoubtedly, the degree of saturation of transferrin with iron determines the extent of iron absorption at least in certain experimental situations (Charley *et al.*, 1963; Cultrera *et al.*, 1962; Beutler *et al.*, 1962; Hyde, 1957; Laurell, 1949; Sölvell, 1960).

The great affinity of transferrin for iron and the great stability of its iron complex allow a gradient for iron to be established from the mucosal cells to the adjoining extracellular tissue spaces, provided that transferrin is present in these spaces (Morgan, 1963). Transferrin influences the absorption process only *indirectly*: it may accelerate or retard the incorporation of iron from the mucosal cells into the organism depending on its degree of saturation with iron (Beutler and Buttenwieser, 1960; Beutler *et al.*, 1962; Fisher and Price, 1963; Hahn *et al.*, 1943; Höglund and Reitzenstein, 1969; Laurell, 1958; Morgan, 1963; Pollack *et al.*, 1963;

Wheby and Jones, 1963; Wheby and Umpierre, 1964; Weintraub *et al.*, 1964). The turnover of transferrin-bound iron may thus act as the determining factor in iron absorption. Unfortunately, there are more theoretical arguments than experimental evidence for this concept (Fletcher and Huehns, 1968).

Why is the absorption of iron increased in cases of "*sideroplastic*" and *hemolytic* anemia although the body's iron stores are full and the plasma iron is high (Bothwell *et al.*, 1958; Brain and Herdan, 1965; Chirasiri and Izak, 1966; Erlandson *et al.*, 1962)? In order to relate this fact to the saturation of transferrin one has to make further assumptions, e.g. to postulate a difference firstly between the availability of the iron attached to the two binding sites of transferrin and secondly between the parts of the transfer system which are thought to be responsible for the *rapid* and the *slow* phase of absorption, demonstrated by Chirasiri and Izak (1966). In summary the *free binding capacity* of transferrin may in certain situations be the limiting factor for the removal of iron from mucosal cells. Transferrin or the degree of its saturation with iron, however, is unlikely to have a direct effect on the transfer process.

Finally it must be added that the plasma iron level is evidently also subject to effects of *sexual hormones*. This is evident from investigations on women treated with contraceptives (Mardell *et al.*, 1969). This treatment leads to an increase of the total iron-binding capacity of the plasma and of the plasma iron level. It is too early to say how significant this observation is for the regulation of the iron metabolism and hence for the absorption of iron in women.

12.4.1.3. *Mucosal factors*

Hahn and his coworkers (Hahn *et al.*, 1939, 1943) were the first investigators to point out that the mucosal epithelium has a special significance in the regulation of iron absorption. These authors concluded from studies in normal and anemic dogs that the extent of absorptive utilization of a single iron dose depends on the degree of saturation of the mucosal cells with iron. Hahn used the expression "mucosal block" in order to describe the reduced absorption of a second iron dose fed after a first one which indicated that the transfer of iron across mucosal cells is saturable. This term, however, turned out to be misleading in as far as it induced a number of objections to assume that after saturation of the mucosal cells with iron absorption ceases altogether (Wöhler *et al.*, 1957; Brown *et al.*, 1958; Smith and Pannacciulli, 1958). It is well known from toxicological evidence that the organism is not protected against oral poisoning with iron (cf. Starkenstein, 1934; Hiyeda, 1939; Bothwell, 1969). Hence, it is doubtful whether the significance of the properties of the mucosal cells described by Hahn is a protective function against an *iatrogenic* or *dietary* iron overload or rather an ability to adapt the absorption to the demand of the organism for iron. Although it is tempting to do so, we shall refrain from following the fate of Hahn's hypothesis in literature (for details see Crosby, 1966).

All the observations which Hahn initially described *in vivo* for dogs (Hahn *et al.*, 1939, 1943) and later for man (Hahn *et al.*, 1951) have been confirmed more recently *in vitro* in non-blood-perfused intestinal segments:

(1) the fractional absorption of iron is greater with smaller than with larger doses (Dowdle *et al.*, 1960; Forth and Rummel, 1965, 1966a);

(2) in gut segments of iron-deficient rats after administration of iron on the mucosal side both the transfer of iron and the iron content in intestinal tissue are greater than in segments prepared from normal animals (Manis and Schachter, 1962a, b; Ruliffson and Hopping, 1963; Forth and Rummel, 1965, 1966a; Helbock and Saltman, 1967);

(3) preloading of the mucosa with iron reduces the transfer of a subsequent dose (Forth, 1963; Forth and Rummel, 1965; Manis and Schachter, 1962a, 1964).

These observations *in vitro* invalidate all speculations about the influence of factors outside the gut regulating the absorption of iron. Instead, they support the view that a system exists in the mucosa which binds iron and regulates the transfer through the mucosal cell.

A schematic representation of the processes involved in the transfer of iron across mucosal cells is given in Fig. 16. Iron can be bound by specific and unspecific binding sites which are located *on the surface* of the mucosal cell—for instance in the brush borders—as well as within the cells. For chemical reasons it is improbable that iron exists to an appreciable degree in the cellular environment as free iron. Under physiological conditions, the small amount of iron contained in normal food is taken up into the pool of rapidly exchangeable iron of the mucosal cells of the duodenum and jejunum. This pool may be identical with the "Fe(II)-pool" of Manis and Schachter (1964).

Iron from this rapidly exchangeable pool can be found by a carrier and transferred rapidly to the basal pole of the mucosal cell. There it is released to transferrin by a still unknown mechanism in which a hypothetical enzyme, iron transferase, may be involved (for references see Pinkerton, 1969). One of the carriers for iron is probably identical

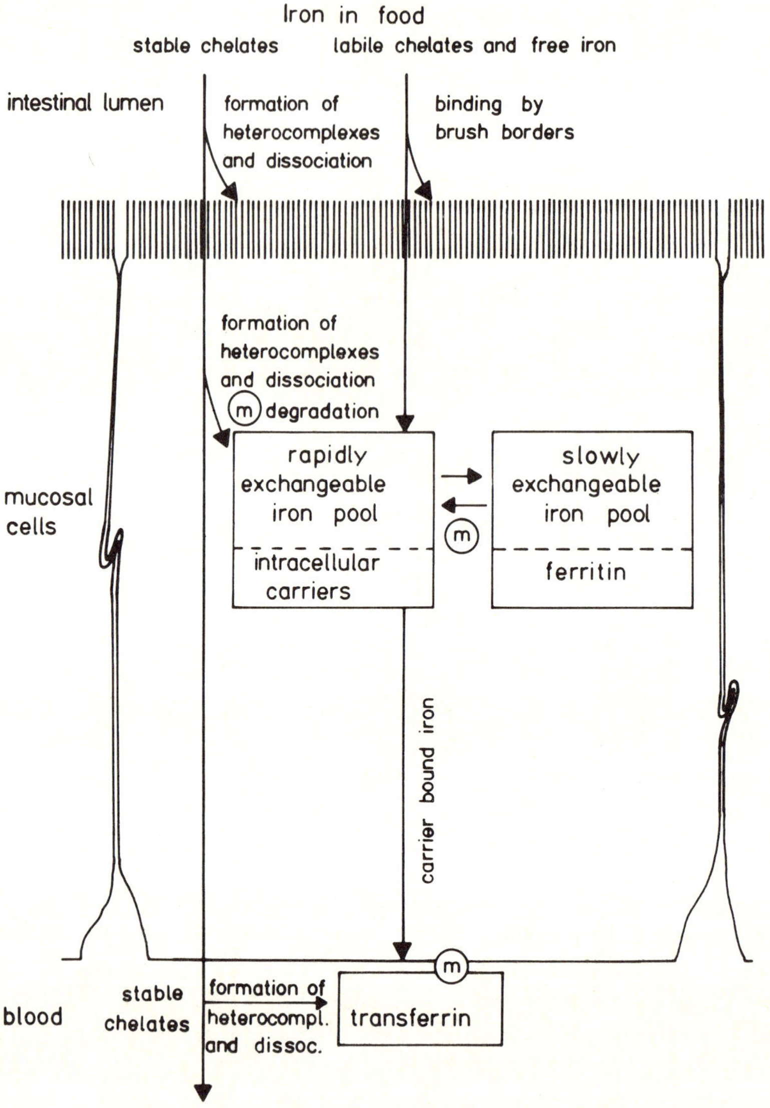

FIG. 16. Schematic representation of the processes involved in iron transfer across duodenal and/or jejunal mucosal cells. (m) = steps which probably depend on metabolism.

with the non-ferritin protein which has been isolated from the mucosal cells of rat jejunum and which is involved in the rapid phase of the transfer process of iron across the mucosal epithelium in iron-deficiency (Hübers *et al.*, 1971b, c, d). It must be remembered that during absorption 95% of the ^{59}Fe in the particle-free fraction of rat mucosal cells are protein-bound and that in iron-deficiency the major fraction of this bound iron is attached to the non-ferritin protein (Hübers *et al.*, 1971b, d).

The difference in iron absorption observed between proximally and distally located segments of the small intestine may possibly be explained by the fact that ileal segments contain less carrier protein (Hübers *et al.*, 1971b) than more proximal segments. In other words, the *duodenum* and the *upper jejunum* are important for the *rapid* phase of absorption whereas the *slow* phase of iron absorption may take place in the *entire small intestine*.

Despite the fact that during absorption only a very small fraction of non-protein-bound iron is present in the particle-free fraction of rat mucosal cells (Hübers *et al.*, 1971b), low molecular carriers for iron such as amino acids or carbonic acids must also be considered. In plants malonic acid and particularly citric acid play an important role in the transport of iron. There, the iron chelates of these compounds appear to be the transport form of iron (Brown and Tiffin, 1965; Palmer *et al.*, 1963; Tiffin, 1966a, b).

Iron which actually is not needed by the organism will be passed from the rapidly exchangeable to the slowly exchangeable pool in which it is—at least in part—*ferritin-bound.* Ferritin-bound iron can be mobilized and incorporated into the organism for the sequestration of iron from ferritin. This process depends on cellular metabolism and requires the presence of reducing agents (for references see Mazur *et al.*, 1958; Mazur and Carleton, 1965) and possibly also the aid of an oxidizing enzyme, ferrioxidase (= ceruloplasmin) prior to the uptake of iron into transferrin (Frieden, 1973). This could happen also within the mucosal cells where the presence of an oxidizing system has been claimed (Manis, 1969); there, the acceptor protein for iron might be the mucosal iron-binding protein 2. Transfer of iron by this process may occur in the slow phase of absorption. Ferritin can provide some protection against excessive iron uptake of the organism in as far as the lifespan of the iron-loaded mucosal cells may be shorter than the release of iron in the second phase of absorption. Thus ferritin-bound iron can be excreted into the intestinal lumen together with exfoliated mucosal cells (Crosby, 1963, 1966, 1968a, b; Conrad and Crosby, 1963). For these reasons it may be concluded that ferritin in the mucosal cells has no greater significance than elsewhere in the organism; ferritin is a storage form of iron which is not needed instantaneously.

In the schematic representation of Fig. 16 the following processes may depend on cellular metabolism: (1) the mobilization of iron from the slowly exchangeable pool, i.e. from ferritin; (2) the release of iron from the carrier protein to transferrin, which is assumed to be catalyzed by iron-transferase (for references see Pinkerton, 1969); (3) the metabolic degradation of stable iron-complexes and chelates.

The iron transfer system can exert a regulative function by ensuring maximal absorptive utilization of food iron according to the requirements of the organism. The efficiency of this transfer system increases with the degree of desaturation of the mucosa. Conversely the efficiency of the system decreases when the iron balance of the organism becomes positive and sufficient metal is present in the food; under these conditions the mucosal cells are loaded with iron.

When the system is overloaded with iron, other factors govern absorption. On exceeding the capacity of the system, i.e. after ingestion of toxic amounts of iron, the absorption increases in direct proportion to the dose unless the solubility of iron becomes a limiting factor. After large iron doses and in cases of poisoning, non-transferrin-bound iron may occur in the portal blood (Wheby and Jones, 1963; Wheby and Umpierre, 1964).

The mechanism of adaptation of the absorptive activity of mucosal cells is still unknown. The number of acceptor sites for iron-binding proteins in mucosal cells of rats increases up to 10 times its normal value, whereas the total protein content of the mucosal cells remains unchanged (Forth and Hübers, unpublished data). In addition, mucosal cells can absorb iron even from such stable chelates as conalbumin (Rummel, 1965) and tris-8-hydroxyquinoline-5-sulfonic acid-Fe(III) (Forth, unpublished data). It is unlikely that either chelate is taken up into the mucosal cells to an appreciable degree. This fact suggests the possibility that the stability of these iron chelates decreases by the formation of heterocomplexes with binding sited at the cellular surface and by the effects of reducing agents derived from the brush borders. This hypothesis remains to be proven experimentally.

12.4.2. ABSORPTION OF COPPER AND ZINC

Copper metabolism is influenced by a number of hormones (androgens, estrogens, ACTH, thyroxine), but it has not been demonstrated in a single case that the gut is the site of the hormonal action (for references see Van Campen, 1971; Evans, 1973). For zinc, indications for a dependence of absorption on circadian rhythms have been obtained in the rat (Heth and Hoekstra, 1965) and in man (Spencer *et al.*, 1965).

The intestine plays a double role in copper and zinc metabolism, serving for both absorption and excretion. Elimination of copper into the gut proceeds mainly via biliary excretion (Van Campen, 1971; Adelstein and Vallee, 1962). For zinc this is not the only route into the gut lumen. Following intravenous administration zinc can be detected in the mucosal cells of the intestine (Vallee, 1962). Whether the metal then enters the gut lumen along with extruded cells or whether a different mechanism secretes zinc into the gut lumen is not yet known. The leading principles for the homoiostasis of the metabolism of copper and zinc are still unknown.

CONCLUDING REMARKS

The differences between the absorption of alkali metals and heavy metals can be attributed to their different chemical properties. With regard to the low solubility of most heavy metals in biological media, their capacity to form complexes and chelates plays an important part. Complex formation with ligands derived from food or digestive secretion is important not only in the intraluminal phase, but also during transfer across the mucosal cells, where chelates may be formed with intracellular ligands.

Several important consequences result with respect to the planning and carrying out of studies on the absorption of heavy metals. Interfering reactions which may intraluminally modify the chemical form of the heavy metal must be eliminated. This requirement cannot be met by feeding heavy metals *in vivo*. Generally, the amount absorbed under these conditions is determined by the availability and not by the absorption process. This process, i.e. the transcellular movement of a heavy metal across the mucosal epithelium, can be investigated only under more or less artificial experimental conditions. With respect to complex formation between heavy metals and intracellular ligands the mucosal cells of different sections of the intestine apparently contain transfer systems for biologically important heavy metals especially for iron and probably also for zinc and copper. These systems are highly specific with regard to the uptake into cells and the transcellular movement of the metals.

As was shown for iron the existence of such transfer systems is also important for regulating absorption.

The existence of binding sites for heavy metals upon and/or within mucosal cells has been found to be important for understanding the absorption of complex-bound heavy metals and for explaining mutual interferences between heavy metals during absorption. A knowledge of these relationships is of practical importance in the physiology of nutrition and in therapeutics.

The investigation of the transfer system of iron, cobalt and zinc by various groups has led to the isolation of protein fractions of mucosal cells capable of binding these heavy metals. This certainly does not rule out a role of low molecular ligands in the transfer of heavy metals.

Confirmation of the participation of specific proteins in the transfer of heavy metals through the mucosal cells may apparently be important not only for the absorption process, but also for the protection of cell metabolism against interfering catalytic heavy metal effects. It is tempting to try to identify such metal proteins in mucosal cells.

REFERENCES

ABERG, B., EKMAN, L., FALK, R., GRETIZ, U., PERSSON, F. and SUIHS, J. O. (1969) Metabolism of methyl mercury (^{203}Hg) compounds in man. *Archs Environm. Health* **19:** 478–484.

ADELSTEIN, S. J. and VALLEE, B. L. (1962) Copper, pp. 385–386. In: *Mineral Metabolism*, II, Part B, COMAR, C. L. and BRONNER, F. (Eds.). Academic Press, New York, London.

ALBERT, A. (1965) *Selective Toxicity*. Methuen, London; Wiley, New York.

ALBERT, A. and REES, C. W. (1956) Avidity of the tetracyclines for the cations of metals. *Nature* **177:** 433–434.

ALLRED, J. B., BRATZER, F. H. and PORTER, O. W. A. (1964) Some factors affecting the *in vitro* binding of zinc by isolated soya bean protein and by α-casein. *Brit. J. Nutr.* **18:** 575–582.

ASHWORTH, A., MILNER, P. F. and WATERLOW, J. C. (1973) Absorption of iron from maize (*Zea mays* L.) and soya beans (*Glycine hispida* Max.) in Jamaican infants. *Brit. J. Nutr.* **29:** 269–278.

AWAI, M. and BROWN, D. B. (1969) Examination of the role of xanthine oxidase in iron absorption by the rat. *J. Lab. Clin. Med.* **73:** 366–378.

BALCERZAK, ST. P., JENSEN, W. N. and POLLACK, S. (1966) Mechanism of action of deferoxamine on iron absorption. *Scand. J. Haemat.* **3:** 205–212.

BALLOU, J. E. and THOMPSON, R. C. (1961) Metabolism of zinc-absorption in the rat. Considerations of permissible exposure limits. *Health Phys.* **6:** 6–18.

BANNERMAN, R. M., EDWARDS, J. A., KREIMAR-BIRNBAUM, M., MCFARLAND, E. and RUSSEL, S. S. (1972) Hereditary microcytic anemia in the mouse; studies in iron distribution and metabolism. *Brit. J. Haemat.* **23:** 235–245.

BANNERMAN, R. M. and MALPASS, J. S. (1965) Studies on desferrioxamine in relation to the absorption of iron. *Brit. J. Haemat.* **11:** 15–20.

BANNERMAN, R. M., PINKERTON, P. H. and EDWARDS, J. A. (1968) Hereditary iron-deficiency anemia due to a specific defect of intestinal absorption. *J. Clin. Invest.* **47:** 5a.

BATES, G. W., BILLUPS, C. and SALTMAN, P. (1967a) The kinetics and mechanism of iron(III) exchange between chelates and transferrin. I. The complexes of citrate and nitrilotriacetic acid. *J. Biol. Chem.* **242:** 2810–2815.

BATES, G. W., BILLUPS, C. and SALTMAN, P. (1967b) The kinetics and mechanism of iron(III) exchange between chelates and transferrin. II. The presentation and removal with ethylenediamine–tetraacetic acid. *J. Biol. Chem.* **242:** 2810–2821.

BATES, G. W., BOYER, J., HEGENAUER, J. C. and SALTMAN, P. (1972) Facilitation of iron absorption by ferric fructose. *Amer. J. Clin. Nutr.* **25:** 983–986.

BEARN, A. G. and KUNKEL, H. G. (1955) Metabolic studies in Wilson's disease using ^{64}Cu. *J. Lab. Clin. Med.* **45:** 623–631.

BECKER, W. M. and HOEKSTRA, W. G. (1966) Effect of vitamin D on ^{65}Cu absorption, distribution and turnover in rats. *J. Nutr.* **90:** 301–309.

BECKER, W. M. and HOEKSTRA, W. G. (1971) The intestinal absorption of zinc, pp. 223–256. In: *Intestinal Absorption of Metal Ions and Radionuclides,* SKORYNA, S. C. and WALDRON-EDWARDS, D. (Eds.). Pergamon Press, Oxford.

BERGHEIM, O. and KIRCH, E. R. (1949) Reduction of iron in the human stomach. *J. Biol. Chem.* **177:** 591–596.

BERGLUND, F. and BERLIN, M. (1969) Risk of methyl mercury cumulation in man and mammals and the relation between body burden of methyl mercury and toxic effects, pp. 258–273. In: *Chemical Fallout*, MILLER, M. and BERG, G. G. (Eds.). C. C. Thomas, Springfield, Ill.

BEUTLER, E. and BUTTENWIESER, E. (1960) The regulation of iron absorption, I. A search for humoral factors. *J. Lab. Clin. Med.* **55:** 274–280.

BEUTLER, E., FAIRBANKS, V. F. and FAHEY, J. L. (1963) *Clinical Disorders of Iron Metabolism,* p. 37. Grune & Stratton, New York.

BEUTLER, E., KELLY, B. M. and BEUTLER, F. (1962) The regulation of iron absorption. II. Relationship between iron dosage and iron absorption. *Am. J. Clin. Nutr.* **11:** 559–567.

BICKEL, M., GÄUMANN, E., KELLER-SCHIERLEIN, W., PRELOG, V., VISCHER, E., WETTSTEIN, A. and ZÄHNER, H. (1960) Über eisenhaltige Wachstumsfaktoren, die Sideramine, und ihre Antagonisten, die eisenhaltigen Antibiotika-Sideromycine. *Experientia* **16:** 129–133.

BIELIG, H. J. and BAYER, E. (1955) Eisenaustausch zwischen Proteinen; Modellversuche zur Eisenresorption. *Naturwissenschaften* **42:** 466.

BIGGS, D. A. E. (1967) The pancreas and iron absorption. *Am. J. Dig. Dis.* **12:** 293–302.

BILLUPS, C., PAPE, L. and SALTMAN, P. (1967) The kinetics and mechanism of iron(III) exchange between chelates and transferrin. III. Amount of iron–ethylenediamine-tetraacetic acid initially bound to protein. *J. Biol. Chem.* **242:** 4284–4286.

BINDER, H. J., FISCHER, D. S., THAYER, W. R., SPENCER, R. P. and SPIRO, H. M. (1966) Effect of iron deficiency on the gastrointestinal tract of the rat. *Gastroenterology* **51:** 364–367.

BLANC, B. (1965) Rôle des protéines impliquées dans la résorption et le métabolisme du fer, pp. 113–121. In: *Radioisotope in der Gastroenterologie*, HOFFMANN, C. and DELALOYE, B. (Eds.). Schattauer, Stuttgart.

BLANC, B. (1967) La lactotransferrine, ses relations avec les aspects physiologiques du métabolisme du fer, pp. 125–132. In: *Protides of the Biological Fluids*, PETERS, H. (Ed.). Elsevier, Amsterdam, London, New York.

BLANC, B. and ISSLIKER, H. (1965) Répartition du fer dans diverses fractions tissulaires de la muqueuse intestinal au cours de l'absorption. Mise en évidence et caracterisation partielle d'une mucoprotéin fixatrice du fer. *Helv. Phys. Acta* **23:** 145–148.

BLOCK, M. (1958) Hemosiderosis and hemochromatosis, pp. 115–130. In: *Iron in Clinical Medicine*, WALLERSTEIN, R. O. and METTIER, ST. R. (Eds.). Univ. of Calif. Press, Berkeley and Los Angeles.

BONNET, J. D., HAGEDORN, A. B. and OWEN, C. A. (1960) A quantitative method for measuring the gastrointestinal absorption of iron. *Blood* **15:** 36–44.

BOTHWELL, TH. H. (1969) Iron overload in the Bantu, pp. 362–373. In: *Iron Metabolism*, GROSS, F. (Ed.). Springer, Berlin, Göttingen, Heidelberg.

BOTHWELL, TH. H. and FINCH, C. A. (1962) Iron excretion, pp. 120–123. In: *Iron Metabolism*, Little, Brown & Co., Boston.

BOTHWELL, TH. H., PIRZIO-BIROLI, G. and FINCH, C. A. (1958) Iron-absorption. I. Factors influencing absorption. *J. Lab. Clin. Med.* **51:** 24–36.

BOWEN, H. J. M. (1966) *Trace Elements in Biochemistry*, p. 114. Academic Press, London and New York.

BRAIN, M. C. and HERDAN, H. (1965) Tissue iron stores in sideroplastic anemia. *Brit. J. Haemat.* **11:** 107–113.

BREMNER, I. (1970) The nature of trace element binding in herbage and gut contents, pp. 366–369. In: *Trace Element Metabolism in Animals*, MILLS, C. F. (Ed.). Livingstone, Edinburgh and London.

BRITTIN, G. M., HALEY, J. and BRECHER, B. (1968) Enhancement of intestinal iron absorption by a humoral factor of hypoxia in parabiotic rats. *Proc. Soc. Exp. Biol. Med.* **128:** 178–184.

BRITTIN, G. M. and RAVAL, D. (1970) Duodenal ferritin synthesis during iron absorption in the iron-deficient rat. *J. Lab. Clin. Med.* **75:** 811–817.

BROCK, J. F. and TAYLOR, E. H. L. (1934) The diffusion of soluble iron compounds *in vitro*. The effect of acids, bases and electrolytes. *Biochem. J.* **28:** 547–555.

BRODAN, V., BRODANOVA, M., KUHN, E., KORDAČ, K. and VÁLEK, J. (1967) Influence of fructose on iron absorption from the digestive system of healthy subjects. *Nutritio Dieta* **9:** 263–270.

BRODAN, V., KUHN, E., MĂSEK, J., KORDAČ, V., BRODANOVA, M. and VÁLEK, J. (1968) The influence of concomitant absorption in the digestive system. *Acta Biol. Med. Germ.* **20:** 597–605.

BROWN, E. B. (1963) The absorption of iron. *Am. J. Nutr.* **12:** 205–213.

BROWN, E. B., DUBACH, R. and MOORE, C. V. (1958) Studies on iron transportation and metabolism. XI. Critical analysis of mucosal block by large doses of inorganic iron in human subjects. *J. Lab. Clin. Med.* **52:** 335–355.

BROWN, E. B., HWANG, YUN-FEI and ALLGOOD, J. W. (1967) Studies on the site of action of deferoxamine. *J. Lab. Clin. Med.* **69:** 382–404.

BROWN, E. B., HWANG, Y.-F. and NICOL, S. (1966) Absorption of hemoglobin iron. *Clin. Res.* **14:** 312.

BROWN, E. B., HWANG, Y.-F., NICOL, S. and TERNBERG, J. (1968) Absorption of radioiron-labeled hemoglobin by dogs. *J. Lab. Clin. Med.* **72:** 58–64.

BROWN, E. B. and JUSTUS, B. W. (1958) *In vitro* absorption of radioiron by everted pouches of rat intestine. *Am. J. Physiol.* **194:** 319–326.

BROWN, E. B. and ROTHER, M. L. (1963a) Studies of the mechanism of iron absorption. I. Iron uptake by the normal rat. *J. Lab. Clin. Med.* **62:** 357–373.

BROWN, E. B. and ROTHER, M. L. (1963b) Studies of the mechanism of iron absorption. II. Influence of iron deficiency and other conditions on iron uptake by rats. *J. Lab. Clin. Med.* **62:** 804–816.

BROWN, J. C. and TIFFIN, L. O. (1965) Iron stress as related to the iron and citrate occurring in stem exudate. *Pl. Physiol.* **40:** 395–400.

BUCHHEIM, R. (1878) *Lehrbuch der Arzneimittellehre*, p. 218. L. Voss, Leipzig.

BÜTTNER, W. and MUHLER, J. C. (1959) Effect of dietary iron on phosphate metabolism. *Proc. Soc. Exp. Biol. Med.* **100:** 440–442.

BYRD, C. A. and MATRONE, G. (1965) Investigations of chemical basis of zinc–calcium–phytate interaction in biological systems. *Proc. Soc. Exp. Biol. Med.* **119:** 347–349.

CALDWELL, J. H. and GREENBERGER, N. J. (1971) Interruption of the enterohepatic circulation of digitoxin by cholestyramine. *J. Clin. Invest.* **50:** 2626–2637.

CALLENDER, S. T. (1964) In: *Iron Metabolism,* GROSS, F. (Ed.), pp. 595–596. Springer, Berlin, Göttingen, Heidelberg.

CALLENDER, S. T., MALLET, B. J. and SMITH, M. D. (1957) Absorption of hemoglobin iron. *Brit. J. Haemat.* **3:** 186–192.

CALLENDER, S. T. and MALPASS, J. S. (1963) Absorption of iron in cirrhosis of liver. *Brit. Med. J.* **2:** 1516–1518.

CALLENDER, S. T. and WARNER, G. T. (1968) Iron absorption from bread. *Am. J. Clin. Nutr.* **21:** 1170–1174.

CARLTON, W. W. and HENDERSON, W. (1965) Studies in chickens fed a copper-deficient diet supplemented with ascorbic acid, reserpine and diethylstilboestrol. *J. Nutr.* **85:** 67–72.

CARTWRIGHT, C. E., HODGES, R. E., GUBLER, C. I., MAHONEY, J. P., DAUM, K., WINTROBE, M. M. and BEAU, W. B. (1954) Studies on copper metabolism. XIII. Hepatolenticular degeneration. *J. Clin. Invest.* **33:** 1487–1501.

CASTLE, W. B. (1968) Gastric intrinsic factor and vitamin B_{12} absorption. *Handbook of Physiol.* sect. 6, vol. III. *Intestinal Absorption*, p. 1529, CODE, C. F. and HEIDEL, W. (Eds.). Am. Physiol. Soc., Washington, D.C.

CATSCH, A. (1964) *Radioactive Metal Mobilization in Medicine.* C. C. Thomas, Springfield, Ill.

CATSCH, A. (1968) *Dekorporierung radioaktiver und stabiler Metallionen.* Thiemig, München.

CHAPMAN, H. L. and BELL, M. C. (1963) Relative absorption and excretion by beef cattle of copper from various sources. *J. Anim. Sci.* **22:** 82.

CHARLEY, P. J., SARKAR, B., STITT, C. F. and SALTMAN, P. (1969) Chelation of iron by sugars. *Biochim. Biophys. Acta* **69:** 313–321.

CHARLEY, P. J., STITT, C., SHORE, E. and SALTMAN, P. (1963) Studies in the regulation of intestinal iron absorption. *J. Lab. Clin. Med.* **61:** 397–410.

CHARLTON, R. W., JACOBS, P., SEFTEL, H. and BOTHWELL, TH. H. (1969) Effect of alcohol on iron absorption. *Brit. Med. J.* **2:** 1427–1429.

CHARLTON, R. W., JACOBS, P., TORRANCE, J. D. and BOTHWELL, TH. H. (1963) The role of ferritin in iron absorption. *Lancet* 762–764.

CHARLTON, R. W., JACOBS, P., TORRANCE, J. D. and BOTHWELL, TH. H. (1965) The role of the intestinal mucosa in iron absorption. *J. Clin. Invest.* **44:** 543–554.

CHENOWETH, M. B. (1956) Chelation as a mechanism of pharmacological action. *Pharmac. Rev.* **8:** 57–87.

CHERNELCH, M., FAWWAZ, R., SARGENT, T. and WINCHELL, H. S. (1970) Effect of phlebotony and pH on iron absorption from the colon. *J. Nucl. Med.* **11:** 25–24.

CHIRASIRI, L. and IZAK, G. (1966) The effect of acute haemorrhage and acute haemolysis on the intestinal iron absorption in the rat. *Brit. J. Haemat.* **12:** 611–622.

CHODOS, R. B., ROSS, I. F., APT, L., POLLYCOVE, M. and HALKELT, R. (1957) The absorption of radioiron-labeled foods and iron salts in normal and iron-deficient subjects and idiopathic hemochromatosis. *J. Clin. Invest.* **36:** 314–326.

CHOW, B. F., YEH, S. D. J. and EBERSPAECHER, H. (1963) Pituitary gland and iron absorption. *Endocrinology* **72:** 871–875.

CLARKSON, T. W. (1971) Epidemiological and experimental aspects of lead and mercury contamination of food. *J. Food Cosmet. Toxic.* **9:** 229–243.

CLARKSON, T. W. and SHAPIRO, R. E. (1971) The absorption of mercury from food, its significance and new methods of removing mercury from the body. *Proc. Symp. Mercury in Man's Environment,* Royal Soc. of Canada, pp. 124–130.
CLARKSON, T. W., SMALL, H. and NORSETH, T. (1971) The effect of a thiol containing resin on the gastrointestinal absorption and fecal excretion of methylmercury compounds in experimental animals. *Fed. Proc.* **30:** 11, p. 543, Nr. 1947 (abstr.).
CLARKSON, TH. W., SMALL, H. and NORSETH, T. (1973) Excretion and absorption of methyl mercury after polythiol resin treatment. *Arch. Environ. Health* **26:** 173–176.
CLETON, F., TURNBULL, A., FINCH, C. A., THOMPSON, L. and MARTIN, J. (1963) Synthetic chelating agents in iron metabolism. *J. Clin. Invest.* **42:** 327–337.
COATES, M. E. and HOLDSWORTH, E. S. (1961) Vitamin D_3 and absorption of calcium in the chick. *Brit. J. Nutr.* **15:** 131–147.
COHEN, D. (1962) Specific binding of rubidium in *Chlorella. J. Gen. Physiol.* **45:** 959–987.
CONRAD, M. E., CORTELL, ST., WILLIAMS, H. L. and FOY, A. L. (1966a) Polymerization and intraluminal factors in the absorption of hemoglobin iron. *J. Lab. Clin. Med.* **68:** 659–663.
CONRAD, M. E. and CROSBY, W. H. (1963) Intestinal mucosal mechanisms controlling iron absorption. *Blood* **22:** 406–415.
CONRAD, M. E. and SCHADE, ST. G. (1968) Ascorbic acid chelates in iron absorption: a role for hydrochloric acid and bile. *Gastroenterology* **55:** 35–45.
CONRAD, M. E., WEINTRAUB, L. R., SEARS, D. A. and CROSBY, W. H. (1966b) Absorption of hemoglobin iron. *Am. J. Physiol.* **211:** 1123–1130.
COOK, I. D., BROWN, G. N. and VALBERG, L. S. (1964) The effect of achylia gastrica on iron absorption. *J. Clin. Invest.* **43:** 1185–1191.
COTZIAS, G. C. (1962) Manganese, pp. 404–442. In: *Mineral Metabolism,* vol. 2, part B, COMAR, C. L. and BRONNER, F. (Eds.). Academic Press, New York.
COTZIAS, G. C., BORG, C. C. and SELLECK, B. (1962) Specificity of zinc pathway through the body: turnover in Zn^{65} in the mouse. *Am. J. Physiol.* **202:** 359–363.
COWAN, B., JOSEPH, S. and SATIJA, V. K. (1966a) The gastric mucosa in anemia in Punjabis. *Gut* **7:** 234–243.
COWAN, J. W., ESFAHAM, M., SALJI, J. P. and AZZAM, S. A. (1966b) Effect of phytate on iron absorption in the rat. *J. Nutr.* **90:** 423–427.
CRAMPTON, R. F., MATTHEWS, D. M. and POISNER, R. (1964) The absorption of copper by sacs of hamster small intestine. *J. Physiol.* (*Lond.*) **170:** 27P.
CRAMPTON, R. F., MATTHEWS, D. M. and POISNER, R. (1965a) Further observations on copper absorption by hamster small intestine. *J. Physiol.* (*Lond.*) **179:** 66P.
CRAMPTON, R. F., MATTHEWS, D. M. and POISNER, R. (1965b) Observations on the mechanism of absorption of copper by the small intestine. *J. Physiol.* (*Lond.*) **178:** 111–126.
CRANE, R. K. (1968) Absorption of sugars, pp. 1323–1352. In: *Handbook of Physiology,* sect. 6, vol. III, *Intestinal Absorption,* CODE, CH. F. and HEIDEL, W. (Eds.). Am. Physiol. Soc., Washington, D.C.
CRESSMAN, W. A., SUGITA, E. T., DOLUISIO, I. T. and N. NIEBERGALL, P. (1966) Complexation of penicillins and penicilloic acids by cupric ions. *J. Pharm. Pharmac.* **18:** 801–808.
CRICHTON, R. R. (1971) Ferritin: structure, synthesis and function. *New Engl. J. Med.* **284:** 1413–1422.
CRICHTON, R. R. (1973) Struktur und Funktion von Ferritin. *Angew. Chemie* **85:** 53–98.
CROSBY, W. H. (1963) The control of iron balance by the intestinal mucosa. *Blood* **22:** 441–449.
CROSBY, W. H. (1966) Mucosal block: an evaluation of concepts relating to control of iron absorption. *Seminars in Hematol.* **3:** 299–313.
CROSBY, W. H. (1968a) Control of iron absorption by intestinal luminal factors. *Am. J. Clin. Nutr.* **21:** 1189–1193.

CROSBY, W. H. (1968b) Iron absorption, pp. 1553–1570. In: *Handbook of Physiol.*, sect. 6, vol. III, CODE, CH. F. and HELDEL, W. (Eds.). Am. Physiol. Soc., Washington, D.C.

CULTRERA, G., RICOTTI, V. and MAGLIULO, E. (1962) Il ruolo della transferrina nell'assorbimento intestinale di Fe^{59} del ratto normale e sidero sico. *Haematologica* **47:** 189–198.

DAVENPORT, H. W. (1961a) Gastrin, pp. 106–108. In: *Physiology of the Digestive Tract,* DAVENPORT, H. W. (Ed.). Year Book Med. Publ. Inc., Chicago.

DAVENPORT, H. W. (1961b) Control of gastric emptying, pp. 50–51. In: *Physiology of the Digestive Tract,* DAVENPORT, H. W. (Ed.). Year Book Med. Publ. Inc., Chicago.

DAVIS, A. E. and BIGGS, J. C. (1967) The pancreas and iron absorption. *Am. J. Dig. Dis.* **12:** 293–302.

DAVIS, G. K. (1966) Factors influencing zinc availability in animals, p. 215. In: *Zinc Metabolism*, PRASAD, A. S. (Ed.). C.C. Thomas, Springfield, Ill.

DAVIS, P. S. and DELLER, D. J. (1966) Prediction and demonstration of iron chelating ability of sugars. *Nature* **212:** 404–405.

DAVIS, P. S. and DELLER, D. J. (1967) Salicylates and iron absorption; competition of salicylate and gastric juice for iron. *Gastroenterology* **52:** 691–694.

DAVIS, P. S., LUKE, C. G. and DELLER, D. J. (1966) Reduction of gastric iron binding protein in haemochromatosis. A previously unrecognized metabolic defect. *Lancet* 1431–1433.

DAVIS, P. S., LUKE, C. G. and DELLER, D. J. (1967) Gastric iron-binding protein in iron chelation by gastric juice. *Nature* **214:** 1126.

DAVIS, P. N., NORRIS, L. C. and KRATZER, F. H. (1962) Interferences of soyabean proteins with the utilization of trace minerals. *J. Nutr.* **77:** 217–228.

DAWSON, R. B., RAFAL, S. and WEINTRAUB, L. (1970) Absorption of hemoglobin iron: the role of xanthine oxidase in the intestinal heme-splitting reaction. *Blood* **35:** 94–103.

DEICHMANN, W. B. and GERARDE, H. W. (1969) *Toxicology of Drugs and Chemicals,* Academic Press, New York and London.

DELALOYE, B., MAGNENAT, P. and BLANC, B. (1966) Considération sur l'absorption intestinale et sur la dynamique du fer alimentaire et inorganique chez l'homme: influence de la mucoprotéine. *Schweiz. Med. Wschr.* **96:** 1252–1256.

DEOBALD, H. J. and ELVEHEJEM, C. A. (1935) The effect of feeding high amounts of soluble iron and aluminum salts. *Am. J. Physiol.* **111:** 118–123.

DICK, A. T. (1956) Molybdenum and copper relationships in animal nutrition, p. 445. In: *In Organic Nitrogen Metabolism,* MCELROY, W. D. and GLASS, B. (Eds.). Johns Hopkins, Baltimore.

DIEZ-EWALD, M., WEINTRAUB, L. R. and CROSBY, W. H. (1968) Interrelationship of iron and manganese metabolism. *Proc. Soc. Exp. Biol. Med.* **129:** 448–451.

DIPALAMO, J. R. (Ed.) in: *Drill's Pharmacology in Medicine*, 1964, p. 879. McGraw-Hill, New York.

DONALDSON, R. M. and BARRERAS, R. F. (1965) Intestinal absorption of trace quantities of chromium. *J. Lab. Clin. Med.* **66:** 866–867.

DONALDSON, R. M. and BARRERAS, R. F. (1966) Intestinal absorption of trace quantities of chromium. *J. Lab. Clin. Med.* **68:** 484–493.

DOWDLE, E. B., SCHACHTER, D. and SCHENKER, H. (1960) Active transport of Fe^{59} by everted segments of rat duodenum. *Am. J. Physiol.* **198:** 609–613.

DOYLE, J. J., PFANDER, W. H., GREBING, S. E. and PIERCE, J. O. (1972) Effects of dietary cadmium on growth and tissue levels in sheep. In: *Trace Substances in Environmental Health*, vol. VI, HEMPHILL, D. D. (Ed.), pp. 181–186. Univ. of Missouri, Columbia, U.S.A.

DREISBACH, R. H. (1966) *Handbook of Poisoning*. Lange Medical Publications, Los Altos, Calif.

DREYFUS, I. C. and SCHAPIRA, G. (1964) The metabolism of iron in hemochromatosis, pp. 296–325. In: *Iron Metabolism*, GROSS, F. (Ed.). Springer, Berlin, Göttingen, Heidelberg.

Dupuis, Y. and Fournier, P. (1963) Lactose and the absorption of calcium and strontium, pp. 277–293. In: *The Transfer of Calcium and Strontium Across Biological Membranes,* Wasserman, R. H. (Ed.). Academic Press, New York.

Durbin, P. W., Scott, K. G. and Hamilton, J. G. (1957) *The Distribution of Radioisotopes of Some Heavy Metals in the Rat.* Univ. Calif. Publ. Pharmac. 3, No. 1, 1, Berkeley.

Duthie, H. L. (1964) The relative importance of the duodenum in the intestinal absorption of iron. *Brit. J. Haemat.* **10:** 59–68.

Dvorak, P. (1970) Hexacyanoferrate(II) als Thallium-Antidote. Herstellung und Eigenschaften. *Arzneimittel Forsch.* **20:** 1886–1888.

Dvorak, P. (1971) Bindung von Thallium(I) durch Hexacyanoferrat(II). *Z. Naturforschung* **26b:** 277–281.

Dwyer, F. P. and Mellor, D. P. (1964) *Chelating Agents and Metal Chelates.* Academic Press, New York and London.

Edwards, J. A. and Bannerman, R. M. (1970a) Hereditary defect in intestinal iron transfer in sex-linked anemia. *Fed. Proc.* **29:** 300.

Edwards, J. A. and Bannerman, R. M. (1970b) Hereditary defect of intestinal iron transport in mice with sex-linked anemia. *J. Clin. Invest.* **49:** 1869–1871.

Edwards, J. A. and Hoke, J. E. (1972) Defect of intestinal mucosal iron uptake in mice with hereditary microcytic anemia. *Proc. Soc. Exp. Biol. Med.* **141:** 81–84.

Eichholtz, F. (1934a) Kupfer, pp. 1958–1959. In: *Handbuch der exp. Pharmakologie,* vol. 3, 2, Heffter, A. and Heubner, W. (Eds.). Springer, Berlin.

Eichholtz, F. (1934b) Zink, p. 1918. In: *Handbuch der exp. Pharmakologie,* vol. 3, 3, Heffter, A. and Heubner, W. (Eds.). Springer, Berlin.

Elwood, P. C., Jacobs, A., Pitman, R. C. and Entwistle, C. C. (1964) Epidemiology of the Paterson–Kelly syndrome. *Lancet* **2:** 716–720.

Elwood, P. C., Newton, D., Eakins, J. D. and Brown, D. A. (1968) Absorption of iron from bread. *Am. J. Clin. Nutr.* **21:** 1162–1169.

Enwonwu, C. O., Monsen, E. R. and Jacobson, K. (1972) Absorption of iron in protein-calorie deficient rats and immediate effects of re-feeding an adequate protein diet. *Amer. J. Dig. Dis.* **17:** 959–968.

Erlandson, M. E., Walden, B., Stern, G., Hilgartner, M. W., Wehman, J. and Smith, C. H. (1962) Studies on congenital hemolytic syndromes. IV. Gastrointestinal absorption of iron. *Blood* **19:** 359–378.

Evans, G. W. (1973) Copper homeostasis in the mammalian system. *Physiol. Rev.* **53:** 535–570.

Everett, N. B., Garrett, W. E. and Simmons, B. S. (1954) Lymphatics in iron absorption and transport. *Am. J. Physiol.* **178:** 45–48.

Ewe, K. (1968) Die Beeinflussung der Eisen-Aufnahme im Dünndarm durch Komplexbildung mit 8-Hydroxychinolin und dessen Sulfonat. Perfusionsuntersuchungen am menschlichen Jejunum. *Klin. Wschr.* **46:** 296–300.

Experts Report on Methyl Mercury in Fish (1971) *Nordisk Hygienisk Tidskrift*, Suppl. 4: Stockholm.

Feaster, J. P., Hansard, S. L., McCall, J. T., Skipper, F. H. and Xavis, G. K. (1954) Absorption and tissue distribution of radiozinc in steers fed high-zinc rations. *J. Anim. Sci.* **13:** 781–788.

Feldman, S., Rachmilewitz, E. A. and Izak, G. (1966) The effect of central nervous system stimulation on erythropoiesis in rats with chronically implanted electrodes. *J. Lab. Clin. Med.* **67:** 713.

Ferguson, W. S., Lewis, A. H. and Watson, S. J. (1938) Action of molybdenum in nutrition of milking cattle. *Nature* **141:** 553.

Fisher, D. S. and Price, D. C. (1963) A possible humoral regulator of iron absorption. *Proc. Soc. Exp. Biol. Med.* **112:** 228–229.

FISHER, R. B. and PARSONS, D. S. (1949) A preparation of surviving rat small intestine for the study of absorption. *J. Physiol.* (*Lond.*) **110:** 36–46.

FISHER, R. B. and PARSONS, D. S. (1950) The gradient of mucosal surface area in the small intestine of the rat. *J. Anat.* **84:** 272–282.

FLETCHER, J. and HUEHNS, E. R. (1968) Function of transferrin. *Nature* **218:** 1211–1214.

FLURY, F. (1934) Blei, p. 1958. In: *Handbuch der exp. Pharmakologie*. vol. 3, 3, HEFFTER, A. and HEUBNER, W. (Eds.). Springer, Berlin.

FOREMAN, H. (1966) The pharmacology of some useful chelating agents, pp. 82–94. In: *Metal-Binding in Medicine,* SEVEN, M. and JOHNSON, L. A. (Eds.). Lippincott, Philadelphia, Montreal.

FOREMAN, H. and TRUJILLO, TH. (1954) The metabolism of C^{14} labeled ethylenediamine-tetraacetic-acid in human beings. *J. Lab. Clin. Med.* **43:** 566–571.

FORRESTER, R. H., CONRAD, M. E. and CROSBY, W. H. (1962) Measurement of total body $iron^{59}$ in animals using whole-body-liquid scintillation detectors. *Proc. Soc. Exp. Biol. Med.* **111:** 115–119.

FORST, A. W. (1935) Wismut, p. 2388. In: *Handbuch der exp. Pharmakologie,* vol. 3, 4, HEFFTER, A. and HEUBNER, W. (Eds.). Springer, Berlin.

FORTH, W. (1963) In: *Radioisotope in der Hämatologie*, pp. 61–63, KEIDERLING, W. and HOFFMANN, G. (Eds.). Schattauer, Stuttgart.

FORTH, W. (1966) Untersuchungen über die Resorption von Eisen und chemisch verwandten Schwermetallen an Därmen normaler und anämischer Ratten *in vivo* und *in vitro*; ein Beitrag zur Frage der Spezifität des eisenbindenden Systems in der Mucosa. *Habil. Schrift,* Homburg/Saar.

FORTH, W. (1968) Eisen- und Kobalt-Resorption am perfundierten Dünndarmsegment, pp. 242–250. In: *Stoffwechsel der isoliert perfundierten Leber,* STAIB, W. and SCHOLZ, R. (Eds.). Springer, Berlin, Heidelberg, New York.

FORTH, W. (1970) Absorption of iron and chemically related metals *in vitro* and *in vivo*; the specificity of an iron binding system in the intestinal mucosa of the rat, pp. 298–310. In: *Trace Element Metabolism in Animals,* MILLS, C. F. (Ed.). Livingstone, Edinburgh and London.

FORTH, W. (1971) Resorption von Eisen und chemisch verwandten Metallen *in vitro* und *in vivo*; die Spezifität des eisenbindenden Systems in der Mucosa des Jejunums von Ratten, pp. 83–103. In: *Frontiers of Nuclear Medicine,* HORST, W. (Ed.). Springer: Berlin, Heidelberg, New York.

FORTH, W. and ANDRES, H. (1969) Methode zur Erzeugung eines Eisenmangels bei Ratten. *Arzlneimittel-Forsch.* **19:** 363–364.

FORTH, W., FURUKAWA, E. and RUMMEL, W. (1969) Intestinale Resorption von Herzglycosiden *in vitro* und *in vivo. Naunyn-Schmiedebergs Arch. exp. Path. Pharmak.* **262:** 53–72.

FORTH, W., HUBERS, H., HUBERS, E. and RUMMEL, W. (1972) Does a transfer system for iron exist in the mucosal cells of the small intestine?, pp. 121–130. In: *Trace Substances in Environmental Health*, vol. VI, HEMPHILL, D. D. (Ed.). Univ. of Missouri, Columbia, Mo.

FORTH, W., LEOPOLD, C. and RUMMEL, W. (1968a) Eisendurchtritt von der Mucosa zur Serosaseite und umgekehrt an isolierten Eisenarmen und normalen Segmenten von Jejunum und Ileum. *Naunyn-Schmiedebergs Arch. exp. Path. Pharmak.* **261:** 434–440.

FORTH, W., LICHTENBERG, H. and RUMMEL, W. (1965a) Zur Beurteilung der Fe-Resorption unter verschiedenen methodischen Bedingungen. *Naunyn-Schmiedebergs Arch. exp. Path. Pharmak.* **250:** 234–235.

FORTH, W., NELL, G. and RUMMEL, W. (1973) Chelating agents and the transfer of heavy metals across the mucosal epithelium. In: *Trace Substances in Environmental Health,* VII; D.D. HEMPHILL (Ed.). Univ. of Missouri, Columbia, Mo.

FORTH, W., PFLEGER, K., ROHNS, G. and RUMMEL, W. (1964) Der Einfluss von Komplexbildern auf die Verteilung intravenös verabreichten Eisens im Organismus. *Proc. der gem. Tagung der deutschen Gesellschaft für Biophysik, der osterr. Gesellschaft für reine und angewandte Biophysik und der Schweizer Gesellschaft für Strahlenbiologie,* pp. 319–326, Vienna.

FORTH, W., PFLEGER, K. and RUMMEL, W. (1963) Zur Wirkung von Komplexbildnern auf die Fe-Resorption der Ratte. *Naunyn-Schmiedebergs Arch. exp. Path. Pharmak.* **245:** 89.

FORTH, W., PFLEGER, K., RUMMEL, W., SEIFEN, E. and RICHMOND, SP. J. (1965b) Der Einfluβ verschiedener Liganden auf Resorption, Verteilung und Ausscheidung von Eisen nach oraler Verabfolgung. *Naunyn-Schmiedebergs Arch. exp. Path. Pharmak.* **252:** 242–257.

FORTH, W. and RUMMEL, W. (1965) Eisen-Resorption an isolierten Dünndarmpräparaten von normalen und anämischen Ratten. *Naunyn-Schmiedebergs Arch. exp. Path. Pharmak.* **252:** 205–223.

FORTH, W. and RUMMEL, W. (1966a) Beziehungen zwischen Eisen-Konzentration und Resorption am isolierten Dünndarm normaler und anämischer Ratten. *Med. Pharmac. Exp.* **14:** 289–296.

FORTH, W. and RUMMEL, W. (1966b) Abhängigkeit der Eisenresorption von der Eisenbindung durch den Darm. *Med. Pharmac. Exp.* **14:** 384–390.

FORTH, W. and RUMMEL, W. (1968) Zur Frage der Regulation der Eisenresorption durch Gastroferrin, ein eisenbindendes Protein des Magensaftes. *Klin. Wschr.* **46:** 1003–1005.

FORTH, W. and RUMMEL, W. (1969) Beziehungen zwischen dem Durchtritt des Eisens durch die Darmwand und seiner Bindung im Gewebe. *Naunyn-Schmiedebergs Arch. exp. Path. Pharmak.* **264:** 230–232.

FORTH, W. and RUMMEL, W. (1971) Absorption of iron and chemically related metals *in vitro* and *in vivo*; the specificity of an iron binding system in the intestinal mucosa of the rat, pp. 173–192. In: *Intestinal Absorption of Metal Ions and Radionuclides,* SKORYNA, S. C. and WALDRON-EDWARD, D. (Eds.). Pergamon Press, Oxford.

FORTH, W. and RUMMEL, W. (1973) Iron absorption. *Physiol. Rev.* **53:** 724–792.

FORTH, W., RUMMEL, W. and BECKER, P. J. (1966) Die vergleichende Prüfung von Bindung und Durchtritt von Eisen, Kobalt und Kupfer durch isolierte Jejunumsegmente normaler und anämischer Ratten. *Med. Pharmac. Exp.* **15:** 179–186.

FORTH, W., RUMMEL, W., CRÜSEMANN, D. and PFLEGER, K. (1967) Die Bedeutung der Bindung in der Zellmembran für die Fe-Aufnahme der Reticulozyten. *Naunyn-Schmiedebergs Arch. exp. Path. Pharmak.* **257:** 275–276.

FORTH, W., RUMMEL, W., CRÜSEMANN, D. and SIMON, J. (1968b) Die Bindung von Eisen und verwandten Schwermetallen in der Membran und ihre Aufnahme in Reticulozyten, pp. 444–446. In: *Metabolism and Membrane Permeability of Erythrocytes and Thrombocytes,* DEUTSCH, E., GERLACH, E. and MOSER, K. (Eds.). G. Thieme, Stuttgart.

FORTH, W., RUMMEL, W. and PFLEGER, K. (1968c) Der Einfluβ von Liganden auf die Retention von Eisen nach oraler Verabfolgung an normale und anämische Ratten. *Naunyn-Schmiedebergs Arch. exp. Path. Pharmak.* **261:** 225–238.

FORTH, W., RUMMEL, W. and SEIFEN, E. (1965c) Der Einfluβ verschiedener Liganden auf Eisendurchtritt und -bindung an isolierten Darmpräparaten normaler und anämischer Ratten. *Naunyn-Schmiedebergs Arch. exp. Path. Pharmak.* **252:** 224–231.

FORTH, W. and SEIFEN, E. (1961) Der Einfluβ von Komplexbildern auf die Fe^{59}-Resorption am isolierten Darm der Ratte. *Naunyn-Schmiedebergs Arch. Exp. Path. Pharmak.* **241:** 55.

FRIEDEN, E. (1973) The ferrous to ferric cycles in iron metabolism. *Nutr. Rev.* **31:** 41–44.

FURCHNER, J. E. and RICHMOND, C. R. (1962) Effect of dietary zinc on the absorption of orally administered Zn^{65}. *Health Phys.* **8:** 35–40.

GALLO, D. G., BAILEY, K. R. and SHEFFNER, A. L. (1965) The interaction between cholestyramine and drugs. *Proc. Soc. Exp. Biol. Med.* **120:** 60–65.

GARVAN, F. L. (1964) Metal chelates of ethylenediaminetetra-acetic acid and related substances, pp. 283–333. In: *Chelating Agents and Metal Chelates*, DWYER, F. P. and MELLOR, D. P. (Eds.). Academic Press, New York and London.

GEHRING, P. I. and HAMMOND, P. B. (1964) The uptake of thallium by rabbit erythrocytes. *J. Pharmac. Exp. Therap.* **145:** 215–221.

GEHRING, P. I. and HAMMOND, P. B. (1967) The interrelationship between thallium and potassium in animals. *J. Pharmac. Exp. Therap.* **155:** 187–201.

GEORGI, J. R. (1964) Absorption of hemoglobin iron-59 in sheep. *J. Vet. Anim. Husb. Res., Mhow* **25:** 952–954.

GERSCHMAN, R., NYE, S. W., GILBERT, D. L., DWYER, P. and FENN, W. O. (1954) Studies on oxygen poisoning: protective effect of β-mercaptoethylamine. *Proc. Soc. Exp. Biol. Med.* **85:** 75–77.

GITLIN, D. and CRUCHAUD, A. (1962) On the kinetics of iron absorption in mice. *J. Clin. Invest.* **41:** 344–350.

GITLIN, D., HUGHES, W. L. and JANEWAY, CH. A. (1960) Absorption and excretion of copper in mice. *Nature* **188:** 150–151.

GOLDBERG, A., LOCKHEAD, A. C. and DAGG, J. H. (1963) Histamine fast achlorhydria and iron absorption. *Lancet* **2:** 848–850.

GOLDBERG, L. and MARTIN, L. E. (1964) The absorption, distribution and utilization of iron in fat-soluble form. *Life Sci.* **3:** 1465–1474.

GORTEN, M. K., HEPNER, R. and WORKMAN, J. B. (1963) Iron metabolism in premature infants. I. Absorption and utilization of iron as measured by isotope studies. *J. Pediat.* **63:** 1063–1071.

GOUCHER, CH. R. and TAYLOR, J. F. (1964) Compounds of ferric iron in the adenosine triphosphate and other nucleoside phosphates. *J. Biochem.* **239:** 2251–2255.

GRANICK, S. (1946) Ferritin IX. *J. Biol. Chem.* **164:** 737–746.

GRANICK, S. (1949) Iron metabolism and hemochromatesis. *Bull. N.Y. Acad. Med.* **25:** 403–428.

GRANICK, S. (1951) Structure and physiological functions of ferritin. *Physiol. Rev.* **31:** 489–511.

GRASSMANN, E. and KIRCHGESSNER, M. (1969) Kupfer-absorption aus Komplexen mit verschiedenen organischen Säuren. *Z. Tierphysiol.* **25:** 125–128.

GREENBERG, D. M., COPP., D. H. and CUTHBERTSON, E. M. (1943) Studies in mineral metabolism with the aid of artificial radioactive isotopes. VII. The distribution and excretion, particularly by way of the bile of iron, cobalt and manganese. *J. Biol. Chem.* **147:** 749–756.

GREENBERG, M. S., WONG, H., MILLER, ST. A., SCARLATTA, R. W. and CHALMERS, TH. C. (1960) Iron absorption and turnover in hypoxia. *J. Clin. Invest.* **39:** 992.

GREENBERGER, N. J. (1973) Effects of antibiotics and other agents on the intestinal transport of iron. *Amer. J. Clin. Nutr.* **26:** 104–112.

GREENBERGER, N. J., BALCERZAK, ST. P. and ACKERMAN, G. A. (1969) Iron uptake by isolated intestinal brush borders: changes induced by alterations in iron stores. *J. Lab. Clin. Med.* **73:** 711–721.

GREENBERGER, N. J. and RUPPERT, R. D. (1966a) Inhibition of protein synthesis: a mechanism for the production of impaired iron absorption. *Science* **153:** 315–316.

GREENBERGER, N. J. and RUPPERT, R. B. (1966b) Tetracycline-induced inhibition of iron absorption. *Clin. Res.* **14:** 432.

GREENBERGER, N. J., RUPPERT, R. D. and CUPPAGE, F. E. (1967) Inhibition of intestinal iron transport induced by tetracycline. *Gastroenterology* **53:** 590–599.

GREENGARD, O., SENTENAC, A. and MENDELSOHN, N. (1964) Phosvitin, the iron carrier of egg yolk. *Biochim. Biophys. Acta* **90:** 406–407.

GROEN, J., VAN DEN BROCK, W. A. and VELDMAN, H. (1947) Absorption of iron compounds from the small intestine in the rat. *Biochim. Biophys. Acta* **1:** 315.

GROSS, P. (1973) Oberflächenbestimmung am Dünndarm von Ratten. Doctoral Thesis, Med. Faculty, Homburg/Saar, W. Germany.

GUGGENHEIM, K. (1964) The role of zinc, copper and calcium in the etiology of the "meat anemia". *Blood* **23:** 786–794.

GUGGENHEIM, K., ILAN, J., FOSTICK, M. and TAL, E. (1963) Prevention of meat anemia in mice by copper and calcium. *J. Nutr.* **79:** 245–250.

GUNN, S. A., GOULD, T. C. and ANDERSON, W. A. D. (1962) Interference with fecal excretion of Zn^{65} by cadmium. *Proc. Soc. Exp. Biol. Med.* **111:** 559–562.

HAGHSHENASS, M., MAHLOUDJI, M., REINHOLD, J. G. and MOHAMMADI, N. (1972) Iron-deficiency anemia in an Iranian population associated with high intakes of iron. *Amer. J. Clin. Nutr.* **25:** 1143–1146.

HAHN, P. F., BALE, W. F., LAWRENCE, E. O. and WHIPPLE, G. H. (1939) Radioactive iron and its metabolism in anemia. *J. Exp. Med.* **69:** 739–753.

HAHN, P. F., BALE, W. F., ROSS, J. F., BALFOUR, W. M. and WHIPPLE, G. H. (1943) Radioactive iron absorption by gastrointestinal tract. *J. Exp. Med.* **78:** 169–188.

HAHN, P. F., CAROTHERS, E. L., DARBY, W. J., MARTIN, M., SHEPPARD, C. W., CANNON, R. O., BEAM, A. S., DENSEN, P. M., PETTERSON, J. C. and MCCLELLAN, G. S. (1951) Iron metabolism in human pregnancy as studied with the radioactive isotope Fe^{59}. *Am. J. Obst. Gyn.* **61:** 477–486.

HAHN, P. F., JONES, E., LOWE, R. C., MENEELY, G. R. and PEACOCK, W. (1945) The relative absorption and utilization of ferrous and ferric iron in anemia as determined with the radioactive isotope. *Am. J. Physiol.* **143:** 191–197.

HALLBERG, L. (1963) Die Eisenresorption, pp. 47–59. In: *Radioisotope in der Hämatologie,* KEIDERLING, W. and HOFFMANN, G. (Eds.). Schattauer, Stuttgart.

HALLBERG, L. and SÖLVELL, L. (1960) Iron absorption during constant intragastric infusion of iron in man. *Acta Med. Scand.* **168:** Suppl. **358:** 43–69.

HALLBERG, L. and SÖLVELL, L. (1964) Absorption of hemoglobin iron in man. *Proc. 10th Congr. Int. Soc. Haematol. Stockholm* F: 5.

HALLIDAY, J. W. and POWELL, L. W. (1973) The use of suspensions of the isolated rat mucosal cells to study mechanisms of iron absorption. *Clin. Chim. Acta* **43:** 267–276.

HARTMAN, R. H., MATRONE, C. and WISE, C. H. (1955) Effect of high dietary manganese on hemoglobin formation. *J. Nutr.* **55:** 429–439.

HATHORN, M. K. S. (1971) The influence of hypoxia on iron absorption in the rat. *Gastroenterology* **60:** 76–81.

HEDENBERG, L. (1969) Studies on iron metabolism with desferrioxamine in man. *Scand. J. Haemat.* Suppl. **6:** 5–86.

HEGSTED, M., FINCH, C. A. and KINNEY, TH. D. (1949) The influence of diet on iron absorption. II. The interrelation of iron and phosphorus. *J. Exp. Med.* **90:** 147–156.

HELBOCK, H. I. and SALTMAN, P. (1967) The transport of iron by rat intestine. *Biochim. Biophys. Acta* **135:** 979–990.

HEMMATI, A. (1968) Die Bestimmung des Resorptionsortes von Eisen in Intestinalkanal mit einer ferngesteurten Darmkapsel. *Dt. Med. Wschr.* **93:** 1468–1472.

HENDRYCH, F. and WEDEN, H. (1934) Kobalt und Nickel, p. 1447. In: *Handbuch der exp. Pharmakologie,* vol. 3, 2; HEFFTER, A. and HEUBNER, W. (Eds.). Springer, Berlin.

HENSCHLER, D. and KIRSCHNER, U. (1969) Zur Resorption und Toxicität von Selensulfid. *Arch. Toxibiol.* **24:** 341–344.

HERNDON, J. F., RICE, E. G., TUCKER, R. G., VAN LOON, E. J. and GREENBERG, S. (1958) Iron absorption and metabolism. III. The enhancement of iron absorption in rats by *d*-sorbitol. *J. Nutr.* **64:** 615–623.

HESSE, E. (1934) Thallium, indium, gallium, p. 2182. In: *Handbuch der exp. Pharmakologie,* vol. 3, 3, HEFFTER, A. and HEUBNER, W. (Eds.). Springer, Berlin.

HETH, D. A., BECKER, W. M. and HOEKSTRA, W. G. (1966) Effect of calcium, phosphorus and zinc on zinc-65 absorption and turnover in rats fed semipurified diets. *J. Nutr.* **88:** 331–337.

HETH, D. A. and HOEKSTRA, W. G. (1965) Zinc-^{65} absorption and turnover in rats. I. A procedure to determine zinc-^{65} absorption and the antagonistic effect of calcium in a practical diet. *J. Nutr.* **85:** 367–374.

HEUBNER, W. (1912) Über Eisenwirkung bei Chlorose. *Therap. Monatshefte,* p. 44. Cit. acc. to TÜRK, H., *Ein Beitrag zur Geschichte der Eisentherapie bei Anämien.* Doctoral Thesis, Med. Fac., Marburg (1944).

HEUBNER, W. (1934) Silber, p. 2104. In: *Handbuch der exp. Pharmakologie,* vol. 3, 3, HEFFTER, A. and HEUBNER, W. (Eds.). Springer, Berlin.

HILL, C. H. (1970) The effect of EDTA on the absorption of zinc from intestinal segments of the chick. *Fed. Proc.* **29:** 298.

HILL, C. H., MATRONE, G., PAGNE, W. L. and BARBER, C. W. (1963) *In vivo* interactions of cadmium with copper, zinc and iron. *J. Nutr.* **80:** 227–235.

HILL, C. H. and STARCHER, B. (1965) Effect of reducing agents on copper deficiency in chicks. *J. Nutr.* **85:** 271–274.

HILL, C. H., STARCHER, B. and MATRONE, G. (1964) Mercury and silver interrelationships with copper. *J. Nutr.* **83:** 107–110.

HIYEDA, K. (1939) The cause of Kashin–Beck's disease. *Jap. J. Med. Sci.* **4:** 91–106.

HOEFER, J. A., MÜLLER, E. R., ULREY, P. E., RITCHIE, H. P. and LUECKE, R. W. (1960) Interrelationships between calcium, zinc, iron and copper in swine feeding. *J. Anim. Sci.* **19:** 249–259.

HOEKSTRA, W. G. (1964) Recent observations on mineral interrelationships. *Fed. Proc.* **23:** 1068–1076.

HOEKSTRA, W. G. (1970) The complexity of dietary factors affecting zinc nutrition and metabolism in chicks and swine, pp. 347–353. In: *Trace Element Metabolism in Animals,* MILLS, C. F. (Ed.). Livingstone, Edinburgh and London.

HÖGLUND, S. and REITZENSTEIN, P. (1969a) Studies in iron absorption. IV. Effect of humoral factors on iron absorption. *Blood* **34:** 488–495.

HÖGLUND, S. and REITZENSTEIN, P. (1969b) Studies in iron absorption. V. Effect of gastrointestinal factors on iron absorption. *Blood* **34:** 496–504.

HOLDSWORTH, E. S. (1965) Vitamin D_3 and calcium absorption in the chick. *Biochem. J.* **96:** 475–483.

HOLDSWORTH, E. S. and WEBLING, D. D. A. (1971) The effect of bile, bile salts and detergents on the absorption of calcium and other cations, pp. 339–358. In: *Intestinal Absorption of Metal Ions and Radionuclides,* SKORYNA, S. C. and WALDRON-EDWARDS, D. (Eds.). Pergamon Press, Oxford.

HOPKINS, L. L. and NOBLE, M. A. (1969) Effect of iron deficiency on orally administered Fe(III) upon the gastrointestinal uptake of ^{51}Cr(III) in rats. *Fed. Proc.* **28:** 299.

HOPPING, J. M. and RULIFFSON, W. S. (1963) Effects of chelating agents on radioiron absorption and distribution in rats *in vivo*. *Am. J. Physiol.* **205:** 885–889.

HOPPING, J. M. and RULIFFSON, W. S. (1966) Roles of citric and asorbic acid in enteric iron absorption in rats. *Am. J. Physiol.* **210:** 1316–1320.

HÜBERS, H., HÜBERS, E., FORTH, W., LEOPOLD, G. and RUMMEL, W. (1971a) Binding of iron and other metals in brush borders of jejunum and ileum of the rat *in vitro*. *Acta Pharm. Toxic.* **29:** Suppl. 4, 22.

HÜBERS, H., HÜBERS, E., FORTH, W. and RUMMEL, W. (1971b) Binding of iron to a nonferritin protein in the mucosal cells of normal and iron-deficient rats during absorption. *Life Sci.* **10:** Part I, 1141–1148.

HÜBERS, H., HÜBERS, E., FORTH, W. and RUMMEL, W. (1972) Iron absorption and cellular transfer protein in the intestinal mucosa of mice with hereditary anemia. *Naunyn-Schmiedebergs Arch. exp. Path. Pharmak.* **274:** R 56.

HÜBERS, H., HÜBERS, E., SIMON, J. and FORTH, W. (1971c) A method for preparing stable density gradients and their application for fractionation of intestinal mucosal cells. *Life Sci.* **10:** Part I, 377–384.

HÜBERS, H., HÜBERS, E., SIMON, J., FORTH, W. and RUMMEL, W. (1971d) The subcellular distribution of ^{59}Fe in mucosal cells of normal and iron-deficient rats during absorption. *Naunyn-Schmiedebergs Arch. exp. Path. Pharmak.* R 65.

HUFF, R. L., LAWRENCE, J. H. and SIN, W. F. (1951) Effect of changes in altitude on hematopoietic activity. *Medicine (Balt.)* **30:** 197–217.

HUNT, C. E. and CARLTON, W. W. (1965) Cardiovascular lesions associated with experimental copper deficiency in the rabbit. *J. Nutr.* **87:** 385–393.

HUSSAIN, R., WALKER, R. B., LAGNISSE, M., CLARK, P. and FINCH, C. A. (1965) Nutritive value of food iron. *Am. J. Clin. Nutr.* **16:** 464–471.

HWANG, Y.-F. and BROWN, E. (1963) Studies of the effect of desferrioxamine on human iron absorption and excretion. *J. Lab. Clin. Med.* **62:** 885.

HWANG, Y.-F. and BROWN, E. B. (1965) Effect of desferrioxamine on iron absorption. *Lancet* **1:** 135–137.

HYDE, A. (1957) Absorption of radioiron perfused through the duodenum of the rat. *Am. J. Physiol.* **191:** 265–270.

IIDA, H., MOORE, E. W., BREITMAN, S. A. and ZAMCHECK, N. (1968) Effect of pH on active transport of D-glucose in the small intestine of hamsters. *Proc. Soc. Exp. Biol. Med.* **127:** 730–732.

JACOBI, H., PFLEGER, K. and RUMMEL, W. (1956a) Einfluβ von Phosphaten auf die enterale Reserption physiologischer Eisenmengen. *Naturwissenschaften* **43:** 354–355.

JACOBI, H., PFLEGER, K. and RUMMEL, W. (1956b) Komplexbildner und aktiver Transport durch die Darmwand. *Naunyn-Schmiedebergs Arch. exp. Path. Pharmak.* **229:** 198–206.

JACOBS, A. (1969) Tissue changes in iron deficiency. *Brit. J. Haemat.* **16:** 1–4.

JACOBS, A., KAYE, M. D. and TREVETT, D. (1969) The chelation of iron during intestinal absorption. *J. Lab. Clin. Med.* **74:** 212–217.

JACOBS, A. and MILES, P. M. (1970) The formation of iron complexes with bile and bile constituents. *Gut* **11:** 732–734.

JACOBS, A. and OWEN, G. M. (1969) Effect of gastric juice on iron absorption in patients with gastric atrophy. *Gut* **10:** 488–490.

JACOBS, A., RHODES, J. and EAKINS, J. P. (1967) Gastric factors influencing iron absorption in anemic patients. *Scand. J. Haemat.* **4:** 105–110.

JACOBS, A., RHODES, J., PETERS, D. K., CAMPBELL, H. and EAKINS, J. D. (1966) Gastric acidity and iron absorption. *Brit. J. Haemat.* **12:** 728–736.

JACOBS, P., BOTHWELL, TH. H. and CHARLTON, R. W. (1964) Role of hydrochloric acid in iron absorption. *J. Appl. Physiol.* **19:** 187–188.

JACOBS, P., CHARLTON, R. W. and BOTHWELL, TH. H. (1968) The influence of gastric factors on the absorption of iron salts. *S. Afr. Med. Sci.* **33:** 53–57.

JANDL, J. H. and KATZ, I. H. (1963) The plasma-to-cell cycle of transferrin. *J. Clin. Invest.* **42:** 314–326.

JOSEPHS, H. W. (1958) Absorption of iron as a problem in human physiology. A critical review. *J. Haematol.* **13:** 1–54.

KAHN, I. (1966) The pancreas and iron absorption. *Gastroenterology* **51:** 736.

KAKEMI, K., ARITA, T., HORI, R., RONISHI, R. and NISHIMURA, K. (1969) Absorption and excretion of drugs. XXXIII. The correlation between the absorption of barbituric acid derivatives from the rat small intestine and their binding to the mucosa. *Chem. Pharm. Bull. Tokyo* **17:** 248–254.

KATO, K. and JOB, V. (1940) Influence of cobalt on iron transportation and storage: a chemical and histologic study. *Am. J. Clin. Pathol.* **10:** 751–761.

KATZ, J. H. and JANDL, J. H. (1964) The role of transferrin in the transport of iron into the developing red cell, pp. 103–117. In: *Iron Metabolism*, GROSS, F. (Ed.). Springer, Berlin, Göttingen, Heidelberg.

KAUFMAN, R. M., POLLACK, S. and CROSBY, W. H. (1966) Iron-deficient diet: effects in rats and human. *Blood* **28:** 726–737.

KAVIN, H., CHARLTON, R. W., JACOBS, P., GREEN, R., TORRANCE, I. D. and BOTHWELL, TH. H. (1967) Effect of the exocrine pancreatic secretions on iron absorption. *Gut* **8:** 556–564.

KEBERLE, H. (1964) The biochemistry of desferrioxamine and its relation to iron metabolism. *Ann. N.Y. Acad. Sci.* **119:** 758–768.

KIMBER, C. and WEINTRAUB, L. R. (1968) Malabsorption of iron secondary to iron deficiency. *New Engl. J. Med.* **279:** 453–459.

KIRCH, E. R., BERGHEIM, O., KLEINBERG, J. and JAMES, S. (1947) Reduction of iron by foods in artificial gastric digestion. *J. Biol. Chem.* **171:** 687–694.

KIRCHGESSNER, M. (1961) Der Einfluβ einer Antibiotikum-Zulage auf die Retention verschiedener Spurenelemente bei wachsenden Schweinen. *Festschrift zum VIII. Intern. Tierzuchtkongress, Hamburg,* pp. 95–97. E. Ulmer, Stuttgart.

KIRCHGESSNER, M. (1965) Availability of some trace elements. *Proc. Nutr. Soc.* **24:** 89–99.

KIRCHGESSNER, M. (1972) *Trace Elements in Nutritional Physiology*, II. Tierernährungskongress Madrid 1972. Vol. IV, pp. 297–317.

KIRCHGESSNER, M. and GRASSMANN, E. (1970a) Copper absorption from Cu(II) amino-acid complexes. 5. Dynamics of copper absorption. *Z. Tierphysiol.* **26:** 3–7.

KIRCHGESSNER, M. and GRASSMANN, E. (1970b) The dynamics of copper absorption, pp. 277–285. In: *Trace Element Metabolism in Animals,* MILLS, C. F. (Ed.). Livingstone, Edinburgh and London.

KIRCHGESSNER, M., HAMPEL, G. and D. A. ROTH-MAIER (1970) Zum Einfluss unterschiedlicher Proetinversorgung und einer $CuSO_4$ Zulage auf die Kupferverwertung bei Mastküken. *Z. Tierphysiol.* **26:** 279–285.

KIRCHGESSNER, M., SCHWARZ, F. J. and GRASSMANN, E. (1973) Intestinal absorption of copper and zinc after dietary depletion. *Bioinorganic Chem.* **2:** 255–262.

KIRCHGESSNER, M. and WESER, U. (1963) Spurenelemente im Stoffwechsel wachsender Schweine bei unterschiedlichen Kupferzulagen. *Z. Tierphysiol.* **18:** 181–186.

KIRCHGESSNER, M. and WESER, U. (1965a) Komplex-Stabilität und Kupfer-Absorption. 4. Mitteilung. *Z. Tierphysiol.* **20:** 44–49.

KIRCHGESSNER, M. and WESER, U. (1965b) Zur Absorption einiger Spurenelemente bei Chlortetracyclinzulagen. *Z. Tierphysiol.* **20:** 317–320.

KIRCHGESSNER, M., WESER, U. and FRIESECKE, H. (1963) Cu und Mo im Stoffwechsel wachsender Schweine. *Z. Tierphysiol.* **18:** 239–242.

KIRCHGESSNER, M., WESER, U. and MÜLLER, H. L. (1967) Absorption einiger mono-oligo-und polymerer Aminosäure-Cu-Komplexe. *Z. Tierphysiol.* **22:** 76–81.

KLAVINS, I. V., KINNEY, T. D. and KAUFMAN, N. (1962) The influence of dietary protein on iron absorption. *Brit. J. Exp. Path.* **43:** 172–180.

KNIFFEN, J. C., NOYES, W. D. and PORTER, F. S. (1970) Iron and cholestyramine in erythropoietic protoporphyria. *Clin. Res.* **18:** 38.

KOEPKE, J. A. and STEWART, W. B. (1964) The role of gastric secretion in iron absorption. *Proc. Soc. Exp. Biol. Med.* **115:** 927–929.

KOIKE, TH. D., KRATZER, F. H. and VOHRA, P. (1964) Intestinal absorption of zinc or calcium–ethylenediaminetetraacetic acid complexes in chicken. *Proc. Soc. Exp. Biol. Med.* **117:** 485–486.

KRANTZ, S., GOLDWASSER, E. and JACOBSON. L. O. (1959) Studies on erythopoiesis, XIV. The relationship of humoral stimulation to iron absorption. *Blood* **14:** 654–661.

KRATZER, F. H. and STARCHER, B. (1963) Quantitative relation of EDTA availability of zinc for turkey poults. *Proc. Soc. Exp. Biol. Med.* **113:** 424–426.

KROE, D., KAUFMAN, N., KINNEY, T. D. and KLAVINS, J. V. (1963a) The effect of histidine on iron absorption. *Fed. Proc.* **23:** 512.

KROE, D., KAUFMAN, N., KINNEY, TH. D. and KLAVINS, J. V. (1964) The influence of histidine on iron and cobalt absorption. *Fed. Proc.* **23:** 511.

KROE, D., KAUFMAN, N., KLAVINS, J. V. and KINNEY, TH. D. (1966) Interrelation of amino acids and pH on intestinal iron absorption. *Am. J. Physiol.* **211:** 414–418.

KROE, D., KINNEY, TH. D., KAUFMAN, N. and KLAVINS, J. V. (1963b) The influence of amino acids on iron absorption. *Blood* **21:** 546–552.

KUNA, S. (1964) The pH of gastric juice in the normal resting stomach. *Arch. Int. Pharmacodyn.* **152:** 79–97.

LANGECKER, H. (1934) Mangan, pp. 1329–1338. In: *Handbuch der exp. Pharmakologie,* Vol. 3, 2. HEFFTER, A. and HEUBNER, W. (Eds.). Springer, Berlin.

LAURELL, C. B. (1949) Studies on the transportation and metabolism of iron in the body with special reference to the iron binding component in human plasma. *Acta Physiol. Scand.,* Suppl. **46:** 1–129.

LAURELL, C. B. (1952) Plasma iron and the transport of iron in the organism. *Pharmac. Rev.* **4:** 371–395.

LAURELL, C. B. (1958) Iron transportation, p. 8. In: *Iron in Clinical Medicine,* WALLERSTEIN, R. O. and METTIER, S. R. (Eds.). Univ. Press, Berkeley, Los Angeles.

LAUTERBACH, F. (1969) Intestinal absorption and metabolism of cardiac glycosides. *Naunyn-Schmiedebergs Arch. exp. Path. Pharmak.* **263:** 26–39.

LAYRISSE, M., MARTINEZ-TORRES, C. and ROCHE, M. (1968) Effect of interaction of various foods on iron absorption. *Am. J. Clin. Nutr.* **21:** 1175–1183.

LAYRISSE, M., MARTINEZ-TORRES, C. and ROCHE, M. (1969) Food iron absorption: a comparison of vegetable and animal foods. *Blood* **33:** 430–443.

LEE, J. C. and RICHTER, W. (1971) Ferritin from different organs of man, rat, rabbit and pig. *Comp. Biochem. Physiol.* **39B:** 325–333.

LEE, R. C., NACHT, S., LUKENS, J. N. and CARTWRIGHT, G. E. (1968) Iron metabolism in copper-deficient mice. *J. Clin. Invest.* **47:** 2058–2069.

LEMBERG, R., LEGGE, J. W. and LOCKWOOD, W. H. (1939) Coupled oxidation of ascorbic acid and haemoglobin. I. *Biochem. J.* **33:** 754–758.

LEMBERG, R., LEGGE, J. W. and LOCKWOOD, W. H. (1941a) Coupled oxidation of ascorbic acid and haemoglobin. II. Formation and properties of choleglobin. *Biochem. J.* **35:** 328–338.

LEMBERG, R., LEGGE, J. W. and LOCKWOOD, W. H. (1941b) Coupled oxidation of ascorbic acid and haemoglobin. III. Quantitative studies of choleglobin formation. Estimation of haemoglobin and ascorbic acid oxidations. *Biochem. J.* **35:** 339–352.

LENGEMANN, F. W. (1963) Overall aspects of calcium and strontium absorption, pp. 85–96. In: *The Transfer of Calcium and Strontium across Biological Membranes,* WASSERMAN, R. H. (Ed.). Academic Press, New York.

LEOPOLD, G., FURUKAWA, E., FORTH, W. and RUMMEL, W. (1968) Vergleichende Untersuchung der Resorption von Schwermetallen *in vivo* und *in vitro*. *Naunyn-Schmiedebergs Arch. exp. Path. Pharmak.* **263:** 275–276.

LEVINE, P. H., LEVINE, A. J. and WEINTRAUB, L. H. (1972) The role of transferrin in the control of iron absorption: studies on a cellular level. *J. Lab. Clin. Med.* **80:** 333–341.

LEVINE, P. H. and WEINTRAUB, L. R. (1969) Transferrin and the control of iron absorption; studies on a cellular level. *Blood* **34:** 854.

LEWIS, K. O. (1973) The nature of copper complexes in bile and their relationship to the absorption and excretion of copper in normal subjects and in Wilson's disease. *Gut* **14:** 221–232.

LEWIS, P. K., HOEKSTRA, W. C. and GRUMMER, R. H. (1957) Restricted calcium feeding versus zinc supplementation for the control of parakeratosis in swine. *J. Anim. Sci.* **16:** 578.

LINSCHEER, W., MOORE, E. and GREENBERG, M. (1963) Iron absorption in the proximal small intestine in cirrhosis. *Clin. Res.* **11:** 186.

LÖFROTH, G. (1972) The mercury problem; a review at midway, pp. 63–70. In: *Trace Substances in Environmental Health,* vol. VI, HEMPHILL, D. D. (Ed.). Univ. of Missouri, Columbia, Mo.

LOSOWSKY, M. S. and WILSON, A. R. (1967) Whole-body counting of the absorption and distribution of iron in haemochromatosis. *Clin. Sci.* **32:** 151–160.

LUKE, C. G., DAVIS, P. S. and DELLER, P. J. (1967) Changes in gastric iron-binding protein (gastroferrin) during iron-deficiency anemia. *Lancet* **2:** 926–927.

LUND, A. (1956) Distribution of thallium in the organism and its elimination. *Acta Pharmac. Toxic.* **12:** 251–259.

MADDAIAH, V. T., KURUICK, A. A. and REID, B. L. (1964) Phytic acid studies. *Proc. Soc. Exp. Biol. Med.* **115:** 391–393.

MAILLIARD, J. A. (1966) Iron deficiency following gastric resection. *Am. J. Gastroenterology* **45:** 109–113.

MANIS, J. (1969) Ferrous iron oxidation by intestinal mucosal homogenates and its possible relation to iron absorption. *J. Clin. Invest.* **48:** 55 A.

MANIS, J. (1970) Active transport of iron by intestine selective genetic defect in mouse. *Nature* **227:** 385–386.

MANIS, J. (1971) Intestinal iron transport defect in the mouse with sex linked anemia. *Am. J. Physiol.* **220:** 135–139.

MANIS J. G. and SCHACHTER, D. (1962a) Active transport of iron by intestine: features of the two-step mechanism. *Am. J. Physiol.* **203:** 73–80.

MANIS, J. G. and SCHACHTER, D. (1962b) Active transport of iron by intestine: effects of oral iron and pregnancy. *Am. J. Physiol.* **203:** 81–86.

MANIS, J. G. and SCHACHTER, D. (1964) Active transport of iron by intestine: mucosal iron pools. *Am. J. Physiol.* **207:** 893–900.

MANIS, J. and SCHACHTER, D. (1965) Fe^{59}-amino acid complexes: are they intermediates in Fe^{59} absorption across intestinal mucosa? *Proc. Soc. Exp. Biol. Med.* **119:** 1185–1187.

MARDELL, M., SIMMONS, C. and ZILVA, J. E. (1969) A comparison of the effect of oral contraceptives, pregnancy and sex on iron metabolism. *J. Clin. Endoc. Metab.* **29:** 1489.

MARSTON, H. R. and ALLEN, S. H. (1967) Function of copper in the metabolism of iron. *Nature* **215:** 645–646.

MARTELL, A. E. and CALVIN, M. (1952) *Chemistry of the Metal Chelate Compounds.* Prentice-Hall, New York.

MARTELL, A. E. and CALVIN, M. (1958) *Die Chemie der Metallechelatverbindungen.* Chemie, Weinheim/Bergstr.

MARTIN, H., NOWICKI, L. and SCHÜTZ, E. (1967) Zur Frage der Resorptionsverhinderung von Nahrungseisen durch orale Desferrioxamin-Gaben. *Dt. med. Wschr.* **92:** 892–894.

MARTINEZ-TORRES, C. and LAYRISSE, M. (1970) Effect of amino acids on iron absorption from a staple vegetable food. *Blood* **35:** 669–682.

MASSON, P. L. and HEREMANS, J. F. (1967) Studies on lactoferrin, the iron-binding protein of secretions, pp. 115–124. In: *Protides of the Biological Fluids*, PETERS, H. (Ed.). Elsevier Publ. Co., Amsterdam, London, New York.

MATRONE, G. (1970) Studies on copper–molybdenum–sulfate interrelationships, pp. 354–361. In: *Trace Element Metabolism in Animals*, MILLS, C. F. (Ed.). Livingstone, Edinburgh and London.

MATRONE, G., HARTMAN, R. H. and CLAWSON, A. J. (1959) Studies of a manganese–iron antagonism in the nutrition of rabbits and piglets. *J. Nutr.* **67:** 309–317.

MAZUR, A., BAEZ, S. and SHORR, E. (1955) The mechanism of iron release from ferritin as related to its biological properties. *J. Biol. Chem.* **213:** 147–160.

MAZUR, A. and CARLETON, S. (1965) Hepatic xanthine oxidase and ferritin iron in the developing rat. *Blood* **26:** 317–322.

MAZUR, A., GREEN, S., SAHA, A. and CARLETON, A. (1958) Mechanism of release of ferritin iron *in vivo* by xanthine oxidase. *J. Clin. Invest.* **37:** 1809–1817.

McCance, R. A., Edgecombe, C. N. and Widdowson, E. M. (1943) Phytic acid and iron absorption. *Lancet* **1**: 126–128.

McCance, R. A. and Widdowson, E. M. (1939) Absorption and excretion of iron. *Lancet* **1**: 680–684.

McDonald, R. A. and Pechet, C. S. (1964) Absorption by rats of iron in wine. *Proc. Soc. Exp. Biol. Med.* **117**: 54–56.

McGowan, J. P. (1930) The absorption and excretion of iron by the intestine and the nutritional and therapeutic value of its salts. *Edin. Med. J.* **37**: 85–96.

McPhersons, A. and Hemingway, R. C. (1965) Effects of protein intake on the storage of copper in the liver of sheep. *J. Sci. Food Agric.* **16**: 220–227.

Mendel, G. A. (1961) Studies on iron absorption. I. The relationship between the rate of erythropoiesis, hypoxia and iron absorption. *Blood* **18**: 727–736.

Mendel, G. A., Weiler, R. J. and Mangalik, A. (1963) Studies on iron absorption. II. The absorption of iron in experimental anemias of diverse etiology. *Blood* **22**: 450–458.

Merkulova, I. S., Soroka, V. R. and Rudenko, N. Z. (1968) Absorption of ionized and complex bound copper in the stomach and small intestine. *Bull. Exp. Biol. Med. U.S.S.R.* **66**: 56–58.

Methfessel, A. H. and Spencer, H. (1966) Intestinal site of absorption and secretion of Ca^{47} and Zn^{65} in adult rats. *Fed. Proc.* **25**: 483.

Methfessel, A. H. and Spencer, H. (1973a) Zinc metabolism in the rat. I. Intestinal absorption of zinc. *J. Appl. Physiol.* **34**: 58–62.

Methfessel, A. H. and Spencer, H. (1973b) Zinc metabolism in the rat. II. Secretion of zinc into the intestine. *J. Appl. Physiol.* **34**: 63–67.

Michaelides, G. I. and Philis, H. Chr. (1959) Pathogenesis and treatment of the anaemia associated with hiatus hernia. *Lancet* 552.

Miettinen, J. K. (1969) Methylmercury as a food chain problem in Scandinavia, p. 96. In: *Chem. and Toxic Aspects of Environm. Qual. Intern. Symp. Munich.*

Milev, N., Sattler, E. L. and Menden, E. (1970) Aufnahme und Einlagerung von Blei im Körper unter verschiedenen Ernährungsbedingungen. *Medizin. Ernähr.* **11**: 29–32.

Miller, I. K. and Cragle, R. C. (1965) Gastrointestinal sites of absorption and endogenous secretion of zinc in dairy cattle. *J. Dairy Sci.* **48**: 370–373.

Miller, I. K. and Jensen, L. S. (1966) Effect of dietary protein source on zinc absorption and excretion along the alimentary tracts of chicks. *Poult. Sci.* **45**: 1051–1053.

Miller, W. I., Martin, Y. C., Gentry, R. P. and Blackmon, D. M. (1968) ^{65}Zn and stable zinc absorption, excretion and tissue concentrations as effected by type of diet and level of zinc in normal calves. *J. Nutr.* **94**: 391–401.

Mills, C. F. (1954) Copper complexes in grassland herbage. *Biochem. J.* **57**: 603–610.

Mills, C. F. (1956) The dietary availability of copper in the form of naturally occurring organic complexes. *Biochem. J.* **63**: 190–193.

Mills, C. F. (1958) Comparative metabolic studies of inorganic and herbage-complex forms of copper in rats and sheep. *Soil Sci.* **85**: 100–105.

Mills, C. F. (1961) *Studies on Copper Metabolism (1952–1960)*. Rowett Research Inst. Collected Papers **17**: 57.

Moeschlin, S. (1972) *Klinik und Therapie der Vergiftungen*. G. Thieme, Stuttgart.

Moeschlin, S. and Schnider, U. (1964) Treatment of primary and secondary haemochromatosis and acute iron poisoning with a new, potent iron-eliminating agent (desferrioxamine B), pp. 525–550. In: *Iron Metabolism*, Gross, F. (Ed.). Springer, Berlin, Göttingen, Heidelberg.

Moore, C. V. (1958) Etiology of iron-deficiency anemia, pp. 133–143. In: *Iron in Clinical Medicine*, Wallerstein, R. O. and Mettier, St. R. (Eds.). Univ. of Calif. Press, Berkeley and Los Angeles.

MOORE, C. V. (1964) Iron nutrition, pp. 241–255. In: *Iron Metabolism*, GROSS, F. (Ed.). Springer, Berlin, Göttingen, Heidelberg.

MOORE, C. V., ARROWSMITH, W. M. R., WELCH, J. and MINNICH, V. (1939) Studies in iron transportation and metabolism. IV. Observations on the absorption of iron from the gastrointestinal tract. *J. Clin. Invest.* **18:** 553–580.

MOORE, C. V. and BROWN, E. B. (1967) Der Eisenstoffwechsel. *Documenta Geigy, Acta Clin.* No. 7.

MOORE, C. V. and DUBACH, R. (1951) Observations on the absorption of iron from foods tagged with radioiron. *Trans. Ass. Am. Physns* **64:** 245–256.

MOORE, C. V., DUBACH, R., MINNICH, V. and ROBERTS, H. K. (1944) Absorption of ferrous and ferric radioactive iron by human subjects and by dogs. *J. Clin. Invest.* **23:** 755–767.

MOORE, E. W., LINSCHEER, W. G. and KEENE, W. R. (1964) Iron absorption kinetic studies in the normal dog. *J. Clin. Invest.* **43:** 1282.

MOORE, T., CONSTABLE, B. I., DAY, K. C., IMPEY, S. C. and SYMONDS, K. R. (1964) Copper deficiency in rats fed upon raw meat. *Brit. J. Nutr.* **18:** 135–146.

MORGAN, E. H. (1963) Exchange of iron and transferrin across endothelial surfaces in the rat and rabbit. *J. Physiol.* **169:** 339–352.

MORGAN, O. S., WEIR, D. G., GATENBY, P. B. B. and SCOTT, I. M. (1969) Studies on an iron binding component in human gastric juice. *Lancet* 861–863.

MULLINS, L. J. and MOORE, R. D. (1960) The movement of calcium ions in muscle. *J. Gen. Physiol.* **43:** 759–773.

MURRAY, M. J. and STEIN, N. (1966) Does the pancreas influence iron absorption? A critical review of information to date. *Gastroenterology* **51:** 694–700.

MURRAY, M. J. and STEIN, N. (1968) The effects on iron absorption of gastrointestinal secretions from patients with iron-deficiency anaemia and haemochromatosis. *Brit. J. Haemat.* **15:** 87–91.

NASSET, E. S. (1968) Emptying of the stomach, p. 424. In: *Medical Physiology*, vol. I, MOUNCASTLE, V. B. (Ed.). Mosby, Saint Louis.

NEUBERG, C. and MANDL, I. (1949) Functions of ATP and other phosphoric acid derivatives. *Archs Biochem.* **23:** 499–501.

NEUMANN, P. Z. and SASS-KORTSAK, A. (1967) The state of copper in human serum: evidence for an amino acid-bound fraction. *J. Clin. Invest.* **46:** 646–658.

NIEBERGALL, P. I., HUSSAR, D. A., CRESSMAN, W. A., SUGITA, E. T. and DOLUISIO, I. T. (1966) Metal binding tendencies of various antibiotics. *J. Pharm. Pharmac.* **18:** 729–738.

NIELSEN, F. H., SUNDE, M. L. and HOEKSTRA, W. C. (1966) Effect of some dietary synthetic and natural chelating agents on the zinc-deficiency syndrome in the chick. *J. Nutr.* **89:** 35–42.

NIELSEN, F. H., SUNDE, M. L. and HOEKSTRA, W. C. (1967) Effect of histamine, histidine and some related compounds on the zinc-deficient chick. *Proc. Soc. Exp. Biol. Med.* **124:** 1106–1110.

NIGROVIC, V. (1965) Retention of radiocaesium by the rat as influenced by Prussian Blue and other compounds. *Physics. Med. Biol.* **10:** 81–89.

NIGROVIC, V. and CATSCH, A. (1965) Tierexperimentelle Untersuchungen zur Behandlung der akuten Eisenvergiftung. *Naunyn-Schmiedebergs Arch. exp. Path. Pharmak.* **251:** 225–232.

NIGROVIC, V., SPRENG, P. and BOHNE, F. (1967) Untersuchungen zur Frage der enteralen Eisenresorption, pp. 147–150. In: *Radioisotope in der Gastroenterologie*, HOFFMANN and DELALOYE (Eds.). Schattauer, Stuttgart.

OBERLEAS, D., MUHRER, M. E. and O'DELL, B. L. (1966a) The availability of zinc from foodstuffs, p. 225. In: *Zinc Metabolism*, PRASAD, A. S. (Ed.). C. C. Thomas, Springfield, Ill.

OBERLEAS, D., MUHRER, M. E. and O'DELL, B. L. (1966b) Dietary metal-complexing agents and zinc availability in the rat. *J. Nutr.* **90:** 56–62.

O'DELL, N. L. and SAVAGE, I. E. (1960) Effect of phytic acid on zinc availability. *Proc. Soc. Exp. Biol. Med.* **103:** 304–306.

O'REILLY, S. and BANK, W. (1966) New oral chelating agents for treatment of Wilson's disease. *Nature* **212:** 1597–1598.

OWEN, CH. A. (1964) Absorption and excretion of Cu^{64}-labeled copper by the rat. *Am. J. Physiol.* **207:** 1203–1206.

PALEY, K. R. and SUSSMAN, E. S. (1963) Absorption of radioactive cobalt chloride in human subjects. *Metabolism* **12:** 975–982.

PALMER, M. J., DE KOCK, P. C. and BACON, J. S. (1963) Changes in the concentrations of malic acid, citric acid, calcium and potassium in the leaves during growth of normal and iron-deficient mustard plants (*Sinapis alba*). *Biochem. J.* **86:** 484–494.

PEARSON, W. N. and REICH, M. (1965) *In vitro* studies of Fe^{59} absorption by everted intestinal sacs of rat. *J. Nutr.* **87:** 117–124.

PEARSON, W. N. and REICH, M. B. (1969) Studies of ferritin and a new iron binding protein found in the intestinal mucosa of the rat. *J. Nutr.* **99:** 137–140.

PEARSON, W. N., SCHWINK, T. and REICH, M. B. (1966) *In vitro* studies of zinc absorption in the rat, p. 239. In: *Zinc Metabolism*, PRASAD, A. S. (Ed.). C. C. Thomas, Springfield, Ill.

PENSACK, J. M., HENSEN, I. N. and BOGDANOFF, P. O. (1958) The effect of calcium and phosphorus on the zinc requirement of growing chicks. *Poult. Sci.* **36:** 1232–1233.

PETERSON, R. E. and MANN, J. D. (1952) Transport of radioactive iron in intestinal lymph. *Am. J. Physiol.* **169:** 763–766.

PHILLIPS, C. S. G. and WILLIAMS, R. J. P. (1965) *Inorganic Chemistry,* vols. I and II. Clarendon Press, Oxford.

PINKERTON, P. H. (1968) Histological evidence of disordered iron transport in the sex-linked hypochromic anemia of mice. *J. Path. Bact.* **95:** 155–165.

PINKERTON, P. H. (1969) Control of iron absorption by the intestinal epithelial cell. Review and hypothesis. *Am. Int. Med.* **70:** 401–408.

PINKERTON, P. H. and BANNERMAN, R. M. (1967) Hereditary defect in iron absorption in mice. *Nature* **216:** 482–483.

PINKERTON, P. H., BANNERMAN, R. M., DOEBLIN, T. D., BENISCH, B. M. and EDWARDS, J. A. (1970) Iron metabolism and absorption studies in sex-linked anemia of mice. *Brit. J. Haemat.* **18:** 211–228.

POLLACK, S. (1968) Iron absorption, p. 1553. In: *Handbook of Physiology,* sect. 6, vol. III, CODE, CH. F. and HEIDEL, W. (Eds.). Published by CROSBY, W. H. (1968), Am. Physiol. Soc., Washington, D.C.

POLLACK, S., BALCERZAK, ST. P. and CROSBY, W. H. (1963) Transferrin and the absorption of iron. *Blood* **21:** 33–38.

POLLACK, S., CAMPANA, TH. and ARCARION, A. (1972) A search for a mucosal iron carrier. Identification of mucosal fractions with rapid turnover of Fe^{59}. *J. Lab. Clin. Med.* **80:** 322–332.

POLLACK, S., GEORGE, J. N., REBA, R. C., KAUFMAN, R. and CROSBY, W. H. (1965) The absorption of nonferrous metals in iron deficiency. *J. Clin. Invest.* **44:** 1470–1473.

POLLACK, S., KAUFMAN, R. M. and CROSBY, W. H. (1964) Iron absorption: effects of sugars and reducing agents. *Blood* **24:** 577–581.

POWELL, C. W., MILLER, W. J. and BLACKMON, D. M. (1967) Effects of dietary EDTA and cadmium on absorption, excretion and retention of orally administered Zn^{65} in various tissues of zinc-deficient and normal goats and calves. *J. Nutr.* **93:** 203–212.

POWELL, C. W., MILLER, W. J., MORTON, J. P. and CLIFTON, C. M. (1964) Influence of dietary cadmium level and supplemental zinc on cadmium toxicity in the bovine. *J. Nutr.* **84:** 205–214.

POWELL, L. W., CAMPBELL, C. B. and WILSON, E. (1970) Intestinal mucosal uptake of iron and iron retention in idiopathic haemochromatosis as evidence for a mucosal abnormality. *Gut* **11:** 727–731.

PRASAD, A. S. and OBERLEAS, D. (1971) Binding of iron to amino acids and serum proteins *in vitro. Proc. Soc. Exp. Biol. Med.* **138:** 932–935.

PRASAD, K. N. and OSBORNE, J. W. (1963) Influence of β-mercaptoethylamine, mesenteric vessel clamping and pH on intestinal absorption of Fe^{59} in rats. *Proc. Soc. Exp. Biol. Med.* **114:** 523–527.

PRINGLE, A., GOLDBERG, A., MACDONAL, E. and JOHNSTON, S. (1962) ^{59}Fe iron sorbitol–citric-acid complex in iron-deficiency anaemia. *Lancet* 749–752.

RAGAN, H. A., NACHT, S., LEE, G. R., BISHOP, C. R. and CARTWRIGHT, G. E. (1969) Effect of ceruloplasmin on plasma iron in copper-deficient swine. *Amer. J. Physiol.* **217:** 1320–1323.

REDDY, B. S., WESTMANN, B. S. and PLEASANTS, J. R. (1965) Iron, copper and manganese in germfree and conventional rats. *J. Nutr.* **86:** 159–168.

REITZENSTEIN, P. G., CRONKITE, E. P., MEYER, L. M. and USENIK, E. A. (1960) Lymphatics in intestinal absorption of vitamin B_{12} and iron. *Proc. Soc. Exp. Biol. Med.* **105:** 233–236.

REYNAFERYE, C. and RAMOS, J. (1962) Influence of plasma filtrate containing erythropoietic factor on intestinal iron absorption in rats. *Proc. Soc. Exp. Biol. Med.* **109:** 868–869.

RICHMOND, C. R., FURCHNER, J. E., TRAFTON, C. A. and LANGHAM, W. H. (1962) Comparative metabolism of radionuclides in mammals. I. Uptake and retention of orally administered Zn^{65} by four mammalian species. *Health Phys.* **8:** 481–489.

RIEBER, E. E., CONRAD, M. and CROSBY, W. H. (1967) Gastrectomy and iron absorption: effects of bleeding, iron loading and ascorbic acid in rats. *Proc. Soc. Exp. Biol. Med.* **124:** 577–580.

ROBERSON, R. H. and SCHAIBLE, P. I. (1960) The availability to the chick of zinc as the sulfate, oxide or carbonate. *Poult. Sci.* **39:** 835–837.

ROBINSON, J. W. L., JEQUIER, J. CL., FELBER, J. P. and MIRKOVITCH, V. (1965) Amino acid absorption by the intestinal mucosa. *J. Surg. Res.* **5:** 150–152.

ROESER, H. P., LEE, G. R. and CARTWRIGHT, G. E. (1970) The role of ceruloplasmin in iron metabolism. *J. Clin. Invest.* **49:** 2408–2417.

RUBINI, M. E., MONTALVO, G., LOCKHART, C. P. and JOHNSON, C. R. (1961) Metabolism of zinc-65. *Am. J. Physiol.* **200:** 1345–1348.

RUDZKI, Z., BAKER, R. J. and DELLER, D. J. (1973) The iron-binding protein in human gastric juice. II. Nature of the interaction of the glycoprotein with iron. *Digestion* **8:** 53–76.

RUDZKI, Z. and DELLER, D. J. (1973) The iron-binding glycoprotein of human gastric juice. I. Isolation and characterization. *Digestion* **8:** 35–52.

RULIFFSON, W. S. and HOPPING, J. M. (1963) Maturation, iron deficiency and ligands in enteric radioiron transport *in vitro. Am. J. Physiol.* **204:** 171–175.

RUMMEL, W. (1965) Enterale Resorptionsvorgange und ihre Beeinflussung. *Naunyn-Schmiedebergs Arch. exp. Path. Pharmak.* **250:** 189–209.

RUMMEL, W. and FORTH, W. (1968) Zur Frage der metabolischen Abhängigkeit von Eisenbindung- und durchtritt durch den isolierten Dünndarm. *Naunyn-Schmiedebergs Arch. exp. Path. Pharmak.* **260:** 50–57.

RUMMEL, W., FORTH, W. and PFLEGER, K. (1967) Der Einfluβ verschiedener Liganden auf die Eisenresorption, pp. 129–134. In: *Radioisotopen in der Gastroenterologie,* HOFFMANN, G. (Ed.). Schattauer, Stuttgart.

RUMMEL, W. and STUPP, F. H. (1960) Der Einfluβ von Kalium und Calcium auf die Salz-, Glucose- und Wasser-Resorption des isolierten Dünndarms. *Naunyn-Schmiedebergs Arch. exp. Path. Pharmak.* **240:** 79–92.

RUSKIN, S. L. and MERRIL, A. T. (1949) Newer studies of iron absorption. *Am. J. Dig. Dis.* **16:** 182–188.

RUSZNYAK, I., GYÖRGY, L., ORMAI, S. and MILLNER, T. (1968) On some potassium-like qualities of the thallium ion. *Experientia* **24:** 809–810.

SAHAGIAN, B. M., HARDING-BARLOW, J. and PERRY, R. M. (1966) Uptakes of zinc, manganese, cadmium and mercury by intestinal strips of rat intestine. *J. Nutr.* **90:** 259–267.

SAHAGIAN, B. M., HARDING-BARLOW, J. and PERRY, H. M. (1967) Transmural movements of zinc, manganese, cadmium and mercury by rat small intestine. *J. Nutr.* **93:** 291–300.

SALTMAN, P., CHARLEY, PH. and SARKAR, B. (1962) Chelation of metal ions by sugars. *Fed. Proc.* **21:** 307.

SARKAR, B. and KRUCK, TH. P. A. (1966) Copper–amino acid complexes in human serum, p. 183. In: *The Biochemistry of Copper,* PEISACH, J., AISEN, PH. and BLUMBERG, W. E. (Eds.). Academic Press, New York and London.

SAUER, J. P., CHAPMAN, CH. W. and GALLAGHER, N. I. (1969) Effects of altered erythropoiesis on iron absorption. *Lab. Invest.* **20:** 558–561.

SAVAGE, I. E., YOHE, I. M., PICKETT, F. E. and O'DELL, B. L. (1964) Zinc metabolism in the growing chick. Tissue concentration and effect of phytate on absorption. *Poult. Sci.* **43:** 420–426.

SAYERS, M. H., LYNCH, S. R., JACOBS, P., CHARLTON, R. W., BOTHWELL, T. H., WALKER, R. B. and MAYETT, F. (1973) The effects of ascorbic acid supplementation on the absorption of iron in maize, wheat and soya. *Brit. J. Haemat.* **24:** 209–218.

SCHADE, A. L. (1967) Non-heme metalloproteins: their distribution, biological function and chemical characteristics, pp. 13–23. In: *Protides of the Biological Fluids,* PETERS, H. (Ed.). Elsevier Publ. Co., Amsterdam, London, New York.

SCHADE, A. L. and CAROLINE, L. (1944) Raw hen egg white and the role of iron in growth inhibition of *Shigella dysenteriae, Staphylococcus aureus, Escherichia coli* and *Saccharomyces cerevesiae. Science* **100:** 14–15.

SCHADE, A. L. and CAROLINE, L. (1946) Iron-binding component in human blood plasma. *Science* **104:** 340–341.

SCHADE, A. L., OYAMA, J., REINHART, R. W. and MILLER, J. R. (1954) Bound iron and unsaturated iron binding capacity of serum and reliable quantitative determination. *Proc. Soc. Exp. Biol. Med.* **87:** 443–448.

SCHADE, ST. C., FELSHER, B. F., BERNIER, C. M. and CONRAD, M. E. (1970a) Interrelationship of cobalt and iron absorption. *J. Lab. Clin. Med.* **75:** 435–441.

SCHADE, ST. C., FELSHER, B. F. and CONRAD, M. E. (1969) An effect of intestinal motility on iron absorption. *Proc. Soc. Exp. Biol. Med.* **130:** 757–761.

SCHADE, ST. C., FELSHER, B. F., GLADER, B. E. and CONRAD, M. E. (1970b) Effect of cobalt upon iron absorption. *Proc. Soc. Exp. Biol. Med.* **134:** 741–743.

SCHÄFER, K. H. (1959) Regulation des Eisenstoffwechsel, pp. 147–153. In: *Eisenstoffwechsel,* KEIDERLING, W. (Ed.). G. Thieme, Stuttgart.

SCHLOSSMANN, H. (1934) Platin und die Metalle der Platin-Gruppe, p. 2170. In: *Handbuch der exp. Pharmakologie,* vol. 3, 3, HEFFTER, A. and HEUBNER, W. (Eds.). Springer, Berlin.

SCHÜBEL, K. (1934) Zinn, p. 1569. In: *Handbuch der exp. Pharmakologie,* vol. 3, 3, HEFFTER, A. and HEUBNER, W. (Eds.). Springer, Berlin.

SCHUBERT, J. (1955) Removal of radioelements from the mammalian body. *Am. Rev. Nucl. Sci.* **5:** 369–412.

SCHUBERT, J. (1964) The chemical basis of chelation, pp. 466–494. In: *Iron Metabolism,* GROSS, F. (Ed.). Springer, Berlin, Göttingen, Heidelberg.

SCHULTZ, ST. G. and CURRAN, P. (1968) Intestinal absorption of sodium chloride and water, pp. 1245–1276. In: *Handbook of Physiol.*, sect. 6, vol. III. *Intestinal Absorption*, CODE, C. F. and HEIDEL, W. (Eds.). Am. Physiol. Soc., Washington, D.C.

SCHULTZE, M. O., ELVEHJEM, C. A. and HART, E. B. (1934) The availability of copper in various compounds as a supplement to iron in hemoglobin formation. *J. Biol. Chem.* **106:** 735–774.

SCHULTZE, M. O., ELVEHJEM, C. A. and HART, E. B. (1936) Further studies on the availability of copper from various sources as supplements to iron in hemoglobin formation. *J. Biol. Chem.* **115:** 453–457.

SCHULZ, J. and SMITH, N. J. (1958) A quantitative study of the absorption of food iron in infants and children. *Am. J. Dis. Child.* **95:** 109–119.

SCHWARZ, F. J., GRASSMANN, E. and KIRCHGESSNER, M. (1973a) Zur Cu-Absorption *in vitro* aus Cu-Aminosäure- und Peptidkomplexen. *Z. Tierphysiol.* **31:** 98–102.

SCHWARZ, F. J. and KIRCHGESSNER, M. (1973) Intestinale Cu-Absorption *in vitro* nach Fe- oder Zn-Depletion. *Z. Tierphysiol.* **31:** 91–98.

SCHWARZ, F. J., KIRCHGESSNER, M. and WEIGAND, E. (1973b) Zum Durchtritt von Kupfer-64 von der Serosa zur Mucosa. *Z. Tierphysiol.* **31:** 103–106.

SCHWARZ, K. (1970) Control of environmental conditions in trace element research: an experimental approach to unrecognized trace element requirements in: *Trace Element Metabolism in Animals* (C. F. MILLS, Ed.). Livingstone; Edinburgh and London.

SCHWARZ, K. (1973) New essential trace elements: Progress report and outlook. *2nd TEMA Symposium on Trace Element Metabolism in Animals* (W. G. HOEKSTRA, Ed.). Univ. of Wisconsin, Madison, Wis.

SCHWARZENBACH, G. (1958) Die Chemie wässeriger Metallsalzlosungen. *Angew. Chemie* **70:** 451–460.

SEELIG, M. S. (1972) Relationships of copper and molybdenum to iron metabolism. *Amer. J. Clin. Nutr.* **25:** 1022–1037.

SEREFIS, S. (1934) Die Resorptionsbedingungen des Wismuts vom Magen-Darm-Kanal aus. *Dt. med. Wschr.* **60:** 1237–1240.

SHARPE, L. M., HARRIS, R. S., PEACADE, W. C. and COOKE, R. C. (1948) Effects of phytate and other food ingredients on the absorption of radioactive iron. *Fed. Proc.* **7:** 298.

SHEEHAN, R. G. and FRENKEL, E. P. (1972) The control of iron absorption by the gastrointestinal mucosal cell. *J. Clin. Invest.* **51:** 224–231.

SILLEN, L. C. and MARTELL, A. E. (1964) *Stability Constants of Metal–Ion Complexes.* The Chemical Society, London.

SKORYNA, ST. C., TANAKA, Y., MOORE, W. JR. and STARA, J. F. (1972) Prevention of gastrointestinal absorption of excessive trace elements intake, pp. 3–14. In: *Trace Substances in Environmental Health*, vol. VI, HEMPHILL, D. D. (Ed.). Univ. of Missouri, Columbia, Mo.

SMITH, D. L., BIERWAGEN, M. E. and EARLY, TH. K. (1957) Effect of environmental oxygen tension on intestinal iron absorption. *Proc. Soc. Exp. Biol. Med.* **94:** 710–711.

SMITH, M. D. and PANNACCIULLI, I. M. (1958) Absorption of inorganic iron from graded doses: its significance in relation to iron absorption tests and the "mucosal block" theory. *Brit. J. Haemat.* **4:** 428–431.

SMITH, N. J. and SCHULZ, J. (1958) The absorption of iron in infants and children, pp. 65–73. In: *Iron in Clinical Medicine,* WALLERSTEIN, R. O. and METTIER, ST. R. (Eds.). Univ. Calif. Press, Berkeley and Los Angeles.

SMITH, P. M., STUDLEY, F. and WILLIAMS, R. (1969) Postulated gastric factor enhancing iron absorption in haemochromatosis. *Brit. J. Haemat.* **16:** 443–449.

SÖLVELL, L. (1960) Effect of iron and transferrin intravenously on iron absorption and turnover in man. *Acta Med. Scand.* **168:** Suppl. **358:** 71–81.

SPENCER, H., VANKINSCOTT, V., LEWIN, I. and SAMACHSON, J. (1965) Zinc-65 metabolism during low and high calcium intake in man. *J. Nutr.* **86:** 169–177.

STARCHER, B. C. (1969) Studies on the mechanism of copper absorption in the chick. *J. Nutr.* **97:** 321–326.

STARKENSTEIN, E. (1934) Eisen, pp. 682–1286. In: *Handbuch der exp. Pharmakologie*, vol. 3, 2, HEFFTER, A. and HEUBNER, W. (Eds.). Springer, Berlin.

STERNLIEB, I., VAN DEN HAMER, C. J. A. and ALPERT, S. (1967) Role of lymphatics in copper absorption. *Nature* **216:** 824.

STEWART, W. B. and GAMBINO, S. R. (1961) Kinetics of iron absorption in normal dogs. *Am. J. Physiol.* **201:** 67–70.

STITT, C., CHARLEY, P. J., BUTT, E. M. and SALTMAN, P. (1962) Rapid induction of iron deposition in spleen and liver with an iron-fructose chelate. *Proc. Soc. Exp. Biol. Med.* **110:** 70–71.

STONE, W. D. (1968) Gastric secretory response to iron therapy. *Gut* **9:** 99–105.

STRAIN, W. H. and PORIES, W. J. (1970) The role of zinc in tissue repair after injury, pp. 77–89. In: *Trace Element Metabolism in Animals*, MILLS, C. F. (Ed.). Livingstone, Edinburgh and London.

STROHMEYER, G. W., MILLER, ST. A., SCARLOTTA, R. W., MOORE, E. W., GREENBERG, M. S. and CHALMERS, TH. C. (1964) Effects of hypoxia on iron absorption and mobilization in the rat. *Amer. J. Physiol.* **207:** 55–61.

SÜLLMANN, H. (1931) Zur Frage der Eisenresorption. *Biochem. Z.* **134:** 241.

SUPPLEE, W. C. (1961) Production of zinc deficiency in turkey poults by dietary cadmium. *Poult. Sci.* **40:** 827–828.

SUSO, F. A. and EDWARDS, H. M. (1968) Influence of various chelating agents on absorption of ^{60}Ca, ^{59}Fe, ^{54}Mn and ^{65}Zn by chickens. *Poult. Sci.* **47:** 1417–1425.

SUSO, F. A. and EDWARDS, H. M. (1969) Studies on the ability of blood plasma and intestinal mucosa extract to bind ^{65}Zn. *Fed. Proc.* **28:** 761.

SUSO, F. A. and EDWARDS, H. M. (1971) Binding capacity of intestinal mucosa and blood plasma for zinc. *Proc. Soc. Exp. Biol. Med.* **137:** 306–308.

SUTTLE, N. F. and MILLS, C. F. (1966) Studies on the toxicity of copper to pigs. 2. Effect of protein source and other dietary components on the response to high and moderate intakes of copper. *Brit. J. Nutr.* **20:** 149–161.

SWINYARD, F. A. (1970) In: *The Pharmacological Basis of Therapeutics*, p. 995, GOODMAN, L. S. and GILMAN, A. (Eds.). Macmillan, New York.

SYDERHELM, R. and TAMMANN, H. (1934) Cit. acc. to STARKENSTEIN, E., Eisen, in: *Handbuch der exp. Pharmakologie*, vol. 3, 2, pp. 1186 ff. HEFFTER, A. and HEUBNER, W. (Eds.). Springer, Berlin.

TANAKA, Y. and SKORYNA, S. C. (1969) The use of acidic polysaccharides as inhibitors of intestinal absorption of metal ions. Abstr. Am. Chem. 158, Meeting Ce 20.

TAPPER, E. J., BUSHI, S., RUPPERT, R. D. and GREENBERGER, N. J. (1967) Effect of acute and chronic ethanol treatment on iron absorption. *Clin. Res.* **15:** 419.

TAPPER, E. J., BUSHI, S., RUPPERT, R. D. and GREENBERGER, N. J. (1968) Effect of accute and chronic ethanol treatment on the absorption of iron in rats. *Am. J. Med. Sci.* **255:** 46–52.

TEALE, F. W. J. (1959) Cleavage of the haem–protein link by acid methylethylketone. *Biol. Biophys. Acta* **35:** 543.

TERATO, K., FUJITA, T. and YOSHINO, Y. (1973a) Studies on iron absorption. I. The role of low molecular polymer in iron absorption. *Amer. J. Dig. Dis.* **18:** 121–128.

TERATO, K., HIRAMATSU, Y. and YOSHINO, Y. (1973b) Studies on iron absorption. II. Transport mechanism of low molecular iron chelate in rat intestine. *Amer. J. Dig. Dis.* **18:** 129–134.

TEXTER, E. C., LAURETA, H. C. and CHOU, CH. CH. (1971) Vascular factors in metal iron absorption, pp. 383–394. In: *Intestinal Absorption of Metal Ions, Trace Elements and Radionuclides*, SKORYNA, S. C. and WALDRON-EDWARDS, D. (Eds.). Pergamon Press, Oxford.

THOMAS, F. B., MCCULLOUGH, F. S. and GREENBERGER, N. J. (1971) Inhibition of the intestinal absorption of inorganic and hemoglobin iron by cholestyramine. *J. Lab. Clin. Med.* **78:** 70–80.

THOMAS, F. B., MCCULLOUGH, F. S. and GREENBERGER, N. J. (1972c) Effect of phenobarbital on the absorption of inorganic and hemoglobin iron in the rat. *Gastroenterology* **62:** 590–599.

THOMAS, F. B., SALSBUREY, D. and GREENBERGER, N. J. (1972b) Inhibition of absorption by cholestyramine. *Dig. Dis.* **17:** 263–269.

THOMSON, A. B. R., OLATUNBOSUN, D. and VALBERG, L. S. (1971c) Interrelation of intestinal transport system for manganese and iron. *J. Lab. Clin. Med.* **78:** 642–655.

THOMSON, A. B. R., SHAVER, CH., LEE, D. J., JONES, B. L. and VALBERG, L. S. (1971b) Effect of varying iron stores on site of intestinal absorption of cobalt and iron. *Am. J. Physiol.* **220:** 674–678.

THOMSON, A. B. R. and VALBERG, L. S. (1971) Kinetics of intestinal iron absorption in the rat: effect of cobalt. *Amer. J. Physiol.* **220:** 1080–1085.

THOMSON, A. B. R. and VALBERG, L. S. (1972) Intestinal uptake of iron, cobalt and manganese in the iron-deficient rat. *Amer. J. Physiol.* **223:** 1327–1329.

THOMSON, A. B. R., VALBERG, L. S. and SINCLAIR, D. G. (1971c) Competitive nature of the intestinal transport mechanism for cobalt and iron in the rat. *J. Clin. Invest.* **50:** 2384–2394.

TIFFIN, L. O. (1966a) Iron translocation. I. Plant culture, exudate sampling, iron citrate analysis. *Plant Physiol.* **41:** 510–514.

TIFFIN, L. O. (1966b) Iron translocation. II. Citrate/iron ratios in plant stem exudates. *Plant Physiol.* **41:** 515–518.

TOMPSETT, S. L. (1940) Factors influencing the absorption of iron and copper from the alimentary tract. *Biochem. J.* **39:** 961–969.

TRIPOD, J. (1964) A pharmacological comparison of the binding of iron and other metals, pp. 503–517. In: *Iron Metabolism,* GROSS, F. (Ed.). Springer, Berlin, Göttingen, Heidelberg.

TRIPOD, J. and KEBERLE, H. (1962) Essais biologiques avec la desferrioxamine. *Helv. Physiol. Acta* **20:** 291–293.

TURK, H. (1940) Ein Beitrag zur Geschichte der Eisentherapie bei Anämien. Doctoral Thesis, Med. Fac., Marburg/Lahn.

TURNBULL, A. L., CLETON, F. and FINCH, C. A. (1962) Iron absorption. IV. The absorption of hemoglobin iron. *J. Clin. Invest.* **41:** 1897–1907.

UNDERWOOD, E. I. (1938) A comparison of ferrous and ferric iron in the nutrition of the rat. *J. Nutr.* **16:** 299–308.

USSING, H. H. (1960) The alkali metal ions in isolated systems and tissues, pp. 45–69. In: *The Alkali Metal Ions in Biology, Handbuch der exper. Pharmakologie,* EICHLER, O. and FARAH, A. (Eds.). Springer, Berlin, Göttingen, Heidelberg.

VALBERG, L. S. (1971) Cobalt absorption, pp. 257–264. In: *Intestinal Absorption of Metal Ions, Trace Elements and Radionuclides,* SKORYNA, S. C. and WALDRON-EDWARDS, D. (Eds.). Pergamon Press, Oxford.

VALBERG, L. S., LUDWIG, J. and OLATUNBOSUN, D. (1969) Alteration in cobalt absorption in patients with disorders of iron metabolism. *Gastroenterology* **56:** 241–251.

VALBERG, L. S. and OLATUNBOSUN, D. (1968) Alteration in cobalt absorption in patients with disorders of iron metabolism. *Gastroenterology* **54:** 1279.

VALLEE, B. L. (1962) Zinc, pp. 463–464. In: *Mineral Metabolism,* vol. II, part B, COMAR, C. L. and BRONNER, F. (Eds.). Academic Press, New York, London.

VAN CAMPEN, D. (1966) Effects of zinc, cadmium, silver and mercury on the absorption and distribution of copper-64 in rats. *J. Nutr.* **88:** 125–130.

VAN CAMPEN, D. (1969) Copper interference with the intestinal absorption of zinc-65 by rats. *J. Nutr.* **97:** 104–108.

VAN CAMPEN, D. (1970) Competition between copper and zinc during absorption, pp. 287–296. In: *Trace Element Metabolism in Animals*, MILLS, C. F. (Ed.). Livingstone, Edinburgh and London.

VAN CAMPEN, D. (1971) Absorption of copper from the gastrointestinal tract, pp. 211–228. In: *Absorption of Radioactive Metals*, SKORYNA, S. C. and WALDRON-EDWARD, E. (Eds.). Pergamon Press, Oxford.

VAN CAMPEN, D. (1973) Enhancement of iron absorption from ligated segments of rat intestine by histidine, cysteine, and lysine: effects of removing ionizing groups and of stereoisomerism. *J. Nutr.* **103:** 139–142.

VAN CAMPEN, D. and GROSS, E. (1968) Influence of ascorbic acid on the absorption of copper by rats. *J. Nutr.* **95:** 617–622.

VAN CAMPEN, D. and GROSS, E. (1969) Effect of histidine and certain other amino acids on the absorption of iron-59 by rats. *J. Nutr.* **99:** 68–74.

VAN CAMPEN, D. R. and KOWALSKI, T. J. (1971) Studies on zinc absorption: ^{65}Zn binding by homogenates of rat intestinal mucosa. *Proc. Soc. Exp. Biol. Med.* **136:** 294–297.

VAN CAMPEN, D. R. and MITCHELL, E. A. (1965) Absorption of Cu^{64}, Zn^{65}, Mo^{99} and Fe^{59} from ligated segments of the rat gastrointestinal tract. *J. Nutr.* **86:** 120–124.

VAN CAMPEN, D. and SCAIFE, P. U. (1967) Zinc interference with copper absorption in rats. *J. Nutr.* **91:** 472–476.

VASSER, PH. S. and TAYLOR, I. M. (1956) Effects of hypoxia on iron absorption. *Proc. Soc. Exp. Biol. Med.* **93:** 504–506.

VENKATACHALAM, P. S., BRADING, I., GEORGE and WALSH, R. J. (1956) An experiment in rats to determine whether iron is absorbed only in the ferrous state. *Austr. J. Exp. Biol. Med. Sci.* **34:** 389–394.

VIAULT, E. (1891) Sur la quantité d'oxygène contenue dans le sang des animaux des hauts plateaux de l'amérique du sud. *C.r. Acad. Sci.* (*Paris*) **112:** 295–298.

VLCEK, B. (1967) Acceleration of metal transport in yeast cells treated with a lipophilic complex. *Experientia* **23:** 1014–1017.

VOHRA, P. and GONZALES, N. (1969) The effect of EDTA on the preferential absorption of zinc than manganese in turkey poults. *Poultry Sci.* **48:** 1509–1510.

VOHRA, P., GRAY, C. A. and KRATZER, F. H. (1965) Phytic acid–metal complexes. *Proc. Soc. Exp. Biol. Med.* **120:** 447–449.

VOHRA, P. and KRATZER, F. H. (1966) Influence of various phosphates and other complexing agents on the availability of zinc for turkey poults. *J. Nutr.* **89:** 106–112.

VOIGT, C. and BRÜSCHKE, G. (1967) Magenschleimhaut und Eisenmangel. *Dt. med. Wschr.* **92:** 1082–1086.

VOLKHEIMER, G., SCHULZ, F. H., LINDENAU, A. and BERTZ, U. (1969) Resorption of metallic iron particles. *Gut* **10:** 32–33.

WACK, J. P. and WYATT, J. P. (1959) Studies on ferrodynamics. I. Gastrointestinal absorption of ^{59}Fe in the rat under differing dietary states. *Pathology* **67:** 237–247.

WALDRON-EDWARD, D., PAUL, T. M. and SKORYNA, S. C. (1966) Effects of the counter ion and pH on intestinal absorption of calcium and strontium. *Proc. Soc. Exp. Biol. Med.* **123:** 532–538.

WALSH, R. J., KALDOR, I., BRADING, J. and GEORGE, E. P. (1955) The availability of iron in meat: some experiments with radioactive iron. *Austr. Ann. Med.* **4:** 272–276.

WALZ, A., PRIBILLA, W., HÄRING, R. and KOEPPE, P. (1970) Gleichzeitige Messung der Vitamin B_{12} nach Eisen-Resorption mit einem Ganzkorper-aktivitätszähler nach Gastrektomie, Magenresection und atrophischer Gastritis. *Dt. med. Wschr.* **95:** 25–30.

WAXMANN, S., PRATT, P. and HERBERT, V. (1968) Malabsorption of hemoglobin iron in pernicious anemia correction with intrinsic factor-containing substances. *J. Clin. Invest.* **47:** 1819–1825.

WEBER, K. M. (1969a) Die Schädigung des Darmes durch ÄDTA und DTPA bei der Ratte. *Z. ges. exp. Med.* **150:** 354–360.

WEBER, K. M. (1969b) Metabolismus and Toxicität therapeutischer Chelatbildner. 6 Mittlg. Die histoautoradiographische Lokalisation von ÄDTA in Organen der Ratte. *Strahlentherapie* **137:** 708–711.

WEBER, K. M., BOHNE, F. and REBE, U. (1970) Decrease of DNA synthesis in duodenal crypt cells of rats treated with Na_3 (Ca-DTPA). *Europ. J. Pharmac.* **11:** 117–118.

WEBER, P. M., O'REILLY, S., POLLYCOVE, M. and SHIPLEY, L. (1969) Gastrointestinal absorption of copper: studies with ^{64}Cu, ^{65}Zn, a whole-body counter and the scintillation camera. *J. Nucl. Med.* **10:** 591–596.

WEBLING, D. D. A. and HOLDSWORTH, E. S. (1965) The effect of bile, bile acids and detergents on calcium absorption in the chick. *Biochem. J.* **97:** 408–421.

WEBLING, D. D. A. and HOLDSWORTH, E. S. (1966a) Bile salts and calcium absorption. *Biochem. J.* **100:** 652–660.

WEBLING, D. D. A. and HOLDSWORTH, E. S. (1966b) Bile and the absorption of strontium and iron. *Biochem. J.* **100:** 661–663.

WEINTRAUB, L. R., CONRAD, M. E. and CROSBY, W. H. (1964) The significance of iron turnover in the control of iron absorption. *Blood* **24:** 19–24.

WEINTRAUB, L. R., CONRAD, M. E. and CROSBY, W. H. (1965a) Absorption of hemoglobin iron by the rat. *Proc. Soc. Exp. Biol. Med.* **120:** 840–843.

WEINTRAUB, L. R., CONRAD, M. E. and CROSBY, W. H. (1965b) Regulation of the intestinal absorption of iron by the rats of erythropoiesis. *Brit. J. Haemat.* **11:** 432–438.

WEINTRAUB, L. R., DAWSON, R. B. and RAFAL, S. (1968a) Absorption of hemoglobin iron: the release of iron from heme by intestinal xanthine oxidase. *J. Clin. Invest.* **47:** 101 a.

WEINTRAUB, L. R., WEINSTEIN, M. B., HUSER, H. J. and RAFAL, S. (1968b) Absorption of hemoglobin iron: the role of heme-splitting substance in the intestinal mucosa. *J. Clin. Invest.* **47:** 531–539.

WELCH, C. ST., WAKEFIELD, E. C. and ADAMS, M. (1936) Function of the large intestine of man in absorption and excretion. *Archs intern. Med.* **58:** 1095–1110.

WESER, U. and KIRCHGESSNER, M. (1965) Dialysegeschwindigkeit freier Kupfer-Ionen bei Zusatz verschiedener anorganischer Liganden. *Z. Tierphysiol.* **20:** 37–40.

WHEBY, M. S. (1966) Site of absorption in man. *Clin. Res.* **14:** 50.

WHEBY, M. S. and CROSBY, W. H. (1963) The gastrointestinal tract and iron absorption. *Blood* **22:** 416–428.

WHEBY, M. S. and JONES, L. C. (1963) Role of transferrin in iron absorption. *J. Clin. Invest.* **42:** 1007–1016.

WHEBY, M. S., JONES, L. G. and CROSBY, W. H. (1964) Studies on iron absorption. Intestinal regulatory mechanism. *J. Clin. Invest.* **43:** 1433–1442.

WHEBY, M. S., SUTTLE, G. E. and FORD, K. T. (1970) Intestinal absorption of hemoglobin iron. *Gastroenterology* **58:** 647–654.

WHEBY, M. S. and UMPIERRE, C. (1964) Effect of transferrin saturation on iron absorption in man. *New Engl. J. Med.* **271:** 1391–1395.

WHITEHEAD, I. S. W. and BANNERMAN, R. M. (1964) Absorption of iron by gastrectomized rats. *Gut.* **5:** 38–44.

WILBRANDT, W. and ROSENBERG, TH. (1961) The concept of carrier transport and its corollaries in pharmacology. *Pharm. Rev.* **13:** 169–183.

WILLIAMS, B. I. P. (1966) The selectivity of metal–protein interactions, pp. 25–36. In: *Protides of the Biological Fluids*, vol. 14, PETERS, H. (Ed.). Elsevier Publ. Co., Amsterdam.

WILSON, T. H. and WISEMAN, C. (1954) The use of sacs of everted small intestine for the study of the transference of substances from the mucosal to the serosal surface. *J. Physiol.* (*Lond.*) **123:** 116–125.

WINNE, D. and REMISCHOWSKY, J. (1971) Der Einfluβ der Durchblutung auf die Resorption von Polyalkoholen aus dem Jenunum der Ratte. *Naunyn-Schmiedebergs Arch. exp. Path. Pharmak.* **270:** 22–40.

WIRTH, W., HECHT, G. and GLOXHUBER, CH. (1967) *Toxikologie Fibel.* G. Thieme, Stuttgart.

WISEMAN, G. (1968) Absorption of amino acids, pp. 1277–1308. In: *Handbook of Physiology*, sect. 6, vol. III, *Intestinal Absorption*, CODE, C. F. and HEIDEL, W. (Eds.). Am. Physiol. Soc., Washington, D.C.

WÖHLER, F. (1964) The treatment of haemochromatosis with desferrioxamine, pp. 551–567. In: *Iron Metabolism*, GROSS, F. (Ed.). Springer; Berlin, Göttingen, Heidelberg.

WÖHLER, F. and EMRICH, D. (1956) Tierexperimentelle Untersuchungen zur Kobaltwirkung auf den Eisenstoffwechsel (Speichereisen). *Naunyn-Schmiedebergs Arch. exp. Path. Pharmak.* **229**: 92–100.

WÖHLER, F., HEILMEYER, L., EMRICH, D. and SHIN HO KANG (1957) Zur Funktion des Ferritins bei der Eisenresorption. *Naunyn-Schmiedebergs Arch. exp. Path. Pharmak.* **230**: 107–124.

WÖHLER, F. and KÖRNIG, D. (1964) Zur Beeinflussung der Eisenresorption durch Ascorbinsäure, Kobalt und Stoffwechselprodukte von Symbionten aus normaler Darmflora. *Arzneimittel-Forsch.* **14**: 953–962

WORWOOD, M., EDWARDS, A. and JACOBS, A. (1971) A non-ferritin protein compound in the rat small intestinal mucosa during iron absorption. *Nature* **229**: 409–410.

WORWOOD, M. and JACOBS, A. (1971a) The subcellular distribution of orally administered ^{59}Fe in rat small intestinal mucosa. *Brit. J. Haemat.* **20**: 587–596.

WORWOOD, M. and JACOBS, A. (1971b) Absorption of ^{59}Fe in the rat: iron binding substances in the soluble fraction of intestinal mucosa. *Life Sci.* **10**: part I, 1363–1373.

WYNTER, C. V. A. and WILLIAMS, R. (1968) Iron-binding properties of gastric juice in idiopathic haemochromatosis. *Lancet* 534–537.

YAMABE, S. (1967) A further study of Cu^{++} chelate of Kanamycin. *Jap. J. Pharmac.* **17**: 120–124.

YEH, S. D. J. and CHOW, B. F. (1965) Iron absorption by bilaterally nephrectomized rats. *Proc. Soc. Exp. Biol. Med.* **119**: 563–565.

YEH, S. D. J. and SHILS, M. E. (1966) Effect of tetracycline on intestinal absorption of various nutrients by the rat. *Proc. Soc. Exp. Biol. Med.* **123**: 367–375.

CHAPTER 13

INHERITED DEFECTS OF INTESTINAL ABSORPTION

K. R. Kerry, *Melbourne, Victoria, Australia*
A. G. F. Davidson, *Vancouver, Canada*
A. Fanconi, *Winterthur, Switzerland*

INTRODUCTION

This review reports on those inborn errors of metabolism where the primary defect is located, or thought to be located, in the mechanisms of intestinal absorption. All known disorders with affected transport into or out from the epithelial cells of the small intestinal mucosa are covered.* Although symptoms, diagnosis, treatment and genetic aspects are described, emphasis has been placed on the intestinal abnormalities.

13.1. DEFECTIVE CARBOHYDRATE ABSORPTION

13.1.1. GLUCOSE–GALACTOSE MALABSORPTION SYNDROME (CONGENITAL GLUCOSE–GALACTOSE MALABSORPTION)

Glucose–galactose malabsorption is a congenital disorder characterized by the inability of the patients to absorb adequately glucose and galactose and also 3-*O*-methylglucose and possibly other sugars of theoretical interest but of no clinical importance (see below). Fructose, however, is absorbed normally.

When patients are fed glucose or galactose either as the free monosaccharides or combined as digestible oligosaccharides or polysaccharides there is no rise in blood-sugar levels, the patients rapidly develop diarrhea and the unabsorbed sugars are excreted with the feces. Prolonged feeding leads to secondary symptoms of dehydration, electrolyte depletion,

*Manuscript completed August 1969; a limited revision was made in July 1971 when some additional references were added. Some additions were also made in proof.

malnutrition and may in the extreme case lead to death from inanition. Symptoms develop shortly after the first milk feedings and persist so long as the offending sugars are fed. Clinical remission follows the removal of carbohydrate from the diet or the substitution of fructose as the carbohydrate source. Patients are treated by keeping them throughout their lives on diets low in glucose and galactose. Diets and problems associated with dietary management of patients have been reviewed by Dahlqvist *et al.* (1968).

The clinical picture resembles that of sucrase or lactase deficiency (see Rey and Frezal, 1967 for review) but patients with glucose–galactose malabsorption may be readily distinguished since they continue to show symptoms when the offending disaccharides in the diet are replaced by their constituent monosaccharides.

Patients may also be distinguished from others suffering from generalized monosaccharide malabsorption (see Burke and Danks, 1966; Zetterstrom and Waldenstrom, 1968) since they absorb fructose normally. Further problems associated with the differential diagnosis of sugar malabsorption syndromes and the clinical management of these patients have been discussed by Dahlqvist *et al.* (1968) and Lindquist and Meeuwisse (1968).

13.1.1.1. *Genetics*

Lindquist and Meeuwisse (1968), Melin and Meeuwisse (1969) reported the pedigrees of several Swedish families with inbred marriages and common ancestors dating from the eighteenth century. These families contain affected children of both sexes. The pedigrees clearly demonstrate an autosomal recessive manner of inheritance. Clinical abnormalities which can be attributed to the disorder alone have not been found in the heterozygotes although the intermittent glucosuria reported in parents may be related. Glucose tolerance tests in these individuals appear clinically normal (Lindquist *et al.,* 1963). Preliminary investigations by Elsas *et al.* (1969a, b) suggest, however, that the rate of glucose absorption may be lower in the parents of patients. Elsas *et al.* (1969a) also report "moderately reduced minimal thresholds for glucose" in both parents of a patient.

13.1.1.2. *Nature of the defect*

Specimens of the intestinal mucosa obtained by per oral biopsy (unlike those from normals) do not accumulate ^{14}C-glucose (Eggermont and Loeb, 1966; Meeuwisse and Dahlqvist, 1968; Abraham *et al.,* 1967) although the accumulation of ^{14}C-alanine (Meeuwisse and Dahlqvist, 1968) and ^{14}C-leucine (Eggermont and Loeb, 1966) is normal. Failure of intestinal biopsy tissue to absorb ^{14}C-galactose was demonstrated also using autoradiography by Schneider *et al.* (1966). Small amounts of sugar, however, do cross the intestinal mucosa *in vivo* since orally administered ^{14}C-glucose, ^{14}C-galactose (Linneweh and Schaumlöffel, 1965) and 3-*O*-methylglucose (Anderson *et al.*, 1965; Abraham *et al.*, 1967; Kerry, 1967) and can be detected in the blood and urine. In the one patient (Abraham *et al.*, 1967) there was no rise in the level of blood insulin following an oral glucose load.

Examination of the intestinal mucosa (obtained by per oral biopsy) by light (Anderson *et al.*, 1965; Schneider *et al.*, 1966) and electron microscopy (Schneider *et al.*, 1966; Meeuwisse and Dahlqvist, 1966) has revealed no gross structural abnormality. Microvilli are present and normal activity of the enzymes associated with the microvillus membrane (maltase, sucrase, lactase, trehalase and alkaline phosphatase) are normal (Anderson *et al.*, 1965; Dubois *et al.*, 1966; Abraham *et al.*, 1967; Meeuwisse and Dahlqvist, 1968). On clinical evidence other transport mechanisms, e.g. for the absorption of amino acids, fat and vitamins, appear normal. The absorption of sodium is normal clinically and experimentally (Meeuwisse and Dahlqvist, 1968). Patients also have Na^+-K^+-activated, ouabain-inhibited adenosine triphosphatase (transport-ATPase) activity.

13.1.1.3. *Localization of the defect*

Since this disorder affects only those sugars which, in the presence of Na^+, are transported against a concentration difference (e.g. glucose, galactose and 3-*O*-methylglucose) the defect is considered to be localized in the mechanism for active intestinal transport. In the normal this mechanism, according to the hypothesis of Crane and associates (see Crane, 1968), is considered to operate in the following manner. The absorption of glucose, galactose and some other sugars is considered to be effected by a specific carrier, moving the hexose across the cell membrane. This step is substrate-specific, sodium-dependent, ATP-independent and results in the rapid equilibration of sugars between the cells and the medium. This carrier system is capable only of equilibration, the asymmetry required to achieve "uphill" accumulation of sugar is ascribed to a gradient of Na^+ concentration "downhill" into the cells, maintained by the operation of the energy-dependent outwardly directed Na^+ pump. Thus the defect in the glucose–galactose malabsorption may be localized in principle at two levels: either at the stage of entry of the sugar (and Na^+) into the cell, i.e. the carrier mechanism, or at the mechanism for pumping sodium from the cells. The evidently normal sodium metabolism, accumulation of L-amino acids and normal pump ATPase activity indicate that the pump mechanism is apparently undamaged and suggest therefore that the fault is in the mechanism of entry into the cells, possibly at the level of the "carrier".

13.1.1.4. *Renal defects*

Some evidence exists that in glucose–galactose malabsorption a similar defect exists in the tubular absorption of glucose in the kidney. Most patients reported have had glucosuria and when the level of blood glucose is raised by intravenous infusion glucose appeared in the urine before the normal threshold level was reached (Anderson *et al.*, 1965; Lindquist and Meeuwisse, 1968; Marks *et al.*, 1966; Meeuwisse, 1970). Compared with intestinal absorption less is known about the mechanism of tubular absorption of glucose but it is thought also to be carrier-mediated and similar to the intestinal system.

13.2. DEFECTIVE AMINO ACID ABSORPTION

13.2.1. HUMAN CYSTINURIA

Cystinuria is an inherited anomaly of intestinal and renal transport of lysine, arginine, cystine, ornithine (Dent and Rose, 1951) and of the mixed disulfide of cysteine and homocysteine (Frimpter, 1961). Early descriptions date from that of Wollaston (1810) who recognized only the excess urinary excretion of cystine which often forms urinary stones because of its low solubility. It was not realized until recent times that the defect was one of renal tubular transport involving other amino acids and that a similar defect was present in the intestine. An important historical review has been presented by Knox (1966). Urinary loss of amino acids averages, for an adult male, approximately 1.0 g cystine, 1.7 g lysine, 1.0 g arginine and 0.4 g ornithine per day in the untreated patient (Colliss *et al.*, 1963). Despite a simultaneous defect in the intestine (see later discussion) the fecal loss of these amino acids is not great and absorption of each is almost complete at normal rates of ingestion (Milne *et al.*, 1961). The clinical consequences of this disorder result from the urinary loss of lysine (an essential amino acid) which has some repercussions on growth (Colliss *et al.*, 1963) and the formation of urinary calculi from cystine which causes renal colic, and obstructions which predispose to urinary tract infection and renal failure.

The problem of stone formation in cystinuria has been investigated in detail by Dent and Senior (1955). Cystine has low solubility in moderately acid or neutral solutions but increases with increasing pH. Solubility is approximately 300 mg/l at pH 5.0 and 400 mg/l at pH 7.0. Since these concentrations are frequently exceeded in the urine of patients, particularly at night when the urine is more concentrated and tends to be more acidic, cystine crystallizes and forms stones. The occurrence of stones in patients seems almost inevitable although the age of the patient at which they first form varies from a few months to 30 years or more. Treatment is directed towards preventing the saturation of urine with cystine. This is done by: (i) encouraging a high fluid intake to promote diuresis, (ii) reducing the formation of cystine by low methionine diets, (iii) maintaining an alkaline urine by frequent use of alkali and an alkaline ash diet and (iv) administering D-penicillamine (D-β-β-dimethylcysteine) (Crawhall *et al.*, 1963) or *N*-acetyl-penicillamine (Stokes *et al.*, 1968). These compounds form mixed disulfides with cysteine which are more soluble than cystine and have been effective in preventing stone formation and dissolving existing stones. *N*-acetyl-penicillamine is to be preferred since toxic side effects of penicillamine (fever, granulocytopenia, thrombocytopenia, proteinuria and a reversible nephrotic syndrome) are minimal with the *N*-acetyl derivative. The problem of medical management of cystinuric patients has been discussed by Frimpter (1968).

13.2.1.1. *Intestinal defects in cystinuria*

The intestinal defect in this disease was first investigated by Milne and colleagues (Milne *et al.*, 1961; Asatoor *et al.*, 1962) who demonstrated defective absorption of lysine, arginine and ornithine. Later, Thier *et al.* (1964), London and Foley (1965), Foley and London (1965) and Rosenberg *et al.* (1965) demonstrated that the absorption of cystine was defective also. Arginine, lysine and ornithine were given orally to patients and the levels of each determined in the plasma, feces and urine. Following the oral ingestion of lysine, arginine or cystine there was a smaller rise than normal in the plasma levels of these amino acids and a large percentage of each dose was recovered in the stools. In addition, compounds produced (or derivatives of these) from each amino acid by colonic bacteria were detected also in the stools and urine of patients, but not normals, at a variable time (usually 8–48 hr) after loading. These included citrulline, putrescine and pyrrolidine from arginine, cadaverine and piperidine from lysine, and inorganic sulfate from cystine. Patients were found also to have a *select* strain of *Escherichia coli* which was particularly efficient in the decarboxylation of these amino acids (Asatoor *et al.*, 1962).

Similarly, oral doses of cystine produced a smaller increase in plasma cystine and cysteine and urinary inorganic sulfate. Pretreatment with neomycin produced a proportionately greater production in post-cystine sulfate excretion in the cystinuric patients than in the normal control subjects, thus indicating that more cystine was degraded to inorganic sulfur compounds by colonic bacteria in cystinuric cases.

The nature of the defect was investigated further using *in vitro* techniques by Rosenberg and colleagues (Rosenberg, 1967; Rosenberg *et al.*, 1966; see also Segal, 1968). Intestinal tissue obtained by per oral biopsy was incubated in a physiological medium containing ^{14}C-lysine or ^{35}S-cystine and the accumulation of these amino acids by the tissue measured in the presence and absence of Na^+, anaerobic conditions and a high concentration of arginine. Sodium depletion or anaerobic conditions inhibit the active accumulation of lysine, cystine and also arginine which is accumulated by the same transport mechanism and acts as a competitive inhibitor of lysine or cystine transport.

On the basis of results obtained, it was found that at least three separate intestinal transport defects exist.

In type I there was no active transport of lysine, arginine or cystine and absorption occurred down a concentration gradient only. In contrast to normal, the rate of absorption of lysine (from a 0.065 mM solution) or cystine (from a 0.03 mM solution) was not influenced by the absence of Na^+, anaerobiosis or the presence of excess arginine (0.8 mM) (a competitive inhabitor of the absorption of these amino acids). The absorption of cysteine, however, was normal and thus indicates that it and cystine are absorbed by different mechanisms.

Those designated as type II cystinurics are represented by a group of only two individuals who have some ability to accumulate cystine but not lysine in the intestinal mucosa above medium concentration; the final tissue/medium ratio for cystine was only 2.4 compared to an average figure of 7 for normals. Following an oral load of cystine (0.05 mc mole/kg) there was no rise in plasma cystine levels and the uptake of cystine by intestinal biopsy tissue was reduced by anaerobiosis (36 %), by Na^+ free medium (21 %) and by 0.8 mM arginine (67 %).

In contrast, active transport of lysine could not be demonstrated and what absorption did occur was not influenced by the absence of Na^+, anaerobic conditions or 0.8 mM arginine.

In type III cystinuria, the defect in absorption of both cystine and lysine was only partial; both these amino acids were absorbed against a concentration gradient and the absorption was affected by anaerobic conditions, the absence of sodium and the presence of L-arginine. A normal rise in plasma cystine occurs following oral loading (0.05 mc mole/kg).

13.2.1.2. *Amino acid transport in the kidney*

Based on the patterns of excretion of amino acids, the defects in renal transport of arginine, lysine, ornithine and cystine show similarities with the intestinal defect although apparently quite different in kind.

Fox *et al.* (1964) studied the absorption of labeled amino acids by kidney slices from normal and cystinuric patients. In normal tissue, arginine, lysine and cystine were all transported against a concentration gradient (cystine always appeared in the tissues as the reduced compound cysteine). Lysine and arginine mutually inhibit the transport of the other but cystine had no effect, nor had these amino acids or ornithine any effect on cystine transport. It appears, therefore, that the mechanisms for the transport of cystine in the kidney is distinct from that for dibasic amino acid transport and that the latter amino acids all compete for a common renal transport mechanism. These findings have been confirmed by using other techniques (Segal *et al.*, 1967).

When similar investigations were performed on kidney biopsy tissue from all three types of cystinuria, it was found that the active accumulation of lysine and arginine occurred at a reduced rate (about 50% normal) but cystine absorption was entirely normal. Thus considerable differences exist between the intestinal and renal defects in cystinuria. Of particular interest is the observation that the absorption of cystine was entirely normal since cystinuria is the feature by which the disease is distinguished. The reason for this apparent anomaly is obscure but the point is, of course, of prime importance in the understanding of the pathology of the disease. Segal (1968) speculates that "it may be related to the fact that the intracellular form of the amino acid is cysteine and that lysine inhibits cystine efflux. This leads to the possibility that cysteine and lysine share a common efflux mechanism. Should this mechanism be defective, then there could be a pile-up of intracellular cystine which results in a failure of cystine being absorbed to be reduced. A mass action effect at the cell membrane may then prevent the cystine moving across the membrane."

13.2.1.3. *Genetics*

After an extensive genetic study of this disorder, Harris and Warren (1953) and Harris *et al.* (1955) recognized that two forms existed, the recessive and the incompletely recessive. These were distinguished on the basis of aminoaciduria in parents and siblings. In the *recessive* form, which was the most common, the presumed heterozygotes were completely normal; in the *incompletely* recessive form, all members of the family showed a continuous variation in the excretion of lysine and cystine but not arginine in the urine, ranging from completely normal to grossly abnormal. In this second type, it was presumed that those individuals with intermediate values were the heterozygotes.

Since parents of patients with the intestinal defect of type I cystinuria showed no cystinuria, the defect in these patients is of the recessive type. Parents and siblings of patients with type II and type III intestinal defects, however, showed aminoaciduria and these are therefore subdivisions of the incompletely recessive cystinuria described by Harris *et al.* (1953). It appears that intestinal transport of cystine and diamino-monocarboxylic acids is under the control of multiple allelic genes and that clinical cystinuria is due to a mutation in one or more of these genes. Therefore, combinations of the various types of cystinuria are possible theoretically and have been summarized by Scriver (1969).

Knox (1966) has summarized the literature on the incidence of cystinuria. Approximately 1% of all urinary calculi are cystine stones; the overall incidence of calculus patients is one in 1000; thus, the incidence of stone-forming cystinuric patients is about one per 100,000 population. A Swedish survey indicated an incidence of one per 200,000.

13.2.2. HYPERDIBASICAMINOACIDURIA WITHOUT CYSTINURIA

Whelan and Scriver (1968) have reported a family in which thirteen of the thirty-three kin have an abnormally high urinary excretion rate for lysine, arginine and ornithine; cystine, however, is excreted normally and thus distinguishes this trait from classical cystinuria. There also is some evidence (plasma lysine levels following loading) for a partial defect in intestinal absorption of lysine but again the absorption of cystine is normal. It was suggested that this trait is dominantly inherited and that affected members of this family are heterozygotes. Homozygotes which have not been detected might be expected to show a complete defect for intestinal and renal absorption of these amino acids. It has been speculated, however, that the syndrome of protein intolerance with dibasic aminoaciduria reported in Finland by Kekomäki and colleagues (see Kekomäki *et al.*, 1968) may be homozygotes to this disorder.

This trait is of considerable theoretical interest since it provides evidence for a genetic control of the membrane transport system shared exclusively by dibasic amino acids.

13.2.3. CYSTINURIA IN NON-HUMAN MAMMALS

Cystinuria with the formation of cystine stones occurs in several varieties of the domestic dog (see Treacher, 1964) and the mink (Oldfield *et al.*, 1956).

Cystinuria in dogs appears similar to the defect of humans and thus has potential as a model for the investigation of the human disorder although it is different in two respects: (a) it is inherited as a sex-linked recessive trait present in male animals only (Brand *et al.*, 1940; Hess and Sullivan, 1942; see also Knox, 1966), and (b) the stones produced are usually impacted in the narrow urethra of the male dog with resultant retention of urine and its consequences (cf. calculus formation in the renal pelvis of human patients). Minor biochemical differences are also found.

As in the human, cystinuric dogs excrete abnormal amounts of lysine, cystine (Crane and Turner, 1956), arginine and ornithine (Treacher, 1962, 1963, 1964) and the cysteine–homocysteine disulfide (Frimpter, 1963) in their urine. In addition, Treacher (1963) reported an abnormally high urinary output of citrulline and threonine; this may, however, be a defect secondary to the main disorder (Milne, 1964).

Evidence also exists for the presence of an intestinal defect of absorption. Oral cystine fed to cystinuric dogs did not increase the urinary output of cystine; this is in contrast to the increased excretion of cystine following the feeding of cysteine or methionine. This suggests normal absorption of cysteine and methionine but not cystine (Hess and Sullivan, 1942). Lysine is also poorly absorbed. Treacher (1963) found that following an oral load of lysine hydrochloride (as two doses of 6 g each given 2 hr apart) there was a rise in urinary piperidine and a smaller rise of pyrrolidine some 17–21 hr later. This is a result similar to that found in cystinuric humans. A similar rise in the excretion of these compounds was not found in the control dogs.

In vitro experiments on intestinal and renal absorption of amino acids have not been performed to date on tissue from cystinuric dogs. It is expected that such experiments would be particularly rewarding in the characterization of both the human and the canine disease and provide further insight into the mechanisms of intestinal and renal tubular absorption of amino acids.

Another kind of cystinuria possibly occurring as a species trait has been recorded in genets, which are small arboreal mongooses, native to Africa. Datta and Harris (1953) reported a urinary cystine level of 1.0–1.5 mg/ml which is at or near the saturation point for cystine in the genet *Genetta tigrina*. In contrast to the cystinuria in man, dog and mink there is no evidence of cystine stones in genets. In an attempt to resolve the anomaly Crawhall and Segal (1965) investigated the urinary amino acids from another *G. tigrina* and a male and a female *G. genetta neumanii* using different methods. They found the urinary excretion of cystine was higher than that normally found in man but not as high as that reported earlier (Datta and Harris, 1953). The discrepancy was partially accounted for by the occurrence of 3-sulfocysteine (cysteine-*S*-sulfonate) which would not have been distinguished from cystine by the methods employed by Datta and Harris (1953). Elliot *et al.* (1968) reported the cystine content of the urine of one genet to be 470 mg/ml. This is 4–5 times that found in the urine from normal humans and is in the range where cystine stones may be expected to occur (Harris and Warren, 1953) (3-sulfocysteine would not be measured by the technique they employed). They suggest genet urine contains a substance which inhibits crystallization.

13.2.4. BLUE-DIAPER SYNDROME. TRYPTOPHAN MALABSORPTION

Two siblings only have been described with this defect, which is apparently localized in the specific mechanism for the intestinal absorption of tryptophan (Michael *et al.*, 1962). Despite similarities in symptoms resulting from the tryptophan malabsorption this disorder is quite distinct from Hartnup disease in most respects. In particular no abnormalities in the intestinal absorption of other amino acids were observed and only normal levels of amino acids were found in the urine.

Both patients presented (at 7 and 9 months of age respectively) with failure to thrive. They had a history of recurrent unexplained fever and infections, marked irritability, constipation and secondary defects in calcium metabolism. Each had extensive nephrocalcinosis associated with hypercalcemia, azotemia, a considerable reduction of glomerular filtration rate and a high phosphate clearance. The hypercalcemia improved and was controlled on a diet low in calcium and vitamin D.

The interrelationship between tryptophan malabsorption and the hypercalcemia is obscure. Possible explanations have been discussed by Drummond *et al.* (1964).

The symptoms of nicotinamide deficiency, psychological disturbances and cerebellar ataxia found in Hartnup disease (see pp. 758–762) were not

TABLE 1. METABOLIC PRODUCTS DERIVED FROM BREAKDOWN OF UNABSORBED AMINO ACIDS BY COLONIC BACTERIA IN DISORDERS OF INTESTINAL ABSORPTION OF AMINO ACIDS

Disorder (syndrome)	Amino acid ingested in excess	Derivatives in feces	Derivatives in urine
Cystinuria	Lysine	Cadaverine Piperidine	Cadaverine (occasionally) Piperidine
	Ornithine	Putrescine Pyrrolidine	Putrescine (occasionally) Pyrrolidine
	Arginine	Citrulline Ornithine Putrescine Pyrrolidine	Citrulline Putrescine (occasionally) Pyrrolidine
"Blue Diaper"		Indole	Indolylacetamide
			Indican (indoxyl sulphate) bis-Indolyl-indoxyl
Hartnup and "Blue Diaper"	Tryptophan	Tryptamine Indolyl-3-acetic acid Indolyl-propionic acid Indolyl-lactic acid	Indolyl-3-acetic acid Indolylacetylglutamine Indolyl-3-acrylic acid Indolylacrylylglycine
Hartnup	Phenylalanine	β-Phenylethyl-amine Benzoic acid	Phenylacetylglutamine Hippuric acid
	Tyrosine	Tyramine	*p*-Hydroxyphenylacetic acid and other phenolic acids
Methionine malabsorption	Methionine	α-Hydroxybutyric acid	

(After Milne, 1964, 1968)

present. The possibility that they may develop with age in these patients still exists. Starting from infancy an unusual bluish coloration of the napkins (diapers) of each child was observed (hence the syndrome name). The dye (indigotin) derives from the oxidative condensation of two molecules of indican which was present in excess in the urine of these patients.

The two patients described were male; a female sibling had intermittent blue staining of the napkins but none of the other symptoms shown by her brothers. The mother showed a high excretion of several metabolites of the kynurenine pathway which were lowered following administration of neomycin (see below).

Evidence for tryptophan malabsorption in these patients is similar to that for the same phenomena in Hartnup patients on a normal diet. Stools contained elevated levels of tryptophan and its metabolites (Table 1). The urine contained normal levels of tryptophan but elevated levels of the indolic metabolites, particularly indican and indole-3-acetic acid. Oral loading with tryptophan caused an increase in the fecal excretion of tryptophan and indoles and an increased urinary excretion of indoles which was particularly marked late in the 24-hr period following administration. The excretion of indolic metabolites was reduced almost to normal following on intravenous neomycin. Plasma levels of tryptophan after oral doses of the amino acid were lower than normal.

There was a striking difference between the effects of oral and intravenous administration of tryptophan on the urinary excretion of metabolites of the kynurenine pathway. In normal infants the excretion is similar for both routes of administration but in a patient the excretion rate of metabolites was several times higher after intravenous loading. This difference in response was not abolished by oral administration of neomycin. From these observations it appears that less tryptophan is available for bodily metabolism (mainly in the liver) when given orally to the patient and is thus further evidence for defective tryptophan absorption. Slightly raised levels of kynurenine pathway intermediates were found when patients were given normal diets, but as these returned to normal after neomycin it is apparent that these metabolites were due to action of colonic bacteria.

13.2.5. HARTNUP DISEASE: DEFECTIVE ABSORPTION OF MONOAMINOMONOCARBOXYLIC ACIDS

Hartnup disease, so named after the family of the first patient (Baron *et al.*, 1956), is a disorder of intestinal and renal tubular transport of tryptophan and other monoaminomonocarboxylic acids. An extensive review was presented by Jepson (1966).

The diagnostic feature of Hartnup disease is the *pattern* of amino-aciduria, as well as the *quantity* of each amino acid excreted. Due to raised renal clearances, alanine, serine, threonine, asparagine, glutamine, valine, leucine, isoleucine, phenylalanine, tyrosine, tryptophan, histidine and citrulline are excreted in excessive amounts (approximately 5–10 times normal). Plasma levels of these amino acids are normal or reduced (Cusworth and Dent, 1960). The excretion of other amino acids is normal and there is no proteinuria. Other manifestations are intermittent and variable. Renal and bladder stones are not found since the amino acids involved are reasonably soluble in urine (cf. cystinuria). Products, principally indoles, arising from the degradation of unabsorbed tryptophan by colonic microorganisms (see below) are found frequently in the urine following high oral intakes of tryptophan (Table 1) (Asatoor *et al.*, 1963). Though suggestive of Hartnup disease, indoluria is not diagnostic as often suggested, since it is found in other disorders, e.g. phenylketonuria (Bessman and Tada, 1960), blue-diaper syndrome (Drummond *et al.*, 1964).

Aminoaciduria presumably occurs from birth, but patients most commonly present when older (although usually before 10 years) with a red scaly rash on exposed surfaces of the skin, similar to that of dietary pellagra. It is cured completely by administering nicotinamide (40–400 mg/day). Other symptoms include headaches, poor concentration, reversible cerebellar ataxia and electroencephalographic abnormalities, as well as psychological changes ranging from emotional instability to delirium. The extent to which these symptoms may be attributed to nicotinamide deficiency or to toxic metabolites is still unclear (see Milne, 1968). Poor diets, exposure to sunlight, fever (Baron *et al.*, 1956), sulfo-namide therapy (Henderson, 1958) and psychologic stress all appear to precipitate the skin and psycho-neurological abnormalities. Several patients are mentally retarded but others have normal intelligence and ability; mental deterioration with age appears to be the exception rather than the rule (Jepson, 1966).

Statistical evidence for reduced stature in Hartnup patients has been reported (Colliss *et al.*, 1963) and poor nutrition has been seen in others. These factors may be due to the wastage of essential amino acids in the stools and urine and nicotinamide deficiency secondary to the loss of tryptophan.

The most effective treatment is simply to maintain an adequate level of nutrition. Apart from providing replacement doses of nicotinamide, administration of additional nicotinamide is of little benefit.

13.2.5.1. *Genetics*

Milne (1969) has collated known cases which total thirty-six. The patients, twenty-three girls and thirteen boys, are from thirty-two families and the number of offspring totals eighty. Several inbred marriages have been recorded (see Jepson, 1966). These family trees strongly suggest an autosomal recessive mode of inheritance.

Gross abnormalities in heterozygotes have not been reported. A normal response to tryptophan loading tests is found (although Wong and Pillai, 1966, have reported an exception). Urinary excretion of amino acids is also normal.

Photosensitivity has been reported in a number of relatives (aunts and uncles) (Weyers and Bickel, 1958; Halvorsen and Halvorsen, 1963; Pomeroy *et al.*, 1968).

13.2.5.2. *Defective intestinal absorption*

Intestinal absorption of tryptophan and other monoaminomonocarboxylic acids is not normal in patients with Hartnup disease although the nature and extent of the defect (i.e. which amino acids are affected) are yet to be determined. Evidence suggesting defective absorption is based on the following observations:

1. Following an oral loading dose of tryptophan, histidine or phenylalanine there was a delayed and incomplete rise in blood levels of these amino acids and increased amounts were found in the stool (Milne *et al.*, 1960; Wong and Pillai, 1966; Navab and Asatoor, 1970).
2. The total amount of free amino acids, particularly tryptophan and phenylalanine, in the stools of patients was many times normal and the pattern of excretion closely mirrored the (abnormal) pattern of amino acids found in the urine of the same patients (Scriver, 1965). The amount of each amino acid excreted is dependent on intake level: on low levels or on an ordinary diet only normal excretion was found (Seakins and Ersser, 1967).
3. Stools and urine of patients contain abnormally high levels of metabolites (summarized in Table 1) ultimately derived from tryptophan, phenylalanine and tyrosine following fermentation by colonic microorganisms, particularly *Escherichia coli*. The pathways by

which these metabolites are produced have been reviewed extensively by Jepson (1966) (see also Milne, 1964, 1968). The metabolites in the urine are absorbed from the colon and excreted intact or else further metabolized by the liver and then excreted. Intravenous loading with tryptophan, for instance, caused no increase in urinary indicans and treatment of patients with orally administered antibiotics such as neomycin (Shaw *et al.*, 1960) or chlortetracycline (Baron *et al.*, 1956) reduced the excretion of these metabolites in urine and feces to normal levels. This suggests that Hartnup patients absorb tryptophan, phenylalanine and tyrosine more slowly from the small intestine than normals, thus allowing more to pass through to the colon for metabolism by microorganisms.

Thus, patients with Hartnup disease have defective intestinal absorption of certain amino acids but it cannot be stated with certainty that this is a primary defect although it is strongly indicated by analogy with the renal tubular defect. Since there is a rise in blood tryptophan following oral loading, some is absorbed. However, this is not necessarily contrary to the hypothesis of a primary defect if it is accepted that two mechanisms exist in the intestinal mucosa (in addition to passive diffusion) for the absorption of tryptophan: the first a specific mechanism for the absorption of tryptophan alone which is defective in "blue-diaper syndrome" (see above) and a second rather non-specific mechanism for monoamino-monocarboxylic acids (including tryptophan) with the latter mechanism only absent in Hartnup patients. Recent investigations of Asatoor and colleagues (Asatoor *et al.*, 1970a, b; Navab and Asatoor, 1970) have shown phenylalanine, tryptophan and histidine are absorbed at rates approaching normal when given orally as the dipeptides phenylalanyl-phenylalanine, glycyl-tryptophan and β-alanyl-L-histidine (carnosine), respectively. The absorption of these peptides is thus by a different mechanism to that for the free amino acids. The relative importance of this mechanism in the absorption of peptides from protein digestion is not known for the normal individuals but it must assume greater importance in Hartnup patients in the absorption of essential amino acids.

In vitro studies on the absorption of amino acids by intestinal biopsy specimens from patients will be of particular interest in pinpointing exactly which amino acids are involved and the degree to which the absorption of each is impaired. The problems of obtaining suitable tissue from, or carrying out further investigations on, patients who are outwardly normal have been outlined by Milne (1968).

Tarlow *et al.* (1970) demonstrated in another Hartnup patient that an "affected" amino acid (in this case tyrosine) is better absorbed when given as the dipeptide (glycyl-L-tyrosine). Further, they demonstrated that the intestinal mucosa obtained by per oral biopsy is able to accumulate histidine for which there is a transport defect when it is presented as the dipeptide. It was found that the uptake of histidine was three times greater when the tissue was incubated in glycylhistidine than in an equivalent concentration of histidine. The tissue concentrations of histidine exceeded the medium concentration only when histidine was present as the dipeptide.

13.2.6. OASTHOUSE SYNDROME: METHIONINE MALABSORPTION

Two patients, both female, with an isolated intestinal defect in methionine absorption have been reported (Smith and Strang, 1958; Hooft *et al.*, 1964, 1965, 1968). Both had white hair and blue eyes and exhibited similar symptoms of severe mental retardation, edema, attacks of hyperpnea, generalized convulsions and episodic diarrhea. The urine had a peculiar but characteristic smell similar to an oast house; the cause was traced to the abnormal presence of alpha-hydroxybutyric acid, a bacterial product resulting from methionine metabolism in the colon. The patient of Smith and Strang (1958) demonstrated deranged phenylalanine metabolism. The ferric chloride test for phenylpyruvic acid was positive and the urine contained elevated levels of phenylalanine, and tyrosine. These features were absent in the patient of Hooft *et al.* (1964) and, as Milne (1968) suggests in retrospect, the former patient possibly had phenylketonuria in addition to methionine malabsorption.

The investigations of Hooft and colleagues have provided considerable insight into the disorder. Symptoms continued while a high intake of methionine was maintained. Large amounts of alpha-hydroxybutyric acid were detected in both urine and feces and methionine and branch chain amino acids in the feces alone. Pathological aminoaciduria was not observed.

After some time on a methionine-poor diet the diarrhea disappeared and the fecal excretion of amino acids and alpha-hydroxybutyric acid returned to normal. During 12 months of the diet there was continuous clinical improvement, diarrhea or convulsions did not recur, the white hair darkened and the electroencephalographic abnormalities improved.

After an oral load of methionine there was profuse diarrhea with an increase in stool weight, the excretion of alpha-hydroxybutyric acids, nitrogen, methionine sulfoxides and a general rise in the level of most amino acids. Two to three days following the loading test there was a rise in both fecal and urinary alpha-hydroxybutyric acids. These changes were not found when a similar dose was given to normal children or children with other disorders such as phenylketonuria, gastroenteritis, mental retardation of unknown origin or when other amino acids were given, particularly those which could theoretically be metabolized to alpha-hydroxybutyrate (glutamic acid, isoleucine, serine, threonine, homoserine and homocysteine). It was concluded that the intestinal defect was specific for the absorption of methionine and the unabsorbed methionine was the source of alpha-hydroxybutyrate found in the feces and urine as a result of its metabolism in the colon.

Some methionine *is* absorbed, however, since there is a normal rise in plasma levels following loading. Whether this indicates a partial defect in a single mechanism for methionine absorption or the presence of a second less active mechanism is not known. There is no evidence that a similar defect is present in the kidney.

13.2.7. INTESTINAL MALABSORPTION OF PROLINE AND HYDROXYPROLINE IN PATIENTS WITH A SPECIFIC RENAL IMINOGLYCINURIA

Iminoglycinuria resulting from a specific defect of renal tubular absorption (not to be confused with hyper-prolinemia; see Efron, 1966) has been reported in six infants (Tada *et al.*, 1965; Morikawa *et al.*, 1966; Scriver and Wilson, 1967; Goodman *et al.*, 1967; Rosenberg *et al.*, 1968). The fact that all patients showed raised renal clearances for glycine, proline and hydroxyproline despite normal plasma levels of these amino acids links these patients together. The pedigrees indicate an autosomal recessive mode of transmission. However, as Rosenberg *et al.* (1968) point out, several clinical and biochemical differences exist between patients and it is probable that future studies will reveal that the abnormal phenotypes may be due to more than a single mutant genotype.

Patients ranged in age from 1 to 42 years of age, were of oriental or caucasian origin and of both sexes. Four of the six had mental retardation although this may be an incidental finding since some patients were detected during routine urine examination in mental institutions. Scriver and Wilson (1967), Goodman *et al.* (1967) and Rosenberg *et al.* (1968) reported that parents or children of affected subjects excreted increased quantities of glycine but not proline or hydroxyproline in the urine.

However, Tada *et al.* (1965) examined the parents of one affected child and found no increase in glycine excretion.

13.2.7.1. *Intestinal defects*

Patients with iminoglycinuria were investigated for intestinal absorption defects, unfortunately with conflicting results. Morikawa *et al.* (1966) investigated absorption of proline, hydroxyproline and glycine in one of their three patients. Each amino acid was tested independently by giving an oral load (0.1 g/kg body weight). In order to minimize bacterial metabolism of any unabsorbed amino acids in the colon, kanamycin was given orally for 5 days prior to and during the test. Following the administration of each amino acid there was a rise in its level in the stools over the next 24 hr. A similar finding was not made in normal controls. The absorption of tyrosine and arginine by patients was normal. There was also a tendency (as seen in the urinary excretion following intravenous loading) for either proline, hydroxyproline or glycine to cause an increase in the fecal excretion of the other two amino acids. Even under basal conditions, slightly elevated levels of fecal proline and glycine (but not hydroxyproline) were found. The latter finding may be due to low levels of hydroxyproline in the Japanese diet.

Goodman *et al.* (1967) observed that there was a small and delayed rise of plasma proline following an oral loading dose (0.1 g proline/kg body weight). Furthermore, when the patient was given a diet (gelatine) with a high content of proline, hydroxyproline and glycine, there was a raised level of proline but not hydroxyproline or glycine in the stools collected over the following 24 hr. These findings suggest an absorption defect for proline, but not of hydroxyproline and glycine. This is in contrast to the results obtained by Morikawa *et al.* (1966). Furthermore, Rosenberg *et al.* (1968) found completely normal intestinal absorption in their patient despite intensive investigations. After oral loads of glycine or proline these amino acids were not detected in the feces and there was a normal rise in the plasma levels of each. A jejunal mucosal specimen obtained by per oral biopsy accumulated glycine-2-^{14}C to concentrations similar to that from a normal control.

The reason for the presence of intestinal defects in some patients and absence in others is unknown. It is possible that the presence of another transport system in the intestine masks the defect, or that more than one type of genetic defect occurs which alters the gene product responsible for the shared transport of glycine and the amino acids (Rosenberg *et al.*, 1967).

13.2.8. DEFECTIVE INTESTINAL TRANSPORT OF LYSINE IN LOWE'S SYNDROME

Since the original description by Lowe *et al.* (1952) more than fifty cases have been reported (see Chutorian and Rowland, 1966) of a syndrome characterized by mental retardation, hypotonia, cataracts, glaucoma, renal disease, metabolic acidosis, proteinuria, generalized hyperaminoaciduria and organicaciduria. The pattern of aminoaciduria is variable and appears to be of the overflow type. The disorder is inherited as a sex-linked trait present in the male only (see, however, reports of presumed diagnosis in three females: Svorc *et al.*, 1967).

Recent investigations of Bartsocas *et al.* (1969) suggest that a partial defect of intestinal absorption of lysine and arginine but not glycine exists in these patients. Lysine and arginine were absorbed against a concentration gradient by intestinal biopsy specimens obtained from two patients by per oral biopsy but the amount accumulated was only 50% that of normal. The absorption of glycine was completely normal. The significance of these intestinal defects is uncertain and they may in fact be secondary or even incidental to the other defects. More patients, particularly the few females reported, need to be investigated before any conclusion can be made.

13.3. DEFECTIVE TRIGLYCERIDE ABSORPTION

13.3.1. DEFECTIVE TRIGLYCERIDE ABSORPTION IN PATIENTS WITH CONGENITAL ABSENCE OF BETA-LIPOPROTEIN (BASSEN–KORNZWEIG SYNDROME; A-BETA-LIPOPROTEINEMIA)

Bassen and Kornzweig (1950) described a syndrome consisting of steatorrhea, atypical retinitis pigmentosa, ataxia, neuropathy and abnormally shaped erythrocytes. Later, Salt *et al.* (1960) reported the associated and extremely important feature of serum lipoprotein deficiency. Reviews of this disorder have been presented by Isselbacher *et al.* (1964), Farquhar and Ways (1966) and Sturman (1968).

13.3.1.1. *Clinical features*

In early childhood, symptoms of fat malabsorption predominate. Steatorrhea is gross and 15–20% of the ingested fat is excreted in the stools. Intestinal lipase and bile salts are normal. Intestinal mucosa obtained by per oral biopsy have villi of normal shape and length but the columnar cells are distended with lipid droplets. Glucose absorption is normal and xylose borderline. The serum is clear; total cholesterol, phospholipid and triglyceride concentrations are very low. Chylomicra do not appear after a meal containing fat. Beta-lipoprotein cannot be detected in the serum (Salt *et al.*, 1960; Mabry *et al.*, 1960) and lipoprotein is reduced to about half its normal concentration. Estimation of individual plasma phospholipids shows a relative decrease in phosphatidyl choline and an increase in sphingomyelin; the amount of linoleic acid in phosphatidyl choline is greatly reduced (Ways *et al.*, 1963; Jones and Ways, 1967). The total concentration on non-esterified fatty acids is normal or slightly reduced (Salt *et al.*, 1960). Vitamin E and the carotenoid pigments, which are transported with the triglycerides, are absent from the serum and vitamin A levels in the serum are low.

Fifty per cent or more of red cells of patients are present as *acanthocytes* (cells with a spiny surface). Their shape prevents rouleaux formation and produces an unusually low sedimentation rate. These cells have a normal or slightly decreased life span, osmotic and acid fragility but increased susceptibility to mechanical trauma and rate of destruction in lysolecithin hemolysis tests. The lipid composition of the red cells is abnormal with a decrease in lecithin and an increase in sphingomyelin content. In addition, the linoleic fraction of the phospholipid fatty acid is markedly reduced (Ways *et al.*, 1963). These findings reflect plasma concentrations. An exchange in lipids between red cells and plasma probably occurs (see Reed, 1959). However, acanthocytes retain their structure when placed in normal serum and similarly normal cells do not become acanthocytes when placed in patient's serum. The structure of acanthocytes, however, can be converted into normal erythrocytes by treatment with nonionic detergents (Switzer and Eder, 1962).

Neurological abnormalities of ataxia, intention tremors, nystagmus and absence of deep tendon reflexes which resemble closely Friedreich's ataxia develop between the ages of 5 and 11 years and become progressively more debilitating with age. These symptoms are associated with degeneration of posterior and lateral columns of spinal chord and spinocerebellar changes (Singer *et al.*, 1952; Schwartz *et al.*, 1963; Sobrevilla *et al.*, 1964).

Progressive retinal abnormalities, affecting the macular and the periphery, usually appear at 11 years or older. These include pigmentary degeneration, impaired dark adapation and abnormal electroretinogram (Kornzweig and Bassen, 1957; Rey, 1961; Wolff *et al.*, 1964; and others).

Diagnosis is made on direct demonstration of absence of serum lipoprotein and the combination of symptoms. No single symptom is pathognomic although a serum cholesterol level of less than 60 mg/100 ml in cases of unexplained steatorrhea, retinitis pigmentosa or Friedreich-like ataxia makes the diagnosis likely (Lloyd, 1968). No known therapy is successful in stemming the neurological disturbances and treatment is restricted to improving the nutritional status of the patient. Generally, patients prefer a low fat diet which in addition is beneficial and helps reduce steatorrhea and improves growth and development (Forsyth *et al.*, 1965). In children or older patients where a higher calorie intake is needed, medium chain triglycerides (which are readily absorbed—see later) may be given as a supplement or replacement for the long chain fats (Isselbacher *et al.*, 1964). Linoleic acid should always be given with medium chain triglycerides as they contain no essential fatty acids. Large doses of water-miscible preparations of vitamin A (20,000 units/day) and vitamin E (1.5 g DL-α-Tocopherol acetate/day) should be given as well as additional vitamin K and vitamin D.

13.3.1.2. *Genetics*

The syndrome of congenital absence of beta-lipoprotein as described is inherited as an autosomal recessive disorder (see Farquhar and Ways, 1966). Heterozygotes have normal levels of beta-lipoprotein and are asymptomatic. No racial predilection is apparent.

In addition to the congenital *absence* of beta-lipoprotein there probably exists a distinct spectrum of conditions with varying degrees of beta-lipoprotein *deficiency* and accompanying symptoms (Kuo and Basset, 1962; Tolentino *et al.*, 1964; Van Buchem *et al.*, 1966). These disorders are probably distinct and patients are not heterozygotes of the above disease. The term Bassen–Kornzweig syndrome is normally restricted to cases where serum beta-lipoprotein is absent.

13.3.1.3. *Intestinal defect*

The defect in fat absorption in these patients is not absolute and 70–80% of ingested fat is absorbed after a normal to high fat meal. However, the constant steatorrhea is distinctly pathological. The malabsorption of fat in these patients is, as discussed below, related to defective transport but why the defect is partial is still not known, although absorption of the medium chain fatty acids via the portal system (not normally functional for the absorption of long-chain triglycerides) explains the absorption of some (see Farquhar and Ways, 1966). It seems likely that this route assumes greater importance for absorption of all fatty acids in patients (Kayden and Medick, 1969).

The defect is thought to be located in the process which translocates reconstituted triglycerides from the absorptive cells of the intestine into the lacteals rather than defective intraluminal digestion of fat or absorption into the epithelial cells. Evidence which suggests this may be summarized as follows:

1. Concentrations of pancreatic lipase and bile salts in intestinal juice are normal and *in vivo* and *in vitro* cause the progressive hydrolysis of triglycerides to monoglycerides and free fatty acids (Salt *et al.*, 1960; Rey, 1961; Lamy *et al.*, 1961).
2. Using ^{14}C-palmitate, Isselbacher *et al.* (1964) demonstrated that this fatty acid, at least, is absorbed and incorporated into triglyceride within the epithelial cell. Whether or not the rate of absorption is normal is not known.
3. Microscopic examination of frozen sections of intestinal mucosa which have been suitably stained show villi of normal shape and length but the epithelial cells are filled with triglyceride droplets, especially at the villous tips. By contrast, practically no fat droplets are found in the intercellular spaces or lacteals of the submucosa or lamina propria (see Isselbacher *et al.*, 1964). These findings differ considerably from other cases of steatorrhea, such as coeliac disease, where partial or total villous atrophy is present but lipid droplets in the mucosal cells are absent.

   Even on normal diets the concentration of fat in the mucosal cells is elevated and tends to remain so even after 14 days on a low fat diet (Saunders *et al.*, 1966; Ways *et al.*, 1967).
4. Following a fat meal, chylomicrons are not found in the serum and no rise in serum lipids occurs. Using the electron microscope, chylomicrons were found to be absent from the intercellular spaces of the absorptive cells, within the lamina propria or the lacteals of the villous cores (Isselbacher *et al.*, 1964; Dobbins, 1966). Therefore, it appears that chylomicrons are not formed. Distension of the Golgi vacuoles with lipophilic material normally seen in similar circumstances was also absent (Dobbins, 1966).

This evidence suggests that the defect is related to the inability of cells to form chylomicrons. Since beta-lipoprotein is absent from the serum of these patients and beta-lipoprotein is a constituent of chylomicrons, fat malabsorption is possibly a secondary phenomenon to the lipoprotein deficiency. Probably, beta-lipoprotein is produced intracellularly as the chylomicrons are formed. Sabesin and Isselbacher (1965) found that puromycin (an inhibitor of protein synthesis) when fed to rats produced symptoms of vacuolization of the intestinal mucosa and a fall in serum triglyceride which were similar to those found in patients. They suggested that the defect may be one of failure to synthesize the protein moiety ("B" protein). However, Lees (1967) found a beta-globulin in serum "B" protein and suggested the alternative hypothesis that the protein molecule is produced but defective. Dole and Hamlin (1962) suggest a defect in the synthetic step which coats the chylomicron with protein. This hypothesis is still tenable.

13.4. DEFECTIVE MINERAL ABSORPTION (CATIONS)

13.4.1. INTESTINAL MALABSORPTION OF MAGNESIUM

Seven cases of hypomagnesemia with a secondary hypocalcemia have been reported where evidence suggests that the disorder is due primarily to a selective intestinal malabsorption of magnesium (Freeman and Pearson, 1966; Paunier *et al.*, 1965, 1968; Salet *et al.*, 1966; Friedman *et al.*, 1967; Skyberg *et al.*, 1967, 1968; Fournet, 1968; Celander *et al.*, 1969). Other known causes of hypomagnesemia have been excluded. The first six patients, which included one set of siblings, were male. This had suggested a possible sex-linked mode of inheritance. The most recent patient, however, was female and the mode of inheritance is now uncertain. The patients presented between 2 and 6 weeks of age with symptoms dominated by tetanic convulsions, low serum calcium and even lower serum magnesium levels. The delay from birth in the onset of symptoms may be due to the time taken to deplete the magnesium stores derived from the mother. Normal calcium and magnesium levels were restored (with concomitant disappearance of symptoms) by administering magnesium parenterally or by giving an oral supplement of 25–30 mEq of Mg^{2+} per day (approximately 3–5 times the normal intake). Symptoms returned after restoring the patients' intake of magnesium to a normal level even after 3 years or more of treatment (Paunier *et al.*, 1968). The hypocalcemia could not be corrected by administration of oral or parenteral calcium alone. Intramuscular parathormone (Skyberg *et al.*, 1968; Fournet, 1968) or vitamin D (Paunier *et al.*, 1965, 1968) raised the level of calcium but not of magnesium. The absorption of fat, glucose, xylose, vitamin B_{12} and calcium by patients was normal (Paunier *et al.*, 1968). Liver damage was reported by Skyberg *et al.* (1968) and some mild histological changes in the kidneys by Paunier *et al.* (1968). These were considered to be secondary to the magnesium deficiency and not the cause of it. Histological examination of intestinal mucosa obtained by per oral biopsy from a patient showed some patches with mild villous atrophy (Skyberg *et al.*, 1968); the findings were probably not significant. Levels of muscle Mg^{2+} and K^+ were lower in a patient than normal (Paunier *et al.*, 1968).

Evidence that the hypomagnesemia is due to an intestinal absorption defect rather than a pathological loss due to urinary or gastrointestinal excretion is based on the observations: (1) that parenterally administered radioactive magnesium (^{28}Mg) is apparently metabolized normally and normal amounts only are excreted by the kidneys or into the gastrointestinal tract (Skyberg, 1968), and (2) that orally administered Mg^{2+} is poorly absorbed by all patients investigated. Skyberg *et al.* (1968b) found that the fecal recovery of labeled magnesium administered orally amounted to 88% as compared with 33% and 29% in two normal controls of the same age. Only 0.2% of the dose appeared in the urine after 4 days whereas the normal control excreted about 10% of the dose. (More detailed work confirming the above findings and additional information on the nature of the disorder have been reported by Stromme *et al.*, 1969.)

The nature and exact location in the intestinal mucosa of the defect are not known. Since the patients are successfully treated by increasing the level of dietary intake of magnesium some absorption takes place but probably by diffusion directed along a concentration gradient. It is interesting to note that the defect is selective for the absorption of magnesium and that the absorption of calcium is apparently unaffected. Experiments in rats, rabbits and guinea pigs have suggested that mechanisms for the absorption of these metals have some step in common or are perhaps identical (Schachter and Rosen, 1959; Alcock and Mac-Intyre, 1960).

13.4.2 COPPER MALABSORPTION: MENKES'S KINKY-HAIR SYNDROME

The syndrome originally described by Menkes *et al.* (1962) and later reported by others (Bray, 1965; Aguilar *et al.*, 1966; Seelenfreund *et al.*, 1968; Wesenberg *et al.*, 1969; Danks *et al.*, 1972a, b) has been shown recently to be due to copper deficiency consequent upon defective intestinal malabsorption of this cation (Danks *et al.*, 1972a, b, 1973).

Menkes's syndrome is inherited as an X-linked recessive trait (Menkes *et al.*, 1962); in Victoria, Australia the incidence was calculated to be approximately 1:35,000 live births (Danks *et al.*, 1972a). The syndrome is characterized by progressive mental deterioration, disturbance of muscle tone, pili torti (kinky hair), hypothermia, scorbutic-like changes in the metaphyses of the long bones and arterial disease. The latter is manifest as arterial tortuosity with fragmentation of the internal elastic lamina and thickening of the intima in the most severely affected vessels. Death usually occurs before 3 years of age. Treatment may be possible with parenteral and perhaps oral copper but research is still needed to determine which compounds are to be administered and at what rate. Danks *et al.* (1972a) point out that early diagnosis and treatment will be required to prevent structural brain damage and that it may be necessary to start treatment before birth since early onset of symptoms suggests these babies lack the large store of copper present in the liver of the newborn.

Patients have low levels of serum, liver and brain copper which are not restored to normal by oral loading with copper. Intravenous copper is apparently handled normally with some clinical improvement. Following an oral dose of radioactive copper (^{64}Cu) there was a subnormal rise in radioactivity in the serum and most was excreted in the stools. Intestinal mucosa obtained by per oral biopsy, however, contained abnormally high levels of copper. While the precise nature of this defect is obscure, these findings suggest that the intestinal defect is localized in the mechanism for translocation from the mucosal cells to other tissues (in this it is reminiscent of iron malabsorption in mice—see section 13.4.3) and not at the point of entry into the epithelial cells.

Cultured fibroblasts from patients and heterozygotes show metachromasia which disappears during continued culture. Danks *et al.* (1973) suggest that this may be "an indication of defective cellular metabolism consequent upon copper deficiency, and is gradually corrected by passive diffusion of copper from the medium during many days of culture". These findings suggest that the defect is present in these cells also and thus provides useful material for the study of this disorder. This finding may also be useful in heterozygote recognition.

13.4.3. IRON: IRON MALABSORPTION IN MICE

Hereditary anemia in mice derived from the male descendants of a daughter of a single X-irradiated male mouse was reported by Falconer and Isaacson (1962). The mutant gene (symbol sla) is carried on the X-chromosome and the anemic mice (hemizygous males and homozygous females) show symptoms of iron deficiency despite an adequate intake of dietary iron.

The anemia, which occurs soon after birth but tends to regress with age, can be treated with parenteral iron. The hematological and biological abnormalities in these mice have been investigated by Bannerman, Pinkerton and colleagues (Bannerman and Pinkerton, 1967; Pinkerton and Bannerman, 1967a, b; Bannerman *et al.*, 1968; Pinkerton, 1968) and the genetics by Grewal (1962).

Mean corpuscular hemoglobin and mean cell volume were markedly reduced, siderocytes and sideroblasts were absent and histochemical studies indicated severe depletion of iron stores, particularly of the spleen. In addition low levels of serum iron, an increased serum iron binding capacity and increased concentrations of free erythrocyte protoporphyrin were found. Radioactive iron given intramuscularly was cleared from the plasma more rapidly than normal and utilization of this tracer as determined by its reappearance in the peripheral blood was also more rapid and more complete.

When given an oral dose as the ferrous salt the mice retain (as measured by whole body counting) less ^{59}Fe than do the homozygous normal (wild type) mice. No reduction in Fe^{2+} absorption was observed in heterozygous carriers. Absorption of radioactive cobalt (^{57}Co), copper (^{64}Cu), zinc (^{65}Zn) and fat (^{131}I-labeled triolein) was normal in anemic mice (Bannerman *et al.*, 1968). An examination of the intestinal mucosa of the anemic mice showed that the gross anatomical appearance of the mucosa was normal but there was clear histological evidence of excessive deposition of iron in the luminal borders of the duodenal and upper jejunal mucosal epithelium (Pinkerton, 1968).

Studies on iron transport by everted sacs from sla mice and suitable controls showed that overall uptake of iron by the mucosa was the same for sla and normal sacs but transport of iron to the inside (serosal surface) of the sac was much decreased in sla (Manis, 1970, 1971). The defect thus appears specific for the absorption of iron and probably involves a single, genetically determined, step in iron absorption. Its exact nature is not known but since large iron deposits were found in the epithelial cells and iron was accumulated by the mucosa of everted sacs but not transported to the serosal medium, the defect is not localized at the point of entry of iron into the cells but in the process for its translocation to other tissues. Manis (1970) speculates on the following explanations for defective serosal transport: (1) the absence of a necessary step in the transport mechanism, (2) the production of a substance which binds iron so effectively so as to make it unavailable for the serosal transfer step, or (3) the production of an inhibitor which decreases the serosal transfer of iron. Elucidation of the underlying defect will greatly increase our knowledge of the mechanism for the intestinal transport of iron.*

A similar disorder in humans has not been reported. Human hypochromic anemias which have points of resemblance to the defect in mice have been discussed by Bannerman and Pinkerton (1967).

13.5. DEFECTIVE MINERAL ABSORPTION (ANIONS)

13.5.1. CHLORIDE: FAMILIAL CHLORIDE DIARRHEA; CHLORIDORRHEA; CONGENITAL ALKALOSIS WITH CHLORIDORRHEA

The characteristic feature of this disorder is the presence of watery diarrhea with an abnormally high concentration of Cl^- in the fecal fluid which exceeds the sum of concentrations of Na^+ and K^+. In most other forms of diarrhea the reverse of this ratio is found (see Evanson and Stanbury, 1965). Known cases (twenty-two in total) have been summarized by Launiala *et al.* (1968) and an autosomal recessive mode of inheritance recorded. The first two patients were reported simultaneously by Darrow (1945) and Gamble *et al.* (1945). The patient originally described by Darrow (1945) still manifests the same metabolic derangements at 11 years of age (Owen, 1964).

Patients are often born prematurely following a pregnancy complicated by hydramnios and suffer considerable weight loss at birth. Diarrhea commences at or soon after birth and persists with varying severity despite any treatment adopted to date. Absence of meconium was reported in some, suggesting the possibility of intrauterine diarrhea (Launiala *et al.*, 1968). The Cl^- concentration of the stools ranges from 30 to 100 mEq/l in the neonatal patient and rises to a rather constant level of 150 mEq/l (approx. $1\frac{1}{2}$ times that of plasma Cl^-) in the elder child. At these concentrations, Cl^- and its accompanying cations act as an osmotic cathartic; a direct relationship is observed between fecal Cl^- content and stool volume (Evanson and Stanbury, 1965). The normal level of Cl^- is approximately 4–38 mEq/l (Wrong and Metcalfe-Gibson, 1965). Hypoelectrolytemia, particularly hypokalemia and hypochloridemia, is present from birth and metabolic alkalosis, often present in the neonate, develops in the first few months of life. These defects are due to the loss of the ions in the feces.

No treatment to date has been successful in stemming the diarrhea

*For further discussion of this topic see Chapter 12, p. 681 (Eds.).

or the chloride loss which continues even after removal of Cl^- from the diet, although one administration of an additional 2–14 mEq/kg body weight/day of KCl usually results in a return to normal of the plasma electrolyte levels and some improvement in growth (Launiala *et al.*, 1968). There is considerable renal involvement although no evidence exists for a defect in renal tubular absorption of Cl^- (see Pasternack and Perheentupa, 1966; Pasternack *et al.*, 1967). Raised levels of urinary K^+ are frequently observed and suggested by Launiala *et al.* (1968) to result from secondary aldosteronism. Vascular and degenerative changes occur and a heavy deposition of calcium is frequent. Cl^- is virtually absent from the urine in the untreated patient but following oral administration (see above) or intravenous infusion of saline the levels of urinary Cl^- return to normal. The urine is usually alkaline with pH between 6 and 8.

The primary defect appears to involve the mechanism which normally reduces the chloride concentration of the colon and rectal contents. Following milk feeding or constant intragastric infusion of a hypotonic solution of NaCl (or KCl) and glucose, there was no net absorption of water or Cl^- and the Cl^- content of the ileal contents was similar to that in the stools. In control infants most Cl^- was absorbed during passage through the ileum. Concentrations of Na^+ and K^+ were similar to normal although net fluxes of these ions were different from controls and presumably due to the lack of net water movement. The ratio $(Na^+) + (K^+)/(Cl^-)$ in the small intestine was 1.0 or less in patients but 1.2–1.4 in normal controls.

This suggests a balance between sodium and potassium ions with the chloride ion whereas in normals other anions were present (Launiala *et al.*, 1968). It is significant, therefore, that the concentrations of intestinal bicarbonate were found to be extremely low in patients and were 1.2–1.8 mEq/l compared to 30–70 mEq/l in normals (Fordtran and Locklear, 1966) and the excretion of bicarbonate in the stools of patients was extremely low and did not exceed 2–4 m mol/day (stool volumes 500–840 ml) (Evanson and Stanbury, 1965) compared to a normal value of approximately 32 mEq/l (Wrong *et al.*, 1965).

Little is known of the mechanisms, particularly in the human, for the intestinal absorption of chloride although there is evidence to suggest "passive" Cl^- as well as "active" Cl^- absorption and secretion in the small intestine. In the large intestine active transport of Cl^- has not been demonstrated and experiments of Curran and Schwartz (1960) have shown that in the rat at least Cl^- transport could be attributed entirely to "passive" diffusion. However, several studies have disclosed an inverse relationship between net Cl^- and net HCO_3^- movements in both small and large intestine which suggests an *exchange* mechanism of absorption and clearly one of these movements must be directed against the transepithelial electrical potential difference. It seems likely that quantitative if not qualitative differences exist in Cl^- transport at different locations in the intestinal tract. Absorption of Na^+, Cl^- and water has been reviewed recently by Shultz and Curran (1968) and Fordtran and Ingelfinger (1968).

The findings of high Cl^- and low HCO_3^- levels in the coronic contents of patients in the presence of normal or near-normal concentration of Na^+, K^+, NH_4^+ and pH are therefore consistent with the hypothesis that the defect is localized at some level of a Cl^-/HCO_3^- exchange mechanism (Evanson and Stanbury, 1965).

Alternatively, Gamble *et al.* (1945), Duyck (1955) and Jeune *et al.* (1967) suggested increased Cl^- section as the underlying defect.

Chloride *can* be absorbed from the gastrointestinal tract, since normal serum chloride levels are restored by the administration of *oral* sodium chloride. When serum chloride levels are raised by parenteral administration there is an increase in fecal chloride. However, these results may also be explained as the result of faulty absorption and of the chloride absorption after oral NaCl being directed down a concentration gradient.

The defect is not a phenomenon secondary to K^+ deficiency (Kelsey, 1954) since restoration of normal serum K^+ levels produced a small but significant change in Cl^- retention but by no means returned Cl^- absorption to normal (Evanson and Stanbury, 1965).

13.5.2. FAMILIAL HYPOPHOSPHATEMIC VITAMIN-D-RESISTANT RICKETS: A PRIMARY DEFECT IN INTESTINAL AND RENAL ABSORPTION OF PHOSPHATE (BY A. FANCONI)*

Defective intestinal absorption of both calcium and phosphate has been proposed as the cause of this still poorly understood disorder. Recent evidence now suggests that impairment of absorption of phosphate rather than of calcium in the renal tubule and intestinal mucosa and possibly other organs may underlie this disease.

The disease has been described by different names such as "familial hypophosphatemia", "idiopathic hypophosphatemic vitamin D refractory rickets", "renal tubular rickets", "familial phosphate diabetes", etc. A recent and extensive review by Williams *et al.* (1966) summarizes current

*Present address: Kinderklinik, Kantonspital, 8400 Winterthur, Switzerland.

opinions about genetic, clinical, pathogenetic and therapeutic aspects of this disorder.

13.5.2.1. *Clinical description*

The first clinical symptoms usually appear at the end of the first year or in the second year of life. Patients are short and have bowed legs and a waddling gait. The longitudinal growth which is usually normal in infancy begins to slow down; the patients never reach a normal adult size. The shortness of stature is nearly entirely limited to the lower extremities (McNair and Stickler, 1969). The femora show an ante- and a laterocurvation. Radiological examination reveals the characteristic metaphyseal lesion of chronic rickets together with a coarse trabecular structure of the long bones. In later years, particularly in untreated cases, the bowing deformities and stunting of the legs increase and often require osteotomy. The head is square-shaped with a prominent forehead. Unlike ordinary vitamin-D-deficiency rickets, there is no muscular weakness or hypotonicity. Tetany never occurs. The general health is not impaired and the patients feel well.

The main *biochemical* finding is a very low serum inorganic phosphorus concentration (usually below 3 mg/100 ml), which is present from infancy, constant in all the cases and necessary for the diagnosis. Urinary phosphorus excretion is relatively increased, resulting in an increased renal phosphate clearance. The serum calcium concentration is always normal, the urinary calcium excretion usually low. There is no proteinuria or hyperaminoaciduria, only exceptionally glucosuria (Dent, 1952) and no further signs of any renal involvement other than the decreased tubular phosphate reabsorption. Plasma pH and electrolytes are normal. The alkaline phosphatase in the serum is elevated as a sign of active rickets.

Hypophosphatemic vitamin-D-resistant rickets has to be distinguished by clinical, radiological and biochemical signs from the following conditions: vitamin-D-deficiency rickets, pseudo-vitamin-D-deficiency rickets, late hypophosphatemic vitamin-D-resistant rickets with hyperglycinuria, hyperazotemic glomerular osteodystrophy, rickets in complex renal tubular disorders as seen in cystinosis, Lowe's syndrome or idiopathic deToni–Debre–Fanconi syndrome, hypophosphatasia, metaphyseal dysostosis.

13.5.2.2. *Genetics*

Although sporadic cases occur, it is well established that vitamin-D-resistant rickets is a hereditary disorder and transmitted by a sex-linked dominant gene (Burnett *et al.*, 1964; Dent and Harris, 1956; Tobler *et al.*, 1956; Williams *et al.*, 1966; Winters *et al.*, 1958).

Affected females are heterozygous, affected males are hemizygous. The ratio of affected females to males is roughly 2:1.

The degree of manifestations varies considerably. The most constant and often only abnormality is hypophosphatemia associated with a diminished renal tubular reabsorption of phosphate. This monosymptomatic form is mainly observed in female patients, particularly in mothers of more severely affected children. In hypophosphatemic males, rickets are nearly always present and the bone deformities are more severe than in females. This resistance of the female to severe bone disease is usually explained by the protective action of the normal allele in the other X-chromosome.

13.5.2.3. *Pathogenetical considerations*

Many balance studies in patients with untreated vitamin-D-resistant rickets (Albright *et al.*, 1937; Dent and Harris, 1956; Royer *et al.*, 1961; Stickler, 1963; and others) show unequivocally that the fecal calcium excretion is strongly increased. The urinary calcium excretion is low. The calcium balance is therefore insufficiently positive for the age of the patient. These changes are identical with those found in untreated vitamin-D-deficiency rickets. The phosphate balance is insufficient also, as increased quantities are excreted both in the feces and the urine. It is generally concluded that the intestinal absorption of calcium and phosphate is impaired. The mechanism of this defect is not known yet.

From these findings, Albright *et al.* (1937) in their original description of the disease, as well as later investigators, postulated the following pathogenesis of this disorder.

The impaired *intestinal calcium absorption* as the primary disturbance leads to a small decrease of the serum calcium concentration which immediately stimulates the secretion of parathyroid hormone. This secondary hyperparathyroidism mobilizes calcium from the bone in order to maintain the serum calcium concentration within the normal range and inhibits the tubular reabsorption of phosphate which lowers the serum phosphate concentration. One of the main arguments in favor of this hypothesis is the hypophosphaturic effect of intravenous infusions of calcium in these patients which has been observed by many investigators (Field and Reiss, 1960; Lafferty *et al.*, 1963; Nigrin *et al.*, 1962; Royer *et al.*, 1961). This effect is generally thought to be produced by a suppression of the increased parathyroid activity. However, Lavender and

Pullman (1963) observed that this suppressive effect on renal phosphate excretion can be achieved by a direct pharmacological action of calcium on the renal tubule, independent of the effect of the serum calcium on the parathyroid glands. There are further strong arguments against the hypothesis of a primary defect of intestinal calcium absorption and secondary hyperparathyroidism:

1. Hypocalcemia is never observed in these patients.
2. Evidence of chronic secondary hyperparathyroidism in the bone is missing.
3. With vitamin D treatment in high doses, the serum phosphate does not reach normal levels, although the intestinal calcium absorption becomes normal in the same way as in vitamin-D-treatment-deficiency rickets.
4. In family members with asymptomatic hypophosphatemia without bone disease, calcium and phosphate balances have been found to be normal (Williams *et al.,* 1966).
5. Serum immunoreactive parathyroid hormone is normal in patients who are not treated with phosphate (Arnaud *et al.,* 1971).

A simpler explanation for the pathogenesis of the constant hypophosphatemia is the hypothesis of a *primary renal tubular defect* of reabsorption of phosphate (Dent, 1952; Fanconi and Girardet, 1952). However, some features of the disease are hardly to be explained by a simple tubular defect, particularly the persistent osteopathy and the failure to grow. An impairment of the intestinal calcium absorption with decreased responsiveness to vitamin D also occurs in chronic hyperazotemic glomerular renal failure. Recent investigations (Avioli *et al.,* 1966; Blunt *et al.,* 1968; DeLuca *et al.,* 1967; Frazer and Kodicek, 1970) on the *metabolism of vitamin D* and the activation of cholecalciferol (vitamin D_3) to 25-OH-cholecalciferol* and 1α, 25-di-OH-cholecalciferol might be able to clarify the mechanism of vitamin D resistance and advance our knowledge about the cause of vitamin-D-resistant rickets.

The complexity of this disease, which affects the renal tubular reabsorption of phosphate, the intestinal absorption of calcium and phosphate, and the texture and growth of bone, points to a more basic and general metabolic defect with a *disturbance of cellular phosphate transport* (Rey and Frezal, 1966), which is supported by the recent investigations by Glorieux and Scriver (1972). They suggest the existence of two components of tubular phosphate reabsorption in the human kidney: a parathyroid hormone-sensitive system which is deficient in hypophosphatemic

*Cf. Chapter 11, pp. 546–547 (Eds.).

resistant rickets, and a parathyroid hormone-resistant but calcium-sensitive system which remains unimpaired. Short *et al.* (1973) demonstrated a similar transport defect for phosphate by the human intestinal mucosa in an *in vitro* incubation study. The primary defect in this disease seems therefore to be an impairment of phosphate transport in the renal tubule, the intestinal mucosa, and possibly other organs.

13.5.2.4. *Treatment*

There is no ideal treatment as yet. Physiological or small therapeutic doses of vitamin D which would cure nutritional rickets are completely ineffective. Since the first description of the disease, *vitamin* D_2, D_3 or *dihydrotachysterol* in pharmacological doses (usually 1 to 3 mg per day) has been given by nearly all authors.* This treatment has a beneficial effect on the radiological and clinical aspect of the rickets, brings the alkaline phosphatase activity in the serum down to normal and normalizes the calcium balance. However, it cannot accelerate growth to a normal rate, normalize the bone structure completely and increase the serum phosphate level to the normal range. The toxic effects of hypercalcemia occur before the serum phosphate becomes normal. Vitamin D treatment can be reduced or even discontinued when growth is completed.

Objections against this treatment have been raised by Nigrin *et al.* (1962) and others because of the dangers of nephrocalcinosis and progressive renal damage, and recently by McNair and Stickler (1969) who also question its therapeutic value. An alternative or additional treatment is the administration of large amounts of neutral phosphate by mouth to increase the intestinal phosphate uptake and the serum phosphate concentration. This therapy has been found useful in adult patients (Nagant de Deuxchaines and Krane, 1967) and in children (Glorieux *et al.,* 1972; McEnery *et al.,* 1972).

13.6. DEFECTIVE VITAMIN ABSORPTION

13.6.1. VITAMIN B_{12}: FAMILIAL SELECTIVE MALABSORPTION OF VITAMIN B_{12} (BY A. G. F. DAVIDSON)†

This rare disorder was first recognized by Gräsbeck *et al.* (1960) and Imerslund (1960), who independently described a syndrome in children

*At present already 1,25-$(OH)_2$-D_3 and related compounds are available for therapeutical purposes (cf. Chapter 11, pp. 546 and 547); these compounds may cause similar hazards as Vitamin D or dihydrotachysterol and, hence, must be dosed most carefully (Eds.).

†Department of Paediatrics, University of British Columbia, Vancouver, Canada.

which was characterized by isolated malabsorption of vitamin B_{12} despite the presence of intrinsic factor, and usually associated with proteinuria. Since that time over fifty additional cases have been reported (see Visakorpi and Furuhjelm, 1968). It is also possible that additional cases have been presented in earlier literature as "pernicious anemia".

Although the classification of vitamin B_{12} deficiency states in childhood is at present not clear, this syndrome can be clearly separated from other B_{12} deficiency states by the demonstration of B_{12} malabsorption despite normal secretion of intrinsic factor and by the absence of other demonstrable small-bowel pathology.

Illness in this syndrome typically starts insidiously, making the exact time of onset difficult to determine. In most cases, anemia was noted in the second year of life, though cases have been reported aged under 6 months (Visakorpi and Furuhjelm, 1968). Frequent symptoms include pallor, weakness, anorexia, vomiting, failure to thrive. Gastrointestinal symptoms are common and the clinical picture may even resemble coeliac disease, but it is felt that these manifestations may be due to the B_{12} deficiency (Visakorpi and Furuhjelm, 1968; Foroozan and Trier, 1967) and that they are not of primary etiological significance. In the Finnish series (Visakorpi and Furuhjelm, 1968), neurological signs were common, especially ataxia and paresthesia, but these are not as prominent in the other cases reported.

Laboratory examinations show typical megaloblastic and macrocytic anemia. Leucopenia and thrombocytopenia are common. Serum B_{12} is low and folic acid normal. The Schilling test shows poor absorption of B_{12} and human or hog intrinsic factor *fails to correct* the absorption defect. Normal activity of intrinsic factor in gastric juice from these patients can be confirmed by administering the juice to patients with true pernicious anemia and observing the normalization of B_{12} absorption which occurs in them. Free gastric acid has been found in almost all cases reported and gastric biopsy is usually normal. Tests for generalized intestinal malabsorption are usually normal.

Slight persistent or intermittent proteinuria is almost invariable and is predominantly due to albumin. No definite cause for this has been found, though there seems to be a high incidence of renal abnormalities found on kidney biopsy or on i.v.p. (Visakorpi and Furuhjelm, 1968). Treatment consists of parenteral administration of vitamin B_{12}.

13.6.1.1. *Genetics*

The first reports on this syndrome noted its familial and congenital nature. Subsequent reports have confirmed its inheritance as an autosomal recessive condition. No abnormalities have been detected in heterozygotes except for one report of slightly decreased B_{12} absorption (Mohamed *et al.*, 1966). A relatively large number of cases have been reported from Scandinavia (Gräsbeck *et al.*, 1960; Imerslund, 1960; Sievens, 1964; Hippe, 1966; Anttila and Salmi, 1967; Visakorpi and Furuhjelm, 1968), which may reflect either increased incidence or increased awareness. A recent report from Israel (Ben-Bassat *et al.*, 1969) has shown an unusually high incidence of 1:1200 among Jews of North African (Sephardim) origin, with a maximum prevalence among 3–15-year-old Israeli Jews of Tunisian origin. Inheritance here also confirmed the autosomal recessive pattern but there was an unusual and unexplained preponderance of males with a male to female ratio of 14:1.

13.6.1.2. *Basic defect*

In normal intestine there is evidence that vitamin B_{12} is absorbed both by the active and passive mechanisms (Herbert, 1968). Passive absorption is probably of insignificant degree and can be considered non-operative with respect to the small amounts present in the usual food sources of B_{12}. Normally, active absorption seems to occur in the ileum in man (Stewart *et al.*, 1967) and to require that the B_{12} be linked to a glycoprotein ("intrinsic factor") which is produced by gastric parietal cells (Moedemaeker *et al.*, 1964). This complex probably consists of a dimer of intrinsic factor containing 2 moles B_{12} per mole of dimer with a molecular weight in the range of 115,000; 97% of the bulk of this complex is due to the intrinsic factor. When the intrinsic factor–B_{12} complex reaches the ileum, it apparently becomes attached to special "receptor sites" on the brush border of the mucosal cells (Herbert *et al.*, 1964). This attachment requires a pH above 5.6 and the presence of ionic calcium (Herbert, 1968). Intrinsic factor alone can also "fit" the receptor sites, but not quite as selectively as does the intrinsic factor–B_{12} complex.

The next stage in B_{12} absorption is not clear but it has been suggested that B_{12} must be split off the intrinsic factor–B_{12} complex (by a "releasing factor") before it is absorbed through the mucosal cell via an active transport process and appears in the portal blood, and that intrinsic factor itself is not normally absorbed (Herbert, 1968; Cooper and Castle, 1960; Highley *et al.*, 1965).

In this syndrome of selective B_{12} malabsorption, intrinsic factor is present and appears to function normally as is evidenced by the ability of gastric juice from these patients to normalize B_{12} absorption in patients with pernicious anemia. The defect therefore seems to lie in the later stages of absorption. Ileal biopsy has failed to show a structural defect (Visakorpi and Furuhjelm, 1968), implying that absorptive failure is at the ultra-structural or the molecular (metabolic) level. The main possibilities seem to be that there is a lack or abnormality of the so-called "receptor sites", or that the splitting of the B_{12}–intrinsic factor complex fails to occur (defect in releasing factor), or that there is some block in the actual B_{12} absorption process.

Antibodies to the intrinsic factor–B_{12} complex have been reported to occur and to cause failure of absorption in an adult with pernicious anemia (Schade *et al.*, 1966) but there is no evidence to suggest that this happens in those patients with selective malabsorption of B_{12} (Editorial in *New Eng. J. Med.*, 1968). Attempts have been made to demonstrate lack of releasing factor in these patients by observing whether normal intestinal juice improves B_{12} absorption, but results have been equivocal (Visakorpi and Furuhjelm, 1968). The lack of positive results here is hardly surprising, however, since if a releasing factor does exist it would not necessarily be found in the intestinal juice but should be located in the cell membrane in a similar manner to the disaccharidases. Finally, a defect at the receptor site or at the membrane transport mechanism was suggested by Gräsbeck and Kvist (1967), because these patients absorb massive oral doses of B_{12} less well than do patients with pernicious anemia.

A recent study (Mackenzie *et al.*, 1972) of ileal mucosal biopsies from one of three brothers with this syndrome has confirmed that ileal mucosa appears normal on light and electron microscopy. Cyanocobalomin uptake studies on homogenates of the biopsies suggest that receptor sites for the *intrinsic factor–B_{12}* complex are normal and that the defect in this syndrome occurs at a stage after the complex attaches to the surface of the ileal cell and before the vitamin appears in the blood. Transcobalamin II levels in the blood were normal, thus also suggesting normal ability of the blood to transport the vitamin.

13.6.2. CONGENITAL MALABSORPTION OF FOLATE

A congenital defect in intestinal absorption of folate was first recorded in a 5-year-old girl (Luhby *et al.*, 1961) and later (Luhby *et al.*, 1965; Luhby and Cooperman, 1967) in her sister. A third case, an 18-year-old girl, was reported by Lanzkowsky *et al.* (1969) and Lanzkowsky (1970).

All patients had symptoms of folic acid deficiency including relapsing megaloblastic anemia and raised urinary levels of formiminoglutamic acid (Figlu) dating from 3 months of age. Patients could not be maintained on a normal diet and required supplements of 10–40 mg folic acid orally or 250 μg intramuscularly per day to achieve hematologic remission. Additional to the defect of intestinal malabsorption of folate all three children had low levels of folic acid in the cerebrospinal fluid which remained low even when serum levels were raised by folate administration. This suggests that a defect in the passage of folate from blood to cerebrospinal fluid is also present. Renal abnormalities have not been reported.

Despite these similarities between patients certain other differences exist which suggest the possibility of different defects of folic acid absorption. The patients of Luhby *et al.* were moderately retarded both physically and mentally and suffered from ataxia and convulsions. Cerebral calcification was not observed. By contrast the patient of Lanzkowsky *et al.* had petit mal and occasional grand mal seizures from 9 years and at 18 years poor articulation and an athetotic movement disorder of the upper limbs resembling extrapyramidal disease but without tremor, ataxia or cerebellar signs. A roentgenogram of the skull showed punctate calcification of the basal ganglia, particularly of the caudate nucleus.

Neurological disorders in the patients of Luhby *et al.* (1961, 1965) were improved by folate administration but the fit frequency in the patient of Lanzkowsky *et al.* (1969) *decreased during folate depletion*. The relationship between folic acid deficiency and mental retardation is uncertain.

Treatment of all patients consisted only of additional folate amounting to 10–40 mg/day given orally or 250 μg/day intramuscularly.

13.6.2.1. *Intestinal defect*

Dietary folate is absorbed primarily from the proximal region of the small intestine in the normal person but how it is absorbed is poorly understood. Current concepts of events occurring during folate absorption have been reviewed recently by Rosenberg and Godwin (1971). A specific, saturable and energy-requiring system has been postulated but conclusive evidence has yet to be obtained. As shown below, patients are unable to absorb "dietary" folates or folic acid in normal amounts although the absorption of all other compounds is outwardly normal. This suggests that absorption of folic acid in the normal is not due to passive diffusion alone and that the patients have a defect in the normal mechanism for absorption.

All three patients failed adequately to absorb pteroylmonoglutamic acid (folic acid) and "dietary" folate (consisting primarily of gamma-glutamyl peptide conjugates of reduced formyl or methyl folates) although metabolism of parenterally administered folic acid was normal. Lanzkowsky *et al.* (1969) demonstrated further that their patient was unable to absorb (in contrast to normal individuals) pteroyl diglutamic acid (diopterin), pteroyltriglutamic acid (teropterin), N^5-formyltetrahydrofolic acid and N^5-methyltetrahydrofolic acid. Lyophilized calf jejunum or pancreas and normal human duodenal juice given with folic acid all failed to enhance its absorption. Other substances, e.g. glucose, xylose, fat, vitamin A and vitamin K, were absorbed normally by all patients. The histology of the jejunal mucosa as observed with light and electron microscopy was also normal.

These findings suggest that the defect is localized in the absorption from the intestinal lumen or its translocation into the portal system and is not due to defective intraluminal hydrolysis of "dietary" folates (by gamma-glutamylcarboxypeptidase), the deficiency of a co-factor, or generalized malabsorption due to a decrease in absorptive area (as occurs in sprue).

Since Lanzkowsky *et al.* (1969) also demonstrated that their patient was unable to absorb N^5-formyltetrahydrofolic acid and N^5-methyltetrahydrofolic acid, the lesion is not localized in the metabolic production of these two compounds (which normally occurs before absorbed folic acid is discharged into the portal system).

The nature of the defect thus remains obscure but it is anticipated that further study on these patients will provide not only an insight into the nature of the lesion but also the mechanism for the transport of folate in the normal.

ACKNOWLEDGEMENTS

I thank Professor G. Semenza for helpful discussions and critically reviewing the manuscript, Dr. G. Davidson, Dr. R. R. W. Townley, Dr. Valerie Burke and Dr. M. Gracey for helpful discussions, Miss Pamela Hore for editorial assistance, and Miss Lynnette Fischer-Jones, Miss Ginia de Vallier, Miss R. Schmid and Miss Kathleen Carmody for preparing the manuscript.

I gratefully acknowledge the assistance given by the Antarctic Division, Department of Supply, Melbourne in allowing the time for the revision and final preparation of the manuscript.

This work was carried out under a grant from the U.S. Air Force under grant EOOAR–68–0017 (to Professor Semenza).

REFERENCES

ABRAHAM, J. M., LEVIN, B., OBERHOLZER, V. G. and RUSSELL, A. (1967) Glucose–galactose malabsorption. *Arch. Dis. Childh.* **42:** 592–597.

AGUILAR, M. J., CHADWICK, D. L., ODUYAMA, K., and KAMOSHITA, S. (1966) Kinky hair disease: I. Clinical and pathological features. *J. Neuropath. Exp. Neuroe.* **25:** 507.

ALBRIGHT, F., BUTLER, A. M. and BLOOMBERG, E. (1937) Rickets resistant to vitamin D therapy. *Am. J. Dis. Child.* **54:** 529–547.

ALCOCK, N. and MACINTYRE, I. (1960) Interrelation of calcium and magnesium absorption. *Biochem. J.* **76:** 19–20.

ANDERSON, C. M., KERRY, K. R. and TOWNLEY, R. R. W. (1965) An inborn defect of intestinal absorption of certain monosaccharides. *Arch. Dis. Childh.* **40:** 1–6.

ANTTILA, R. and SALMI, H. A. (1967) Selektiv malabsorption av vitamin B_{12} med proteinuri hos barn. Beskrivning av tva fall. *Abst. XV Nord. Ped. Kong.*, p. 46 (cited VISAKORPI and FURUHJELM, 1968).

ARNAUD, C., GLORIEUX, F., and SCRIVER, C. (1971) Serum parathyroid hormone in X-linked hypophosphatemia. *Science* **173:** 845.

ASATOOR, A. M., BANDOH, J. K., LANT, A. F., MILNE, M. D. and NAVAB, F. (1970a) Intestinal absorption of carnosine and its constituent amino acids in man. *Gut* **11:** 250–254.

ASATOOR, A. M., CHENG, B., EDWARDS, K. D. G., LANT, A. F., MATTHEWS, D. M., MILNE, M. D., NAVAB, F. and RICHARDS, A. J. (1970b) Intestinal absorption of two dipeptides in Hartnup disease. *Gut* **11:** 380–387.

ASATOOR, A. M., CRASKE, J., LONDON, D. R. and MILNE, M. D. (1963) Indole production in Hartnup disease. *Lancet* **1:** 126–128.

ASATOOR, A. M., LACEV, B. W., LONDON, D. R. and MILNE, M. D. (1962) Amino-acid metabolism in cystinuria. *Clin. Sci.* **23:** 285–304.

AVIOLI, L. V., MCDONALD, J. E. and WILLIAMS, T. F. (1966) Abnormal metabolism of vitamin D_3 in vitamin D-resistant rickets and familial hypophosphatemia. *J. Clin. Invest.* **45:** 982.

BANNERMAN, R. M. and PINKERTON, P. H. (1967) X-linked hypochromic anaemia of mice. *Brit. J. Haemat.* **13:** 1000–1013.

BANNERMAN, R. M., PINKERTON, P. H. and EDWARDS, J. A. (1968) Hereditary iron-deficiency anaemia due to a specific defect of intestinal absorption. *J. Clin. Invest.* **47:** 5a.

BARON, D. N., DENT, C. E., HARRIS, H., HART, E. W. and JEPSON, J. B. (1956) Hereditary pellagra-like skin rash with temporary cerebellar ataxia, constant renal amino-aciduria and other bizarre biochemical features. *Lancet* **2:** 421–428.

BARTSOCAS, C. S., LEVY, H. L., CRAWFORD, J. D. and THIER, S. O. (1969) A defect in intestinal amino-acid transport in Lowe's syndrome. *Am. J. Dis. Child.* **117:** 93–95.

BASSEN, F. A. and KORNZWEIG, A. L. (1950) Malformation of the erythrocytes in a case of atypical retinitis pigmentosa. *Blood* **5:** 381–387.

BEN-BASSAT, I., FEINSTEIN, A. and RAMOT, B. (1969) Selective vitamin B_{12} malabsorption with proteinuria in Israel. Clinical and general aspects. *Israel J. Med. Sci.* **5:** 62–68.

BESSMAN, S. P. and TADA, K. (1960) Indicanuria in phenylketonuria. *Metabolism* **9:** 377–385.

BILLING, D. M. and DEGNAN, M. (1971) Kinky hair syndrome: A new case and a review. *Amer. J. Dis. Child.* **121:** 447.

BLUNT, J. W., DELUCA, H. F. and SCHNOES, H. K. (1968) 25-Hydroxycholecalciferol: a biologically active metabolite of cholecalciferol. *Chem. Comm.* **14:** 801.

BRAND, E., CAHILL, G. F. and KASSELL, B. (1940) Canine cystinuria: family history of two cystinuric Irish terriers and cystine determinations in dog urine. *J. Biol. Chem.* **133:** 431–436.

BRAY, P. F. (1965) Sex-linked neurodegenerative disease associated with monilethrix. *Pediatrics* **36:** 417.

BURKE, V. and DANKS, D. M. (1966) Monosaccharide malabsorption in young infants. *Lancet* **1:** 1177–1180.

BURNETT, CH. H., DENT, C. E., HARPER, C. and WARLAND, B. J. (1964) Vitamin D-resistant rickets. *Am. J. Med.* **36:** 222–232.

CELANDER, O., MACDOWALL, J. and LUNDGREN, S. (1969) Personal communication.

CHUTORIAN, A. and ROWLAND, L. P. (1966) Lowe's syndrome. *Neurology* **16:** 115–122.

COLLISS, J. E., LEVI, A. J. and MILNE, M. D. (1963) Stature and nutrition in cystinuria and Hartnup disease. *Brit. Med. J.* **1:** 590–592.

COOPER, B. A. and CASTLE, W. B. (1960) Sequential mechanisms in the enhanced absorption of vitamin B_{12} by intrinsic factor in the rat. *J. Clin. Invest.* **39:** 199–214.

CRANE, C. W. and TURNER, A. W. (1956) Amino-acid patterns of urine and blood plasma in a cystinuric Labrador dog. *Nature* (*Lond.*) **177:** 237–238.

CRANE, R. K. (1968) Absorption of sugars, pp. 1323–1351. In: *Handbook of Physiology,* CODE, C. F. (Ed.), sect. 6, vol. III. American Physiological Society, Washington, D.C.

CRAWFORD, T. B. B., ASHCROFT, G. W., ECCLESTON, D. and SMITH, A. N. (1965) Some observations on the metabolism of indoles in two patients with the carcinoid syndrome. *Gastroenterology* **48:** 745–752.

CRAWHALL, J. C. and SEGAL, S. (1965) Sulphocysteine in the urine of the blotched Kenya genet. *Nature* (*Lond.*) **208:** 1320–1322.

CRAWHALL, J. C., SCOWDEN, E. F. and WATTS, R. W. E. (1963) Effect of penicillamine on cystinuria. *Brit. Med. J.* **1:** 588–590.

CURRAN, P. F. and SCHWARTZ, G. F. (1960) Na, Cl, and water transport by rat colon. *J. Gen. Physiol.* **43:** 555–571.

CUSWORTH, D. C. and DENT, C. E. (1960) Renal clearances of amino acids in normal adults and patients with aminoaciduria. *Biochem. J.* **74:** 550–561.

DAHLQVIST, A., LINDQUIST, B. and MEEUWISSE, G. (1968) Disturbances of the digestion and absorption of carbohydrates, pp. 199–222. In: *Carbohydrate Metabolism and its Disorders,* vol. II, DICKENS, F., RANDLE, P. J. and WHELAN, W. J. (Eds.). Academic Press.

DANKS, D. M., CAMPBELL, P. E., STEVENS, B. J., MAYNE, V. and CARTWRIGHT, E. (1972a) Menkes' kinky hair syndrome. An inherited defect in copper absorption with widespread effects. *Pediatrics* **50:** 188–201.

DANKS, D. M., CARTWRIGHT, E., STEVENS, B. J. and TOWNLEY, R. R. W. (1973) Menkes' kinky hair disease: Further definition of the defect in copper transport. *Science* **179:** 1140–1142.

DANKS, D. M., STEVENS, B. J., CAMPBELL, P. E., GILLESPIE, J. M., WALKER-SMITH, J., BLOMFIELD, J. and TURNER, J. (1972b) Menkes' kinky-hair syndrome. *Lancet* **1:** 1100–1103.

DARROW, D. C. (1945) Congenital alkalosis with diarrhoea. *J. Pediat.* **26:** 519–532.

DATTA, S. P. and HARRIS, H. (1953) Urinary amino-acid patterns of some mammals. *Ann. Eugen.* **18:** 107–116.

DeLuca, H. F., Lund, J., Rosenbloom, A. and Lobeck, C. C. (1967) Metabolism of tritiated vitamin D_3 in familial vitamin D-resistant rickets with hypophosphataemia. *J. Ped.* **70:** 828–832.

Dent, C. E. (1952) Rickets and osteomalacia from renal tubule defects. *J. Bone Jt. Surg.* **34-B:** 266–274.

Dent, C. E. and Harris, H. (1956) Hereditary forms of rickets and osteomalacia. *J. Bone Jt. Surg.* **38-B:** 204–226.

Dent, C. E. and Rose, G. A. (1951) Amino-acid metabolism in cystinuria. *Q. J. Med.* **20:** 205–219.

Dent, C. E. and Senior, B. (1955) Studies on the treatment of cystinuria. *Brit. J. Urol.* **27:** 316–332.

Dobbins, W. O. (1966) An ultrastructural study of the intestinal mucosa in congenital β-lipoprotein deficiency with particular emphasis upon the intestinal absorptive cell. *Gastroenterology* **50:** 195–210.

Dole, V. P. and Hamlin, J. T. (1962) Particulate fat in lymph and blood. *Physiol. Rev.* **42:** 674–701.

Drummond, K. N., Michael, A. F., Ulstrom, R. A. and Good, R. A. (1964) The blue diaper syndrome: familial hypercalcemia with nephrocalcinosis and indicanuria. A new familial disease, with definition of the metabolic abnormality. *Am. J. Med.* **37:** 928–948.

Dubois, R., Loeb, H., Eggermont, E. and Mainguet, P. (1966) Etude clinique et biochimique d'un cas de malabsorption congénitale du glucose et du galactose. *Helv. Paediat. Acta* **21:** 577–587.

Duyck, E. M. R. A. (1955) L'alcalose congénitale avec diarrhée. Aspect du métabolisme minéral. Thèse (Stenfert Kroese, Leyden). Cited Launiala *et al.* (1968).

Editorial (1968) Selective malabsorption of vitamin B_{12}. *New Engl. J. Med.* **279:** 433–434.

Edwards, J. A. and Bannerman, R. M. (1970) Hereditary defect of intestinal iron transport in mice with sex-linked anaemia. *J. Clin. Invest.* **49:** 1869–1871.

Efron, M. (1966) Disorders of proline and hydroxyproline metabolism, pp. 376–392. In: *The Metabolic Basis of Inherited Disease,* 2nd ed., Stanbury, J. B., Wyngaarden, J. B. and Fredrickson, D. S. (Eds.). McGraw-Hill, N.Y.

Eggermont, E. and Loeb, H. (1966) Glucose–galactose intolerance. *Lancet* **2:** 343–344.

Elliot, J. S., Ribeiro, M. E. and Eusebio, E. (1968) Cystinuria in the blotched genet. *Invest. Urol.* **5:** 568–571.

Elsas, L. G., Hillman, R. E., Patterson, J. N. and Rosenberg, L. E. (1969a) Renal and intestinal hexose transport in the glucose–galactose malabsorption syndrome. Abstract. *Clin. Res.* **17:** 28.

Elsas, L. G., Hillman, R. E., Patterson, J. N. and Rosenberg, L. E. (1969b) The glucose–galactose malabsorption syndrome (GGMS): a genetic analysis of renal and intestinal transport, pp. 38–39. In: *Excerpta Medica Int. Cong.* Series 3, No. 191, Frazer, E. C. (Ed.).

Evanson, J. M. and Stanbury, S. W. (1965) Congenital chloridorrhoea or so-called congenital alkalosis with diarrhoea. *Gut* **6:** 29–38.

Falconer, D. S. and Isaacson, J. H. (1962) The genetics of sex-linked anaemia in the mouse. *Genet. Res.* **3:** 248–250.

Fanconi, G. and Girardet, P. (1952) Familiärer persistierender Phosphatdiabetes mit D-vitamin-resistenter Rachitis. *Helv. Paediat. Acta* **7:** 14–41.

Farquhar, J. W. and Ways, P. (1966) A-beta-lipoproteinaemia, pp. 509–522. In: *The Metabolic Basis of Inherited Disease,* 2nd ed., Stanbury, J. B., Wyngaarden, J. B. and Fredrickson, D. S. (Eds.). McGraw-Hill, N.Y.

Field, M. H. and Reiss, E. (1960) Vitamin D-resistant rickets: the effect of calcium infusion on phosphate reabsorption. *J. Clin. Invest.* **39:** 1807–1817.

FOLEY, T. H. and LONDON, D. R. (1965) Cysteine metabolism in cystinuria. *Clin. Sci.* **29:** 549–554.

FORDTRAN, J. S. and INGELFINGER, F. J. (1968) Absorption of water, electrolytes, and sugars from the human gut, pp. 1457–1490. In: *Handbook of Physiology,* CODE, C. F. (Ed.). American Physiological Society, Washington, D.C.

FORDTRAN, J. S. and LOCKLEAR, T. W. (1966) Ionic constituents and osmolality of gastric and small-intestinal fluid after eating. *Am. J. Dig. Dis.* **11:** 503–521.

FOROOZAN, P. and TRIER, J. S. (1967) Mucosa of the small intestine in pernicious anemia. *New Engl. J. Med.* **277:** 553–559.

FORSYTH, C. C., LLOYD, J. K. and FOSBROOKE, A. S. (1965) A-β-lipoproteinaemia. *Arch. Dis. Childh.* **40:** 47–52.

FOURNET, J. P. (1968) Le métabolisme du magnésium et sa pathologie en pédiatrie. Thesis (Paris).

FOX, M., THIER, S., ROSENBERG, L., KISER, W. and SEGAL, S. (1964) Evidence against a single renal transport defect in cystinuria. *New Engl. J. Med.* **270:** 556–561.

FRAZER, D. R. and KODICEK, E. (1970) Unique biosynthesis by kidney of a biologically active vitamin D metabolite. *Nature* **228:** 764.

FREEMAN, R. M. and PEARSON, E. (1966) Hypomagnesaemia of unknown etiology. *Am. J. Med.* **41:** 645–656.

FRIEDMAN, M., HATCHER, G. and WATSON, L. (1967) Primary hypomagnesaemia with secondary hypocalcaemia in an infant. *Lancet* **1:** 703–705.

FRIMPTER, G. W. (1961) The disulfide of L-cysteine and L-homocysteine in urine of patients with cystinuria. *J. Biol. Chem.* **236:** PC51–PC53.

FRIMPTER, G. W. (1963) Cystinuria: metabolism of the disulfide of cysteine and homocysteine. *J. Clin. Invest.* **42:** 1956–1964.

FRIMPTER, G. W. (1968) Medical management of cystinuria. *Am. J. Med. Sci.* **255:** 348–357.

GAMBLE, J. L., FAHEY, K. R., APPLETON, J. and MACLACHLAN, E. (1945) Congenital alkalosis with diarrhoea. *J. Pediat.* **26:** 509–518.

GLORIEUX, F. and SCRIVER, C. R. (1972) Loss of a parathyroid hormone sensitive component of phosphate transport in X-linked hypophosphatemia. *Science* **175:** 997.

GLORIEUX, F., SCRIVER, C. R., READE, T. M., GOLDMAN, H., and ROSEBOROUGH, A. (1972) Use of phosphate and vitamin D to prevent dwarfism and rickets in X-linked hypophosphatemia. *New Eng. J. Med.* **287:** 481.

GOLDBERG, L. S. and FUDENBERG, H. H. (1968) Familial selective malabsorption of vitamin B_{12}. Re-evaluation of an *in vivo* intrinsic-factor inhibitor. *New Engl. J. Med.* **279:** 405–407.

GOODMAN, S. I., MCINTYRE, C. M. and O'BRIEN, D. (1967) Impaired intestinal transport of proline in a patient with familial iminoaciduria. *J. Pediat.* **71:** 246–249.

GRÄSBECK, R. and KVIST, G. (1967) Observations on patients with the syndrome "selective vitamin B_{12} malabsorption and proteinuria". *Scand. J. Clin. Lab. Invest.* **19:** Suppl. **95:** 38–39.

GRÄSBECK, R., GORDIN, R., KANTERO, I. and KUHLBÄCK, B. (1960) Selective vitamin B_{12} malabsorption and proteinuria in young people: a syndrome. *Acta Med. Scand.* **167:** 289–296.

GREWAL, M. S. (1962) A sex-linked anaemia in the mouse. *Genet. Res.* **3:** 238–247.

HALVORSEN, K. and HALVORSEN, S. (1963) Hartnup disease. *Pediatrics* **31:** 29–38.

HARRIS, H. and WARREN, F. L. (1953) Quantitative studies on the urinary cystine in patients with cystine stones and their relatives. *Ann. Eugenics* **18:** 125–171.

HARRIS, H., MITTWOCH, U., ROBSON, E. B. and WARREN, F. L. (1955) Phenotypes and genotypes in cystinuria. *Ann. Human Genet.* **20:** 57–91.

HAVERBACK, B. J., DYCE, B. and THOMAS, H. V. (1960) Indole metabolism in the malabsorption syndrome. *New Engl. J. Med.* **262:** 754–757.

HENDERSON, W. (1958) A case of Hartnup disease. *Arch. Dis. Childh.* **33:** 114–117.

HERBERT, V. (1968) Absorption of vitamin B_{12} and folic acid. *Gastroenterology* **54:** 110–115.

HERBERT, V., STREIFF, R. R. and SULLIVAN, L. W. (1964) Notes on vitamin B_{12} absorption; autoimmunity and childhood pernicious anaemia; relation of intrinsic factor to blood group substance. *Medicine* **43:** 679–687.

HESS, W. C. and SULLIVAN, M. X. (1942) Canine cystinuria. The effect of feeding cystine, cysteine, and methionine at different dietary protein levels. *J. Biol. Chem.* **143:** 545–550.

HIGHLEY, D. R., STEIFF, R. R., ELLENBOGEN, L., HERBERT, V. and CASTLE, W. B. (1965) Releasing factor and endogenous vitamin B_{12}. *Proc. Soc. Exp. Biol. Med.* **119:** 565–570.

HIPPE, E. (1966) Malabsorption of vitamin B_{12}. Report of a case in a one-year-old boy, including studies of the absorption of B_{12}. *Acta Paediat. Scand.* **55:** 510–516.

HOOFT, C. and ANTENER, I. (1968) Methionine malabsorption syndrome, pp. 127–136. In: *Intestinal Absorption and Malabsorption*, SHMERLING, D. H., BERGER, H. and PRADER, A. (Eds.). *Modern Problems in Pediatrics*, vol. 11, Karger, Basel.

HOOFT, C., CARTON, D., SNOECK, J., TIMMERMANS, J., ANTENER, I., VAN DEN HENDE, CH. and OYAERT, W. (1968) Further investigations in the methionine malabsorption syndrome. *Helv. Paediat. Acta* **23:** 334–349.

HOOFT, C., TIMMERMANS, J., SNOECK, J., ANTENER, I., OYAERT, W. and VAN DEN HENDE, CH. (1964) Methionine malabsorption in a mentally defective child. *Lancet* **2:** 20.

HOOFT, C., TIMMERMANS, J., SNOECK, J., ANTENER, I., OYAERT, W. and VAN DEN HENDE, CH. (1965) Methionine malabsorption syndrome. *Ann. Paediat.* (*Basel*) **205:** 73–104.

IMERSLUND, O. (1960) Indiopathic chronic megaloblastic anaemia in children. *Acta Paediat. Scand.* **49:** Suppl. **119:** 1–115.

ISSELBACHER, K. J., SCHEIG, R., PLOTKIN, G. R. and CAULFIELD, J. B. (1964) Congenital β-lipoprotein deficiency: an hereditary disorder involving a defect in the absorption and transport of lipids. *Medicine* **43:** 347–361.

JEPSON, J. B. (1966) Hartnup disease, pp. 1283–1299. In: *The Metabolic Basis of Inherited Disease,* 2nd ed., STANBURY, J. B., WYNGAARDEN, J. B. and FREDRICKSON, D. S. (Eds.). McGraw-Hill, N.Y.

JEUNE, M., HERMIER, M., HARTEMANN, E., LORAS, B., HAOUR, F., COTTON, J. B. and COLLOMBEL, C. (1967) Diarrhée chlorée congénitale avec alcalase métabolique. *Pédiatrie* (*Lyon*) **22:** 663.

JONES, J. W. and WAYS, P. (1967) Abnormalities of high density lipoproteins in abetalipoproteinaemia. *J. Clin. Invest.* **46:** 1151.

KAYDEN, H. J. and MEDICK, M. (1969) The absorption and metabolism of short and long chain fatty acids in puromycin-treated rats. *Biochem. Biophys. Acta* **176:** 37–43.

KEKOMÄKI, M., TOIVAKKA, E., HÄKKINEN, V. and SALASPURO, M. (1968) Familial protein intolerance with deficient transport of basic amino acids. *Acta Med. Scand.* **183:** 357–359.

KELSEY, W. M. (1954) Congenital alkalosis with diarrhoea. *Am. J. Dis. Child.* **88:** 344–347.

KERRY, K. R. (1967) Normal and abnormal digestion and absorption of carbohydrates in infancy and childhood. Doctoral Thesis, University of Melbourne.

KNOX, W. E. (1966) Cystinuria, pp. 1262–1282. In: *The Metabolic Basis of Inherited Disease*, 2nd ed., STANBURY, J. B., WYNGAARDEN, J. B. and FREDRICKSON, D. S. (Eds.). McGraw-Hill, N.Y.

KORNZWEIG, A. L. and BASSEN, F. A. (1957) Retinitis pigmentosa, acanthrocytosis and heredodegenerative neuromuscular disease. *Arch. Ophthal.* **58:** 183–192.

KUO, P. T. and BASSET, D. R. (1962) Blood and tissue lipids in a family with hypo-betalipoproteinemia. *Circulation* **26:** 660.

LAFFERTY, F. W., HERNDON, C. H. and PEARSON, O. H. (1963) Pathogenesis of vitamin D-resistant rickets and the response to a high calcium intake. *J. Clin. Endocr. Metab.* **23:** 903–917.

LAMY, M., FREZAL, J., POLONOVSKI, C. and REY, J. (1961) L'absence congénitale de béta-lipoproteins. *Presse Méd.* **69:** 1511–1514.

LANZKOWSKY, P. (1970) Congenital malabsorption of folate. *Am. J. Med.* **48:** 580–583.

LANZKOWSKY, P., ERLANDSON, M. E. and BEZAN, A. I. (1969) Isolated defect of folic acid absorption associated with mental retardation and cerebral calcification. *Blood* **34:** 452–465.

LAPLANE, R., POLONOVSKI, C., ETIENNE, M., DEBRARY, P., LODS, J. C. and PISSARRO, B. (1962) L'intolérance aux sucres à transfert intestinal actif. Ses rapports avec l'intolérance au lactose et le syndrome céliaque. *Arch. Franç. Pédiat.* **19:** 895–944.

LAUNIALA, K., PASTERNACK, A., PERHEENTUPA, J. and HALLMAN, N. (1967) Familial chloride diarrhoea (Congenital alkalosis with diarrhoea). *Acta Paediat. Scand.* **56:** 320.

LAUNIALA, K., PERHEENTUPA, J., PASTERNACK, A. and HALLMAN, N. (1968) Familial chloride diarrhoea—chloride malabsorption, pp. 137–149. In: *Intestinal Absorption and Malabsorption*, SHMERLING, D. H., BERGER, H. and PRADER, A. (Eds.). *Modern Problems in Pediatrics*, vol. 11, Karger, Basel.

LAVENDER, A. R. and PULLMAN, T. N. (1963) Changes in inorganic phosphate excretion induced by renal arterial infusion of calcium. *Am. J. Physiol.* **205:** 1025–1032.

LEES, R. S. (1967) Immunological evidence for the presence of B protein (apoprotein of β-lipoprotein) in normal and abetaliproteinemic plasma. *J. Lipid Res.* **8:** 396–405.

LINDQUIST, B. and MEEUWISSE, G. W. (1962) Chronic diarrhoea caused by monosaccharide malabsorption. *Acta Paediat. Scand.* **51:** 674–685.

LINDQUIST, B. and MEEUWISSE, G. W. (1963) Intestinal transport of monosaccharides in generalised and selective malabsorption. *Acta Paediat. Scand.* Supp. **146:** 110–115.

LINDQUIST, B. and MEEUWISSE, G. W. (1968) Glucose–galactose malabsorption, pp. 92–100. In: *Intestinal Absorption and Malabsorption*, SHMERLING, D. H., BERGER, H. and PRADER, A. (Eds.). *Modern Problems in Pediatrics*, vol. 11, Karger, Basel.

LINDQUIST, B., MEEUWISSE, G. W. and MELIN, K. (1963) Osmotic diarrhoea in genetically transmitted glucose–galactose malabsorption. *Acta Paediat. Scand.* **52:** 217–219.

LINNEWEH, F., SCHAUMLÖFFEL, E. and BARTHELMAI, W. (1965) Angeborene Glucose- und Galaktose-Malabsorption. *Klin. Wschr.* **43:** 405–409.

LLOYD, J. K. (1968) Disorders of the serum lipoproteins I. Lipoprotein deficiency states. *Arch. Dis. Childh.* **43:** 393–403.

LONDON, D. R. and FOLEY, T. H. (1965) Cystine metabolism in cystinuria. *Clin. Sci.* **29:** 129–141.

LOWE, C. U., TERREY, M. and MACLACHLAN, E. A. (1952) Organicaciduria, decreased renal ammonia production, hydrophthalmos, and mental retardation. A clinical entity. *Am. J. Dis. Child.* **83:** 164–184.

LUHBY, A. L. and COOPERMAN, J. L. (1967) Congenital megaloblastic anemia and progressive central nervous system degeneration. Further clinical and physiological characterization and therapy of syndrome due to inborn error of folate transport. American Pediatric Society Inc. Annual Meeting, Atlantic City. Cited LANZKOWSKY *et al.*, 1970.

LUHBY, A. L., COOPERMAN, J. L. and PESCI-BOUREL, A. (1965) A new inborn error of metabolism: folic acid responsive megaloblastic anemia, ataxia, mental retardation and convulsions. American Pediatric Society Inc., Annual Meeting, Philadelphia. Cited LANZKOWSKY *et al.*, 1970.

LUHBY, A. L., EAGLE, F. J., ROTH, E. and COOPERMAN, J. M. (1961) Relapsing megaloblastic anaemia in an infant due to a specific defect in gastrointestinal absorption of folic acid. *Am. J. Dis. Child.* **102:** 482–483.

MABRY, C. C., DIGEORGE, A. M. and AURBACH, V. H. (1960) Studies concerning the defect in patients with acanthrocytosis. *Clin. Res.* **8:** 371.

MACKENZIE, I. L., DONALDSON, R. M., TRIER, J. S. and MATHAN, V. I. (1972) Ileal mucosa in familial selective vitamin B_{12} malabsorption. *New Eng. J. Med.* **286:** 1021–1025.

MANIS, J. (1970) Active transport of iron by intestine: Selective genetic defect in the mouse. *Nature (Lond.)* **227:** 385–386.

MANIS, J. (1971) Intestinal iron-transport in the mouse with sex-linked anemia. *Am. J. Physiol.* **220:** 135–139.

MARKS, J. F., NORTON, J. B. and FORDTRAN, J. S. (1966) Glucose–galactose malabsorption. *J. Pediat.* **69:** 225–228.

MCCARTHY, C. F., BORLAND, J. L., LYNCH, H. J., OWEN, E. E. and TYOR, M. P. (1964) Defective uptake of basic amino acids and L-cystine by intestinal mucosa of patients with cystinuria. *J. Clin. Invest.* **43:** 1518–1524.

MCENERY, P. T., SILVERMAN, F. N. and WEST, C. D. (1972) Acceleration of growth with combined vitamin D–phosphate therapy of hypophosphatemic resistant rickets. *J. Pediat.* **80:** 763.

MCNAIR, S. L. and STICKLER, G. (1969) Growth in familial hypophosphatemic vitamin D-resistant rickets. *New Engl. J. Med.* **281:** 511–516.

MEEUWISSE, G. W. (1970a) Renal glucosuria in glucose–galactose malabsorption. *Acta Paediat. Scand.* **59:** 456.

MEEUWISSE, G. W. (1970b) Glucose–galactose malabsorption. Studies on renal glucosuria. *Helv. Pediat. Acta* **25:** 13–24.

MEEUWISSE, G. W. (1970c) Glucose–galactose malabsorption. A study on the transfer of glucose across the red cell membrane. *Scand. J. Clin. Lab. Invest.* **25:** 145–149.

MEEUWISSE, G. W. and DAHLQVIST, A. (1966) Glucose–galactose malabsorption. *Lancet* **21:** 858.

MEEUWISSE, G. W. and DAHLQVIST, A. (1968) Glucose–galactose malabsorption. A study with biopsy of the small intestinal mucosa. *Acta Paediat. Scand.* **57:** 273–280.

MEEUWISSE, G. W. and LINDQUIST, B. (1970) Glucose–galactose malabsorption. Studies on the intermediate carbohydrate metabolism. *Acta Paediat. Scand.* **59:** 74–79.

MELIN, K. and MEEUWISSE, G. W. (1969) Glucose–galactose malabsorption: A genetic study. *Acta Paediat. Scand.* Suppl. **188:** 19–24.

MENKES, J. H., ALTER, M., STEIGLEDER, G. K., WEAKLEY, D. R. and SUNG, J. H. (1962) A sex-linked recessive disorder and retardation of growth, peculiar and focal cerebral and cerebellar degeneration. *Pediatrics* **29:** 764.

MICHAEL, A. F., DRUMMOND, K. N., ULSTROM, R. A. and GOOD, R. A. (1962) The blue diaper syndrome: familial hypercalcemia of infancy associated with abnormal tryptophan metabolism. *Am. J. Dis. Child.* **104:** 510–511.

MILNE, M. D. (1964) Disorders of amino-acid transport. *Brit. Med. J.* **1:** 327–336.

MILNE, M. D. (1968) Genetic disorders of intestinal amino acid transport, pp. 1309–1321. In: *American Handbook of Physiology,* vol. 6, No. III, CODE, C. (Ed.). American Physiological Society, New York.

MILNE, M. D. (1969) Hartnup disease. *Biochem. J.* **111:** 3P–4P.

MILNE, M. D., ASATOOR, A. M., EDWARDS, K. D. G. and LOUGHRIDGE, L. W. (1961) The intestinal absorption defect in cystinuria. *Gut* **2:** 323–337.

MILNE, M. D., CRAWFORD, M. A., GIRAÕ, C. B. and LOUGHRIDGE, L. W. (1960) The metabolic disorder in Hartnup disease. *Quart. J. Med.* **29:** 407–421.

MOEDEMAEKER, P. J., ABELS, J., WACHTERS, J. J., ARENDS, A. and NIEWEG, H. O. (1964) Investigations about the site of production of Castle's gastric intrinsic factor. *Lab. Invest.* **13:** 1394–1399.

MOHAMED, S. D., MCKAY, E. and GALLOWAY, W. H. (1966) Juvenile familial megaloblastic anemia due to selective malabsorption of vitamin B_{12}. *Quart. J. Med.* **35:** 433–453.

MORIKAWA, T., TADA, K., ANDO, T., YOSHIDA, T., YOKOYAMA, Y. and ARAKAWA, T. (1966) Prolinuria: defect in intestinal absorption of amino acids and glycine. *Tohoku J. Exp. Med.* **90:** 105–116.

NAGANT DE DEUXCHAINES, C. and KRANE, S. M. (1967) The treatment of adult phosphate diabetes and Fanconi syndrome with neutral sodium phosphate. *Am. J. Med.* **43:** 508–543.

NAVAB, F. and ASATOOR, A. M. (1970) Studies on intestinal absorption of amino acids and a dipeptide in a case of Hartnup disease. *Gut* **11:** 373–379.

NIGRIN, G., COCHRANE, W. A., JANNIGAN, D. and ERNST, A. (1962) Results of calcium infusion and renal biopsy studies in refractory rickets. *Am. J. Dis. Child.* **104:** 478–479.

OLDFIELD, J. E., ALLEN, P. H. and ADAIR, J. (1956) Identification of cystine calculi in mink. *Proc. Soc. Exp. Biol. Med.* **91:** 560–562.

OWEN, G. M. (1964) Metabolic alkalosis with diarrhoea and chloride-free urine. *J. Pediat.* **65:** 849–857.

PASTERNACK, A. and PERHEENTUPA, J. (1966) Hypertensive angiopathy in familial chloride diarrhoea. *Lancet* **2:** 1047–1049.

PASTERNACK, A., PERHEENTUPA, J., LAUNIALA, K. and HALLMAN, N. (1967) Kidney biopsy findings in familial chloride diarrhoea. *Acta Endocr. Kobh.* **55:** 1–9.

PAUNIER, L., RADDE, I. C., KOOH, S. W., CONEN, P. E. and FRASER, D. (1968) Primary hypomagnesemia with secondary calcemia in an infant. *Pediatrics* **41:** 385–402.

PAUNIER, L., RADDE, I. C., KOOH, S. W. and FRASER, D. (1965) Primary hypomagnesemia with secondary hypocalcemia. *J. Pediat.* **67:** 945.

PERHEENTUPA, J., EKLUND, J. and KOJO, N. (1965) Familial chloride diarrhoea ("Congenital alkalosis with diarrhoea"). *Acta Paediat. Scand.* Suppl. **159:** 119–120.

PINKERTON, P. H. (1968) Histological evidence of disordered iron transport in the X-linked hypochromic anaemia of mice. *J. Path. Bact.* **95:** 155–165.

PINKERTON, P. H. and BANNERMAN, R. M. (1966) X-linked hypochromic anemia of mice—a disorder of iron metabolism. *Blood* **28:** 987.

PINKERTON, P. H. and BANNERMAN, R. M. (1967a) Hereditary defect in iron absorption in mice. *Nature* **216:** 482–483.

PINKERTON, P. H. and BANNERMAN, R. M. (1967b) The hereditary anaemias of mice. *Hemat. Rev.*

POMEROY, J., EFRON, M. L., DAYMAN, J. and HOEFNAGEL, D. (1968) Hartnup disorder in a New England family. *New Engl. J. Med.* **278:** 1214–1216.

REED, C. F. (1959) Studies of *in vivo* and *in vitro* exchange of erythrocyte and plasma phospholipids (abstract). *J. Clin. Invest.* **38:** 1032–1033.

REY, J. (1961) *L'Absence congénitale de béta-lipoproteines.* R. Foulon et Cie, Paris.

REY, J. and FREZAL, J. (1966) Pathogénie du rachitisme vitamino-résistant hypophosphatémique familial. *Rev. Franç. Etudes Clin. Biol.* **11:** 771–776.

REY, J. and FREZAL, J. (1967) Les anomalies des disaccharidases. *Arch. Franç. Pédiat.* **24:** 65–101.

ROSENBERG, I. H. and GODWIN, H. A. (1971) The digestion and absorption of dietary folate. *Gastroenterology* **60:** 445–463.

ROSENBERG, L. E. (1968) Genetic heterogeneity in cystinuria, pp. 341–353. In: *Aminoacid Metabolism and Genetic Variation,* NYHAN, W. L. (Ed.). McGraw-Hill, N.Y.

ROSENBERG, L. E., CRAWHALL, J. C. and SEGAL, S. (1967) Intestinal transport of cystine and cysteine in man: evidence for separate mechanisms. *J. Clin. Invest.* **46:** 30–34.

ROSENBERG, L. E., DOWNING, S., DURANT, J. L. and SEGAL, S. (1966) Cystinuria: Biochemical evidence for three genetically distinct diseases. *J. Clin. Invest.* **45:** 365–371.

ROSENBERG, L. E., DOWNING, S. J. and SEGAL, S. (1962) Competitive inhibition of dibasic amino acid transport in rat kidney. *J. Biol. Chem.* **237:** 2265–2270.

ROSENBERG, L. E., DURANT, J. L. and ELSAS, L. J. (1968) Familial iminoglycinuria: an inborn error of renal tubular transport. *New Engl. J. Med.* **278:** 1407–1413.

ROSENBERG, L. E., DURANT, J. L. and HOLLAND, J. M. (1965) Intestinal absorption and renal extraction of cystine and cysteine in cystinuria. *New Engl. J. Med.* **275:** 1239–1245.

ROYER, P., LESTRADET, H., FREDERICH, A. and DARTOIS, A. M. (1961) Les rachitismes vitaminorésistants hypophosphatémiques idiopathiques de l'enfant. (Essai de dissociation de deux maladies différentes par l'étude clinique, radiologique, biologique et génétique). *Arch. Franç. Pédiat.* **18:** 41–64.

SABESIN, S. M. and ISSELBACHER, K. J. (1965) Protein synthesis inhibition: mechanism for the production of impaired fat absorption. *Science* **147:** 1149–1151.

SALET, J., POLONOVSKI, C., DEGOUYON, F., PEAN, G., MELEKIAN, B. and FOURNET, J. P. (1966) Tétanie hypocalcémique récidivante par hypomagnésemie congénitale. Une maladie métabolique nouvelle. *Arch. Franç. Pédiat.* **23:** 749–768.

SALT, H. B., WOLFE, O. H., LLOYD, J. K., FOSBROOKE, A. S., CAMERON, A. H. and HUBBLE, D. V. (1960) On having no beta-lipoprotein. A syndrome comprising a-beta-lipoproteinaemia, acanthocytosis and steatorrhoea. *Lancet* **2:** 325–329.

SAUNDERS, D. R., WAYS, P. O., PARAMENTIER, C. M. and RUBIN, C. E. (1966) Studies on the lipid composition of human small bowel mucosa. *J. Clin. Invest.* **45:** 1516–1525.

SCHACHTER, D. and ROSEN, S. M. (1959) Active transport of Ca^{45} by the small intestine and its dependence on vitamin D. *Am. J. Physiol.* **196:** 357–362.

SCHADE, S. C., FEICK, P., MUCKERHEIDE, M. and SCHILLING, R. F. (1966) Occurrence in gastric juice of antibody to a complex of intrinsic factor and vitamin B_{12}. *New Engl. J. Med.* **275:** 528–531.

SCHNEIDER, A. J., KINTER, W. B. and STIRLING, C. E. (1966) Glucose–galactose malabsorption. Report of a case with autoradiographic studies of a mucosal biopsy. *New Engl. J. Med.* **274:** 305–312.

SCHWARTZ, J. F., ROWLAND, L. P., EDER, H., MARKS, P. A., OSSERMAN, E. F., HIRSHBERG, E. and ANDERSON, H. (1963) Bassen–Kornzweig syndrome: deficiency of serum β-lipoprotein. *Arch. Neurol.* **8:** 438–454.

SCRIVER, C. R. (1961) Abnormalities of tryptophan metabolism in a patient with malabsorption syndrome. *J. Lab. Clin. Med.* **58:** 908–919.

SCRIVER, C. R. (1965) Hartnup disease. A genetic modification of intestinal and renal transport of certain neutral alpha amino-acids. *New Engl. J. Med.* **273:** 530–532.

SCRIVER, C. R. (1967) Membrane transport in disorders of imino-acid metabolism. *Am. J. Dis. Child.* **113:** 170–173.

SCRIVER, C. R. (1969) Use of human genetic variation to study membrane transport of amino acids in kidney. *Am. J. Dis. Child.* **117:** 4–12.

SCRIVER, C. R. and WILSON, O. H. (1967) Amino acid transport: evidence for genetic control of two types in human kidney. *Science* **155:** 1428–1430.

SEAKINS, J. W. T. and ERSSER, R. S. (1967) Effects of amino acid loads on a healthy infant with the biochemical features of Hartnup disease. *Arch. Dis. Childh.* **42:** 682–688.

SEELENFREUND, M. H., GARTNER, S. and VINGER, P. F. (1968) *Arch. Ophthal.* **80:** 718.

SEGAL, S. (1968) Tissue transport defects of dibasic amino acids, pp. 56–71. In: *Intestinal Absorption and Malabsorption,* SHMERLING, D. H., BERGER, H. and PRADER, A. (Eds.). *Modern Problems in Pediatrics,* vol. 11, Karger, Basel.

SEGAL, S., SCHWARTZMAN, L., BLAIR, A. and BERTOLI, D. (1967) Dibasic amino acid transport in rat-kidney cortex slices. *Biochem. Biophys. Acta* **135:** 127–135.

SHAW, K. N. F., REDLICH, D., WRIGHT, S. W. and JEPSON, J. B. (1960) Dependence of urinary indole excretion in Hartnup disease upon gut flora. *Federation Proc.* **19:** 194.

SHORT, E. M., BLINDER, H. J. and ROSENBERG, L. E. (1973) Familial hypophosphatemic rickets: Defective transport of inorganic phosphate by intestinal mucosa. *Science* **179:** 700–702.

SHULTZ, S. G. and CURRAN, P. F. (1968) Intestinal absorption of sodium chloride and water, pp. 1245–1275. In: *Handbook of Physiology,* sect. 6, vol. III, CODE, C. F. (Ed.). American Physiological Society, Washington, D.C.

SIEVENS, C. J. (1964) Megaloblastic anaemia in a 3-year-old child. *Blood* **23:** 547.

SINGER, K., FISHER, B. and PERLSTEIN, M. A. (1952) Acanthrocytosis, a genetic erythrocyte malformation. *Blood* **7**: 577–591.

SKYBERG, D., STROMME, J. H., NESBAKKEN, R. and HARNAES, K. (1967) Congenital primary hypomagnesaemia an inborn error of metabolism. *Acta Paediat. Scand.* Suppl. **177**: 26–27.

SKYBERG, D., STROMME, J. H., NESBAKKEN, R. and HARNAES, K. (1968a) Neonatal hypomagnesaemia with selective malabsorption of magnesium—a clinical entity. *Scand. J. Lab. Invest.* **21**: 355–363.

SKYBERG, D., STROMME, J. H., NORMAN, T., JOHANNESSEN, B. K. and SEIP, M. (1968b) (manuscript) Presented at Meeting of the Society of Inborn Errors of Metabolism, Zurich, 1968.

SMITH, A. J. and STRANG, L. B. (1958) An inborn error of metabolism with the urinary excretion of α-hydroxy-butyric acid and phenylpyruvic acid. *Arch. Dis. Childh.* **33**: 109–113.

SOBREVILLA, L. A., GOODMAN, M. L. and KANE, C. A. (1964) Demyelinating central nervous system disease, muscular atrophy and acanthocytosis (Bassen–Kornzweig Syndrome). *Am. J. Med.* **37**: 821–828.

STEWART, J. S., POLLACK, D. J., HOFFBRAND, A. V., MOLLIN, D. L. and BOOTH, C. C. (1967) A study of proximal and distal intestinal structure and absorptive function in idiopathic steatorrhoea. *Quart. J. Med.* **36**: 425–444.

STICKLER, G. B. (1963) External calcium and phosphorus balances in vitamin D-resistant rickets. A comparative review. *J. Pediatrics* **63**: 942–948.

STOKES, G. S., POTTS, J. T., LOTZ, M. and BARTTER, F. C. (1968) New agent in the treatment of cystinuria: *N*-acetyl-D-penicillamine. *Brit. Med. J.* **1**: 284–288.

STROMME, J. H., NESBAKKEN, R., NORMAN, T., SKJORTEN, F., SKYBERG, D. and JOHANNESSEN, B. (1969) Familial hypomagnesemia. Biochemical, histological and hereditary aspects studied in two brothers. *Acta Paediat. Scand.* **58**: 433–444.

STROMME, J. H., SKYBERG, D. and NESBAKKEN, R. (1967) A selective intestinal malabsorption of magnesium in an infant. *Scand. J. Clin. Lab. Invest.* Suppl. **100**: 103P.

STURMAN, R. M. (1968) The Bassen–Kornzweig Syndrome: 18 years in evolution. *J. Mount Sinai Hosp.* **35**: 489–517.

SVORC, J., MASOPUST, J., KOMARKOVA, A., MACEK, M. and HYANEK, J. (1967) Oculocerebrorenal syndrome in a female child. *Am. J. Dis. Child.* **114**: 186–190.

SWITZER, S. and EDER, H. A. (1962) Interconversion of acanthocytes and normal erythrocytes with detergents. *J. Clin. Invest.* **41**: 1404.

TADA, K., MORIKAWA, T., ANDO, T., YOSHIDA, T., and MINAGAWA, A. (1965) Prolinuria: a new renal tubular defect in transport of proline and glycine. *Tohoku J. Exp. Med.* **87**: 133–143.

TARLOW, M. J., SEAKINS, J. W. T., LLOYD, J. K., MATTHEWS, D. M., CHENG, B. and THOMAS, A. J. (1970) Intestinal absorption and biopsy transport of peptides and amino acids in Hartnup disease. *Clin. Sci.* **39**: 18P–19P.

THIER, S., FOX, M., SEGAL, S. and ROSENBERG, L. E. (1964) Cystinuria: *In vitro* demonstration of an intestinal transport defect. *Science* **143**: 482–484.

TOBLER, R., PRADER, A. and TAILLARD, W. (1956) Die familiäre primäre Vitamin-D-resistente Rachitis (Phosphatdiabetes). *Helv. Paediat. Acta* **11**: 209–255.

TOLENTINO, P., SPIRITO, L. and JANNUZZI, C. (1964) Celiac syndrome, retinal dystrophy and acanthocytosis, without defect of beta-lipoprotein. *Ann. Paediat.* (*Basel*) **203**: 178–186.

TREACHER, R. J. (1962) Amino-acid excretion in canine cystine-stone disease. *Vet. Record* **74**: 503–504.

TREACHER, R. J. (1963) The aminoaciduria of canine cystinestone disease. *Res. Vet. Sci.* **4**: 556–567.

TREACHER, R. J. (1964) The aetiology of canine cystinuria. *Biochem. J.* **90**: 494–498.

TREACHER, R. J. (1965) Intestinal absorption of lysine in cystinuric dogs. *J. Comp. Path.* **75:** 309–322.

VAN BUCHEM, F. S. P., POL, G., DE GIER, J., BOTTCHER, C. J. F. and PRIES, C. (1966) Congenital β-lipoprotein deficiency. *Am. J. Med.* **40:** 794–804.

VISAKORPI, J. K. and FURUHJELM, U. (1968) Selective malabsorption of vitamin B_{12}, pp. 150–160. In: *Intestinal Absorption and Malabsorption,* SHMERLING, D. H., BERGER, H. and PRADER, A. (Eds.). *Modern Problems in Pediatrics,* vol. 11, Karger, Basel.

WAYS, P. O., PARMENTIER, C. M., KAYDEN, H. J., JONES, J. W., SAUNDERS, D. R. and RUBIN, C. E. (1967) Studies on the absorptive defect for triglyceride in abetalipoproteinemia. *J. Clin. Invest.* **46:** 35–46.

WAYS, P., REED, C. F. and HANAHAN, D. J. (1963) Red-cell and plasma lipids in acanthocytosis. *J. Clin. Invest.* **42:** 1248–1260.

WESENBERG, R. L., GWINN, J. L., and BARNES, G. R. (1969) Radiological findings in the kinky-hair syndrome. *Radiology* **92:** 500.

WEYERS, H. and BICKEL, H. (1958) Photodermatose mit Aminoacidurie, Indolaceturie und cerebralen Manifestationen (Hartnup-syndrom). *Klin. Wchnschr.* **36:** 893–897.

WHELAN, D. T. and SCRIVER, C. R. (1968) Hyperdibasicaminoaciduria: An inherited disorder of amino acid transport. *Pediat. Res.* **2:** 525–534.

WILLIAMS, T. F., WINTERS, R. W. and BURNETT. CH. H. (1966) Familial (hereditary) vitamin D-resistant rickets with hypophosphatemia, pp. 1179–1204. In: *The Metabolic Basis of Inherited Disease,* 2nd ed., STANBURY, J. B., WYNGAARDEN, J. B. and FREDRICKSON, D. S. (Eds.). McGraw-Hill, N.Y.

WINTERS, R. W., GRAHAM, J. B., WILLIAMS, T. F., MCFALLS, V. W. and BURNETT, CH. H. (1958) A genetic study of familial hypophosphatemia and vitamin D resistant rickets with a review of the literature. *Medicine* **37:** 97–142.

WOLFF, O. H., LLOYD, J. K. and TONKS, E. L. (1964) A-betalipoproteinaemia with special reference to the visual defect. *Exp. Eye Res.* **3:** 439.

WOLLASTON, W. H. (1810) On cystic oxide, a new species of urinary calculus. *Trans. Roy. Soc. London* **100:** 223–230.

WONG, P. W. K., and PILLAI, P. M. (1966) Clinical and biochemical observations in two cases of Hartnup disease. *Arch. Dis. Childh.* **41:** 383–388.

WRONG, O. A. and METCALFE-GIBSON, A. (1965) The electrolyte content of faeces. *Proc. Roy. Soc. Med.* **58:** 1007–1009.

WRONG, O., METCALFE-GIBSON, A., MORRISON, R. B. I., NG, S. I. and HOWARD, A. V. (1965) *In vivo* dialysis of faeces as a method of stool analysis. I. Technique and results in normal subjects. *Clin. Sci.* **28:** 357–375.

YSSING, M. and FRIIS-HANSEN, B. (1966) Congenital alkalosis with diarrhoea. *Acta Paediat. Scand.* **55:** 341–344.

ZETTERSTROM, R. and WALDENSTROM, J. (1968) Familial monosaccharide malabsorption, pp. 101–112. In: *Intestinal Absorption and Malabsorption,* SHMERLING, D. H., BERGER, H. and PRADER, A. (Eds.). *Modern Problems in Pediatrics,* vol. 11, Karger, Basel.

CHAPTER 14

METHODS FOR THE INVESTIGATION OF ABSORPTION IN ANIMALS

K. Pfleger

Homburg/Saar, Federal Republic of Germany

INTRODUCTION

A comprehensive and historical review of the methods for studying absorption from the alimentary canal has recently been published by Parsons (1968). We shall, therefore, only describe and evaluate commonly used methods.

In any study of absorption, the two most interesting problems are (1) the dependence of absorption upon time and concentration, i.e. the kinetics of absorption, and (2) the processes responsible for absorption, such as 'facilitated diffusion', 'carrier-mediated transport' or 'active transport', i.e. the problem of the mechanism of absorption.*

From the technical point of view, the first question should be more easily answered than the second, for which a solution may only be found by using a combination of several methods.

As a rule, it is necessary to trace the substances under study either in the body of the experimental animal, or in the excretion products (urine and feces). If the absorption of metals or organometallic compounds is being studied, it is advisable to use radioactive isotopes, which are now commercially available for nearly all elements. These investigations are particularly simple when γ-emitting radioisotopes may be used, because γ-radiation may be directly and quantitatively determined using commercial scintillation counters and whole-body measuring devices, without any additional processing of the analysis material. Absorption studies of organic compounds are more complex; for carbon, hydrogen and sulfur the only isotopes that may be used are those emitting soft β-radiation. In order to trace soft β-radiation, the analysis samples and experi-

*For definitions see Chapter 2, p. 87 and Chapter 4, p. 250 (Eds.).

mental animals must first be processed using combustion methods, or extraction methods appropriate to the substance being investigated. Nitrogen-15 would also be suitable for absorption studies, but the mass spectrometers required for identification are still too expensive, and there are few ^{15}N-labeled compounds commercially available.

When radioactive isotopes cannot be used for studying absorption, it is necessary to identify the substance by one of the conventional chemical or physicochemical methods. It is advisable to check the efficiency of the method chosen before starting absorption studies, because in most cases the methods have been developed for pharmaceutical purposes only, and are liable to fail in the presence of biological material.

14.1. *IN VIVO* INVESTIGATIONS

14.1.1. INVESTIGATION WITH UNANESTHETIZED INTACT ANIMALS

14.1.1.1. *Experimental animals*

Leaving aside the problems of nutrition physiology, absorption conditions in the intestine of the experimental animal should correspond as much as possible to those in man. For this reason, dogs, cats and rats are preferable to pure herbivores, such as rabbits and guinea-pigs.

For a number of reasons, the size of the experimental animal is a determining factor. It is easier to collect the excretion products of each animal in suitable metabolic cages in the case of dogs, cats and rabbits than in that of smaller animals. The disadvantage of big animals, however, is that the substances have to be administered in quantities that are 10–100 times as large as in small animals. This may cause considerable expense, for example when ^{14}C-labeled compounds are used. There is also the further problem of disposal of the bodies when radioisotopes are used.

14.1.1.2. *Administration of substances*

The aim must be to administer the substance under investigation as far as possible in the same form and manner as it is applied under therapeutic conditions, i.e. as tablets, pills or fluid together with food and drink. It is, however, often necessary to abandon this procedure, because the results must be quantitatively reliable. As a rule, preference is then given to administration of the substance in dissolved form, or as a suspension, by means of the gastric tube. This technic has been described in detail by Ther (1965).

14.1.1.3. *Collection of feces and urine*

For balance investigations, it is essential to collect urine and feces separately. Even then, however, only quantitative information on absorption will be obtained, unless simultaneous determination of excretion is made with the aid of a biliary fistula.

Many methods have been devised for the separate collection of urine and feces. The following procedure has proved useful for rats (Fig. 1). The animals are placed in cages (for dimensions see figure) separately or in groups. The floor of the cage, a plastic surface covered with filter paper of high absorptive quality, is placed at an angle of about 40°. Nigrovic and Mohr (1966) have used commercially available cages of macrolon to which they added a floor of glass rods. The sheet of filter paper is folded so that a duct forms at the lower end in which the feces are collected. Urine is absorbed by the paper, and drying of the urine may be accelerated by a fan. The degree of contamination of the filter paper by feces, and of feces with urine, depends upon the substance tested. Contamination cannot be completely prevented by any method; however, in our experience, it amounts to less than 1 % provided that the animals produce solid feces.

For determination of the excreted substance and its metabolites, feces and filter paper are extracted. If γ-emitting radioisotopes were used for labeling, feces and paper can be placed directly into the radiation measuring device. The application of the method is limited in so far as organic

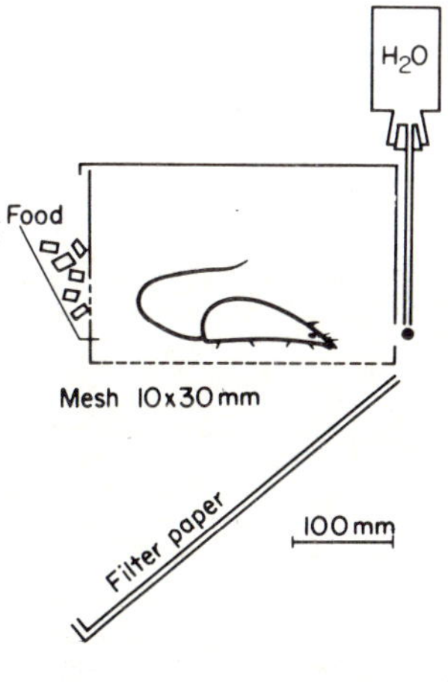

FIG. 1. Cross-section through a device for separate collection of urine and feces.

substances are frequently altered by bacteria in feces even outside the body (Pfleger and Dörr, unpublished data).

Harned *et al.* (1949) and Gross and Connell (1923) described a somewhat more complicated method. Suitable metabolic cages are marketed by Süsee and Schmidt KG, 35 Kassel (West Germany), Maybachstr. 1–7. Urine is separated from feces by a spindle down which the urine flows into the vessel. The spindle and urine vessel are arranged above the pot for collection of feces. Food is administered to the animals either in solid form so that they only nibble at it but are unable to scatter the food, or in semi-liquid form through a hole which is so small that they cannot get at the food with their paws. This method, however, does not give better results than the before-mentioned less complicated one.

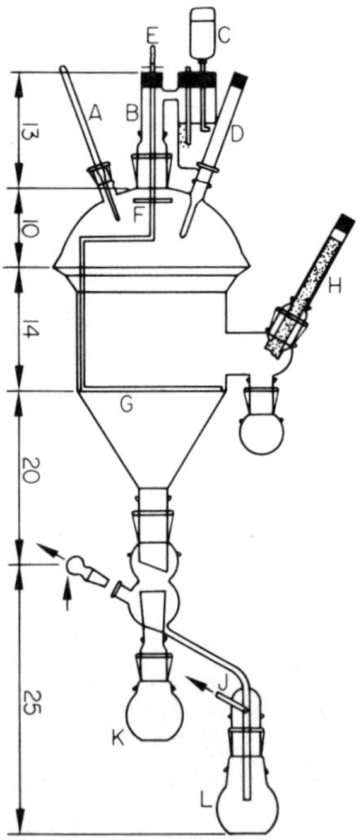

FIG. 2. Metabolic cage for separation of urine, feces and respiration air. A = thermometer, B = adaptor for water connection, C = vessel for automatic control of water level in water seal, D = saturating tube, E = support of top section of vertical part of floor unit, F = plastic disc to distribute air flow along cage walls, G = plastic floor unit, H = feeding tube, I = aperture for withdrawing air, J = tube for ventilating urine flask when cage is cleaned, K = feces flask, L = urine flask.

For investigations where it is also necessary to collect the expired $^{14}CO_2$ or volatile compounds, completely closed metabolic cages of the kind shown in Fig. 2 must be used. The cage illustrated is marketed by Altromin GmbH, 491 Lage (Lippe) (West Germany). A sufficient air stream (500 ml/min) is drawn first through the metabolic cages and then through a wash bottle containing a suitable absorption medium. For $^{14}CO_2$, 150 ml, 25% ethanolamine (changed every 6–12 hr) has proved satisfactory; 0.1 to 1.0 ml ethanolamine is measured with 10–20 ml dioxane scintillator in the liquid scintillation counter. Glycerin can be used as an absorption medium for water or volatile organic compounds.

Larger metabolic cages for rabbits, dogs and cats have been described (cf. Ther, 1965). The tests are so complicated that as a rule only a few metabolic cages can be used at a time.

14.1.1.4. *Observation period*

The residence time in various parts of the intestine plays a major part in the absorption of a substance. It depends upon the environmental conditions and the feeding of the experimental animals used, and it must, if necessary, be determined by suitable labeling. Investigations with barium sulfate have shown that, in the rat, the first white colored material appears in the feces after an average of 4 hr (Haas and Forth, 1956). In fasting animals the residence time is doubled. After the addition of small quantities of ^{59}Fe to the food, the results are similar (Forth *et al.*, 1965). After 6 hr, about 20%; after 12 hr, 35%; after 18 hr, 45% of the iron administered is excreted in the feces. Excretion does not increase much after 24 hr. Consequently, an observation time of 24–48 hr is probably sufficient for rats. The process of excretion can be checked by fractionated collection of feces.

The residence time differs in various sections of the intestine. In the rat, it has been investigated with ^{91}Y particles. The half-time of the residence time in the stomach was 60 min, in the duodenum 6 min, in the upper jejunum 18 min, in the distal jejunum 72 min and in the ileum 102 min (Lengemann, 1963). Dissolved yttrium passed through the stomach and the distal jejunum about twice as quickly as particles.

14.1.2. INVESTIGATIONS ON INTESTINAL LOOPS

The investigation with tied-off intestinal segments has the following advantages:

1. Absorption can be investigated independently of the stomach

emptying time or of the time of passage through the intestine;
2. it is possible to compare different sections of the gastrointestinal tract;
3. it is possible, whenever necessary, to avoid or investigate interference of entero-hepatic circulation.

14.1.2.1. *Intestinal loops in unanesthetized animals*

The most common method is the so-called Thiry–Vella fistula of the dog. The technique of the operation is relatively simple. Using conventional surgical techniques, a loop of the small intestine, having a length of up to 120 cm, is removed from the intestine, and both ends are sewn into the midline of the abdominal wall (Cramer and Dueck, 1962). The two ends of the remaining intestine are connected. Parenteral feeding of the animals is advisable for a few days; 18 days after the operation, the dogs can be used for absorption studies. Generally the loops are perfused during the absorption investigations. Johnston (1932) describes a suitable closure mechanism. The method has also been applied to the rat (Haberich *et al.*, 1968).

14.1.2.2. *Intestinal loops in anesthetized animals*

The method can be practiced in a simple manner on the rat, guinea-pig, rabbit, cat and dog. The animals are anesthetized by i.p. administration of a suitable long-acting anesthetic pentobarbital (Nembutal®, 50 mg/kg). The operation can be started about 15 min after the injection. The anesthesia lasts approximately 3 hr. For larger animals, chloralose–urethane (5% chloralose dissolved hot in 25% urethane, 75–100 mg chloralose per kg administered i.v.) and halothane together with a conventional vaporizer after intubation have also proved useful. Rummel and Seifen (1964) list also other narcotics.

Since only homologous segments may be compared, exact anatomic orientation is essential. The important reference points include the flexura duodenojejunalis (in the rat) and the valvula ileocoecalis. The measurement of the distance in cm between the loop and the reference point provides a suitable standard of comparison.

When applying ligatures between the arches of vessels, care must be taken to ensure that no ischemic region is formed in the segment prepared for the absorption test. The fluid to be investigated is injected through a thin cannula inserted into the lumen of the intestinal loop. The cannula is inserted at one end of the loop and the ligature is tightened around the cannula. In this way it is possible to prevent fluid from passing into the peritoneal cavity. The volume of fluid introduced into the intestinal loop must be adapted to the capacity of the segment. On the one hand, the loop must not be distended; otherwise blood circulation will be restricted. On the other hand, the volume must be sufficient to allow the entire surface of the mucosa to be in contact with the fluid. In the case of rats weighing 200 g, 2 ml fluid can be introduced into a loop of 15–20 cm length.

In most cases, the substances to be tested are administered in a physiological NaCl solution or Tyrode solution (Ther, 1965); a buffer is added when necessary. Although the pH of the solution administered differs markedly from the physiological intraluminal pH of the segment, a rapid adaptation will occur (cf. Chapter 12, p. 621).

It must be remembered that the concentration of the substance to be investigated may change considerably during the test period due to water absorption, particularly in the case of slow absorption of the substance (Kausch, 1969). Water absorption varies in different sections of the gastrointestinal tract, depending on the species, as Table 1 shows. A substantial net absorption of water from the intestine can be prevented using isotonic choline–chloride solution. Because of the excretion of fluid into the intestinal lumen its content increases by 0.1–0.2 ml within 1 hr.

In small animals, the body temperature drops rapidly during narcosis. It is therefore advisable to keep these animals in a chamber at about 34°C during the test.

At the end of the test, the fluid volume in the loop is measured

TABLE 1. ABSORPTION OF WATER IN DIFFERENT PARTS OF THE SMALL INTESTINE OF RATS *in vivo*. Experimental conditions: tied-off loops *in vivo* (operation in ether anesthesia). The loops were filled initially with 2 ml Tyrode solution. The numbers indicate the residual fluid in the loops one hour later in percent of the volume administered ± SEM; $n = 8$–10. Negative sign means fluid transfer from the lumen to blood; positive sign means fluid transfer from blood to lumen (Forth, unpublished data)

RAT	
Stomach[a]	±140 (±16)
Jejunum[b]	− 85 (±17)[e]
Ileum[c]	− 34 (± 7)
Colon[d]	− 48 (± 5)

[a] Entire stomach.
[b] 20 cm length, starting with the flexura duodenojejunalis.
[c] 20 cm length, starting with the valvula ileocoecalis.
[d] Entire colon, 10 cm length.
[e] Guinea-pig: + 70 (± 10).

gravimetrically or with the help of an admixed, non-absorbable marker. Suitable markers are methyl-cellulose (Berger *et al.*, 1959) which can easily be determined by spectrophotometry or ^{14}C-labeled polyethylene glycol 4000 (Schedl, 1966; Soergel, 1968). Inulin-^{14}C and hemoglobin are less suited because they are apparently degraded by the digestive juices (Berger *et al.*, 1959; Soergel, 1968) or contain impurities in the form of low molecular fractions which may be absorbed (Lauterbach and Witte, 1973). The results are probably more accurate if a marker is used, because a residue remains in the lumen during the discharging and weighing of the contents of the intestine. After discharging, the loop is opened opposite to the mesenteric end, rinsed with isotonic solution, dabbed gently with filter paper. Then the segments can be subjected to a suitable method for determining the quantity of the substance in the intestinal wall.

The methods for the analysis of the contents of the intestine and the intestinal wall depend upon the substances investigated. The use of γ-emitting radioisotopes offers the additional advantage that the carcass of the animal after removal of the intestinal loop can be used for determination of absorption by measurement in the whole-body counter.

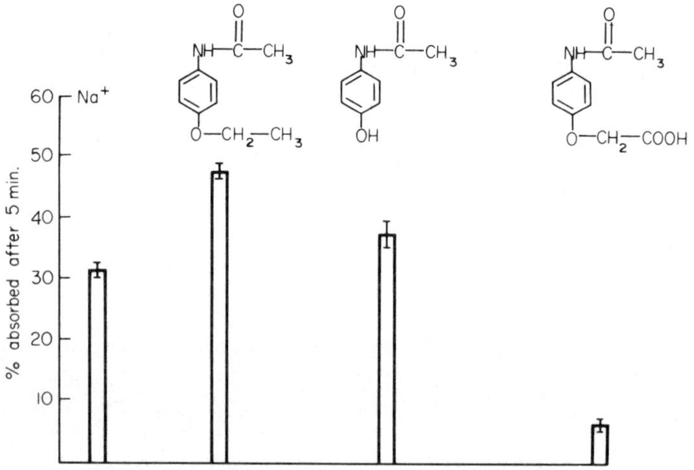

FIG. 3. Absorption of aniline derivatives in comparison with sodium ions from rat tied-off jejunal loops. Length of segments: 20 cm, starting with the flexura duodenojejunalis. Body weight of the rats: 200 g. 2 ml isotonic choline–chloride solution were administered containing 6 mcM of the substances ($n \leq 6$). Na was determined by radiometry, the aniline derivatives by spectrophotometry. (Pfleger and Häuser, unpublished data.)

In some cases, the concentration of the absorbed substance in the blood can be taken as indicator of the absorption rate (Jacobi *et al.*, 1956). Blood samples are taken from larger animals during the test, or, in the smaller animals, blood is obtained by puncture of the heart before removal of the intestinal loop.

To give an idea of the rate at which, under the conditions described, substances disappear from the intestinal lumen, Fig. 3 presents a homologous series of aniline derivatives with ^{22}Na as a standard. Thirty percent of the Na administered disappeared from the jejunum after 5 min; the corresponding quantity of phenacetin amounts to 45%, whereas of the homologous acid, only somewhat more than 5% is absorbed during the same period. About 37% of the *N*-acetylparaaminophenol was absorbed after 5 min. The sequence corresponds to theoretical expectation according to which the absorption rate declines with increasing polarity of the compounds (Pfleger and Häuser, unpublished data).

14.1.2.3. *Luminal circulation of intestinal loops in anesthetized animals*

In the preceding section it has already been pointed out that both the volume of the intestinal content and the concentration of the constituents of the content change when tied-off loops are used. These raise considerable problems as far as the mathematical calculations of the experimental data are concerned. The change of concentration in the luminal fluid can be prevented if the loops are circulated from a fluid reservoir which contains a large volume as compared to the volume absorbed. When recirculating the fluid from a reservoir along the lumen of an intestinal segment the secretion from blood to lumen can also be investigated.

The surgical procedures are the same as described on pp. 802–803. The only additional equipment required is a small thermostat for warming the perfused fluid up to 37°C, and a controllable fluid pump. When recirculation is not required, the pump may be replaced by a hydrostatic pressure device.

14.1.3. INVESTIGATIONS OF ABSORPTION IN DEPENDENCE OF BLOOD PERFUSION

To understand the pharmaco-kinetics one should know whether a substance enters the blood or lymph unaltered, or whether it undergoes a metabolic change during the passage through the mucosal epithelium. Although it is possible to take blood directly from the vena portae even in small animals, this method does not always produce clear results, because recirculation may interfere.

The fraction incorporated via the lymph can be measured by introducing a cannula into the mesenterial lymph vessels or the ductus thoracicus. This technique is simple, when applied in larger animals such as dogs or cats, but it has also been performed in rats (Bollman, 1948; Gallo-Torres and Miller, 1969). Although it is well established that substances enter the organism via the lymph (Paldine and Hyman, 1964; DeMarco and Levine, 1969; Levine, 1971), we must remember that absorption via the lymph is quantitatively insignificant since the ratio of the flow volumes of portal vein to lymph is 600–700:1 (Forth *et al.*, 1969; Levine, 1971; for further references see Wilson, 1962). A further point to be kept in mind is that there is interference with the fraction which recirculates and emerges from the capillaries as an ultrafiltrate (Forth *et al.*, 1969); this may lead to misinterpretation. Lastly, lympho-venous anastomoses are present in the area of the intestine (Paldine and Hyman, 1964). The role of the lymph is discussed in detail in Chapters 2 and 4.

A further point of interest in many problems is the effect on absorption of blood flow.

There are two possible methods for dealing with this problem. The circulation of the experimental animal may be used directly or the intestinal loop is perfused with blood or an artificial medium using a perfusion apparatus.

14.1.3.1. *Perfusion with blood of intestinal loops in animals with intact systemic circulation*

In principle, the blood flowing from the intestinal loops is obtained by placing a cannula in the vein which comes from the loop. In the dog, for example, the quantity of blood supplied by the arteries (Williams *et al.*, 1964) is varied with the aid of a peristaltic pump (sigma), which is interposed between the right femoral artery and the cranial mesenteric artery. The same principle can be applied to the rat. In a method recently developed for the rat (Ochsenfahrt and Winne, 1969) the blood pressure is varied by infusion of blood into the vena jugularis. In dogs, the blood flow in the arteria mesenterica cranialis amounted to 65 ml/min (Williams *et al.*, 1964). Data for the intestinal blood flow in rats range between 0.7 and 1.5 ml/g tissue (Takacs and Vajda, 1963; Csernay *et al.*, 1965; Ross *et al.*, 1966).

14.1.3.2. *Artificial perfusion with blood of intestinal loops*

Perfusion of intestinal loops can be carried out also with the help of

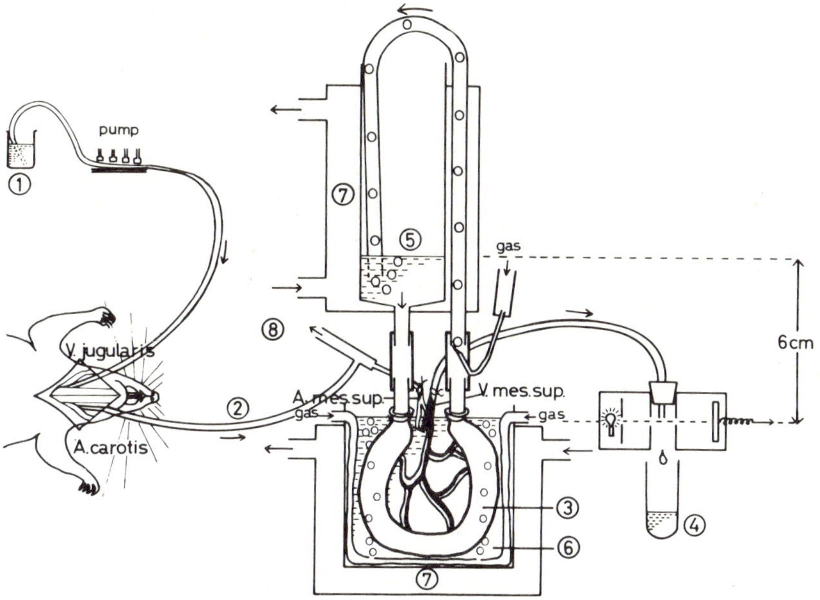

FIG 4. Schematic diagram of a combined intraluminal circulation and vascular perfusion technique in an isolated rat jejunal loop. The arterial blood is supplied by a donor rat in which the blood loss is substituted by a continuous blood infusion. The blood flow can be stopped by clamping the arterial supply. 1 = reservoir containing heparinized rat blood, 2 = arterial blood supply, 3 = isolated jejunal loop (6–8 cm), 4 = venous outflow, 5 = intraluminal circulation fluid (initial volume 10 ml), 6 = serosal bath (initial volume 35 ml), 7 = water jacket, 8 = blood pressure recording. Gas = 95% O_2 and 5% CO_2. (From Ochsenfahrt, 1971.)

artificial circulation *in vitro*. Methods have been developed, and successfully applied using intestinal segments of cold-blooded animals (Parsons and Prichard, 1968), of dogs (Varro *et al.*, 1969), of rabbits (Hohenleitner and Senior, 1969) and of rats (Gerber and Remy-Defraigne, 1966; Jacobs *et al.*, 1957, 1966; Forth, 1968; Lee and Duncan, 1968; For further references see Ross, 1972.)

The composition of the perfusion solution is the most difficult problem. Blood often contains vaso-active substances which make the perfusion impossible. Vasoconstriction can be avoided by adding 100 mg/l of papaverine-hydrochloride to a perfusion medium of the composition specified by Forth (1968).

A way of removing the vaso-active substances is to pass the blood through a second animal before supplying it to the intestinal loop

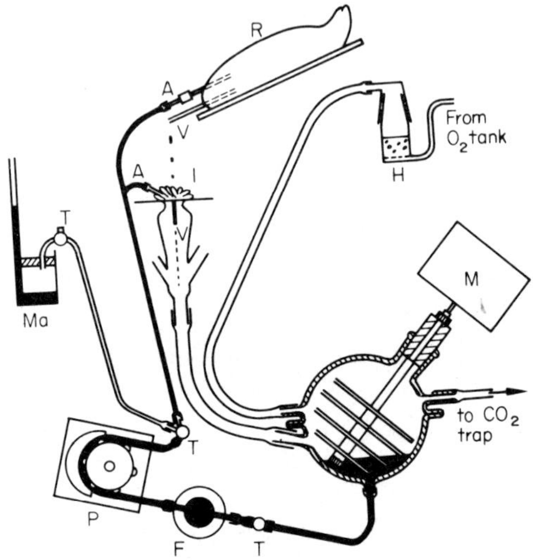

FIG. 5. Apparatus for perfusion of intestinal loops in rats. Method I: the perfused intestinal segment remains in the rat. Method II: the intestinal segment is removed from the rat. A = Inflow cannula, F = filter, H = humidifier, M = motor, Ma = manometer, P = pump, R = rat (method I), T = three-way stop cock, V = outflow cannula, I = intestine (method II). (Gerber and Remy-Defraigne, 1966.)

(Ochsenfahrt and Winne, 1969). The method is substantially the same as that shown in Fig. 4.

It is an empirical fact that in the perfused loop, the intra-luminally supplied quantity of fluid often does not decrease, but increases. The reason for this is not yet clear. It is possible, however, to prevent an increase in luminal volume by addition of oncotically active polymers, such as dextrane, polyvinyl pyrrolidone or albumin, to the perfusion fluid. It must be remembered in this context that dextrane releases 5-hydroxytryptamine in the rat, and polyvinyl pyrrolidone releases histamine in the dog. Apart from its relatively high price albumin is exceptionally suitable, since on the one hand it prevents aggregation of erythrocytes and, on the other hand, has a coating effect on capillaries. Particularly suitable oxygen-carriers are washed cattle erythrocytes because they have a low aggregate-forming tendency. Fluid outflow from the blood into the lumen could be prevented by the addition of an antihistaminic drug (promethazin 40 mg/l) to the blood suspension (Forth, 1968).

Because it is difficult in general to furnish large volumes of blood for perfusion, in Fig. 5 a perfusion device is shown which allows the perfusion with small volumes (Gerber, 1965). In this device the perfused segment may either remain in the animal (method I, Fig. 5) or can be removed and placed into a wet chamber (method II, Fig. 5).

An interesting model of artificial blood perfused rat intestinal segment was described recently by Ochsenfahrt (1971). This preparation allows absorption to be studied under varying blood supply and even without blood flow (Fig. 4).

14.2. *IN VITRO* INVESTIGATIONS

14.2.1. ISOLATED SEGMENTS OF THE SMALL INTESTINE

This method is carried out on segments without blood supply. The situation thus becomes exceptionally clear and analysis samples are easy to obtain, although the substances to be tested must pass from the mucosal cells through the lymph and blood vessels to the serosal side (Lee, 1965). Ochsenfahrt (1971) showed that without blood supply the absorption rates of antipyrine and salicylic acid are 50% lower than that obtained with blood perfusion. For practical purposes mainly two methods are used, the "everted sac" (Wilson and Wiseman, 1954) and the intestinal loop, which is circulated at the mucosal side by a buffer solution (Fisher and Parsons, 1949).

Figure 6 shows the histological picture of an everted rat jejunal segment after 5 min (a, b) and 2 hr (c, d) incubation time. (a) and (b): the intercellular spaces of the epithelium are enlarged at the level of the villi; individual cells are extruded without any disruption of continuity. The lamina propria and the lower layers of the intestinal wall scarcely differ from the normal picture. (c) and (d): the intercellular spaces of the epithelium become widened while the cells shrink. Extrusion of cells is increased and the epithelium of the villus flanks and crypts dissociates. In the area of the villus tip, the connective tissue shows edema. The basal membrane is raised clear of the pellicle of the capillary. The essential point appears to be that no disruption of continuity can be detected even 2 hr after the beginning of the experiment. A similar histological picture as shown here was obtained with intestinal sections perfused according to the method of Fisher and Parsons (1949). For the sake of completeness it must be added that Levine *et al.* (1970) failed to show histological integrity of intestinal everted sacs. This may be due to differences in histological technique.

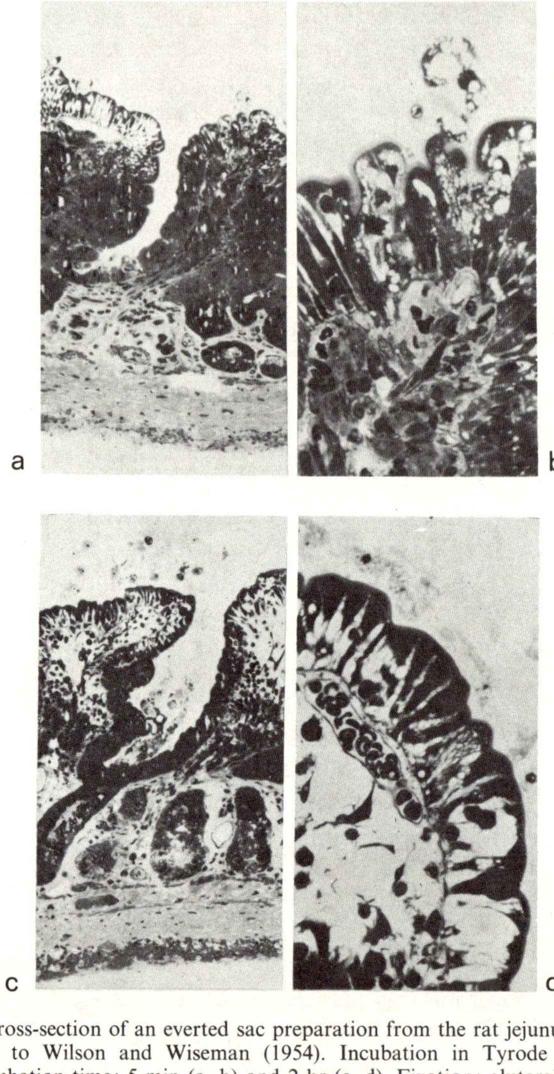

FIG. 6. Cross-section of an everted sac preparation from the rat jejunum. Method according to Wilson and Wiseman (1954). Incubation in Tyrode solution at 37°C. Incubation time: 5 min (a, b) and 2 hr (c, d). Fixation: glutaraldehyde and osmium tetroxide; potting: araldite; thickness of cut: 1 mcm; staining: borax-azure II-methylene blue; scales: (a) 175: 1; (b) 700: 1; (c) 175: 1; (d) 700: 1. The functional integrity of the preparations shown here may be taken from Fig. 7, p. 811. (From Specht and Kulenkampff, unpublished data.)

The functional integrity of the preparations can best be assessed by studying absorption of an actively absorbed substance. Figure 7 shows

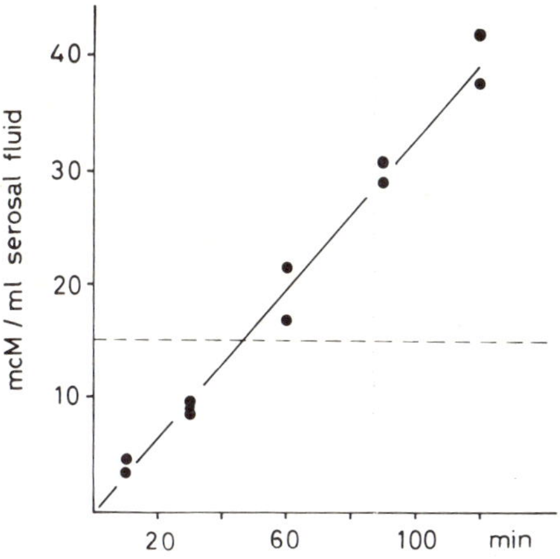

FIG. 7. Uphill transport of glucose across the intestinal wall of jejunal everted sacs of rats. Glucose-concentration at the mucosal side 15 mcM/ml. Mucosal fluid: 12 ml Tyrode solution. Serosal fluid: 0.7 ml Ringer solution. Concentration equilibrium of glucose in mucosal and serosal fluid is reached at the crossing point of the unbroken and the broken lines. Length of the segments: 6 cm, starting with the flexura duodenojejunalis. Two segments were prepared in each rat. Each point represents the value of one segment. The histological integrity of the everted sacs used in this experiment may be taken from Fig. 6, p. 810. (Forth and Nell, unpublished data.)

that concentration of glucose increases linearly with time at the serosal side for a period of up to 2 hr. The sugar is transported uphill; concentration balance between the mucosal and serosal sides is obtained after 45 min at 15 mcM.

In assessing the results, it must be remembered that in the preparations not subjected to blood flow, the substances must pass through the muscle layers of the intestinal wall. It should therefore be checked to what extent the substances investigated are taken up into the intestinal wall.

14.2.2. MEMBRANES OF MUCOSAL EPITHELIUM

The use of membranes consisting entirely of the mucosal epithelium and the lamina propria avoids the disadvantage of long diffusion pathways through muscle cell layers. Methods have been developed for the intestine of the tortoise (Baillien and Schoffeniels, 1960, 1961), piked dogfish (Carlisky and Huang, 1962), dog (Parsons and Paterson, 1965), rabbit (Fromm *et al.*, 1969), rat and guinea-pig small intestine (Lauterbach, 1970), dog (Hakim *et al.*, 1963) and rat colon (Parsons and Paterson, 1965).

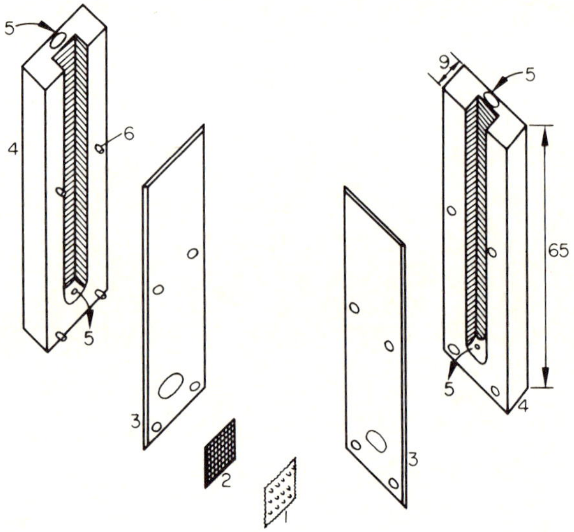

FIG. 8. Diagram showing arrangement of chambers, foils, nylon gauze and tissue for studying passage through the mucosa. 1 = mucosa, 2 = nylon gauze, 3 = partitions, 4 = plexiglass walls, 5 = oxygenation duct, 6 = fixing pins. All components are compressed using a hose clamp in the sequence indicated (dimensions in millimeters). (From Lauterbach, 1969.)

According to Lauterbach (1969) mucosal cell specimens of about 7 mm edge length are cut with a razor from an open piece of small intestine placed on a flat base, and applied to nylon gauze. The nylon gauze with the mucosal membrane attached is mounted as a window between two chambers which are filled with 0.2 ml of warmed incubation fluid (Fig. 8). In a water bath, the chambers are kept at the desired temperature. Leakiness of the mucosal membrane may be checked by adding polyvinyl pyrrolidone Mg 11,500 to the fluid of one chamber.

14.2.3. INTESTINAL RINGS

The question of possible uptake of substances by the mucosal cells can be answered by using intestinal rings (Skala and Hruba, 1964; Boass and Wilson, 1962; Crane and Mandelstam, 1960; Agar *et al.*, 1954).

The test procedure does not differ from the everted sac method except that the intestinal sections are cut into pieces 0.5–1 cm long, and agitated in a suitable oxygenized suspension. Since the muscles of the intestinal specimens immediately contract, the villi of the small intestine come to lie on the outside and are well distended.

14.2.4. MUCOSAL CELL SUSPENSIONS

The only advantage these have over intestinal rings is that their use avoids uptake of substances into the tissues not participating in absorption, such as muscle, connective tissue cells, etc.

Respective methods are described by Hashim and Clark (1969); Søgnen (1967); Perris (1966); Stern and Jensen (1966); Stern and Reilly (1965); Clark and Porteous (1965); Harrer *et al.* (1964); Rasmussen *et al.* (1963); Paterson and Sbarsky (1958).

This advantage is, however, minimized by a number of major disadvantages. The preparation technique is relatively complicated. Since the cells stick together, incubation is difficult. In order to verify whether the cells are damaged during preparation or not, dyes such as thymol blue may be used; living cells do not take up the dye. Apparently it is possible to obtain cells which are morphologically and functionally intact, as was shown for rabbit parietal cells of the stomach (Waldner and Lunseth, 1963) and for chicken intestinal cells (Kimmich, 1970).

14.2.5. SUBCELLULAR FRACTIONS

Brush borders can be obtained from isolated mucosal cells (section 14.2.4) by differential and gradient centrifugation with high velocity centrifuges (Miller and Crane, 1961; Boyd *et al.*, 1968; Forstner *et al.*, 1968). It must be pointed out, however, that the brush borders obtained in this way contain a large fraction of "terminal web" which must be allotted to the cell interior and not to the cell membrane.

The brush borders obtained in this manner have been investigated chiefly for their enzyme content and their ability to form selective bonds with certain substances. With the aid of TRIS buffers which have a specific molarity and pH, they can be divided into even smaller fragments (TRIS-disruption, Eichholtz and Crane, 1965).

Separation of *subcellular fractions* of mucosal cells have been described for rabbits and guinea-pigs (Hübscher *et al.*, 1965; Porteous and Clark, 1965; Takesue and Sato, 1968) and for rats (Clark and Porteous, 1965; Robinson, 1963; Worwood and Jacobs, 1971). The main difficulty in fractionating rat mucosal cells is the large amount of mucus. This difficulty can be overcome using the method of Hübers *et al.* (1971) who introduced a gradient centrifugation in polyvinyl pyrrolidone medium. By this method a total fractionation of mucosal cells into brush borders and nuclei, mitochondria, microsomes and particle-free supernatant can be achieved within 3 hr only.

REFERENCES

AGAR, W. T., HIRD, F. J. R. and SIDHU, G. S. (1954) The uptake of amino acids by the intestine. *Biochim. Biophys. Acta* **14:** 80–84.

BAILLIEN, M. and SCHOFFENIELS, E. (1960) Un nouvel appareil destiné à mesurer le flux des ions à travers la muqueuse intestinal isolée. *Arch. Int. Physiol. Biochem.* **68:** 710–712.

BAILLIEN, M. and SCHOFFENIELS, E. (1961) Le transport actif d'acides amines au niveau de l'epithélium intestinal isolé de la tortue grecque. *Biochim. Biophys. Acta* **53:** 521–536.

BERGER, E., KANTAI, G., HOMER, M. G. and STEELE, J. M. (1959) Simultaneous flux of sodium into and out of the dog intestine. *Am. J. Physiol.* **196:** 74–82.

BOASS, A. and WILSON, T. H. (1962) Development of mechanisms for intestinal absorption of B_{12} in the growing rat. *Fedn Proc.* **21:** 469.

BOLLMAN, J. L. (1948) Cage which limits activity of rats. *J. Lab. Clin. Med.* **33:** 1348.

BOYD, C. A. R., PARSONS, D. S. and THOMAS, A. V. (1968) The presence of K^+ dependence phosphatase in intestinal epithelial cell brush borders isolated by a new method. *Biochim. Biophys. Acta* **150:** 723–726.

CARLISKY, N. J. and HUANG, K. C. (1962) Glucose transport by the intestinal mucosa of the dog fish. *Proc. Soc. Exp. Biol.* (*N.Y.*) **109:** 405–408.

CLARK, B. and PORTEOUS, W. (1965) The isolation and properties of epithelial cell "ghosts" from rat small intestine. *Biochem. J.* **96:** 539–551.

CLARKSON, T. W. and ROTHSTEIN, A. (1960) Transport of cations by the isolated small intestine of the rat. *Am. J. Physiol.* **199:** 898–906.

CRAMER, C. G. and DUECK, J. (1962) *In vivo* transport of calcium from healed Thiry–Vella fistulas in dogs. *Am. J. Physiol.* **202:** 161–164.

CRANE, R. K. and MANDELSTAM, P. (1960) The active transport of sugars by various preparations of hamster intestine. *Biochem. Biophys. Acta* **45:** 460–476.

CSERNAY, L., WOLF, F. and VARRO, V. (1965) Der Kreislaufgradient im Dünndarm. *J. Gastroenter.* **3:** 261–265.

DE MARCO, TH. J. and LEVINE, R. R. (1969) Role of lymphatics in the intestinal absorption and distribution of drugs. *J. Pharmac. Exp. Therap.* **169:** 142–151.

DIAMOND, L., DOLUISIO, J. T. and CROUTHAMEL, W. G. (1970) Physiological factors affecting intestinal drug absorption. *Europ. J. Pharmac.* **11:** 109–114.

EICHHOLTZ, A. and CRANE, R. K. (1965) Studies on the organisation of the brush borders in intestinal epithelial cells. I. Tris disruption of isolated hamster brush borders and density gradient separation of fractions. *J. Cell. Biol.* **26:** 687–691.

FISHER, R. B. and PARSONS, D. S. (1949) A preparation of surviving rat small intestine for the study of absorption. *J. Physiol.* (*Lond.*) **110:** 36–46.

FORSTNER, G. G., SABESIN, S. M. and ISSELBACHER, K. J. (1968) Rat intestinal microvillous membranes, purification and biochemical characterization. *Biochem. J.* **106:** 381–390.

FORTH, W. (1968) Eisen- und Kobalt-Resorption am perfundierten Dünndarmsegment, pp. 242–250. In: *Stoffwechsel der isoliert perfundierten Leber*, STAIB, W. and SCHOLZ, R. (Eds.). Springer-Verlag, Berlin–Heidelberg–New York.

FORTH, W., FURUKAWA, E. and RUMMEL, W. (1969) Die Bestimmung der intestinalen Resorption von Herzglykosiden durch Messung der ^{3}H-markierten Glykosiden im Portal-Venenblut und in der Darmlymphe bei Katzen. *Naunyn-Schmiedebergs Arch. exp. Path. Pharmak.* **264:** 406–419.

FORTH, W., PFLEGER, K., SEIFEN, E. and RICHMOND, I. SP. (1965) Der Einfluβ verschiedener Liganden auf Resorption, Verteilung und Ausscheidung von Eisen nach oraler Verabfolgung. *Naunyn-Schmiedebergs Arch. exp. Path. Pharmak.* **252:** 242–257.

FROMM, D., FIELD, M. and SILEN, W. (1969) Effect of insulin on sugar and amino acid transport across isolated small intestine. *Am. J. Physiol.* **217:** 53–57.

GALLO-TORRES, H. E. and MILLER, O. N. (1969) A modified Bollman's technique for canulation of the rat's thoracic duct: lymph flow standardization. *Proc. Soc. Exp. Biol.* **130:** 552–555.

GERBER, G. B. (1965) An efficient oxygenator for organ perfusion. *J. Appl. Physiol.* **20:** 159–160.

GERBER, J. B. and REMY-DEFRAIGNE, J. (1966) DNA-metabolism in perfused organs. II. Incorporation into DNA and catabolism of thymidine at different levels of substrate by normal and X-irradiated liver and intestine. *Archs. Int. Physiol. Biochem.* **74:** 785–806.

GROSS, L. and CONNELL, S. J. B. (1923) Separation of excreta from rats. *J. Physiol.* **57:** *l*x–*l*xii.

HAAS, H. and FORTH, W. (1956) Ein Beitrag zur Analyse der zentral erregenden Wirkungskomponenten einiger sympathomimetischer Amine. *Arzneimittelforschung* **6:** 436–445.

HABERICH, F. J., HERZER, R., AZIR, O. and DEMHARDL, R. (1968) Resorptions- und Sekretionsstudien am Darm. I. *Zschrft. f. d. gesam. exp. Med.* **148:** 223–237.

HAKIM, A., LESTER, R. G. and LIFSON, H. (1963) Absorption by an *in vitro* preparation of dog intestinal mucosa. *J. Appl. Physiol.* **18:** 409–413.

HARNED, B. K., CUNNINGHAM, R. W. and GILL, E. R. (1949) A metabolism cage for small animals. *Science* **109:** 489–490.

HARRER, D. S., STERN, B. K. and REILLY, E. W. (1964) Removal and dissociation of epithelial cells from the rodent gastrointestinal tract. *Nature* **205:** 319–320.

HASHIM, G. and CLARK, J. (1969) Studies on the effect of vitamin D on calcium absorption and transport. *Biochem. J.* **112:** 275–283.

HOHENLEITNER, F. J. and SENIOR, J. R. (1969) Metabolism of canine small intestine vascularly perfused *in vitro*. *J. Appl. Physiol.* **26:** 119–128.

HÜBERS, H., HÜBERS, E., SIMON, J. and FORTH, W. (1971) A method for preparing stable density gradients and their application for fractionations of intestinal mucosal cells. *Life Sci.* **10:** part II, 377–384.

HUBSCHER, G., WEST, G. R. and BRINDLEY, D. N. (1965) Studies on the fractionation of mucosal homogenates from the small intestine. *Biochem. J.* **97:** 629–642.

JACOBI, H., PFLEGER, K. and RUMMEL, W. (1956) Komplexbildner und aktiver Eisentransport durch die Darmwand. *Arch. exp. Path. Pharmak.* **229:** 198–206.

JACOBS, F. A. and LUPER, M. (1957) Intestinal absorption by perfusion *in situ*. *J. Appl. Physiol.* **11:** 136–138.

JACOBS, P., BOTHWELL, T. A. and CHARLTON, R. W. (1966) Intestinal ion transport studies using a loop of gut with an artificial circulation. *Am. J. Physiol.* **210:** 694–700.

JOHNSTON, C. G. (1932) A method for making quantitative intestinal studies. *Proc. Soc. Exp. Biol. Med.* **30:** 193–196.

KAUSCH, O. (1969) Dissertation. Med. Fakultät der Universität des Saarlandes, Homburg/Saar, W. Germany.

KIMMICH, G. A. (1970) Preparation and properties of mucosal epithelial cells isolated from small intestine of chicken. *Biochem. J.* **9:** 3659–3667.

LAUTERBACH, F. (1969) Metabolismus und enterale Resorption herzwirksamer Glykoside. *Naunyn-Schmiedebergs Arch. exp. Path. Pharmak.* **263:** 26–39.

LAUTERBACH, F. and WITTE, E.-A. (1973) Absorption of drugs by intestinal filtration. *Naunyn-Schmiedebergs Arch. exp. Path. Pharmak.* **277:** R 42.

LEE, J. S. (1961) Flows and pressure in lymphatic and blood vessels of intestine water absorption. *Am. J. Physiol.* **200:** 979–983.

LEE, J. S. (1965) Motility, lymphatic contractility and distension pressure in intestinal absorption. *Am. J. Physiol.* **208:** 621–627.

LEE, J. S. and DUNCAN, K. M. (1968) Lymphatic and venous transport of water from rat jejunum. *Gastroenterology* **54:** 559–567.

LENGEMANN, E. V. (1963) Over-all aspects of calcium and strontium absorption, pp. 85–96. In: *The Transfer of Calcium and Strontium Across Biological Membranes,* WASSERMAN, R. H. (Ed.). Academic Press, New York–London.

LEVINE, R. R. (1971) Intestinal absorption, pp. 28–95. In: *Absorption Phenomena,* RABINOWITZ, J. L. and MYERSON, R. M. (Eds.). J. Wiley: London, New York, Sydney, Toronto.

LEVINE, R. R., MCNAVY, W. F., KORNYUK, PH. J. and LE BLANC, R. (1970) Histological re-evaluation of everted gut technique for studying intestinal absorption. *Europ. J. Pharmac.* **9:** 211–219.

MILLER, D. and CRANE, R. K. (1961) A procedure for the isolation of the epithelial brush border membrane of hamster small intestine. *Anal. Biochem.* **2:** 284–286.

NIGROVIC, V. and MOHR, TH. (1966) Ein neuer Stoffwechselkäfig für Arbeiten mit Radionukliden. *Strahlentherapie* **130:** 314–316.

OCHSENFAHRT, H. (1971) The mucosal-serosal transfer of drugs in the rat jejunum with and without blood flow. *Naunyn-Schmiedebergs Arch. exp. Path. Pharmak.* R 102.

OCHSENFAHRT, H. and WINNE, D. (1969) Der Einfluβ der Durchblutung auf die Resorption von Arzneimitteln aus dem Jejunum der Ratte. *Naunyn-Schmiedebergs Arch. exp. Path. Pharmak.* **264:** 55–57.

OHNELL, R. (1939) The artificially perfused mammalian intestine as a useful preparation for studying intestinal absorption. *J. Cell. Comp. Physiol.* **13:** 155–159.

PALDINE, R. L. and HYMAN, CH. (1964) Relationship between lymphatic and blood flow in various structures in the abdominal cavity. *Proc. Soc. Exp. Biol. Med.* **117:** 904–910.

PARSONS, D. S. (1968) Methods for investigation of intestinal absorption, pp. 1177–1216. In: *Handbook of Physiology*, sect. 6, CODE, CH. F. (Ed.). Am. Physiol. Soc., Washington.

PARSONS, D. S. and PATERSON, C. R. (1960) Fluid and solute transport across rat colonic mucosa. *Quart. J. Exp. Physiol.* **50:** 220–231.

PARSONS, D. S. and PRICHARD, J. S. (1965) Hydrolysis of disaccharides during absorption by the perfused small intestine of amphibia. *Nature* **208:** 1097–1098.

PARSONS, D. S. and PRICHARD, J. S. (1968) A preparation of perfused small intestine for the study of absorption in amphibia. *J. Physiol.* (*Lond.*) **198:** 405–434.

PATERSON, A. R. P. and SBARSKY, S. A. (1958) Purine synthesis in suspensions of mucosa from the small intestine of the rat. *Can. J. Biochem.-Physiol.* **36:** 755–770.

PERRIS, A. D. (1966) Isolation of the epithelial cells of the rat small intestine. *Can. J. Biochem.* **44:** 687–693.

PORTEOUS, J. N. and CLARK, B. (1965) The isolation and characterization of subcellular components of the epithelial cells of rabbit's small intestine. *Biochem. J.* **96:** 159–171.

RASMUSSEN, H., WALDOFF, A., DZIEWIATKOWSKI, D. E. and DELUCA, H. F. (1963) Calcium exchange in isolated intestinal villi. *Biochim. Biophys. Acta* **75:** 250–256.

ROBINSON, G. B. (1963) The distribution of peptides in subcellular fractions from the mucosa of the small intestine of the rat. *Biochem. J.* **88:** 162–168.

ROSS, B. D. (1972) Perfusion techniques in biochemistry; a laboratory manual, pp. 356–394. *Intestine.* Clarendon Press, Oxford.

ROSS, G., WHITE, F. N., BROWN, D. W. and KOLIN, A. (1966) Regional blood flow with rat. *J. Appl. Physiol.* **21:** 1273–1275.

RUMMEL, W. and SEIFEN, E. (1964) Narkose, Injektion und Blutentnahme bei Versuchstieren, pp. 324–329. In: *Biochem. Taschenbuch* (1964) Teil II, RAMEN, H. M. (Ed.). Springer Verlag, Berlin–Göttingen–Heidelberg–New York.

RUMMEL, W. and STUPP, H. F. (1964) Die resorptive Aktivität verschiedener Dunndarmabschnitte der Ratte and ihre Beeinflussung durch Mersalyl. *Naunyn-Schmiedebergs Arch. exp. Path. Pharmak.* **248:** 552–560.

SCHAUBNER, L. S., TOCCO, D. J., BRODIE, B. B. and HOGBEN, C. A. M. (1958) Absorption of drugs from the rat small intestine. *J. Pharmac. Exp. Therap.* **123:** 81–88.

SCHEDL, H. P. (1966) Use of polyethylene glycol and phenol red as unabsorbed indicators for intestinal absorption studies in man. *Gut* **7:** 159–163.

SHEFF, M. F. and SMYTH, D. H. (1955) An apparatus of the study of *in vivo* intestinal absorption in the rat. *J. Physiol.* (*Lond.*) **128:** 67.

SJÖSTRAND, F. S. (1968) A simple and rapid method to prepare dispersion of columnar epithelial cells from the rat intestine. *J. Ultrastructure Res.* **22:** 424.

SKALA, I. and HRUBA, F. (1964) Accumulation of vitamin A by small intestine of the rat *in vitro*. *Am. J. Physiol.* **206:** 458–460.

SÖGNEN, E. (1967) A method for the preparation of suspensions of intestinal mucosal cells by means of Ca-chelators. *Acta Vet. Scand.* **8:** 76–82.

SOERGEL, K. H. (1968) Inert markers. *Gastroenterology* **54:** 449–452.

STERN, B. K. and JENSEN, W. E. (1966) Active transport of glucose suspensions of isolated rat intestinal cells. *Nature* **209:** 789–790.

STERN, B. K. and REILLY, R. W. (1965) Some characteristics of the respiratory metabolism of suspensions of rat intestinal cells. *Nature* **205:** 563–565.

TAKACS, L. and VAJDA, V. (1963) Effect of serotonin on cardiac output and organ blood flow of rats. *Am. J. Physiol.* **204:** 301–303.

TAKESUE, Y. and SATO, R. (1968) Enzyme distribution in subcellular fractions of the intestinal cells. *J. Biochem.* (*Tokyo*) **64:** 873–883.

THER, L. (1965) *Grundlagen der experimentellen Arzneimittelforschung*, Wissenschaftl. Verlagsgesellschaft, Stuttgart.

VARRO, V., CSERNAY, L., GLAHO, G. and SZYTVAS, F. (1969) A simple method for the simultaneous recording of blood flow and absorption in isolated segments of dog intestine. *Am. J. Dig. Dis.* **9:** 138–144.

WALDNER, A. I. and LUNSETH, J. B. (1963) A technic for separation of the cells of the gastric mucosa. *Proc. Soc. Exp. Biol. Med.* **112:** 494–496.

WILLIAMS, J. H., MAGER, M. and JACOBSON, E. D. (1964) Relationship of mesenteric blood flow to intestinal absorption of carbohydrates. *J. Lab. Clin. Med.* **63:** 853–863.

WILSON, T. H. (1956) A modified method for study of intestinal absorption *in vitro*. *J. Appl. Physiol.* **9:** 137–140.

WILSON, T. H. (1962) *Intestinal Absorption*. W. B. Saunders, Philadelphia.

WILSON, T. H. and WISEMAN, G. (1954) The use of sacs of everted small intestine for the study of the transference of substances from the mucosal to the serosal surface. *J. Physiol.* (*Lond.*) **123:** 116–125.

WORWOOD, M. and JACOBS, A. (1971) The subcellular distribution of orally administered ^{59}Fe in rat small intestinal mucosa. *Brit. J. Haemat.* **20:** 587–597.

CHAPTER 15

CLINICAL METHODS FOR MEASURING GASTROINTESTINAL ABSORPTION*

G. Sladen and A. Dawson

London, U.K.

INTRODUCTION

There are many reasons for studying the absorption of pharmacologically active agents in man and it is important to select the appropriate method for the individual study. Such reasons may vary from the need to know the total amount of substance absorbed, its rate of absorption and tissue and blood levels attained during and after absorption or an assessment of the actual absorptive mechanisms involved. The present review deals with the various techniques and their limitations, which have been used to study absorption in man. Not all have, as yet, been applied to the study of drug absorption.

It is necessary to define some terms which will be used frequently. Absorption means the transport of a substance out of the intestinal lumen into blood or lymph. Secretion refers to movement in the opposite direction and may take place via the various intestinal secretory glands or may occur across the intestinal mucosa. No specific mechanisms, such as active transport, are implied by the use of these terms. If a substance moves freely in both directions, a distinction has to be made between net and unidirectional movement. The semantics of these processes have led to some confusion in the literature. Code (1962) has attempted to clarify the matter, but his terminology is not, as yet, in general use.

*This review was completed in 1968.

15.1. METHODS APPLICABLE TO NORMAL CONSCIOUS MAN

15.1.1. METHODS DEPENDING ON THE MEASUREMENT OF APPEARANCE OF THE SUBSTANCE OR ITS METABOLITES IN BODY FLUIDS OR TISSUES

15.1.1.1. *Appearance in blood and urine*

The most widely used method of assessing absorption, especially of drugs, is to measure the appearance of the substance in the blood or urine following the ingestion of a single oral dose. Repeated blood sampling can give information about both the appearance and subsequent disposal of the substance, and cumulative urinary excretion can be used as an index of the total amount absorbed. Many tests of this type have been devised for the investigation of malabsorption in man, for example glucose tolerance (Gaddie *et al.*, 1957), xylose tolerance (Benson *et al.*, 1957; Christiansen *et al.*, 1953), vitamin A tolerance as an indication of fat absorption (Legerton *et al.*, 1953), folic acid absorption based on blood levels (Butterworth *et al.*, 1957; Baker *et al.*, 1968) and on urinary excretion (Girdwood, 1953), and the excretion of radioactive vitamin B_{12} in the urine (Schilling, 1953). For fuller accounts of the use of these and other tests in clinical practice the reader is referred to the report of Doig and Girdwood (1960) and the review by Dawson (1965).

The appearance of test substance in blood and urine depends upon many factors, which may affect both its rate of absorption and its subsequent disposal. These will now be considered in detail.

Gastric emptying. Certain gastrointestinal factors will affect the speed with which the substance reaches its site of absorption. These factors may profoundly affect the rate of absorption, especially if the absorptive process itself is relatively rapid. Gastric emptying is the most important of these factors and, for example, it is well known that the rapid emptying after a partial gastrectomy is associated with an abnormally rapid rise of blood glucose in the glucose tolerance test (Phear, 1962). Very slow emptying could theoretically be responsible for "flat" tolerance curves, erroneously implying impaired absorption. Test *et al.* (1956) found that 25% of normal subjects in a large series had flat glucose tolerance curves (i.e. a rise of blood glucose of less than 20 mgm %), but they were unable to demonstrate that this was due to delayed gastric emptying. However, they used rather crude radiological techniques to measure emptying. Recently, Holdsworth and Besser (1968), using an elegant external scanning technique, have demonstrated an inverse relationship between the peak rise of blood sugar and the half-time of gastric emptying in a series of patients with thyroid disease, before and after treatment.

The factors affecting gastric emptying have been reviewed by Thomas (1957) and by Hunt (1959). The rate of emptying is related to the volume of gastric contents and the stomach empties in an exponential fashion after food (Griffith *et al.*, 1966). In normal subjects, food empties from the stomach with a half-time of between 60 and 80 min. This time is shorter in patients with duodenal ulcer (40–60 min) and very variable in patients with a gastric ulcer (50–120 min). These figures are quoted from the paper of Griffith *et al.* (1966). Using a fluid meal, Holdsworth and Besser (1968) found emptying half-times of 40–70 min in patients with hyperthyroidism compared with 60–200 min in hypothyroid patients. Gastric emptying rates may, therefore, vary widely in health and disease and the volume of fluid given with a test substance or the presence of food may greatly influence the rate of appearance of the test substance in blood or urine. For example, it was found in an animal study that a dilute solution of a barbiturate had a greater hypnotic effect than a smaller volume of concentrated drug and this was due to the more rapid gastric emptying of the former (Moore *et al.*, 1960). Most tolerance

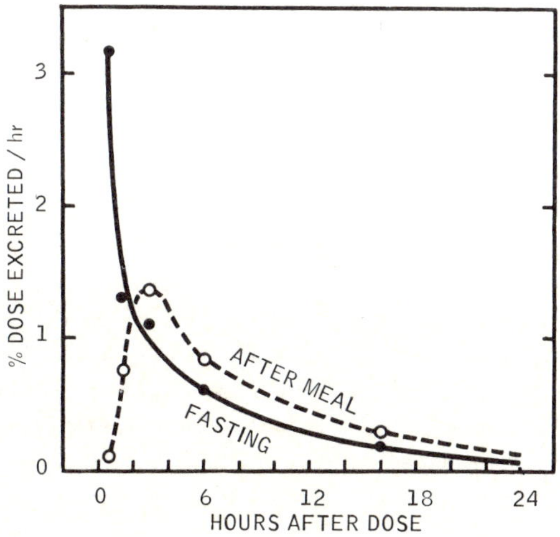

FIG. 1. Fractional urinary excretion of ^{14}C bretylium in a patient who showed a rapid initial excretion after a fasting dose and was given a second dose after a meal (from Dollery *et al.*, 1960).

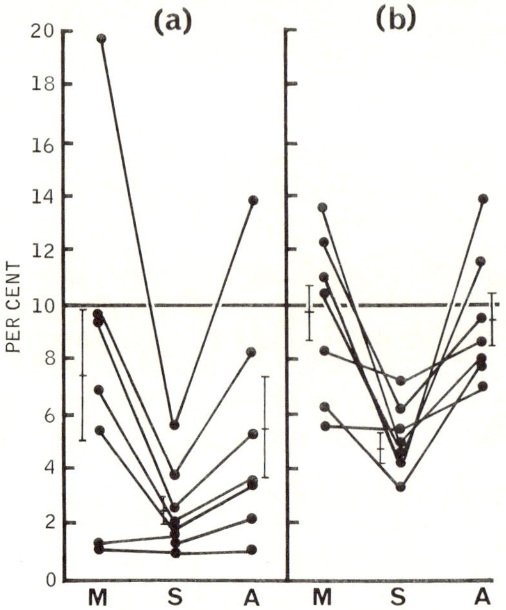

FIG. 2. 24-hour urinary radioactivity as a per cent of 1 mcg $^{58}Co\text{-}B_{12}$ given with a "B_{12}-free" meal (M), fasting ("standard" S) and after histamine ("augmented" A) in two groups of patients who have had a Polya partial gastrectomy: (a) those with overt megaloblastic anemia and (b) those with minor hematological abnormalities and a low serum B_{12}. Each set of three points refers to one individual. The 10% line represents the lower limit of normal (after Turnbull, 1967).

tests are performed on an empty stomach and this may yield misleading information, especially in the case of drugs which are normally taken with meals. Food may delay the absorption of drugs (Harington, 1953; Dollery *et al.*, 1960), Fig. 1, and it is well known that food greatly diminishes the absorption of inorganic iron (Josephs, 1958). Similarly the absorption of inorganic calcium salts is reduced if milk is fed simultaneously (Deller *et al.*, 1965). Delayed gastric emptying may be an important effect of food, but food may also bind to the test substance or interfere mechanically with its access to the intestinal mucosa.

There are situations in which food enhances absorption. For example, after partial gastrectomy vitamin B_{12} absorption is enhanced by food and by histamine (Deller *et al.*, 1961; Turnbull, 1967), Fig. 2. It is presumed that food and histamine stimulate the secretion of intrinsic factor by the remnant of gastric mucosa. This may have been responsible for the non-reproducibility of the Schilling test of vitamin B_{12} absorption in individual subjects after partial gastrectomy (Adams and Cartwright, 1963). A recent study, using the hepatic uptake method (refer to pp. 827, 833), showed that vitamin B_{12} absorption studies gave reasonably consistent results when performed on non-fasting subjects (Townsend *et al.*, 1968). The nature of the food may be important, because fat is known to be a particularly potent inhibitor of gastric emptying. However, if fat-soluble substances are being tested, then fat or oil is usually given as a vehicle, as in the vitamin A test (Legerton *et al.*, 1953; Althausen *et al.*, 1960). The influence of various foods in promoting the appearance of beta-carotene in the blood provides a striking example of some of these effects (Cornwell *et al.*, 1962), Fig. 3.

The other factor which greatly influences the rate of gastric emptying is the tonicity of gastric contents. In general terms, increasing tonicity is associated with delayed gastric emptying. In the case of sodium chloride solutions, and some other simple salts, emptying is also delayed by hypo-tonicity relative to plasma. The studies of Hunt and his colleagues, comparing the effects of monosaccharides and polysaccharides, suggest

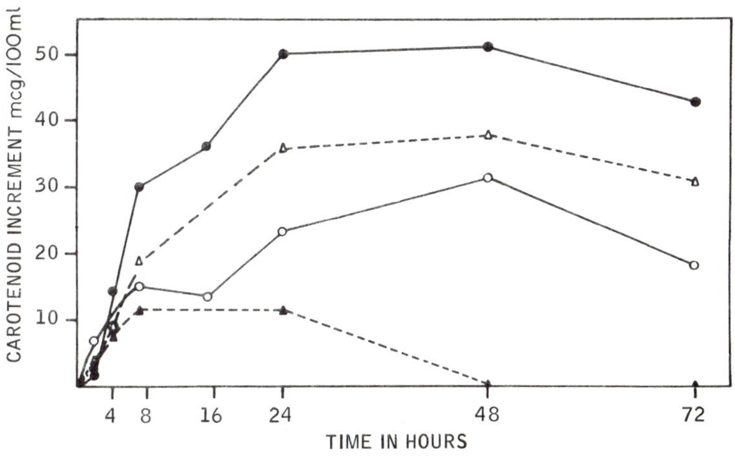

FIG. 3. Mean serum increments in β-carotene for subjects with different test regimens: five subjects with aqueous dispersion β-carotene and lipid test meal (o); two subjects with lipid dispersion β-carotene and lipid test meal (o); two subjects with aqueous dispersion β-carotene and a protein–carbohydrate test meal (△); two subjects with aqueous dispersion β-carotene and no test meal (▲) (from Cornwell *et al.*, 1962).

the presence of osmo-receptors in the duodenal or jejunal mucosa deep to the site of membrane hydrolysis (Hunt, 1956; Hunt and Pathak, 1960; Hunt, 1960; Elias *et al.*, 1968). This factor should be considered when tolerance tests of the absorption of monosaccharides and polysaccharides (Macdonald and Turner, 1968) or amino acids and peptides (Craft *et al.*, 1968) are compared.

In practice, it seems that variations in gastric emptying rates seldom give rise to difficulty in the interpretation of absorption studies of this type. If for any reason it seems important to exclude this factor, it may be necessary to use subjects who have undergone gastric surgery resulting in by-pass of the pylorus, as illustrated in the study of Craft *et al.* (1968). Alternatively, the test substance may be administered directly into the small intestine by means of duodenal intubation. It should be added, for completeness, that many drugs, as opposed to substances of nutritional importance, can be absorbed from the stomach (Hogben *et al.*, 1957).

Intestinal transit. Intestinal motility will affect both the time taken to reach the absorbing site and also the contact time available for absorption. It has been shown, for example, that atropine or a slow rate of delivery will increase the total amount of xylose absorbed and alter the blood curves (Fordtran *et al.*, 1962), Table 1. However, propanthaline (Pro-

TABLE 1. EFFECT OF ATROPINIZATION ON TWENTY-FOUR-HOUR URINARY PENTOSE RECOVERY AFTER THE ADMINISTRATION OF 25 g OF D-XYLOSE IN 500 ml OF WATER[a]

Xylose administration	No. of paired studies	Atropine	Mean 24-hr urinary pentose recovery (g)	Mean difference (g)	SD of difference	P value of difference
30-min jejunal infusion	10	—	6.8	3.7	1.9	0.01
		+	10.5			
Oral	10	—	8.6	2.7	1.2	0.01
		+	11.3			
2-hr jejunal infusion	7	—	10.1	1.9	1.7	0.05
		+	12.0			

[a]Only studies done in same subjects compared with each other.

(From Fordtran *et al.*, 1962)

Banthine®) reduces the rate of appearance of ^{22}Na in the blood after duodenal infusion and this coincides with its inhibitory effect on intestinal motility (Higgins *et al.*, 1956; Groisser and Farrar, 1962). Xylose is absorbed slowly and incompletely, so that the increased mucosal contact time may promote absorption. $Sodiums^{22}$ is absorbed very rapidly and the mechanism of the propantheline effect is obscure. Mechanical spreading of isotope over the intestinal mucosa did not accelerate absorption in the presence of propantheline (Groisser and Farrar, 1962) and perhaps there is actual interference with the sodium-absorbing mechanism.

Finally, the actual site of absorption may affect the appearance of blood curves. The peak appearance of radioactive vitamin B_{12} is reached about 8 hr after its ingestion in physiological doses (Booth and Mollin, 1956). A much earlier peak was found in the studies of Ross *et al.* (1954) who used pharmacological doses of the vitamin. This indicates both the distal site and the complex, time-consuming process involved in the absorption of small doses of vitamin B_{12}.

Site of blood sampling. Following absorption most substances, apart from fat, enter the portal circulation and pass through the liver. Metabolism within the intestinal mucosa and by the liver may affect the shape of peripheral blood curves. In a few cases, portal blood has been sampled and absorption curves have been obtained (Sherlock and Walshe, 1946; Bean *et al.*, 1951; Holdsworth and Dawson, 1965a). The methods used will be referred to later. It was shown, for example, that a marked portal blood curve of thiamine was associated with a flat systemic blood curve, presumably as a result of hepatic uptake (Bean *et al.*, 1951).

However, normally only the systemic blood is available for sampling. The sampling of arterial rather than venous blood will obviate the theoretical problem of local tissue uptake of the test substance. This is, probably, rarely of practical importance, but it has been shown that arterio-venous difference may be responsible for some misleadingly flat glucose (Test *et al.*, 1956) and disaccharide (Newcomer and McGill, 1967) tolerance curves.

Distribution and disposal—comparison of oral and parenteral administration. Tolerance curves and urinary excretion studies are greatly affected by the fate of the substance after absorption has taken place. The volume of distribution and the speed with which distribution equilibrium is reached will influence the early blood concentrations. Subsequent metabolism and excretion will determine the shape of the blood curve during absorption and after this is complete, and also the timing and magnitude of urinary excretion. These factors can be separately assessed by following the fate of parenterally administered test substance, and indeed it is only possible to quantitate absorption rates in studies of this type if the effect of oral and parenteral administration on blood levels and urine excretion are compared. There are many examples of the use of this kind of approach, especially in the study of drug absorption (for example, Dominguez and Pomerone, 1945; Nelson and Schaldemore, 1959; Swintosky, 1956; Levy and Hollister, 1964). Theoretical and mathematical considerations are discussed in detail by Wagner (1961), Wagner and Nelson (1963) and Parsons (1968) and a simplified mathematical approach is to be found as an appendix to this chapter. However, at this stage, some of the problems and assumptions involved will be discussed in qualitative terms.

It has to be assumed that the distribution and fate of orally and parenterally administered test substance are identical. It is now known that this is definitely not the case as far as glucose is concerned. The intestinal absorption of glucose is associated with a greater stimulus to insulin production than occurs after a comparable intravenous injection (McIntyre *et al.*, 1964; Dupre *et al.*, 1968). The metabolic fate of glucose, therefore, clearly depends upon its route of administration. In their studies of the absorption of ^{59}Fe in patients with hemochromatosis, Losowsky and Wilson (1967) found differences in the distribution of iron after oral and intravenous administration. Josephs (1958) also quotes evidence to suggest that the fate of labeled iron depends on the route of administration.

The disposal kinetics of certain drugs are not necessarily constant in an individual subject. For example, the disposal half-life may depend on the initial concentration, usually being longer at high initial concentration (Swintosky, 1956; Dayton *et al.*, 1963). This means that oral and parenteral doses of such drugs should be so adjusted that closely comparable peak blood concentrations are produced. It should also be remembered, when numbers of individuals are studied, that there are genetic variations in the rate of disposal of various drugs. The example of isoniazide (isonicotinic acid hydrazide) is particularly well known (Biehl, 1956) and the subject has recently been reviewed by Clarke *et al.* (1968).

In kinetic studies it is usually assumed that the distribution of test substance is very rapid and that a single body compartment is involved. In the case of substances which are absorbed extremely rapidly, it may be that the rate of distribution rather than metabolism determines the shape of blood curves. This is illustrated by the studies of Scholer and Code (1954) on the absorption of isotopic water (D_2O) after direct infusion into the small intestine. They calculated absorption rates of D_2O by integrating blood curves obtained after intestinal and intravenous administration, the latter indicating the rate of attainment of distribution equilibrium. The kinetics of intravenous D_2O disposal were those of a two-compartment system. These workers have studied the absorption of ^{22}Na in the same way (Reitmeyer *et al.*, 1957) and have also used two isotopes of water and sodium simultaneously (Higgins *et al.*, 1957). The calculations involved in these studies were rather tedious, and in recent years computers have been used increasingly in studies of this type (Garrett *et al.*, 1960; Silverman and Burgen, 1961; Wagner and Nelson, 1963).

Such elaborate information may not be required. The comparison of oral and parenteral administration can also be used to estimate the percentage absorption of a substance, rather than its absorption rate. For example, cumulative urinary excretion (Harington, 1953; Harington *et al.*, 1958; Young *et al.*, 1959) or peak blood levels (Dollery *et al.*, 1961) can be compared. If two isotopes are available, they can be given by the two routes simultaneously and the activities of each can be measured in tissue, blood or urine. The percentage absorption can be calculated from the ratios of activities administered and the ratios of activities measured in the blood or tissue. This is the basis of various double isotope techniques used, for example, in studies of iron absorption (Saylor and Finch, 1953; Bothwell *et al.*, 1958; Hallberg and Sölvell, 1960), vitamin B_{12} absorption using the hepatic uptake technique (Weisberg and Glass, 1966) and thyroxine absorption (Hays, 1968). In view of the possibility that the fate of the test substance may be affected by the route of administration, these methods should be checked by more direct assessment, such as fecal excretion.

Renal excretion. The disposal of test substance will often depend upon the adequacy of renal function and on the nature of its handling by the kidneys. This is of great practical importance in the assessment of malabsorption in the individual patient and is of relevance to the problem of drug dosage in patients with renal failure. Renal dysfunction may both enhance the level of test substance in the blood and delay or reduce its excretion in the urine, so that these measurements may give misleading information about absorption.

The urinary excretion of D-xylose and of radioactive vitamin B_{12} (the Schilling test) are widely used clinically in the investigation of malabsorption. The renal clearance of xylose is closely dependent on the glomerular filtration rate both in adults (Dominguez and Pomerone, 1934; Thaysen and Müllertz, 1962) and in infants (Meeuwisse and Dano, 1965). Urinary excretion of xylose is both reduced and delayed in patients with renal impairment and also with increasing age (Fowler and Cooke, 1960; Texter *et al.*, 1964), Fig. 4. It is assumed, but not proved, that the effect of age is caused by gradual impairment of renal function, although impaired absorption of xylose with increasing age has not apparently been

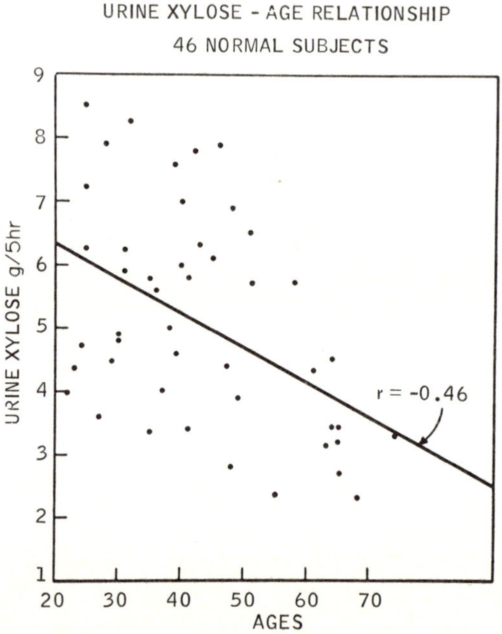

FIG. 4. Plot of urinary excretion of xylose (g/5 hr) as a function of age in years ($p < 0.005$) after administration of 25 g of D-xylose orally (from Texter *et al.*, 1964).

excluded. In doubtful cases it is necessary, therefore, to measure blood levels of xylose as an index of absorption and it is also sometimes helpful to prolong the urinary collection for 24 hr instead of the customary 5 hr (Thaysen and Müllertz, 1962). It should be added that in some cases delayed, as opposed to reduced, xylose excretion is caused by delayed absorption as in a recent personal case of gross intestinal stasis. A comparison of oral and parenteral administration should elucidate the cause of delayed urinary excretion of xylose (Wyngaarden *et al.*, 1957).

The urinary excretion of unbound radioactive vitamin B_{12} compares very closely with that of inulin and it can be used as a measure of glomerular filtration rate (Nelp *et al.*, 1964). The Schilling test is, therefore, similarly affected by impairment of renal function (Rath *et al.*, 1957). In such patients, prolonged urinary collection may reveal that much of the dose is excreted after the first 24 hr, whereas in normal subjects excretion is usually complete within 24 hr (McIntyre *et al.*, 1956).

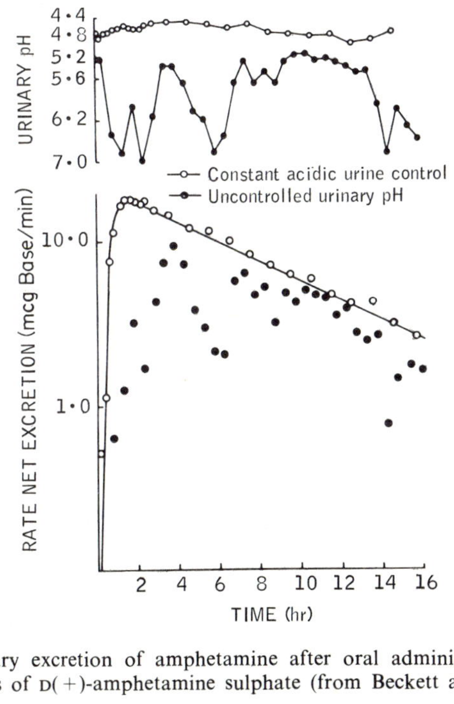

FIG. 5. Urinary excretion of amphetamine after oral administration of 15 mg solution doses of D(+)-amphetamine sulphate (from Beckett and Tucker, 1967).

The excretion of many drugs in normal subjects depends on both glomerular and tubular function. The degree of ionization of weak acids and bases will depend on the pH of the urine. Drugs are reabsorbed

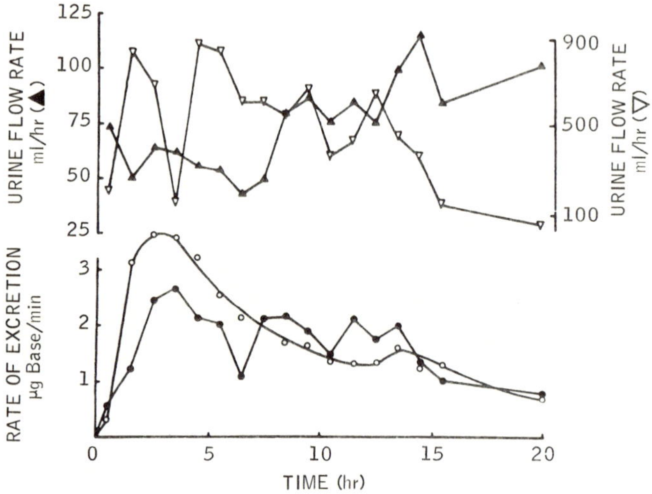

FIG. 6. The rate of excretion of chlorphenamine and corresponding urine flow rates in one subject: conditions of normal flow rates (solid symbols) and high flow rates (open symbols). Urine pH 5.00 ± 0.50 (from Beckett and Tucker, 1967).

effectively by the tubules only in the unionized form (reviewed by Weiner and Mudge, 1965) and so the pH of the urine may have a great influence on the urinary excretion pattern. If appreciable tubular reabsorption takes place, the rate of urine flow will also influence the total amount excreted, because more reabsorption will occur at low rates than at high rates of flow. If the pH of the urine can be adjusted so that reabsorption is virtually prevented, then urinary excretion will be independent of the rate of urine flow. These factors are well illustrated by the studies of Beckett and Rowland (1965) and Beckett and Tucker (1967) on the effects of pH and urine flow on the renal excretion of amphetamine and other drugs. Controlled urinary acidification to pH 4.8 can virtually prevent the tubular reabsorption of amphetamine (Fig. 5), for example, whereas with a drug like chlorphenamine (Chlor-Trimeton®), a fast urine flow rate has to be used to minimize reabsorption (Fig. 6). The kinetics of urinary excretion can best be quantitated when reabsorption is minimized and the decay in excretion rate conforms to a simple exponential function, as illustrated in Fig. 5. This is amplified in the Appendix (p. 856). Beckett and Tucker (1967) have used a simple buccal absorption test to indicate the effects of pH on drug absorption and to predict the ideal conditions for studying urinary excretion patterns. The effects of urine pH on the excretion and pharmacological effect of pempidine (Perolysen®) in hypertensive subjects are strikingly demonstrated in the report of Harington *et al.* (1958). The practical significance of high rates of urine flow and high urine pH in promoting the renal excretion of barbiturates is emphasized by Lassen (1960).

Saturation—the problem of tissue and plasma binding. A factor which may influence blood levels and urinary excretion patterns is that of tissue storage or plasma binding of the absorbed substance. Appreciable blood curves or urinary excretion may only occur when all the potential binding sites are saturated. This is the principle of the familiar saturation test of vitamin C deficiency (Harris, 1942) and it would be necessary to saturate a subject with vitamin C before absorption studies could be performed using blood levels or urine excretion. Similarly, Girdwood (1953) showed that the urinary excretion of folic acid may be greatly reduced in severely depleted patients, even if absorption is adequate. However, Butterworth *et al.* (1957) produced rather contradictory evidence on this matter in their study of tropical sprue patients and, recently, Baker *et al.* (1968) have shown that nutritionally folate-deficient subjects absorbed folic acid normally as judged by blood curves, without any prior loading of the tissues with folic acid. It may depend very much on the dose of folic acid given and the degree of the tissue deficiency. Baker *et al.* (1968) used the pharmacological dose of 5 mg, whereas physiological doses are considered to be of the order of 100–200 mcg. Another problem is that folic acid is ordinarily ingested in the form of polyglutamates and that free folic acid is liberated by the action of an intestinal conjugase (Hoffbrand and Necheles, 1968; Rosenberg *et al.*, 1968). This illustrates the general principle that a clear distinction must be made between pharmacological and physiological dosage on the one hand, and, in the case of substances of nutritional importance, the chemical form administered must be taken into account. Furthermore, in considering the genesis of a nutritional deficiency one cannot extrapolate from results obtained when inappropriate forms of, for example, vitamins are administered.

The use of isotopes enables small physiological doses of various vitamins to be studied, but urinary excretion is usually negligible unless a large dose of non-radioactive material is given at about the same time. This so-called "flushing dose" is usually followed by the rapid excretion of the absorbed radioactive material and presumably produces its effect by blocking all the available binding sites. The best-known example of this is the Schilling test of vitamin B_{12} absorption (Schilling, 1953), and the effects of the timing of the flushing dose are demonstrated in the paper of McIntyre *et al.* (1956). Similar flushing doses are required in absorption studies of isotopically labeled pyridoxine (Brain *et al.*, 1963) and folic acid (Anderson *et al.*, 1960).

Plasma binding of drugs may produce a similar effect on their excretion patterns. Brodie (1964) cites the example of phenylbutazone, which was found clinically to be relatively much less effective in high dosage. The plasma disappearance and urinary excretion were greatly accelerated by high dosage, presumably because the plasma binding sites were fully saturated. This phenomenon may apply to many drugs which are normally firmly bound to tissues or to plasma proteins.

In the interpretation of "flat" blood curves or low urinary excretion rates, it may be important to repeat the observations after the subject has been saturated with the test substance. In this way, Popper *et al.* (1943) showed that the flat vitamin A tolerance curves in liver disease could not be attributed to excessive tissue uptake.

Conclusions. Blood levels and urinary excretion studies can give useful qualitative information about both absorption rates and the total quantities absorbed. For comparative purposes, measurement of the area under a tolerance curve can be used as a very approximate quantitative index of absorption (for example, Tidwell, 1950). The advantage of these methods is that they are usually simple, provided the test substance can be measured with reasonable ease, and they represent a normal method of administration. Blood levels after drug ingestion are clearly of value in estimating the efficacy and required frequency of oral dosage, provided the effects of food and fasting are taken into account. However, the nutritional significance of many of the tests, especially those using vitamins, must be doubtful, because no information about physiological absorption from food is obtained.

The chief disadvantage of the methods is the lack of quantitation of absorption, because so many variables, other than absorption itself, can affect the results. Information about the fate of the test substance after parenteral administration can be used to quantitate both absorption rates and total quantities absorbed, but many assumptions and over-simplifications are required (see Appendix).

Finally, it should be added that these methods can also be applied to the measurement of absorption from the rectum. For example, Samelius and Astrom (1958) have investigated the blood curves of various drugs after administration as suppositories, and Sampson and Brooke (1963) showed that there is appreciable absorption of hydrocortisone by both the normal and the inflamed colonic mucosa when given as an enema.

15.1.1.2. *Appearance in other tissues*

The appearance of certain substances in particular tissues can be used to assess absorption. These methods are not generally applicable, but will be described in brief outline.

The most important example is the measurement, by scanning, of hepatic uptake of radioactive vitamin B_{12} (Glass *et al.*, 1954). Time has to be allowed for the fecal excretion of unabsorbed vitamin, and this is usually expedited by means of purges. The scans can be roughly quantitated for comparative purposes, but of course only qualitative information about absorption rates can be obtained. Compared with the Schilling test, this method has the advantage that accurate urine collections are unnecessary and that a flushing dose of non-radioactive vitamin B_{12} is not required. A double-isotope technique has been devised on this principle (Weisberg and Glass, 1966) and the fractional absorption of an oral dose can be calculated from the activity ratios of the two isotopes.

The measurement of radioactive CO_2 in the breath has been used as an index of absorption, following the ingestion of ^{14}C labeled test substance. The absorption of labeled fats has been studied in this way (Schwabe *et al.*, 1962; Kaihara and Wagner, 1968) and a preliminary report has appeared of a similar study of the absorption of labeled lactose (Salmon *et al.*, 1968). This is an indirect approach, because one is really measuring metabolism rather than absorption. There are several theoretical objections to this type of method, but for convenience these will be deferred to a general consideration of the use of isotopic methods at the end of the chapter. Experience with such methods is minimal and their possible application would seem very limited.

Iodine absorption could be assessed by thyroid uptake of radioactive iodine, but this is ordinarily used as an index of thyroid function. When the absorption of radio-iodinated materials such as trolein, albumin and thyroxine is studied, thyroid uptake has to be blocked by the prior administration of iodine.

Potassium iodide absorption has been assessed by measuring its appearance in the saliva (Small *et al.*, 1961).

15.1.2. METHODS DEPENDING ON THE MEASUREMENT OF DISAPPEARANCE OF SUBSTANCE FROM THE GUT

15.1.2.1. *Whole gut—balance methods*

The principle of these methods is simple, in that absorption is measured as the difference between oral ingestion and fecal excretion. This is the most direct approach to the study of absorption and is more amenable to quantitation than the previously described methods. There are however two major complicating factors. First, secretion of test substance into the intestinal lumen, for example in bile, will underestimate absorption and, in these circumstances, it is necessary to distinguish between net and unidirectional absorption. Secondly, colonic bacteria may degrade the unabsorbed substance or may synthesize it. Thus, carbohydrates are degraded in the colon to various fatty acids and so balance studies are impracticable. Similarly, vitamin A is degraded by colonic contents and balance studies using the radioactive vitamin would be unreliable (Gagnon and Dawson, 1968). Colonic bacteria synthesize many members of the vitamin B group (Denko *et al.*, 1946) and it is therefore necessary to use isotopically labeled B vitamin to measure the fecal excretion of unabsorbed material, as in the vitamin B_{12} excretion test of Heinle *et al.* (1952).

Balance studies have been widely used in the assessment of many aspects of absorption in man and very detailed accounts are given in the papers of Riefenstein *et al.* (1945) and Comfort *et al.* (1953). More recently, the use of isotopically labeled test substances has simplified excretion measurements of, for example, iron (Moore and Dubach, 1951; Bothwell *et al.*, 1958) and vitamin B_{12} (Heinle *et al.*, 1952; Baker and Mollin, 1955).

A distinction must first be made between the administration of a single dose of test substance and continuous ingestion. In the former situation, stools must be collected until all the unabsorbed material has been voided. In the latter situation, a steady state can theoretically develop, in which daily ingestion, excretion and absorption rates are constant. During the steady state, absorption can be calculated as the difference between daily ingestion and excretion. The main difficulty in the former method is the complete and accurate collection of stools and the repeated measurements required to ensure that excretion is complete. The latter method requires both the establishment of a steady state and accurate daily stool collections. Feces are unpleasant to handle and liable to get mislaid or lost on toilet paper. Much co-operation is required by the patients or subjects and their attendant nursing staff. However, another major source of difficulty is the completeness and regularity of colonic emptying.

Colonic physiology. The contents of the terminal ileum are normally liquid or semi-solid and transit to the colon after a meal is usually complete within 4–6 hr. This can be deduced from the intubation studies of Borgström *et al.* (1957), in which meals containing a marker were sampled at different sites in the small intestine. Marker contained in liquid meals appears much more quickly in ileostomy effluent and its excretion is complete within 1–2 hr (Soergel and Hogan, 1967). It is believed that the ascending colon acts as a mixing chamber, where most of the colonic absorption of fluid and electrolytes takes place, and that only subsequently do portions of formed stool move on to the rectum like "cars on a track" (Alvarez and Freedlander, 1924).

Early radiological studies with barium indicated that the colon evacuated the unabsorbed residue of a meal within 24–48 hr, but barium is heavy and unphysiological and may affect intestinal motility. Alvarez and Freedlander (1924) measured the appearance of coloured glass beads in the stool and showed that 80% of the food residue from 1 day was normally excreted within the subsequent 4 days. By using beads of different colors on consecutive days, they showed that there might be considerable mixing of food residues from different days. Beads may also be criticized as unphysiological, but more recently it has been shown that various colored markers, mixed with meals, may take on average 4–5 days to be completely voided (Lutwak and Burton, 1964). Using radioactive chromic oxide as a marker, Hansky and Connell (1962) found that 76% of the marker was excreted on average within 4 days, but their total recoveries were rather low. It must be concluded that colonic passage of food residue is a leisurely and variable process and that prolonged stool collections may be required in the single dose type of balance study. For example, Baker and Mollin (1955), measuring the absorption of vitamin B_{12}, had to continue stool collections for 7 days or more until the daily stool activity was less than 1% of the ingested dose. The need for such prolonged collections suggests that some re-entry of absorbed vitamin into the gut lumen may have taken place.

In continuous ingestion studies, it may be necessary to separate stools into periods that correspond exactly to particular ingestion periods, especially when different substances or doses are being investigated serially. The use of colored markers to indicate stool separation was introduced by Riefenstein *et al.* (1945), who used carmine. Some of the difficulties and variability of stool separation are illustrated by the studies of Lutwak and Burton (1964) who fed carmine and brilliant blue every 6 days alternately during continuous balance studies. The pattern of marker excretion varied both within and between individuals, but generally stool collections from 6-day metabolic periods could be adequately separated. Similarly, Dick (1967) found 6-day metabolic periods satisfactory in his calcium balance studies, in which the periods were separated by carmine markers.

The recent investigations of Davignon *et al.* (1968) have produced much valuable information about patterns of normal colonic emptying and the difficulties inherent in the attainment of a truly steady state in accurate balance studies. They used chromic oxide as an inert internal marker and the use of markers of this type will be discussed in detail in the next section. They found that, on average, about 10 days were required before the fecal excretion of marker bore a constant relation to the intake. However, five of their thirty-five subjects failed to achieve such a state and continued to retain marker for often surprisingly long periods. These people would presumably be quite unsuitable for balance studies,

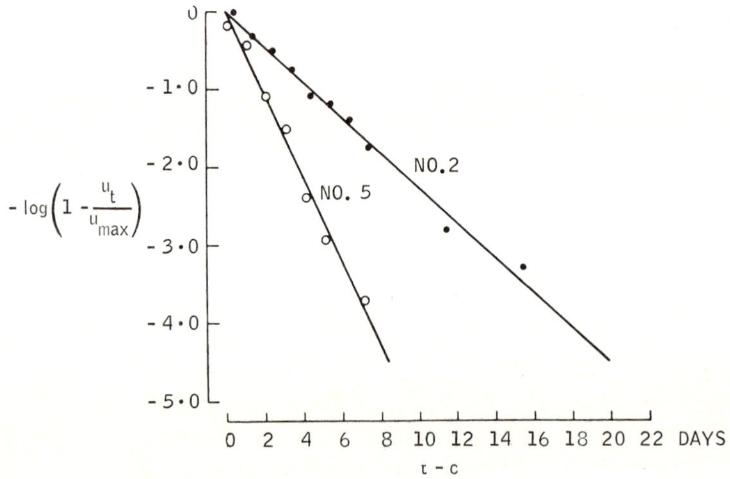

FIG. 7. First-order kinetics of $^{51}Cr_2O_3$ excretion in two patients with low and high fecal Cr_2O_3 turnover rates. Patients (2 and 5) given 10 mcC of $^{51}Cr_2O_3$ by mouth 19 and 96 days respectively after the start of daily administration of 300 mg of unlabeled Cr_2O_3. After correction of t for the transit time c, the plotted times intersected the zero ordinate. U_t = amount of $^{51}Cr_2O_3$ excreted by time t: U_{max} = total amount of $^{51}Cr_2O_3$ recovered. For fuller details see the original paper (from Davignon *et al.*, 1968).

although their bowel habits were apparently normal. During the steady state, Davignon *et al.* (1968) stopped marker ingestion and awaited its complete evacuation. They were then able to calculate the fecal "pool size" and the fractional daily excretion of marker. They also labeled this pool uniformly with isotopically labeled marker and showed that the rate of evacuation bore a simple direct relationship to the pool size. In other words, the pool behaved as a single compartment emptying according to the laws of first-order kinetics (Fig. 7). The fractional daily evacuation of colonic contents varied from 20 % to nearly 100 % in different individuals, but intra-individual differences were not studied. These different emptying patterns bore no apparent relationship to the subjects' bowel habits. In view of these great individual differences, it is necessary to test the validity of the steady state in each individual continuous balance study and to recognize that some individuals may never attain such a steady state, within reasonable time periods.

The use of markers. The other major difficulty in balance studies is the completeness and accuracy of stool collection. Unabsorbed markers can be used to correct for incompleteness of stool collection and were introduced by Edin in 1918 (quoted by Schürch *et al.*, 1950) into animal husbandry. For many years, the literature on this subject was restricted to the use of such markers in assessing the "digestibility" of foodstuffs in farm animals. In the last 20 years, there has been an increasing interest in the use of these markers in human balance studies. The required properties of such markers are that they should be inert and entirely unabsorbed. They should mix uniformly with intestinal contents and should be measurable with ease and accuracy in the stools. Chromic oxide has been the most widely used marker in both animal studies (Kane *et al.*, 1950; Schurch *et al.*, 1950; Mueller, 1956) and in human subjects (Kruela, 1947; Irwin and Crampton, 1951; Stanley and Cheng, 1957; Whitby and Lang, 1960; Nakayama *et al.*, 1960; Rose, 1964; Davignon *et al.*, 1968). There are difficulties and dangers inherent in its chemical analysis (Whitby and Lang, 1960) and the use of isotopic chromic oxide (Hansky and Connell, 1962) may be advantageous. Other markers have been assessed in animal studies (for example, Knapka *et al.*, 1967) and, in man, barium sulfate has been used successfully (Seife, 1962; Boender *et al.*, 1967; Dick, 1967). In intubation studies of intestinal absorption other more soluble markers, such as polyethylene glycol, are widely used and will be discussed in detail later.

Markers can be used in both single-dose studies and in the steady-state

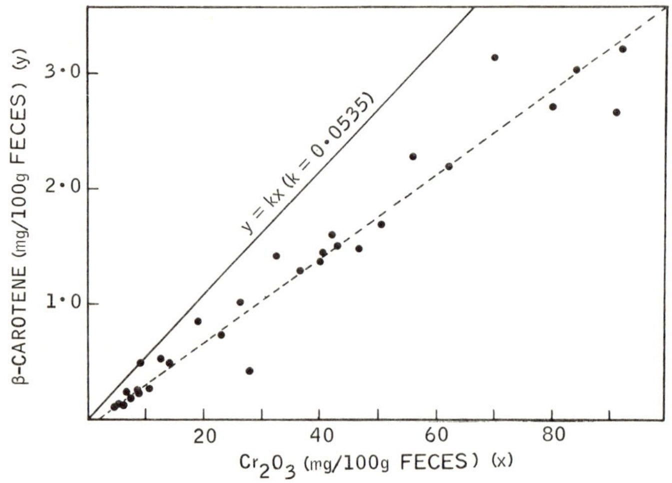

FIG. 8. Regression of fecal β-carotene on fecal Cr_2O_3 after a single oral dose of both. The full line ($y = kx$) is where the regression would have been expected to lie if all the carotene had appeared in the feces (from Owen *et al.*, 1959).

situation. In the former, a known ratio of marker and test substance is ingested and the ratio of substance and marker is measured in the stools. If this ratio remains constant in successive stool collections, then it is valid to assume that unabsorbed substance and marker remain uniformly mixed throughout their transit (Fig. 8). The fractional absorption of test substance can be calculated from the ingested and excreted ratios, and theoretically only one stool specimen need be analyzed. Boender *et al.* (1967) studied iron absorption in this way, in man, using ^{59}Fe and $^{131}BaSO_4$ as the marker. The ratio ^{59}Fe:^{131}Ba in the stools initially was used to indicate the fractional absorption or iron. After 2–3 days the ratio rose because some ^{59}Fe is taken up by mucosal cells and re-enters the lumen as these cells are shed. Subsequent ratios or the final cumulative excretion can be used to calculate fractional retention as opposed to fractional absorption. Stanley and Cheng (1957) measured unidirectional absorption of ^{14}C-labeled cholesterol using chromic oxide in this way. Cholesterol is excreted into the gut in the bile and net absorption was measured by using non-radioactive cholesterol and a steady-state situation. This paper illustrates the use of both types of balance study and the use of isotopes in situations where bidirectional movements of test substance take place.

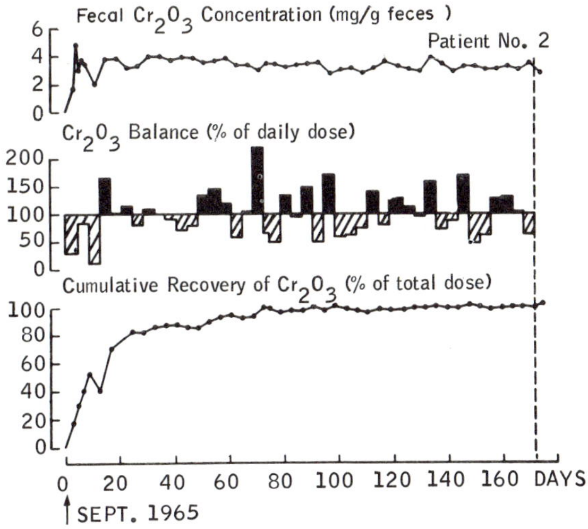

FIG. 9. Excretion pattern of Cr_2O_3 administered daily in an "ideal" patient. The patient, given 300 mg of Cr_2O_3 per day, had a transit time of 2 days and rapidly attained a plateau of fecal concentration of Cr_2O_3 (4 days): the balance data showed that the steady state was reached by 16 days (from Davignon *et al.*, 1968).

In the steady-state situation marker must be fed at regular intervals and it is essential that the daily marker consumption should be accurately known—this is apparently the major difficulty of the technique (Whitby and Lang, 1960). The steady-state must be validated by comparing input and output of marker in short (usually 2–3-day) collection periods and, ideally, output should represent at least 90–95% of input. Figure 9 illustrates the attainment of such a state in an "ideal" subject. It should be noted that in many of the earlier studies much shorter, and probably unsatisfactory, equilibration periods were allowed (for example, Kruela, 1947; Irwin and Crampton, 1951). In the steady state, excretion of test substance can be calculated from the concentrations of marker and substance in a pooled stool collection, which need not represent the complete output. Fecal outputs can be corrected for variations in excretion patterns and completeness of collection, and examples of such correction can be found in the papers of Whitby and Lang (1960), Rose (1964) and Dick (1967). The effects of marker corrections on 6-day collections in calcium balance studies are shown in Fig. 10. Again, theoretically only a single stool need be analyzed and in practice this may occasionally be satisfactory (Rose, 1964). However, in view of the fact

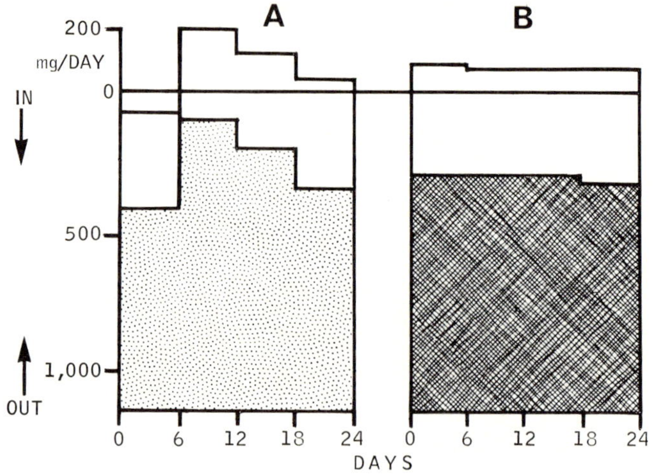

FIG. 10. Calcium balance (A) without and (B) with $BaSO_4$ corrections. Fecal excretion shaded. Urinary excretion unshaded. Intake is represented downwards from zero. Output is represented upwards from the bottom. Net balance is shown by the relation of the uppermost bar to the zero line (from Dick, 1967).

that the steady state is rarely ideal from stool to stool, it is usually recommended that the pooled stools of several days be analyzed.

In their paper, Whitby and Lang (1960) discuss the possibility that chromic oxide might be absorbed by the pathological bowel and that, especially in states of intestinal hurry, a non-uniformity of colonic contents might develop with the relatively dense marker tending to remain behind on the mucosa. There is some evidence that the uniformity of mixing may depend on whether the chromic oxide is given in capsules or mixed in the diet. This is discussed, in relation to animal studies, in the paper of Owen *et al.* (1959). There have been no reports to indicate that these theoretical problems actually occur in human studies.

Application of balance techniques. These methods tend to be avoided because of the many practical difficulties involved. They are particularly suited, however, to the study of substances which are excreted unchanged in appreciable amounts in the feces—for example, calcium, iron, and vitamin B_{12}. As Josephs (1958) emphasized in connection with iron studies, these methods provide the most direct quantitative assessment of absorption, with which other indirect methods can be compared and thus validated.

Balance methods have been traditionally used in the study of fat and nitrogen absorption in man, although now it is not thought necessary to do formal accurate balances in the ordinary clinical assessment of fat malabsorption (Dawson, 1965).

Few drugs have been studied by these methods, but there is, for example, evidence that tetracycline may be excreted in large and very variable amounts in the feces following the oral ingestion of a single dose (Sweeney *et al.*, 1957). Accurate balance studies were not described in this report. The investigations of Maynard *et al.* (1953) suggested that at least 25% of orally administered tetracycline is lost in the stools.

The use of isotopes of both test substance and marker may give balance methods a much greater appeal. However, there are many additional inherent assumptions in such methods and these will be reviewed later in the text.

15.1.2.2. *Segmental studies—the use of intubation methods*

Balance methods cannot be applied to substances which are absorbed completely by upper regions of the small intestine, such as simple sugars, peptides, water and electrolytes and many drugs. Ordinarily these substances make little or no contribution to the composition of stools, as has been demonstrated by the use of fecal dialysis bags (Wrong *et al.*, 1965; Metcalfe-Gibson *et al.*, 1967). Intubation methods allow segmental absorption studies to be made at various levels of the gastrointestinal tract. Absorption is measured as the difference between the amount of substance introduced into the gut and the amount subsequently recovered from the lumen.

Early methods and the use of markers. Long rubber intestinal tubes were introduced by Abbott and Miller in 1936 and they were used to study both gastric and small intestinal absorption. Later, fine polythene tubes were allowed to pass the whole length of the gut, so that all regions could be studied (Blankenhorn *et al.*, 1955). In the early studies test segments were blocked off by inflatable balloons (Abbott *et al.*, 1937) or a single distal balloon was used to permit recovery of unabsorbed material (Groen, 1937). Various early modifications included a continuous infusion method with a non-occlusive distal balloon (Nicholson and Chornock, 1942). The chief disadvantages of these methods were the probable unreliability of the occlusive balloons and the inability to guarantee rapid and complete recovery of unabsorbed material. The introduction of non-absorbed markers into intubation studies was a great advance, because it meant that quantitative recovery of luminal contents was no longer essential. Chromic oxide was unsuitable because it is relatively insoluble in water. The first satisfactory marker, polyethylene glycol (PEG), was used in human studies by Borgstrom *et al.* (1957) and it has been the most widely used marker ever since. It was found to be satisfactory in rat perfusion studies by Fordtran *et al.* (1963) and a rapid recovery of, on average, 97% of ingested PEG was found in patients with established ileostomy (Soergel and Hogan, 1967). Other markers have been tried but are generally considered less reliable. Phenolsulphthalein (Soergel and Hogan, 1967) is absorbed to a slight extent and the same applies to phenol red (Schedl, 1966). The absorption of phenol red may take place in the stomach at low pH as shown in studies on dogs (Bloom *et al.*, 1967), although this does not apply to rats (Schanker *et al.*, 1957); ^{131}I-labeled polyvinylpyrrolidone may become adherent to intestinal mucus and is, therefore, probably an unsatisfactory marker (Schedl and Clifton, 1962). Labeled vitamin B_{12} has also been advocated (Schütz and Reizenstein, 1963) but its use does not appear to have been used by others. The whole problem of the use of markers in studies of this type has been reviewed by Fordtran (1966). This subject will not be discussed in detail, but certain reports of particular interest will be mentioned.

One study of the use of PEG in rats (Dahlqvist and Thomson, 1963) indicated that it might be difficult to recover all the unabsorbed marker from the lumen, because it remained adherent to the intestinal wall. The marker was fed by mouth, whereas in the studies of Fordtran *et al.* (1963) a fast flow perfusion system was used. This means that PEG recoveries may be inadequate unless a fast flow of intestinal contents is produced and this casts some doubt on the original feeding method of Borgström *et al.* (1957).

It is essential that marker and test substance should have the same solubility properties, for it has been shown that PEG is unsuitable for studies of fat absorption (Wiggins and Dawson, 1961). The availability of a suitable lipid soluble marker is keenly awaited. Furthermore, PEG interferes with the action of lipase *in vitro* (Vavrinkova and Krondl, 1965) and, of course, it is essential to know that a marker does not interfere with the digestion or absorption of a test substance.

The studies of Worning and Andrup (1965) suggested that the whole concept of uniform mixing of markers within the lumen might be invalid. They perfused rat duodena with solutions containing radioactive chromium as a marker and examined transverse sections of the excised intestine by autoradiography. It certainly appeared that the marker was not uniformly mixed. However, in these studies bile and pancreatic juice entered the duodenum freely and this was probably responsible for the poor mixing. This does not apply to perfusions of more distal sites and so does not invalidate marker techniques generally.

Single dose methods. As with balance studies, single dose methods and steady-state perfusion systems may be used. In the former method, the marker and test substance are usually fed by mouth and intestinal contents are sampled at different sites distally. If the unabsorbed substance and marker remain uniformly mixed in the lumen and if the sampled fluid is representative of all the fluid passing the sampling site, then it is possible to calculate fractional absorption from the initial and sampled concentration ratios of test substance and marker. The actual concentrations in the samples will depend upon the time of sampling relative to ingestion, but the ratios should remain constant. Hogben *et al.* (1957) used this method in their well-known studies of drug absorption by the human stomach, and it should be pointed out that they used phenol red as a marker but did not assess its validity in man. Borgström *et al.* (1957) studied the magnitude and site of absorption of fats, carbohydrates and protein in this way using PEG, but, as has already been pointed out, PEG is not suitable for fat absorption studies and may remain adherent to the mucosa in these circumstances. A recent study of vitamin B_{12} absorption has confirmed its predominantly ileal site of absorption in this way (Rønnov-Jessen and Hansen, 1965). An alternative single dose method is to introduce marker and test solute into a gut segment isolated between two balloons, and to withdraw the solution after an absorptive period. This method has been used in a recent study of the intestinal absorption of calcium (Ewe, 1968a) and is particularly suited to slowly absorbed substances.

Perfusion methods. In the steady-state technique an open-ended segment of gut is perfused continuously through a proximal orifice and unabsorbed material is sampled at a distal site. Originally trans-intestinal single lumen tubing was used, the tube being blocked for a length which represented the study segment (Schedl and Clifton, 1961, 1963). Subsequently, multi-lumen tubes were introduced, which enabled the sampled material to be retrieved through an additional lumen and obviated the need for intubating the entire intestine (Fordtran *et al.*, 1961; Holdsworth and Dawson, 1964), Fig. 11. Perfusion studies can also be performed

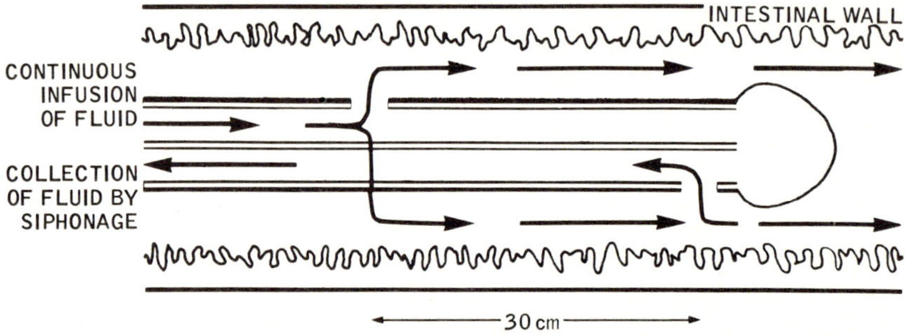

FIG. 11. Diagram of the two-lumen perfusion method for studying small intestinal absorption in man (from Sladen and Dawson, 1968b).

on the colon, unabsorbed fluid being obtained by means of a rectal tube (Levitan *et al.*, 1962).

During the steady state the amounts of PEG entering and leaving the segment should be equal. From the initial and sampled marker concentration, the distal flow rate and hence the fluid absorption rate can be calculated. Similarly, solute absorption rates can be calculated from the change in solute concentration along the segment. The details of the methods and of the calculations involved are fully described in the references quoted above. It should be stressed that this situation is quite different from that of the closed loop, because concentrations of marker and solute vary with distance along the segment and not with time.

In practice it is impossible to achieve a truly steady state, because there are many uncontrollable variables such as intestinal motility, mucosal blood flow, irregular pooling of fluid and alteration of the shape of the gut segment relative to the tube. This means that the absorption rates of water and solute are likely to vary from moment to moment. It is, therefore, necessary to allow both an equilibration period in order to reach an approximately steady state and to continue collection of pooled samples for a prolonged period, so as to minimize the effects of this variation. Equilibration and collection periods of 30–60 min have been recommended by various workers (Cooper *et al.*, 1966; Whalen *et al.*, 1966). The adequacy of the steady state has been judged by comparing marker concentrations in serially collected samples. Fordtran *et al.* (1961) found that there was a variation of approximately $\pm$ 10% of the mean PEG concentration in serial 5-min samples. A more rigorous method is to compare solute absorption rates calculated from serial samples, because this takes into account the relative concentrations of marker and solute. Holdsworth and Dawson (1964) found a mean discrepancy of 10% between pairs of glucose absorption rates. Sladen and Dawson (1968a) estimated a variation of ± 10 % of the mean between triplicate glucose absorption rates for short segments and ± 15 % for longer segments. Undoubtedly the length of the perfused segment and the infusion rate of fluid are important considerations, because longer equilibration times are required for long segments and slow flow rates. This subject has been reviewed in more detail recently (Sladen, 1968). In general terms, adequacy of the steady state should be assessed in any experimental situation and the time periods involved greatly limit the number of observations that can be made on even the most cooperative subject.

The major theoretical disadvantage of the simple double-lumen tube is that it makes no allowance for endogenous gut secretions, which may contaminate the perfusion zone from above, even in the fasting state. Significant contamination would result in underestimation of solute and water absorption rates, depending on the solute concentration in the contaminating fluid and on the mean contamination rate. This is theoretically a major problem in studies of absorption of water and electrolytes, such as sodium, chloride, bicarbonate and, probably, calcium and magnesium. Solutes such as glucose and amino acids are present in small concentration in fasting intestinal contents (Whalen *et al.*, 1966; Adibi and Gray, 1967) and are absorbed avidly, so that contamination is not a serious problem. As far as drugs are concerned, recycling of absorbed drug into the lumen via the upper gastrointestinal secretions may be an important practical difficulty. Furthermore, drugs may be secreted into the stomach as a result of pH gradients across the gastric mucosa. Zawoiski *et al.* (1958) demonstrated such a phenomenon in the case of mecamylamine. The practical significance of such possibilities remains to be seen, because so few drugs have been studied in this way.

Various methods have been introduced to obviate the problem of contamination, but each has its disadvantages and the practical importance of excluding these contaminations has not been demonstrated directly. The three-lumen tube (Cooper *et al.*, 1966; Whalen *et al.*, 1966) incorporates a proximal mixing segment which allows infused and contaminating fluids to mix and be sampled before entry into the distal study segment, Fig. 12. If mixing is complete, the exact composition and flow rate of fluid reaching the distal segment is known. Variable absorption of solute and water by the mixing segment does, however, mean that

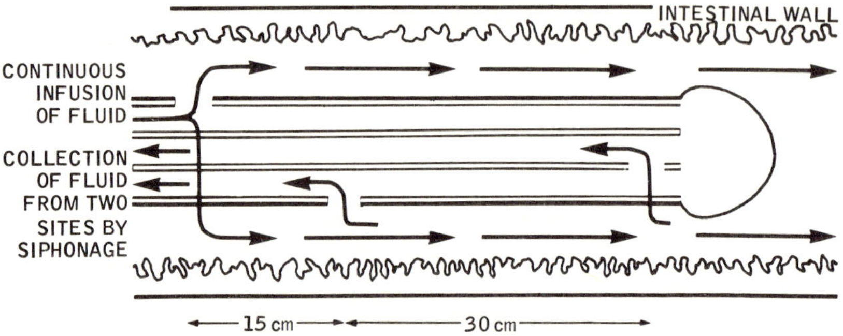

FIG. 12. Diagram of the three-lumen tube perfusion system: a mixing segment of 15 cm and a study segment of 30 cm (from Sladen and Dawson, 1968b).

the composition and flow rate of fluid entering the study segment is difficult to control. In many experimental situations this may be of little practical importance, but in detailed kinetic absorption studies such control is essential.

An alternative approach is the use of a proximal occlusive balloon as described by Phillips and Summerskill (1966) and Ewe (1968b). This has the great advantage of avoiding a mixing segment and would seem to be the more suitable method for kinetic studies. However, it is open to the theoretical objection that an inflated balloon may affect gut motility and mucosal blood flow to such an extent that segmental absorption rates are affected.

In view of these uncertainties and difficulties, the authors have compared the various perfusion techniques in an attempt to define the indications for each method. A comparison of the double- and triple-lumen tube methods (Sladen and Dawson, 1968b) showed no significant difference between mean water and sodium absorption rates from isotonic saline and glucose–saline solutions. This suggests that either contamination rates obtained by others (Whalen *et al.*, 1966) have been exaggerated, or there has been a fortuitous cancelling out of the opposing factors of contamination and proximal backwash of infused fluid (Fordtran, 1966). The balloon technique has been assessed by comparing absorption periods with and without a balloon inflated (Sladen and Dawson, to be published). These studies suggest that the inflated balloon does not seriously interfere with the absorption of glucose, water or electrolytes and they help to quantitate the amounts of contamination and backwash that may occur. As far as water and sodium absorption is concerned, the mean results are not significantly affected by inflation of the balloon. Individual variation of absorption rates is, however, somewhat reduced by inflating the balloon. Under the conditions studied by these authors, the greatest individual variation was found using the three-lumen tube technique.

In summary, it may be concluded that the simple two-lumen tube technique gives reliable results, when mean values of a series of observations are required and when the length of the perfusion segment is immaterial. This applies especially to absorption of substances, which are not ordinarily present in high concentration in the fasting intestinal contents, such as glucose (Whalen *et al.*, 1966), some amino acids (Adibi and Gray, 1967) and probably many drugs. However, accurate information in individual subjects can best be obtained if errors due to variable contamination and backwash are reduced to a minimum. For this purpose the three-lumen tube is the simplest method, but is unsuitable for kinetic studies. The balloon technique is the most difficult practically, but probably reduces individual variation to a minimum and is ideal for kinetic studies.

Application of perfusion methods. These methods, although tedious and time-consuming, do give the most direct information about rates of absorption, as opposed to total or fractional absorption. They have been used particularly in quantitative and kinetic studies of sugar and amino-acid absorption. The effects of solute concentration and perfusion rate on absorption and mutual competition between monosaccharides and amino acids for absorption have been investigated (Schedl and Clifton, 1961; Holdsworth and Dawson, 1964; Fleshler *et al.*, 1966). The kinetics of hydrolysis and absorption of disaccharides have also been studied (Gray and Ingelfinger, 1965, 1966; McMichael *et al.*, 1967). This information is of great physiological interest and enables comparison to be made with results of studies on animal preparations. Information about possible absorption mechanisms is also obtained, but should be interpreted with caution. For example, it is commonly found that a saturable relationship exists between the luminal concentration of a solute and its absorption rate. This may be considered analogous to the kinetics of enzyme–substrate interactions and reciprocal plots can be used to obtain values of V_{max} (maximum theoretical absorption rate) and K_m (solute concentration required to half-saturate the absorption process), according to the method of Lineweaver and Burk (1934). However, it should be stressed that such a relationship does not mean that a saturable carrier is the rate-limiting step of transport. Physical adsorption to membranes or pores could produce the same relationship. Furthermore, the absolute values of K_m and V_{max} vary widely depending partly upon the experimental design of the investigation, as discussed in detail by Sladen (1968).

Regional absorption rates of fluids and electrolytes can only be studied satisfactorily in intact man by perfusion methods and a number of reports have now appeared on absorption by the small intestine (Fordtran *et al.*, 1961; Cooper *et al.*, 1966; Whalen *et al.*, 1966; Phillips and Summerskill, 1967) and by the colon (Levitan *et al.*, 1962; Levitan and Ingelfinger, 1965; Shields *et al.*, 1968). The use of isotopes to measure bidirectional fluxes of water and electrolytes will be discussed in detail in a later section. The movement of fluid in response to osmotic gradients across the intestinal mucosa has been used to measure the permeability properties of different regions of the intestine and to estimate the size of the hypothetical water-filled pores (Fordtran *et al.*, 1965).

A few investigations of pathological absorption processes have been made. For example, various studies on groups of patients with the sprue syndrome (Holdsworth and Dawson, 1965b; Schedl *et al.*, 1968), infantile diarrhea (Torres-Pinedo *et al.*, 1966) and infantile protein-calorie malnutrition (James, 1968) may be quoted. It should be mentioned that the jejunal mucosa is in a secretory state in sprue (Fordtran *et al.*, 1967) and, therefore, contamination by intestinal secretions may cause difficulty. Holdsworth and Dawson (1965b) found far greater discrepancies in their duplicate glucose absorption rates in these patients than in normal subjects.

Very few studies of drug absorption have been made with these methods, but noteworthy examples are those of cortisol absorption by Schedl and Clifton (1963) and of folic acid absorption by Hepner *et al.* (1968), but some of the quantitative interpretations in the latter paper have been seriously criticized (Scott and Orsi, 1968; Helbock, 1968).

In conclusion, it may be stated that, theoretically, the absorption of any water-soluble substance can be studied in this way and the same may apply, in the future, to fat-soluble substances if a marker becomes available. However, in view of its complexity and the wide range of most reported results, the perfusion method is essentially a research procedure and probably little useful information will be obtained from the investigation of individual subjects.

15.1.3. MEASUREMENT OF RETENTION WITHIN THE BODY: USE OF WHOLE-BODY COUNTER

This relatively new method depends entirely on the measurement of the isotopic content of the body, by means of whole-body counting techniques. Although there are many technical problems involved, it would seem to offer a simple and practicable method of measuring the fractional retention of a substance within the body, provided a suitable isotope is available. In principle, a single dose of the labeled substance is ingested and after a short time interval the total whole-body activity is measured and this count is taken as 100%. After this, the activity will decrease as unabsorbed material is excreted in the feces. A steady plateau is reached when all the unabsorbed material is evacuated and this will give a direct estimate of the fractional retention within the body. This can be confirmed by measuring the total output in the feces. The main practical disadvantage is that the time for complete fecal evacuation may be as much as 14 days, as already discussed, but otherwise the method has the great advantage of avoiding fecal collections, multiple blood sampling or intubation. It has been used particularly in studies of iron (van Hoek and Conrad, 1961; Heinrich *et al.*, 1966; Losowsky and Wilson, 1967) and calcium (Kehayoglou *et al.*, 1968; Deller *et al.*, 1965) retention and these papers should be consulted for practical details.

Certain practical considerations should be mentioned here. It seems that the activity of the whole body will depend upon whether the labeled substance is uniformly distributed throughout the body or is residing mainly in the gut. This can be shown by comparing the activity soon after oral and parenteral administration and correction factors may have to be introduced (Pollack *et al.*, 1966). Of more immediate concern here is the possible application of these methods to other substances. The method would not be suitable for any substance that is excreted or metabolized rapidly after absorption. Interpretation would be difficult because the distribution of activity throughout the body would change continuously and would quickly be concentrated in the bladder, breath or even gut, depending upon the mode of excretion. The method can, therefore, only be used for substances which are retained in the body in a structurally unaltered form for prolonged periods. This applies particularly to calcium, iron and vitamin B_{12} but to few, if any, drugs. It should also be stressed, again, that the method measures fractional retention only and gives no information about absorption rates or recycling into the gut lumen.

15.2. METHODS APPLICABLE TO CONSCIOUS BUT ABNORMAL MAN

15.2.1. USE OF LYMPH FISTULA

In experimental studies of fat absorption in animals much use has been made of the collection of lymph from the thoracic duct. This is the most direct method of investigating the products of absorption of fat and fat-soluble vitamins. The thoracic duct can be cannulated in man (Bierman *et al.*, 1953) and several reports have appeared describing the use of this technique in the study of the absorption of fat (Kayden *et al.*, 1967), cholesterol (Hellman *et al.*, 1960) and vitamin A (Blomstrand and Werner, 1967). Good lymph flows can be maintained for 20–40 hr and considerable quantitites of fluid, electrolytes and protein may have to be replaced. However, it is known that alternative lymph pathways exist and lymphaticovenous connections do occur at various sites (Mayerson, 1963). Probably, therefore, thoracic duct cannulation will not yield all the lymph draining the intestine.

In pathological situations communications may develop between the lymphatic system and, for example, the bladder. Patients with chyluria have been used to investigate certain aspects of fat and cholesterol absorption (Blomstrand and Ahrens, 1958a, b; Peterson, 1963). Lymph recovery from the urine will be incomplete and so only qualitative information about absorption processes can be obtained. A lymph fistula in the leg has been used for similar purposes (Munk, 1891, quoted by Parsons, 1968).

15.2.2. SAMPLING OF PORTAL VENOUS COLLATERAL VESSELS

In portal hypertension, collateral venous connections develop between the abdominal wall and the portal venous system. Sherlock and Walshe (1946) first described the cannulation of such vessels for absorption studies and rather more extensive investigations were reported later by Bean *et al.* (1951). A comparison of absorption curves in portal and systemic blood gave some information about hepatic uptake, but in these patients liver function was often abnormal, because nearly all the patients had cirrhosis. Few other uses of this technique have been reported and it must have a very limited application. Portal vein cannulation via the obliterated umbilical vein has been described recently as a method for the radiological investigation of the portal venous system (Lavoie *et al.*, 1967), but it has not yet been used for absorption studies.

After a porto-caval anastomosis, performed for bleeding oesophageal varices, much or all of the portal blood by-passes the liver and can be sampled directly in the peripheral vessels. A comparison of absorption curves before and after such an operation has not been reported, but might also indicate the effects of hepatic uptake. Again, liver function will be abnormal in the majority of cases.

15.2.3. USE OF EXCLUDED SEGMENTS OF INTESTINE

In the classical methods of Thiry and Vella, segments of intestine are excluded and exteriorized, so that substance can be introduced and recovered through the abdominal wall (reviewed by Parsons, 1968). Occasionally, in man such a situation may exist as a result of a surgical procedure and these patients have been used for absorption studies. Shields *et al.* (1966) investigated the effects of aldosterone on fluid and electrolyte absorption by the excluded colon of one patient who was undergoing reconstructive surgery after resection of an oesophageal carcinoma. The excluded colon in patients with a colostomy has been used in the investigation of absorption of short-chain fatty acids (Dawson *et al.*, 1964) and of the effects of aldosterone on the electrolyte composition of colonic fluid (Wrong, 1968). It is uncertain to what extent the excluded gut retains its functional integrity and the completeness of recovery of unabsorbed material must be rigorously assessed in studies of this type.

15.2.4. USE OF PATIENTS WITH ILEOSTOMY

Few absorption studies have been reported in fit patients with established ileostomies. Balance studies should be much simpler than in normal subjects, because the problem of colonic emptying is obviated. However, it is possible that the ileum adapts in some way to the absence of a colon, especially in relation to fluid and electrolyte absorption, but there is no direct evidence to confirm or refute this.

Most studies on ileostomized patients have been concerned with fluid and electrolyte losses and compensatory homeostatic mechanisms. These patients are often on the verge of fluid and sodium depletion (Gallaher *et al.*, 1962) and have a limited capacity to conserve sodium (Kramer, 1966). The effect of salt-retaining steroids on the electrolyte composition of ileostomy fluid has been investigated (Goulston *et al.*, 1963). These patients absorb normal amounts of protein and fat, as judged by nitrogen and fat outputs while on ordinary diets (Kramer *et al.*, 1963). Drug absorption has not been studied in these subjects. It should perhaps be added that the delicate balance of normal ileostomy function may be easily upset by gross alterations in the diet.

15.3. METHODS APPLICABLE TO ANESTHETIZED MAN

15.3.1. CLOSED INTESTINAL LOOPS

During the course of abdominal operations closed loops of intestine with blood supply intact have been used for absorption studies, with subsequent restoration of gut continuity. Water and electrolyte absorption by normal and pathological small intestine has been investigated in this way (Duthie and Atwell, 1963; Atwell and Duthie, 1964). McColl and his colleagues have studied vitamin B_{12} disappearance from closed loops and they concluded that the vitamin could be absorbed equally from jejunum and ileum and that intrinsic factor was not apparently required (McColl *et al.*, 1967; Gazet and McColl, 1967). These reports suffer from the fact that adsorption to the intestinal mucosa cannot be excluded. They demonstrated subsequent hepatic uptake of radioactive B_{12}, but absorption could have occurred later from the ileum. This illustrates a general difficulty in interpreting absorption by disappearance methods. The effects of certain laxatives on intestinal transport processes have also been studied in this way (Hart and McColl, 1968).

15.3.2. PORTAL VEIN SAMPLING

Holdsworth and Dawson (1965a) investigated the absorption of fructose from intestinal loops at operation by sampling the portal vein. They showed that little conversion of fructose to glucose or lactic acid took place in the intestinal mucosa and that most of the fructose appeared unchanged in the portal blood. This differs from what is known about fructose absorption in various animals (Wilson, 1962, pp. 91–94).

15.4. METHODS APPLICABLE TO *IN VITRO* INTESTINE

15.4.1. MUCOSAL BIOPSY SPECIMENS

Intestinal mucosa can be obtained with relative ease by means of various biopsy capsules. Mucosal uptake studies have been performed on a number of test substances and the general problems of methodology are similar to those that apply to animal studies. A few examples of these studies will be quoted. Mucosal accumulation of various monosaccharides and amino acids has been investigated in patients with primary glucose–galactose malabsorption by Meeuwisse and Dahlqvist (1968). The cellular transport and oxidation of lactose ^{14}C was studied in normal subjects and in patients with isolated lactase deficiency by London *et al.* (1967). The kinetics and mutual inhibition of amino acid uptake by the intestinal mucosa of patients with cystinuria has been reported by McCarthy *et al.* (1964) and Thier *et al.* (1965), and the interrelationships between cystine and cysteine transport in these patients and normal subjects was studied by Rosenberg *et al.* (1967).

15.4.2. INTESTINE REMOVED AT OPERATION

Segments of intestine removed at operation have been used in various ways for investigating certain aspects of absorption. Loran *et al.* (1961) used an *in vitro* perfusion system for studying vitamin A transport by isolated human ileum. The electrical properties of isolated sheets of intestine have been correlated with net sodium transport, as measured by bidirectional ionic fluxes, and used in an investigation of possible effects of the cholera toxin on the sodium transporting mechanism (Grady *et al.*, 1967). The intrauterine development of such electrical activity in human fetal intestine and its relationship to the development of absorptive processes in general has been reported by Levin *et al.* (1968).

In vitro methods of this type have been used mainly with animal preparations and have so far found little application to human absorption studies. For this reason, a critical assessment of these methods will not be attempted here and the reader is referred to the reviews of Wilson (1962, pp. 20–30) and Parsons (1968).

15.5. GENERAL CONSIDERATIONS ABOUT THE USE OF ISOTOPES IN ABSORPTION STUDIES

The use of isotopes may obviate the requirement for difficult chemical analyses, so that absorption tests are greatly simplified. Isotopic measurements in conjunction with chemical analysis may be used in the study of bidirectional movements of test substance across the gut mucosa, so that a distinction can be made between net and unidirectional absorption.

Furthermore, isotopic methods have the great advantage that small physiological doses of nutritionally important substances, such as vitamin B_{12} and folic acid, can be used. Hence information about nutritional as opposed to pharmacological absorption can be obtained.

15.5.1. USE OF ISOTOPES AS AN ALTERNATIVE TO CHEMICAL ANALYSIS

The various tests of absorption of labeled iron, calcium, vitamin B_{12} and folic acid have already been discussed. Other examples are the measurement of blood levels of tritiated vitamin D (Thomson *et al.*, 1966), of ^{46}Ca (Avioli *et al.*, 1965) and the use of ^{131}I-labeled fats and fatty acids in the study of both fat absorption and pancreatic lipase activity (Shingleton *et al.*, 1957; McKenna *et al.*, 1957; Sie *et al.*, 1967). In all these methods it is assumed that labeled and unlabeled substances are handled in exactly the same way by the gut mocosa and by subsequent metabolic pathways. However, when, for example, oleic acid is labeled with ^{131}I the molecular weight is greatly increased and there is evidence that its metabolism is altered (van Handel and Zilversmit, 1958). Similarly, leveling of human serum albumin with ^{131}I or ^{51}Cr may result in denaturation of the protein so that the biological half-lives in the body are greatly shortened. This depends on the method of labeling and it is possible to prepare highly purified ^{131}I-labeled plasma proteins with negligible denaturation (McFarlane, 1956). The studies of Kerr *et al.* (1967) demonstrate the very different biological half-lives of ^{131}I and ^{51}Cr-labeled albumin. The subject has been reviewed by McFarlane (1964). Commercially available ^{131}I-labeled triolein contains many impurities and this may result in misleadingly high absorption rates of isotope in patients with undoubted fat malabsorption (Tuna *et al.*, 1963; Kennedy and Kinloch, 1964). The more recent studies of Sie *et al.* (1967) suggest that purified ^{131}I-triolein may be satisfactory for fat absorption studies, at least in the rat if fecal radioactivity is used as the index of absorption.

Following absorption it is only necessary to follow the fate of the isotope in blood and urine to obtain qualitative information about total absorption. However, the subsequent metabolic handling and excretion of the isotope may be different from that of the test substance and it may be necessary to separate these fractions chemically, if the fate of the test substance itself is to be quantitated. This is illustrated by the different decay curves of total blood ^{3}H and chloroform-extractable vitamin D_3–^{3}H after the intravenous injection of tritiated vitamin D (Avioli *et al.*,

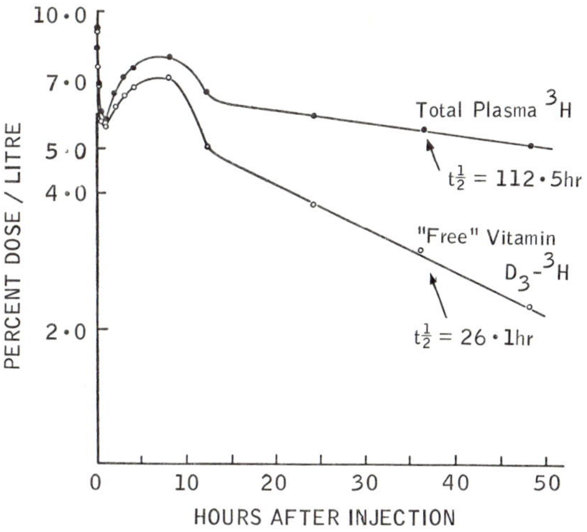

FIG. 13. Total plasma ^{3}H and direct chloroform-extractable vitamin D_3–^{3}H ("free") in plasma after infusion of vitamin D_3–^{3}H into normal subjects (from Avioli *et al.*, 1967).

1967), Fig. 13. Thus it would be impossible to analyze the kinetics of vitamin D_3–^{3}H absorption using the method of Thomson *et al.* (1966) in which whole blood activity was counted. The total amount absorbed can be assessed in this way, provided that the tritiated vitamin is absorbed intact.

Bacterial action in the colon on undigested material may result in the liberation and subsequent absorption of isotope, with consequent invalidation of the test as a measure of absorption. This criticism would probably apply to the studies of Salmon *et al.* (1968) using ^{14}C-lactose, already referred to, but the details of their findings have not yet been published. The studies of Gagnon and Dawson (1968) ^{14}C–vitamin A acetate in rats show that colonic bacteria may degrade this substance into water-soluble metabolites. For this reason, absorption of vitamin A using this isotope could probably only be assessed if the lipid-extractable component of the blood were counted.

Finally, in the case of ^{131}I the free label may be excreted into the gut lumen via the saliva and gastric juice. This might also invalidate absorption studies based on the use of this isotope and was responsible for some of the difficulties in the interpretation of the ^{131}I–albumin-resin test for the assessment of gut losses of protein (Jeejeebhoy and Coghill, 1961; Freeman and Gordon, 1964).

15.5.2. USE OF ISOTOPE IN ADDITION TO CHEMICAL ANALYSIS

The work of Visscher and his colleagues clearly established that water and some electrolytes move freely in both directions across the canine ileal mucosa (Visscher *et al.*, 1944a, b). This has been confirmed in man using perfusion methods with isotopic water and electrolytes at all levels of the gastrointestinal tract (Fordtran *et al.*, 1961; Whalen *et al.*, 1965; Phillips and Summerskill, 1967; Shields *et al.*, 1968). These fluxes are generally two or more times greater than the net absorption measured simultaneously.

In these studies, it is assumed that absorbed isotope is rapidly diluted to negligible specific activity in a large body pool, and that the specific activity of substance passing from blood to lumen can be discounted. The disappearance of isotope will then indicate the unidirectional flux from lumen to blood, while net absorption is measured by chemical analysis. Unidirectional flux from blood to lumen can then be calculated simply by subtraction. Any re-entry of isotope into the lumen will result in the underestimation of fluxes in both directions. The possible magnitude of such underestimation may be indicated by measurement of blood specific activity, representing the pool of distribution, but such observations were not reported in the studies, referred to above. The actual calculations of bidirectional fluxes are rather complex. The early method of Fordtran *et al.* (1961) is oversimplified, as admitted by Fordtran himself (see Fordtran and Ingelfinger, 1968, p. 1460). The main difficulty is in the assessment of the specific activity of the absorbed isotope and some form of mean luminal specific activity has to be used. This problem is discussed at some length in the paper of Shields *et al.* (1966) and Soergel *et al.* (1968).

15.6. MATHEMATICAL APPENDIX: THE QUANTITATION OF ABSORPTION RATES FROM BLOOD CURVES AND URINARY EXCRETION

It is assumed that the absorbed substance is rapidly distributed, after absorption, throughout a single-body compartment—volume V. The rate of disposal of the substance, by both metabolism and excretion, is assumed to be directly proportional to the total amount of substance present in the body tissues at any time.

$$\text{Rate of disposal} = K.V.C_t \tag{1}$$

where C_t = concentration in the blood or plasma at time t.

Finally, it is assumed that, following parenteral administration, a constant fraction (f) of the dose administered is excreted in the urine:

$$\begin{aligned}\text{Rate of urinary excretion} &= f \times \text{rate of overall disposal}\\ &= f.K.V.C_t \end{aligned}\tag{2}$$

The values f and V can only be obtained from a study of the disappearance of parenterally administered substance. K can be obtained similarly from log plots of plasma decay, if the assumption of eqn. (1) holds good, i.e. a first-order kinetic process in a single-body compartment. K can also be obtained from the latter part of blood curves after oral ingestion, when absorption has ceased and the curve represents disposal only. If these values can be measured, the following calculations may be performed.

A. *From the blood curves* (Fig. A.1)

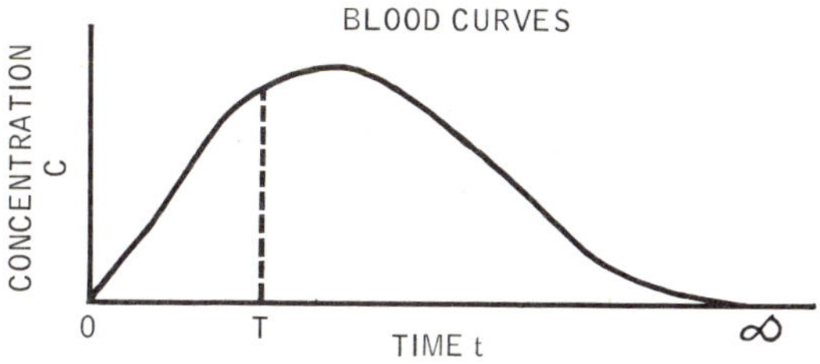

FIG. A.1. Diagram of typical blood absorption curve.

1. Total absorption by time T = Amount present at time T + Amount disposed of by time T

$$= V.C_T + K.V\int_0^T C\,dt^* \tag{3}$$

2. Total absorption ($t = \infty$) = Total disposal

$$= KV\int_0^\infty C\,dt^* \tag{4}$$

*The integral terms can be obtained from the areas under the curve.

3. Rate of absorption at time T = Rate of appearance at time T + Rate of disposal at time T

$$= V\left(\frac{dc}{dt}\right)_T + K.V.C_T \qquad (5)$$

B. *From the urinary excretion data* (Fig. A.2)

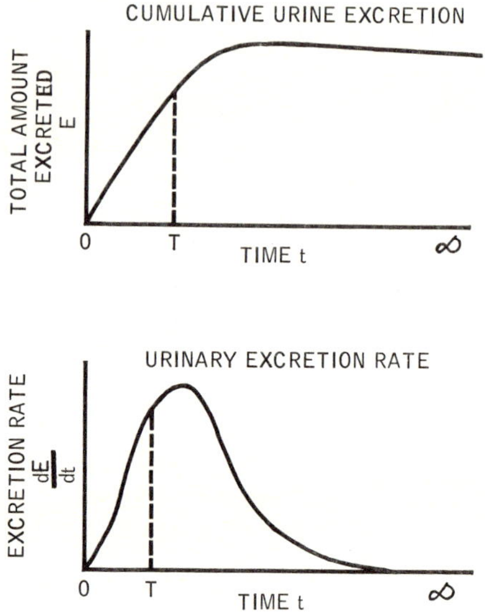

FIG. A.2. Diagram of a cumulative urinary excretion study and a study in which serial excretion rates are calculated.

1. Total absorption by time T = Amount present at time T + Total disposal by time T

$$= \left(\frac{dE}{dt}\right)_T . \frac{1^*}{f.K} + E_T . \frac{1}{f} \qquad (6)$$

2. Total absorption ($t = \infty$) = Total disposal

$$= E_\infty . \frac{1}{f} \qquad (7)$$

*This term is derived from eqn. (2) and equals (VC_T).

3. Rate of absorption at time T = Rate of appearance at time T + Rate of disposal at time T

$$= \left(\frac{d^2E}{dt^2}\right)_T \cdot \frac{1^*}{f.K} + \left(\frac{dE}{dt}\right)_T \cdot \frac{1}{f} \quad (8)$$

These equations indicate the way in which absorption rates may be quantitated in the simplest possible situation and the sort of assumptions and measurements which have to be made. In compiling these equations the following references were found helpful and were used freely: Dominguez and Pomerone (1945), Nelson and Schaldemose (1959), Wagner and Nelson (1963) and Parsons (1968). Examples of the use of these calculations in practice are given in the first two of these papers and also in the following: Swintosky (1956), Levy and Hollister (1964). The early studies of McCance and Madders (1930) on pentose absorption were based on the measurement of f and the use of eqns. (6) and (7). The use of computers in facilitating these calculations was referred to earlier in the text.

REFERENCES

ABBOTT, W. O. and MILLER, T. G. (1936) Intubation studies of the human small intestine. III. A technic for the collection of pure intestinal secretion and for the study of intestinal absorption. *J. Am. Med. Ass.* **106:** 16–18.

ABBOTT, W. O., KARR, W. G. and MILLER, T. G. (1937) Intubation studies of the human small intestine. VII. Factors concerned in absorption of glucose from the jejunum and ileum. *Am. J. Dig. Dis.* **4:** 742–752.

ADAMS, J. F. and CARTWRIGHT, E. J. (1963) The reliability and reproducibility of the Schilling test in primary malabsorptive disease and after partial gastrectomy. *Gut* **4:** 32–36.

ADIBI, S. A. and GRAY, S. J. (1967) Intestinal absorption of essential aminoacids in man. *Gastroenterology* **52:** 837–845.

ALTHAUSEN, T. L., UYEYAMA, K. and LORAN, M. R. (1960) Effects of alcohol on absorption of vitamin A in normal and in gastrectomised subjects. *Gastroenterology* **38:** 942–945.

ALVAREZ, W. C. and FREEDLANDER, B. L. (1924) The rate of progress of food residues through the bowel. *J. Am. Med. Ass.* **83:** 576–580.

ANDERSON, B., BELCHER, E. H., CHANARIN, I. and MOLLIN, D. L. (1960) The urinary and fecal excretion of radioactivity after oral doses of ^{3}H-folic acid. *Brit. J. Haemat.* **6:** 439–455.

ATWELL, J. D. and DUTHIE, H. L. (1964) The absorption of water, sodium and potassium from the ileum of humans showing the effects of regional enteritis. *Gastroenterology* **46:** 16–22.

AVIOLI, L. V., LEE, S. W., MCDONALD, J. E., LUND, J. and DELUCA, H. F. (1967) Metabolism of vitamin D_3–^{3}H in human subjects: distribution in blood, feces and urine. *J. Clin. Invest.* **46:** 983–992.

AVIOLI, L. V., MCDONALD, J. E. and LEE, S. W. (1965) The influence of age on the intestinal absorption of ^{47}Ca in women and its relation to ^{47}Ca absorption in post-menopausal osteoporosis. *J. Clin. Invest.* **44:** 1960–1967.

*This term is obtained by differentiation of eqn. (2) and equals $V\left(\frac{dc}{dt}\right)_T$.

BAKER, H., FRANK, O., ZIFFER, H., FEINGOLD, S. and CINTRON-RIVERA, A. A. (1968) Reversal of folate malabsorption in tropical and non-tropical sprue by calf jejunum. *Brit. Med. J.* **3:** 472–474.

BAKER, S. J. and MOLLIN, D. L. (1955) The relationship between intrinsic factor and the intestinal absorption of vitamin B_{12}. *Brit. J. Haemat.* **1:** 46–51.

BEAN, W. B., FRANKLIN, M., EMBICK, J. F. and DAUM, K. (1951) Absorption studies using portal anastomotic veins. *J. Clin. Invest.* **30:** 263–273.

BECKETT, A. H. and ROWLAND, M. (1965) Urinary excretion kinetics of amphetamine in man. *J. Pharm. Pharmac.* **17:** 628–639.

BECKETT, A. H. and TUCKER, G. T. (1967) Problems in the *in vivo* evaluation of drug preparations and the interpretation of *in vivo* data. *J. Mond. Pharm.* **3:** 181–202.

BENSON, J. A., CULVER, P. J., RAGLAND, S., JONES, C. M., DRUMMEY, G. D. and BOUGAS, E. (1957) The d-xylose absorption test in malabsorption syndromes. *New Engl. J. Med.* **256:** 335–339.

BIEHL, J. P. (1956) The role of the dose and the metabolic fate of isoniazid in the emergence of isoniazid resistance. *Trans. 15th Conf. Chemother. Tuberc.*, pp. 279–282.

BIERMAN, H. R., BYRON, R. L. JR., KELLY, K. H., GILFILLAN, R. S., WHITE, L. P., FREEMAN, N. E. and PETRAKIS, N. L. (1953) The characteristics of thoracic duct lymph in man. *J. Clin. Invest.* **32:** 637–649.

BLANKENHORN, D. H., HIRSCH, J. and AHRENS, E. H. JR. (1955) Transintestinal intubation: technic for measurement of gut length and physiologic sampling at known loci. *Proc. Soc. Exp. Biol. Med.* **88:** 356–362.

BLOMSTRAND, R. and AHRENS, E. H. JR. (1958a) The absorption of fats studied in a patient with chyluria. II. Palmitic and oleic acids. *J. Biol. Chem.* **233:** 321–326.

BLOMSTRAND, R. and AHRENS, E. H. JR. (1958b) Absorption of fats studied in a patient with chyluria. *J. Biol. Chem.* **233:** 327–330.

BLOMSTRAND, R. and WERNER, B. (1967) Studies on the intestinal absorption of radioactive β-carotene and vitamin A in man. *Scand. J. Clin. Lab. Invest.* **19:** 339–345.

BLOOM, D. S., JACOBSON, E. D. and GROSSMAN, M. I. (1967) Validation of dilution indicators in the stomach. *Gastroenterology* **52:** 205–210.

BOENDER, C. A., MULDER, E., PIOEM, J. E., DEWAAL, J. and VERLOOP, M. C. (1967) Iron absorption and retention in man. *Nature* (*Lond.*) **213:** 1236–1237.

BOOTH, C. C. and MOLLIN, D. L. (1956) Plasma, tissue and urinary radioactivity after oral administration of ^{56}Co-labeled vitamin B_{12}. *Brit. J. Haemat.* **2:** 223–236.

BORGSTRÖM, B., DAHLQVIST, A., LUNDH, G. and SJOVALL, J. (1957) Studies of intestinal digestion and absorption in the human. *J. Clin. Invest.* **36:** 1521–1536.

BOTHWELL, T. H., PIRZIO-BIROLI, G. and FINCH, C. A. (1958) Iron absorption. I. Factors influencing absorption. *J. Lab. Clin. Med.* **51:** 24–36.

BRAIN, M. C., STEWART, S. J. and BOOTH, C. C. (1963) The absorption of tritiated pyridoxine in man. *Radioaktive Isotope in Klinik und Forschung* **5:** 475–483, FELLINGER, K. and HÖFER, R. (Eds.). Urban and Schwarzenberg, Munich and Berlin.

BRODIE, B. B. (1964) Distribution and fate of drugs: therapeutic implications, pp. 238–248. In: *Absorption and Distribution of Drugs*, BINNS, T. B. (Ed.). E. and S. Livingstone, Ltd., Edinburgh and London.

BUTTERWORTH, C. E., NADEL, H., PERES-SANTIAGO, E., SANTINI, R. and GARDNER, F. H. (1957) Folic acid absorption, excretion and leucocyte concentration in tropical sprue. *J. Lab. Clin. Med.* **50:** 673–681.

CHRISTIANSEN, P. A., KIRSNER, J. B. and ABLAZA, J. (1959) D-xylose and its use in the diagnosis of malabsorptive states. *Am. J. Med.* **27:** 443–453.

CLARKE, C. A., PRICE EVANS, D. A., HARRIS, R., MCCONNELL, R. B. and WOODROW, J. C. (1968) Genetics in medicine: a review. Part II. Pharmacogenetics. *Quart. J. Med.* (new series) **37:** 183–219.

CODE, C. F. (1962) Normal rates of absorption of water, sodium, and potassium in man and animal. *Am. J. Dig. Dis.* (new series) **7:** 50–56.

COMFORT, M. W., WALLAEGER, E. E. and TAYLOR, A. B. (1953) Non-tropical sprue: observations on absorption and metabolism. *Gastroenterology* **23:** 155–178.

COOPER, H., LEVITAN, R., FORDTRAN, J. S. and INGELFINGER, F. J. (1966) A method of studying absorption of water and solute from the human small intestine. *Gastroenterology* **50:** 1–7.

CORNWELL, D. G., KRUGER, F. A. and ROBINSON, H. B. (1962) Studies on the absorption of beta-carotene and the distribution of total carotenoid in human serum lipoproteins after oral administration. *J. Lipid. Res.* **3:** 65–70.

CRAFT, I. L., GEDDES, D., HYDE, C. W., WISE, I. J. and MATTHEWS, D. M. (1968) Absorption and malabsorption of glycine and glycine peptides in man. *Gut* **9:** 425–437.

DAHLQVIST, A. and THOMSON, D. L. (1963) The digestion and absorption of sucrose by the intact rat. *J. Physiol.* (*Lond.*) **167:** 193–209.

DAVIGNON, J., SIMMONDS, W. J. and AHRENS, E. H. JR. (1968) Usefulness of chromic oxide as an internal standard for balance studies in formula-fed patients and for assessment of colonic function. *J. Clin. Invest.* **47:** 127–138.

DAWSON, A. M. (1965) Malabsorption. *Abstr. Wld. Med.* **38:** 361–381.

DAWSON, A. M., HOLDSWORTH, C. D. and WEBB, J. (1964) Absorption of short cnain fatty acids in man. *Proc. Soc. Exp. Biol. Med.* **117:** 97–100.

DAYTON, P. G., YU, T. F., CHEN, W., BERGER, L. and GUTMAN, A. B. (1963) The physiological disposition of probenecid, including renal clearance, in man, studied by an improved method for its estimation in biological material. *J. Pharm. Exp. Therap.* **140:** 278–286.

DELLER, D. J., GERMAR, H. and WITTS, L. J. (1961) Effect of food on absorption of radioactive vitamin B_{12}. *Lancet* **1:** 574–577.

DELLER, D. J., WORTHLEY, B. W. and MARTIN, H. (1965) Measurement of calcium-47 absorption by whole-body gamma spectrometry. *Austral. Ann. Med.* **14:** 223–231.

DENKO, C. W., GRUNDY, W. E., WHEELER, N. C., HENDERSON, C. R., BERRYMAN, G. H., FRIEDEMANN, T. E. and YOUMANS, J. B. (1946) The excretion of β-complex vitamins by normal adults on a restricted diet. *Arch. Biochem.* **11:** 109–117.

DICK, M. (1967) The use of barium sulphate as a continuous market for faeces. *J. Clin. Path.* **20:** 216–217.

DOIG, A. and GIRDWOOD, R. H. (1960) The absorption of folic acid and labeled cyanocobalamin in intestinal malabsorption. *Quart. J. Med.* (new series) **29:** 333–374.

DOLLERY, C. T., EMSLIE-SMITH, D. and MCMICHAEL, J. (1960) Bretylium tosylate in the treatment of hypertension. *Lancet* **1:** 296–299.

DOLLERY, C. T., EMSLIE-SMITH, D. and MUGGLETON, D. F. (1961) Action of chlorothiazide on the distribution, excretion and hypotensive effect of pempidine in man. *Brit. J. Pharmacol.* **17:** 488–506.

DOMINGUEZ, R. and POMERONE, E. (1934) On the renal excretion of xylose. *J. Clin. Invest.* **13:** 753–766.

DOMINGUEZ, R. and POMERONE, E. (1945) Calculation of the rate of absorption of exogenous creatinine. *Proc. Soc. Exp. Biol. Med.* **60:** 173–181.

DUPRE, J., CURTIS, J. D., WADDELL, R. W. and BECK, J. C. (1968) Regulation of pancreatic endocrine function by gastrointestinal hormones. *Proc. Roy. Soc. Med.* **61:** 815–816.

DUTHIE, H. L. and ATWELL, J. D. (1963) The absorption of water, sodium and potassium in the large intestine with particular reference to the effects of villous papillomas. *Gut* **4:** 373–377.

ELIAS, E., GIBSON, G. J., GREENWOOD, L. F., HUNT, J. N. and TRIPP, J. H. (1968) The slowing of gastric emptying by monosaccharides and disaccharides in test meals. *J. Physiol.* (*Lond.*) **194:** 317–326.

EWE, K. (1968a) Resorption und Sekretion von Calcium im menschlichen Jejunum. *Klin. Wschr.* **46:** 661–666

EWE, K. (1968b) Die Beeinflussung der Eisenaufnahme im Dünndarm durch Komplexbildung mit 8-Hydroxychinolin und dessen Sulfonat. Perfusionsuntersuchungen im menschlichen Jejunum. *Klin. Wschr.* **46:** 296–300.

FLESHLER, B., BUTT, J. H. and WISMAR, J. D. (1966) Absorption of glycine and L-alanine by the human jejunum. *J. Clin. Invest.* **45:** 1433–1441.

FORDTRAN, J. S. (1966) Marker perfusion techniques for measuring intestinal absorption in man. *Gastroenterology* **51:** 1089–1093.

FORDTRAN, J. S. and INGELFINGER, F. J. (1968) Absorption of water, electrolytes and sugars from the human gut, p. 1460. In: *Handbook of Physiology,* Sect. 6, *Alimentary Canal,* vol. III. *Intestinal Absorption,* CODE, C. F. (Ed.). American Physiological Society, Washington, D.C.

FORDTRAN, J. S., LEVITAN, R., BIKERMAN, V., BURROWS, B. A. and INGELFINGER, F. J. (1961) The kinetics of water absorption in the human small intestine. *Trans. Ass. Am. Physcns* **74:** 195–206.

FORDTRAN, J. S., RECTOR, F. C., EWTON, M. F., SOTER, N. and KINNEY, J. (1965) Permeability characteristics of the human small intestine. *J. Clin. Invest.* **44:** 1935–1944.

FORDTRAN, J. S., RECTOR, F. C., LOCKLEAR, T. W. and EWTON, M. F. (1967) Water and solute movement in the small intestine of patients with sprue. *J. Clin. Invest.* **46:** 287–298.

FORDTRAN, J. S., SOERGEL, K. H. and INGELFINGER, F. J. (1962) Intestinal absorption of D-xylose in man. *New Engl. J. Med.* **267:** 274–279.

FOWLER, D. and COOKE, W. T. (1960) Diagnostic significance of D-xylose excretion test. *Gut* **1:** 67–70.

FREEMAN, T. and GORDON, A. H. (1964) The measurement of albumin leak into the gastro-intestinal tract using ^{131}I-albumin and iron-exchange resin by mouth. *Gut* **5:** 155–157.

GADDIE, R., THOMAS, G., SMITH, N. and FRENCH, J. M. (1957) The value of the oral glucose test in the diagnosis of pancreatic from idiopathic steatorrhoea. *Quart. J. Med.* (new series) **26:** 121–130.

GAGNON, M. and DAWSON, A. M. (1968) The effect of bile of vitamin A absorption in the rat. *Proc. Soc. Exp. Biol. Med.* **127:** 99–102.

GALLAHER, N. D., HARRISON, D. D. and SKYRING, A. P. (1962) Fluid and electrolyte disturbances in patients with long-established ileostomies. *Gut* **3:** 219–223.

GARRETT, E. R., THOMAS, R. C., WALLACH, D. P. and ALWAY, C. D. (1960) Psicofuranine: kinetics and mechanisms *in vivo* with the application of the analog computer. *J. Pharm. Exp. Therap.* **130:** 106–118.

GAZET, J. C. and MCCOLL, I. (1967) Absorption of vitamin B_{12} from the small intestine. Study in man, monkey, cat and dog. *Brit. J. Surg.* **54:** 128–131.

GIRDWOOD, R. H. (1953) A folic-acid excretion test in the investigation of intestinal malabsorption. *Lancet* **2:** 53–63.

GLASS, C. G. J., BOYD, L. J., GELLIN, G. A. and STEPHANSON, L. (1954) Uptake of radioactive vitamin B_{12} by the liver in humans: test of measurement of intestinal absorption of vitamin B_{12} and intrinsic factor activity. *Arch. Biochem. Biophys.* **51:** 251–257.

GOULSTON, K., HARRISON, D. D. and SKYRING, A. P. (1963) Effect of mineralocorticoids on the sodium/potassium ratio of human ileostomy fluid. *Lancet* **2:** 541–542.

GRADY, G. F., MADOFF, M. A., DUHAMEL, R. C., MOORE, E. W. and CHALMERS, T. C. (1967) Sodium transport by human ileum *in vitro* and its response to cholera enterotoxin. *Gastroenterology* **53:** 737–744.

GRAY, G. M. and INGELFINGER, F. J. (1965) Intestinal absorption of sucrose in man: the site of hydrolysis and absorption. *J. Clin. Invest.* **44:** 390–398.

GRAY, G. M. and INGELFINGER, F. J. (1966) Intestinal absorption of sucrose in man: interrelation of hydrolysis and monosaccharide product absorption. *J. Clin. Invest.* **45:** 1433–1441.

GRIFFITH, G. H., OWEN, G. M., KIRKMAN, S. and SHIELDS, R. (1966) Measurement of rate of gastric emptying using chromium-51. *Lancet* **1:** 1244–1245.

GROEN, J. (1937) The absorption of hexoses from the upper part of the small intestine in man. *J. Clin. Invest.* **16:** 245–255.

GROISSER, V. W. and FARRAR, J. T. (1962) Effects of intestinal motility on the absorption of sodium in man. *Am. J. Dig. Dis.* (new series) **7:** 57–68.

HALLBERG, L. and SÖLVELL, L. (1960) Determination of the absorption rate of iron in man. *Acta Med. Scand.* in Supplement **358:** 3–9.

HANSKY, J. and CONNELL, A. M. (1962) Measurement of gastrointestinal transit using radioactive chromium. *Gut* **3:** 187–188.

HARINGTON, M. (1953) The absorption and excretion of hexamethonium salts. *Clin. Sci.* **12:** 183–198.

HARINGTON, M., KINCAID-SMITH, P. and MILNE, M. D. (1958) Pharmacology and clinical use of pempidine in the treatment of hypertension. *Lancet* **2:** 6–11.

HARRIS, L. J. (1942) Vitamin C levels of schoolchildren and students in wartime. *Lancet* **1:** 642–644; and Critique of the saturation method for determining vitamin C levels. *ibid.*, pp. 644–646.

HART, S. L. and MCCOLL, I. (1968) The effect of the laxative oxyphenisatin on the intestinal absorption of glucose in rat and man. *Brit. J. Pharmac.* **32:** 683–686.

HAYS, M. T. (1968) Absorption of oral thyroxine in man. *J. Clin. Endocr.* **28:** 749–756.

HEINLE, R. W., WELCH, A. D., SCHARF, V., MEACHAM, G. C. and PRUSOFF, W. H. (1952) Studies of excretion (and absorption) of Co^{60} labeled vitamin B_{12} in pernicious anemia. *Trans. Ass. Am. Physcns* **65:** 214–222.

HEINRICH, H. C., GABBE, E. E., MEINEKE, B. and WHANG, D. H. (1966) Die empfindliche und präzise Bestimmung der intestinalen Eisenresorption beim Menschen durch ^{59}Fe-Gesamptkorper-Retentionsmessung in einem 4π Grossraum-Radioactivitäts-Detektor. *Klin. Wschr.* **44:** 827–833.

HELBOCK, H. J. (1968) Folic-acid absorption in man. *Lancet* **2:** 775–776.

HELLMAN, L., FRAZELL, E. L. and ROSENFELD, R. S. (1960) Direct measurement of cholesterol absorption via the thoracic duct in man. *J. Clin. Invest.* **39:** 1288–1294.

HEPNER, G. W., BOOTH, C. C., COWAN, J., HOFFBRAND, A. G. and MOLLIN, D. L. (1968) Absorption of crystalline folic acid in man. *Lancet* **2:** 302–306.

HIGGINS, J. A., CODE, C. F. and ORVIS, A. L. (1956) The influence of motility on the rate of absorption of sodium and water from the small intestine of healthy persons. *Gastroenterology* **31:** 708–716.

HIGGINS, J. A., LEE, P. R., SCHOLER, J. F., REITEMEIER, R. J., CODE, C. F. and WOLLAEGER, E. E. (1957) Absorption of water and sodium from the small intestine of patients with non-tropical sprue. *J. Clin. Invest.* **36:** 265–269.

HOFFBRAND, A. V. and NECHELES, T. F. (1968) Mechanism of folate deficiency in patients receiving phenytoin. *Lancet* **2:** 528–530.

HOGBEN, C. A. M., SCHANKER, L. S., TOCCO, D. J. and BRODIE, B. B. (1957) Absorption of drugs from the stomach. *J. Pharm. Exp. Therap.* **120:** 540–545.

HOLDSWORTH, C. D. and BESSER, G. M. (1968) Influence of gastric emptying-rate and of insulin response on oral glucose tolerance in thyroid disease. *Lancet* **2:** 700–702.

HOLDSWORTH, C. D. and DAWSON, A. M. (1964) The absorption of monosaccharides in man. *Clin. Sci.* **27:** 371–379.

HOLDSWORTH, C. D. and DAWSON, A. M. (1965a) Absorption of fructose in man. *Proc. Soc. Exp. Biol. Med.* **118:** 142–145.

HOLDSWORTH, C. D. and DAWSON, A. M. (1956b) Glucose and fructose absorption in idiopathic steatorrhoea. *Gut* **6:** 387–391.

HUNT, J. N. (1956) Some properties of an alimentary osmoreceptor mechanism. *J. Physiol.* (*Lond.*) **132:** 267–288.

HUNT, J. N. (1959) Gastric emptying and gastric secretion in man. *Physiol. Rev.* **39:** 491–533.

HUNT, J. N. (1960) The site of receptors slowing gastric emptying in response to starch in test meals. *J. Physiol.* (*Lond.*) **154:** 270–276.

HUNT, J. N. and PATHAK, J. D. (1960) The osmotic effects of some simple molecules and ions on gastric emptying. *J. Physiol.* (*Lond.*) **154:** 254–269.

IRWIN, M. L. and CRAMPTON, E. W. (1951) The use of chromic oxide as an index material in digestion trials with human subjects. *J. Nutr.* **43:** 77–85.

JACOBSON, E. D., BONDY, D. C., BROITMAN, S. A. and FORDTRAN, J. S. (1963) Validity of polyethylene glycol in estimating intestinal water volume. *Gastroenterology* **44:** 761–767.

JAMES, W. P. T. (1968) Intestinal absorption in protein–calorie malnutrition. *Lancet* **1:** 333–335.

JEEJEEBHOY, K. N. and COGHILL, N. F. (1961) The measurement of gastrointestinal protein loss by a new method. *Gut* **2:** 123–130.

JOSEPHS, H. W. (1958) Absorption of iron as a problem in human physiology. *Blood* **13:** 1–54.

KAIHARA, S. and WAGNER, H. N. (1968) Measurement of intestinal fat absorption with carbon-14 labeled tracers. *J. Lab. Clin. Med.* **71:** 400–411.

KANE, E. A., JACOBSON, W. C. and MOORE, L. A. (1950) A comparison of techniques used in digestibility studies with dairy cattle. *J. Nutr.* **41:** 583–596.

KAYDEN, H. J., SENIOR, J. R. and MATTSON, F. H. (1967) The monoglyceride pathway of fat absorption in man. *J. Clin. Invest.* **46:** 1695–1703.

KEHAYOGLOU, A. K., HOLDSWORTH, C. D., AGNEW, J. E., WHELTON, M. J. and SHERLOCK, S. (1968) Bone disease and calcium absorption in primary biliary cirrhosis. *Lancet* **1:** 715–719.

KENNEDY, J. A. and KINLOCH, J. D. (1964) The impurity of radioiodinated triolein. *J. Clin. Path.* **17:** 160–162.

KERR, R. M., DUBOIS, J. J. and HOLT, P. R. (1967) Use of ^{125}I- and ^{51}Cr-labeled albumin for the measurement of gastrointestinal and total albumin catabolism. *J. Clin. Invest.* **46:** 2064–2082.

KNAPKA, J. J., BARTH, K. M., BROWN, D. G. and CRAGLE, R. G. (1967) Evaluation of polyethylene, chromic oxide and cerium-144 as digestibility indicators in burros. *J. Nutr.* **92:** 79–85.

KRAMER, P. (1966) The effect of varying sodium loads on the ileal excreta of human ileostomised subjects. *J. Clin. Invest.* **45:** 1710–1718.

KRAMER, P., KEARNEY, M. M. and INGELFINGER, F. J. (1963) The effect of specific foods and water loading on the ileal excreta of ileostomised human subjects. *Gastroenterology* **42:** 535–546.

KRUELA, M. S. (1947) Absorption of carotene from carrots in man and the use of the quantitative chromic oxide indicator method in absorption experiments. *Biochem. J.* **41:** 269–273.

LASSEN, N. A. (1960) Treatment of severe acute barbiturate poisoning by forced diuresis and alkalinisation of the urine. *Lancet* **2:** 338–342.

LAVOIE, P., LEGARE, A. and VIALLET, A. (1967) Portal catheterisation via the round ligament of the liver. *Am. J. Surg.* **114:** 822–830.

LEGERTON, C. W. JR., TEXTER, E. C. JR., RUFFIN, J. M. (1953) Observations on the vitamin A tolerance curve as an index of the degree of fat absorption. *Gastroenterology* **23:** 477–481.

LEVIN, R. J., KOLDOVSKY, O., HOSKOVA, J., JIRSOVA, V. and UHER, J. (1968) Electrical activity across human foetal small intestine associated with absorption processes. *Gut* **9:** 206–213.

LEVITAN, R., FORDTRAN, J. S., BURROWS, B. A. and INGELFINGER, F. J. (1962) Water and salt absorption in the human colon. *J. Clin. Invest.* **41:** 1754–1759.

LEVITAN, R. and INGELFINGER, F. J. (1965) Effect of δ-aldosterone on salt and water absorption from the intact human colon. *J. Clin. Invest.* **44:** 801–808.

LEVY, G. and HOLLISTER, L. E. (1964) Inter- and intrasubject variations in drug absorption kinetics. *J. Pharm. Sci.* **53:** 1446–1452.

LINEWEAVER, H. and BURK, D. (1934) Determination of enzyme dissociation constants. *J. Am. Chem. Soc.* **56:** 658–666.

LONDON, D. R., CUATRECASAS, P., BIRGE, S. J. JR. and SEGAL, S. (1967) Metabolism of lactose by intestinal mucosa from normal and lactase-deficient subjects. *Lancet.* **1:** 524–526.

LORAN, M. R., ALTHAUSEN, T. L., SPICER, F. W. and GOLDSTEIN, W. I. (1961) Transport of vitamin A across human intestine *in vitro*. *J. Lab. Clin. Med.* **58:** 622–626.

LOSOWSKY, M. S. and WILSON, A. R. (1967) Whole-body counting of the absorption and distribution of iron in haemochromatosis. *Clin. Sci.* **32:** 151–160.

LUTWAK, L. and BURTON, B. T. (1964) Fecal dye markers in metabolic balance studies. The use of brilliant blue and methylcellulose for accurate separation of stool periods. *Am. J. Clin. Nutr.* **14:** 109–111.

MACDONALD, I. and TURNER, L. J. (1968) Serum-fructose levels after sucrose or its constituent monosaccharides. *Lancet* **1:** 841–843.

MAYERSON, H. S. (1963) The physiologic importance of lymph, pp. 1035–1073. In: *Handbook of Physiology,* Sect. 2, *Circulation,* vol. II, HAMILTON, W. F. and DOW, P. (Eds.). American Physiological Society, Washington, D.C.

MAYNARD, A. DE L., ANDRIOLA, J. C. and PIGOT, A. (1953–4) Tetracycline hydrochloride: studies on absorption, diffusion, excretion and clinical trial, pp. 102–107. In: *Antibiotics Annual 1953–4*. Medical Encyclopaedia Inc.

MCCANCE, R. A. and MADDERS, K. (1930) The comparative rates of absorption of sugars from the human intestine. *Biochem. J.* **24:** 795–804.

MCCARTHY, C. F., BORLAND, J. L., LYNCH, H. L., OWEN, E. E. and TYOR, M. P. (1964) Defective uptake of basic amino-acids and L-cystine by intestinal mucosa of patients with cystinuria. *J. Clin. Invest.* **43:** 1518–1524.

MCCOLL, I., ANDREWS, D., GAZET, J. C., RAVEN, J. L. and STREEK, S. (1967) Effect of intrinsic factor on absorption of vitamin B_{12} from small intestine. *Lancet* **1:** 544–545.

MCFARLANE, A. S. (1956) Labeling of plasma proteins with radioactive iodine. *Biochem. J.* **62:** 135–143.

MCFARLANE, A. S. (1964) Metabolism of plasma proteins. Chapter 8 in vol. I of *Mammalian Protein Metabolism,* MUNRO, H. N. and ALLISON, J. B. (Eds.). New York, Academic Press Inc.

MCINTYRE, N., HOLDSWORTH, C. D. and TURNER, D. S. (1964) New interpretation of oral glucose tolerance. *Lancet* **2:** 20–21.

MCINTYRE, P. A., SACHS, M. V., KREVANS, J. R. and CONLEY, G. L. (1956) Pathogenesis and treatment of macrocytic anaemia. Information obtained with radioactive vitamin B_{12}. *Arch. Int. Med.* **98:** 541–549.

MCKENNA, R. D., BOURNE, R. H. and MATZKO, A. (1957) The use of I^{131} labeled fat in the study of fat digestion and absorption in normal individuals and in patients with diseases of fat absorption. *Gastroenterology* **32:** 17–24.

MCMICHAEL, H. B., WEBB, J. and DAWSON, A. M. (1967) The absorption of maltose and lactose in man. *Clin. Sci.* **33:** 135–145.

MEEUWISSE, G. W. and DAHLQVIST, A. (1968) Glucose–galactose malabsorption. *Acta Paed. Scand.* **57:** 273–280.

MEEUWISSE, G. W. and DANO, G. (1965) The xylose absorption test in infancy. *Acta Paed. Scand.* **54:** 33–42.

METCALFE-GIBSON, A., ING, T. S., KUIPER, J. J., RICHARDS, P., WARD, E. E. and WRONG, O. M. (1967) *In vivo* dialysis of feces as a method of stool analysis. II. The influence of diet. *Clin. Sci.* **33:** 89–100.

MOORE, C. V. and DUBACH, R. (1951) Observations on the absorption of iron from foods tagged with radioactive iron. *Trans. Am. Ass. Physcns* **64:** 245–256.

MOORE, P. F., YIM, G. K. W. and MIYA, T. S. (1960) Effect of concentration on oral toxicity of drugs. *Fed. Proc.* **19:** 390 (abstract).

MUELLER, W. J. (1956) Feasibility of the chromic oxide and the lignin indicator methods for metabolism experiments with chicks. *J. Nutr.* **58:** 29–36.

NAKAYAMA, K., NAKAMURA, T., YAMAMOTO, K. and TAMIYA, T. (1960) Evaluation of intestinal absorption after total gastrectomy: chromic oxide indicator method. *Gastroenterology* **38:** 946–953.

NELP, W. B., WAGNER, H. N. JR. and REBA, R. C. (1964) Renal excretion of vitamin B_{12} and its use in measurement of glomerular filtration rate in man. *J. Lab. Clin. Med.* **63:** 480–491.

NELSON, E. and SCHALDEMOSE, I. (1959) Urinary excretion kinetics for evaluation of drug absorption. I. Solution rate limited and nonsolution rate limited absorption of aspirin and benzyl penicillin: absorption rate of sulphaethylthiadiazole. *J. Am. Pharm. Ass.* **48:** 489–495.

NEWCOMER, A. D. and MCGILL, D. B. (1967) Disaccharidase activity in the small intestine: prevalence of lactase deficiency in 100 healthy subjects. *Gastroenterology* **53:** 881–889.

NICHOLSON, J. T. L. and CHORNOCK, F. W. (1942) Intubation studies of the human small intestine. XXII. An improved technic for the study of absorption; its application to ascorbic acid. *J. Clin. Invest.* **21:** 505–509.

OWEN, E. C., DARROCH, R. A. and PROUDFOOT, R. (1959) Studies of the rate of passage and disappearance in the intestine of the goat of carotene dissolved in fat and mixed with chromium sesquioxide. *Brit. J. Nutr.* **13:** 26–37.

PARSONS, D. S. (1968) Methods for investigations of intestinal absorption, pp. 1177–1216. In: *Handbook of Physiology,* Sect. 6, *Alimentary Canal,* vol. III. *Intestinal Absorption,* CODE, C. F. (Ed.). American Physiological Society, Washington, D.C.

PETERSON, M. L. (1963) On the re-esterification of fatty acids during absorption of fat: studies in patients with chyluria. *Gastroenterology* **44:** 774–786.

PHEAR, D. N. (1962) The normal and diabetic patterns of insulin response to glucose. *Lancet* **2:** 955–958.

PHILLIPS, S. F. and SUMMERSKILL, W. H. J. (1966) Occlusion of the jejunum for intestinal perfusion in man. *Mayo Clin. Proc.* **41:** 224–231.

PHILLIPS, S. F. and SUMMERSKILL, W. H. J. (1967) Water and electrolyte transport during maintenance of isotonicity in human jejunum and ileum. *J. Lab. Clin. Med.* **70:** 686–698.

POLLACK, S., BALCERZAK, S. P. and CROSBY, W. H. (1966) Fe^{59} absorption in human subjects using total-body counting technique. *Blood* **28:** 94–97.

POPPER, H., STEIGMANN, F. and ZEVIN, S. (1943) On the variations of the plasma vitamin A level after the administration of large doses of vitamin A in liver disease. *J. Clin. Invest.* **22:** 775–783.

RATH, C. E., MCCURDY, P. R. and DUFFY, B. F. (1957) Effect of renal disease on the Schilling test. *New Engl. J. Med.* **256:** 111–114.

REITEMEYER, R. J., CODE, C. F. and ORVIS, A. L. (1957) Comparison of rate of absorption of labeled sodium and water from upper small intestine of healthy human beings. *J. Appl. Physiol.* **10:** 256–260.

RIEFENSTEIN, E. C., ALBRIGHT, F. and WELLS, S. L. (1945) The accumulation, interpretation and presentation of data pertaining to metabolic balances, notably those of calcium, phosphorus and nitrogen. *J. Clin. Endoc.* **5:** 367–395.

RØNNOV-JESSEN, V. and HANSEN, J. (1965) The site of absorption of Co^{58}-labeled vitamin B_{12} in man. *Blood* **25:** 224–230.

ROSE, G. A. (1964) Experiences with the use of interrupted carmine red and continuous chromium sesquioxide marking of human faeces with reference to calcium, phosphorus and magnesium. *Gut* **5:** 274–279.

ROSENBERG, I. H., GODWIN, H. A., STREIFF, R. R. and CASTLE, W. B. (1968) Impairment of intestinal deconjugation of dietary folate. *Lancet* **2:** 530–532.

ROSENBERG, L. E., CRAWHALL, J. C. and SEGAL, S. (1967) Intestinal transport of cystine and cysteine in man: evidence for separate mechanisms. *J. Clin. Invest.* **46:** 30–34.

ROSS, G. I. M., MOLLIN, D. L., COX, E. V. and UNGLEY, C. C. (1954) Haematologic responses and concentration of vitamin B_{12} in serum and urine following oral administration of vitamin B_{12} without intrinsic factor. *Blood* **9:** 473–488.

SALMON, P. R., MCCARTHY, C. F. and READ, A. E. (1968) An isotope technique for estimating disaccharidases. *Gut* **9:** 365 (abstract).

SAMELIUS, U. and ASTROM, A. (1958) The absorption of an *N*-methylated barbiturate and acetylsalicylic acid from different suppository masses. *Acta Pharm. Toxicol.* **14:** 240–250.

SAMPSON, P. A. and BROOKE, B. N. (1963) Absorption of hydrocortisone from the large bowel. *Lancet* **1:** 701–702.

SAYLOR, L. and FINCH, C. A. (1953) Determination of iron absorption using two isotopes of iron. *Am. J. Physiol.* **172:** 372–376.

SCHANKER, L. S., SHORE, P. A., BRODIE, B. B. and HOGBEN, C. A. M. (1957) Absorption of drugs from the stomach. I. The rat. *J. Pharm. Exp. Therap.* **120:** 528–539.

SCHEDL, H. P. (1966) Use of P.E.G. and phenol red as unabsorbed indicators for intestinal absorption studies in man. *Gut* **7:** 159–163.

SCHEDL, H. P. and CLIFTON, J. A. (1961) Kinetics of intestinal absorption in man: normal subjects and patients with sprue. *J. Clin. Invest.* **40:** 1079 (abstract).

SCHEDL, H. P. and CLIFTON, J. A. (1962) Polyvinylpyrrolidine-I^{131} as an indicator of net intestinal water flux: its binding by intestinal mucus. *Proc. Soc. Exp. Biol. Med.* **110:** 381–384.

SCHEDL, H. P. and CLIFTON, J. A. (1963) Cortisol absorption in man. *Gastroenterology* **44:** 134–145.

SCHEDL, H. P., PIERCE, C. E., RIDER, A. and CLIFTON, J. A. (1968) Absorption of L-methionine from the human small intestine. *J. Clin. Invest.* **47:** 417–425.

SCHILLING, R. F. (1953) Intrinsic factor studies. II. The effect on the urinary excretion of radioactivity after the oral administration of radioactive vitamin B_{12}. *J. Lab. Clin. Med.* **42:** 860–866.

SCHOLER, J. F. and CODE, C. F. (1954) Rate of absorption of water from stomach and small bowel of human beings. *Gastroenterology* **27:** 565–577.

SCHÜRCH, A. F., LLOYD, L. E. and CRAMPTON, E. W. (1950) Use of chromic oxide as an index for determining the digestibility of a diet. *J. Nutr.* **41:** 629–636.

SCHÜTZ, H. B. and REIZENSTEIN, P. (1963) Radiovitamin B_{12} as a dilution indicator in gastrointestinal research. *Am. J. Dig. Dis.* (new series) **8:** 904–907.

SCHWABE, A. D., COZETTO, F. J., BENNETT, L. R. and MELLINKOFF, S. M. (1962) Estimation of fat absorption by monitoring of expired radioactive carbon dioxide after feeding a radioactive fat. *Gastroenterology* **42:** 285–291.

SCOTT, J. M. and ORSI, B. A. (1968) Folic-acid absorption in man. *Lancet* **2:** 775.

SEIFE, B. (1962) Radioactive inert-indicator method for intestinal absorption using differential counting. *J. Lab. Clin. Med.* **59:** 513–519.

SHERLOCK, S. and WALSHE, V. (1946–8) The use of a portal anastomotic vein for absorption studies in man. *Clin. Sci.* **6:** 113–121.

SHIELDS, R., MILES, J. B. and GILBERTSON, C. (1968) Absorption and secretion of water and electrolytes by the intact colon in a patient with primary aldosteronism. *Brit. Med. J.* **1:** 93–96.

SHIELDS, R., MULHOLLAND, A. T. and ELMSLIE, R. G. (1966) Action of aldosterone upon the intestinal transport of potassium, sodium and water. *Gut* **7:** 686–696.

SHINGLETON, W. W., BAYLIN, G. J., ISLEY, J. K., SANDERS, A. P. and RUFFIN, J. M. (1957) The evaluation of pancreatic function by use of I^{131} labeled fat. *Gastroenterology* **32:** 28–32.

SIE, H. G., VALKEMA, A. J. and LOOMEIJER, F. J. (1967) Re-evaluation of radio-iodinated triolein as a test fat in fat absorption studies. *J. Lab. Clin. Med.* **70:** 121–128.

SILVERMAN, M. and BURGEN, A. S. V. (1961) Application of analogue computer to measurement of intestinal absorption rates with tracers. *J. Appl. Physiol.* **16:** 911–913.

SLADEN, G. E. (1968) Perfusion studies in relation to intestinal absorption. *Gut.*

SLADEN, G. E. and DAWSON, A. M. (1968a) Effects of flow rate on the absorption of glucose in a steady state perfusion system in man. *Clin. Sci.*

SLADEN, G. E. and DAWSON, A. N. (1968b) An evaluation of perfusion techniques in the study of water and electrolyte absorption in man: the problem of endogenous secretions. *Gut* **9:** 530–535.

SMALL, M. D., BEZMAN, A., LONGARINI, A. E., FENNELL, A. and ZAMCHECK, N. (1961) Absorption of potassium iodide from gastrointestinal tract. *Proc. Soc. Exp. Biol. Med.* **106:** 450–452.

SOERGEL, K. H. and HOGAN, W. J. (1967) On the suitability of poorly absorbed markers as dilution indicators in the gastrointestinal tract. *Gastroenterology* **52:** 1056–1057.

SOERGEL, K. H., WHALEN, G. E. and HARRIS, J. A. (1968) Passive movement of water and sodium across the human small intestinal mucosa. *J. Appl. Physiol.* **24:** 40–48.

STANLEY, M. M. and CHENG, S. H. (1957) Excretion from the gut and gastrointestinal exchange. Studied by means of the inert indicator method. *Am. J. Dig. Dis.* (new series) **2:** 628–648.

SWEENEY, W. M., HARDY, S. M., DORNBUSH, A. C. and RUEGSEGGER, J. M. (1957) Absorption of tetracycline in human beings as affected by certain excipients. *Antibiotic Med. Clin. Ther.* **4:** 642–656.

SWINTOSKY, J. (1956) Illustrations and pharmaceutical interpretations of first-order drug elimination rate from the bloodstream. *Am. J. Pharm. Ass.* **45:** 395–400.

TEST, C. E., NICHOLS, R. L., LANDAU, R. L., RICKETTS, H. T. and LONGHEAD, R. (1956) A study of the "flat" oral glucose tolerance curve and its relation to rate of emptying of the stomach. *Am. J. Med. Sci.* **231:** 69–74.

TEXTER, E. C., COOPER, J. A. D., VIDINLI, M. and FINLAY, J. M. (1964) Laboratory procedures in the diagnosis of malabsorption. *Med. Clin. N. America* **48:** 117–136.

THAYSEN, E. H. and MÜLLERTZ, S. (1962) The d-xylose absorption tolerance test. *Acta Med. Scand.* **171:** 521–529.

THIER, S. O., SEGAL, S., FOX, M., BLAIR, A. and ROSENBERG, L. E. (1965) Cystinuria: defective intestinal transport of dibasic amino acids and cystine. *J. Clin. Invest.* **44:** 442–448.

THOMAS, J. E. (1957) Mechanics and regulation of gastric emptying. *Physiol. Rev.* **37:** 453–474.

THOMSON, G. R., LEWIS, B. and BOOTH, C. C. (1966) Absorption of vitamin D_3-^{3}H in control subjects and patients with intestinal malabsorption. *J. Clin. Invest.* **45:** 94–102.

TIDWELL, H. C. (1950) Mechanism of fat absorption as evidenced by chylomicrographic studies. *J. Biol. Chem.* **182:** 405–414.

TORRES-PINEDO, R., RIVERA, C. L. and FERNANDEZ, S. (1966) Studies on infant diarrhea. II. Absorption of glucose and net fluxes of water and sodium chloride in a segment of the jejunum. *J. Clin. Invest.* **45:** 1916–1922.

TOWNSEND, J. D., SMITH, T. and LANGMAN, M. J. S. (1968) Reproducibility of the hepatic uptake test of vitamin B_{12} absorption. *Gut* **9:** 199–202.

TUNA, N., MANGOLD, H. K. and MOSSER, D. G. (1963) Re-evaluation of the I^{131}-triolein absorption test. *J. Lab. Clin. Med.* **61:** 620–628.

TURNBULL, A. L. (1967) Absorption of vitamin B_{12} in patients with anemia after Polya partial gastrectomy. *Brit. J. Haemat.* **13:** 752–763.

VAN HANDEL, E. and ZILVERSMIT, D. B. (1958) Limitation of radio-iodine as a label for fat. *J. Lab. Clin. Med.* **52:** 831–839.

VAN HOEK, R. and CONRAD, M. E. JR. (1961) Iron absorption measurement of ingested $iron^{59}$ by a human whole-body liquid scintillation counter. *J. Clin. Invest.* **40:** 1153–1159.

VAVRINKOVA, H. and KRONDL, A. (1965) Use of polyethylene glycol in investigations of absorption of fat. *Nature (Lond.)* **208:** 293–294.

VISSCHER, M. B., FLETCHER, E. S., CARR, C. W., GREGOR, H. P., BUSHEY, M. S. and BARKER, D. E. (1944a) Isotopic tracer studies on the movement of water and ions between intestinal lumen and blood. *Am. J. Physiol.* **142:** 550–575.

VISSCHER, M. B., VARCO, R. H., CARR, C. W., DEAN, R. B. and ERIKSON, D. (1944b) Sodium ion movement between the intestinal lumen and the blood. *Am. J. Physiol.* **141:** 488–505.

WAGNER, J. G. (1961) Biopharmaceutics: absorption aspects. *J. Pharm. Sci.* **50:** 359–387.

WAGNER, J. G. and NELSON, E. (1963) Per cent absorbed time plots derived from blood level and/or urinary excretion data. *J. Pharm. Sci.* **52:** 610–611.

WEINER, I. M. and MUDGE, G. H. (1965) Renal tubular mechanisms for excretion of organic acids and bases. *Am. J. Med.* **36:** 743–762.

WEISBERG, H. and GLASS, G. B. J. (1966) A rapid quantitative method for measuring intestinal absorption of vitamin B_{12} in man using a double label hepatic uptake technique. *J. Lab. Clin. Med.* **68:** 163–172.

WHALEN, G. E., HARRIS, J. A., GEENEN, J. E. and SOERGEL, K. H. (1966) Sodium and water absorption from the human small intestine. The accuracy of the perfusion method. *Gastroenterology* **51:** 975–984.

WHALEN, G. E., HARRIS, J. A. and SOERGEL, K. H. (1965) Bidirectional flux of sodium and water in the human small intestine. *Gastroenterology* **48:** 859 (abstract).

WHITBY, L. G. and LANG, D. (1960) Experience with the chromic oxide method of fecal marketing in metabolic balance investigations on humans. *J. Clin. Invest.* **39:** 854–863.

WIGGINS, H. S. and DAWSON, A. M. (1961) An evaluation of unabsorbable markets in the study of fat absorption. *Gut* **2:** 373–376.

WILSON, T. H. (1962) *Intestinal Absorption.* W. B. Saunders Co., Philadelphia and London.

WORNING, H. and ANDRUP, E. (1965) Experimental studies on the value of the reference substances polyethylene glycol, bromsulphthalein and ^{51}Cr as indicators of fluid content of the intestinal lumen. *Gut* **6:** 487–493.

WRONG, O. (1968) Aldosterone and electrolyte movements in the colon. *Brit. Med. J.* **1:** 379–380.

WRONG, O., METCALFE-GIBSON, A., MORRISON, R. B. I., NG, S. T. and HOWARD, A. V. (1965) *In vivo* dialysis of feces as a method of stool analysis. Technique and results in normal subjects. *Clin. Sci.* **28:** 357–375.

WYNGAARDEN, J. B., SEGAL, S. and FOLEY, J. B. (1957) Physiological disposition and metabolic fate of infused pentoses in man. *J. Clin. Invest.* **36:** 1395–1407.

YOUNG, D. S., FORRESTER, T. M. and MORGAN, T. N. (1959) A comparison of the diuretic action of the chlorothiazide analogues. *Lancet* **2:** 765–768.

ZAWOISKI, E. J., BAER, J. E., BRAUNSCHWEIG, L. W., PAULSON, S. F., SHERMER, A. and BEYER, K. H. (1958) Gastrointestinal secretion and absorption of 3-methylamino-isocamphane hydrochloride (mecamylamine). *J. Pharm. Exp. Therap.* **122:** 442–448.

AUTHOR INDEX

SUBJECT INDEX